HUMAN-ANIMAL MEDICINE

Clinical Approaches to Zoonoses, Toxicants, and Other Shared Health Risks

HUMAN-ANIMAL MEDICINE

Clinical Approaches to Zoonoses, Toxicants, and Other Shared Health Risks

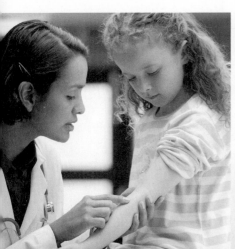
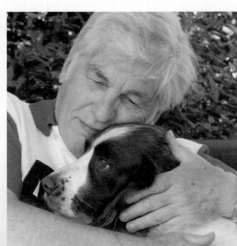
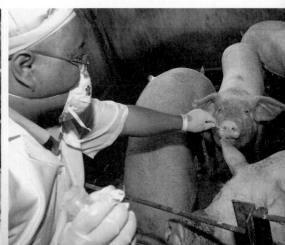

PETER M. RABINOWITZ, MD, MPH
Associate Professor of Medicine
Director of Clinical Services
Yale Occupational and Environmental Medicine Program
Yale University School of Medicine
New Haven, Connecticut

LISA A. CONTI, DVM, MPH, DACVPM, CEHP
Director
Division of Environmental Health
Florida Department of Health
Tallahassee, Florida

with more than 400 illustrations

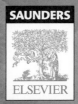

SAUNDERS

ELSEVIER

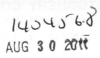

SAUNDERS
ELSEVIER

3251 Riverport Lane
Maryland Heights, Missouri 63043

HUMAN-ANIMAL MEDICINE: CLINICAL APPROACHES TO ZOONOSES,   ISBN 978-1-4160-6837-2
TOXICANTS, AND OTHER SHARED HEALTH RISKS

Notice

Knowledge and best practice in this field are constantly changing. As new research and experience broaden our knowledge, changes in practice, treatment and drug therapy may become necessary or appropriate. Readers are advised to check the most current information provided (i) on procedures featured or (ii) by the manufacturer of each product to be administered, to verify the recommended dose or formula, the method and duration of administration, and contraindications. It is the responsibility of the practitioner, relying on their own experience and knowledge of the patient, to make diagnoses, to determine dosages and the best treatment for each individual patient, and to take all appropriate safety precautions. To the fullest extent of the law, neither the Publisher nor the Editors assume any liability for any injury and/or damage to persons or property arising out of or related to any use of the material contained in this book.

The Publisher

Library of Congress Cataloging-in-Publication Data
Rabinowitz, Peter MacGarr.
    Human-animal medicine: clinical approaches to zoonoses, toxicants, and other shared health risks /
Peter M. Rabinowitz, Lisa A. Conti.
       p. ; cm.
    Includes bibliographical references.
    ISBN 978-1-4160-6837-2 (hardcover : alk. paper)
1. Zoonoses. 2. Environmental health. I. Conti, Lisa A. II. Title.
[DNLM: 1. Communicable Diseases–epidemiology. 2. Bonding, Human-Pet. 3. Communicable Diseases–veterinary. 4. Environmental Monitoring–methods. 5. Sentinel Surveillance–veterinary. 6. Zoonoses–epidemiology. WC 100 R116h 2010]
RA639.R33 2010
614.5′6–dc22

                                                                                    2009040249

Cover image (woman with cat) © Inti St. Clair/Corbis.
Internal images © Graham Bell/Corbis; Shutterstock; and AFI/Getty Images.

Vice President and Publisher: Linda Duncan
Senior Acquisitions Editor: Anthony Winkel
Developmental Editor: Maureen Slaten
Publishing Services Manager: Patricia Tannian
Project Manager: Carrie Stetz
Designer: Jessica Williams

Printed in the United States of America

Last digit is the print number: 9 8 7 6 5 4 3 2 1

This book is dedicated to Ronald M. Davis, MD (1956-2008), immediate past president of the American Medical Association and Director of the Center for Health Promotion and Disease Prevention at the Henry Ford Health System in Detroit. Dr. Davis was a One Health champion, a public health advocate, and an inspiration to all his friends and colleagues. His work established a standard of excellence and collaboration for generations to come.

Contributors

Matthew S. Alkaitis
Dartmouth College
Hanover, New Hampshire
Zoonoses: Orf

Lorraine C. Backer, PhD, MPH
Team Leader
National Center for Environmental Health
Centers for Disease Control and Prevention
Atlanta, Georgia
Toxic Exposures: Harmful Algae Blooms

Carina Blackmore, MS VetMed, PhD, DACVPM
State Public Health Veterinarian
State Environmental Epidemiologist
Chief, Bureau of Environmental Public Health Medicine
Division of Environmental Health
Florida Department of Health
Tallahassee, Florida
Zoonoses: Influenza, West Nile Virus and Other Arbovirus Infections

Roger I. Ceilley, MD
Dermatology and Syphology
The University of Iowa
Iowa City, Iowa
Zoonoses: Scabies

Lisa A. Conti, DVM, MPH, DACVPM, CEHP
Director
Division of Environmental Health
Florida Department of Health
Tallahassee, Florida
Legal and Ethical Issues in Human-Animal Medicine
Establishing a New Approach to Clinical Health History
Sentinel Disease Signs and Symptoms
The Built Environment and Indoor Air Quality
Toxic Exposures: Healthy Homes, Carbon Monoxide, Lead,
  Pesticides, Envenomations
Zoonoses: Overview, Anthrax, Bartonella Infections,
  Brucellosis, Campylobacteriosis, Chlamydophila Psittaci
  and Related Infections, Cryptosporidiosis, Dermatophytosis,
  Dipylidiasis, Echinococcosis, Ehrlichioses and Anaplasmosis,
  Escherichia Coli Infection, Giardiasis, Hantavirus Infections,
  Hookworm Infection, Leishmaniasis, Leptospirosis,
  Lyme Disease, Methicillin-Resistant Staphylococcus
  Aureus Infection, Orf, Plague, Q fever, Rabies, Rocky
  Mountain Spotted Fever and Other Rickettsial Infections,
  Salmonellosis, Toxocara Infestation, Toxoplasmosis,
  Transmissible Spongiform Encephalopathies, Tularemia
Infectious Disease Scenarios
Foodborne Illness
Occupational Health of Animal Workers
Public Health and Human-Animal Medicine
Shared Strategies to Maximize Human and Animal Health

Russell W. Currier, DVM, MPH, DACVPM
Executive Vice President
American College of Veterinary Preventive
  Medicine
Des Moines, Iowa
Zoonoses: Scabies

Tracy DuVernoy, DVM
Veterinary Medicine Officer, Food and Drug Administration
  Center for Food Safety and Applied Nutrition
College Park, Maryland
Zoonoses: Rift Valley Fever

Lora E. Fleming, MD, PhD
Professor
Departments of Epidemiology & Public Health and Marine
  Biology & Fisheries
Miller School of Medicine and Rosenstiel School of Marine
  and Atmospheric Sciences
Miami, Florida
Toxic Exposures: Harmful Algae Blooms

Elena Hollender, MD
Director of Clinical Services
A.G. Holley State Tuberculosis Hospital
Lantana, Florida;
Voluntary Assistant Professor of Medicine
Division of Pulmonary and Critical Care Medicine
Miller School of Medicine
University of Miami
Miami, Florida;
Courtesy Assistant Professor of Medicine
Southeastern National Tuberculosis Center at the University
  of Florida
Department of Medicine
School of Medicine
Gainesville, Florida;
Courtesy Assistant Professor
Department of Epidemiology and Biostatistics
College of Public Health and Health Professions
University of Florida
Gainesville, Florida
Zoonoses: Tuberculosis and Other Mycobacterial
  Infections

Rebecca A. Johnson, PhD, RN, FAAN
Millsap Professor of Gerontological Nursing
Director, Research Center for Human-Animal
  Interaction
College of Veterinary Medicine
University of Missouri
Columbia, Missouri
Psychosocial and Therapeutic Aspects of Human-Animal
  Interaction

Laura H. Kahn, MD, MPH, MPP, FACP
Research Staff
Program on Science and Global Security
Woodrow Wilson School of Public and International Affairs
Princeton University
Princeton, New Jersey
The Convergence of Human and Animal Medicine

Bruce Kaplan, DVM, DAVES (Hon)
Sarasota, Florida
The Convergence of Human and Animal Medicine

Hugh M. Mainzer, MS DVM, DACVPM
Captain, U.S. Public Health Service
Chief Veterinary Officer, U.S. Public Health Service
Division of Emergency and Environmental Health Services
Centers for Disease Control and Prevention
Atlanta, Georgia
Public Health and Human-Animal Medicine

Clifford S. Mitchell, MS, MD, MPH
Director, Environmental Health Coordination & Preventive
    Medicine Residency Programs
Maryland Department of Health and Mental Hygiene
Baltimore, Maryland
The Built Environment and Indoor Air Quality
Allergic Conditions

Ben Hur P. Mobo, Jr., MD
Assistant Professor of Medicine
WHVAMC
West Haven, Connecticut
Occupational Health of Animal Workers

Thomas P. Monath, MD
Partner
Kleiner Perkins Caufield & Byers
Pandemic & Biodefense Fund
Harvard, Massachusetts
The Convergence of Human and Animal Medicine

Lynda U. Odofin, DVM, MSPH
Yale School of Public Health
Yale University
New Haven, Connecticut
Zoonoses: Lymphocytic Choriomeningitis

Natasha Rabinowitz
Mount Holyoke College
South Hadley, Massachusetts
Zoonoses: Orf

Peter M. Rabinowitz, MD, MPH
Associate Professor of Medicine
Director of Clinical Services
Yale Occupational and Environmental Medicine
Yale University School of Medicine
New Haven, Connecticut
Legal and Ethical Issues in Human-Animal Medicine

Establishing a New Approach to Clinical Health History
Sentinel Disease Signs and Symptoms
The Built Environment and Indoor Air Quality
Allergic Conditions
Toxic Exposures: Healthy Homes, Carbon Monoxide, Lead,
    Pesticides, Envenomations
Zoonoses: Overview, Anthrax, Bartonella Infections,
    Brucellosis, Campylobacteriosis, Chlamydophila
    Psittaci and Related Infections, Cryptosporidiosis,
    Dermatophytosis, Dipylidiasis, Echinococcosis, Ehrlichioses
    and Anaplasmosis, Escherichia Coli Infection, Giardiasis,
    Hantavirus Infections, Hookworm Infection, Influenza,
    Leishmaniasis, Leptospirosis, Lyme Disease, Methicillin-
    Resistant Staphylococcus Aureus Infection, Orf, Plague,
    Q fever, Rabies, Rocky Mountain Spotted Fever and Other
    Rickettsial Infections, Salmonellosis, Toxocara Infestation,
    Toxoplasmosis, Transmissible Spongiform Encephalopathies,
    Tuberculosis and Other Mycobacterial Infections,
    Tularemia
Infectious Disease Scenarios
Foodborne Illness
Occupational Health of Animal Workers
Public Health and Human-Animal Medicine
Shared Strategies to Maximize Human and Animal Health

Carol Norris Reinero, DVM, PhD, DACVIM
Assistant Professor, Small Animal Internal Medicine
Department of Veterinary Medicine and Surgery
College of Veterinary Medicine
University of Missouri
Columbia, Missouri
The Built Environment and Indoor Air Quality
Allergic Conditions

Judy Sparer, CIH, MSCE
Industrial Hygienist
Yale Occupational and Environmental Medicine Program
Yale University School of Medicine
New Haven, Connecticut
The Built Environment and Indoor Air Quality

Oyebode A. Taiwo, MD, MPH
Assistant Professor of Medicine
Director, Occupational and Environmental Medicine
    Fellowship Training
Yale Occupational and Environmental Medicine Program
Yale University School of Medicine
New Haven, Connecticut
Occupational Health of Animal Workers

Julia Zaias, DVM, PhD
Research Assistant Professor, Comparative Pathology
Department of Pathology
Miller School of Medicine
University of Miami
Miami, Florida
Toxic Exposures: Harmful Algae Blooms

Reviewers

Alina Alonso, MD
Medical Director
Palm Beach County Health Department
West Palm Beach, Florida

Larry Anderson, DVM, MD
Family Practitioner
Family Care Center
Wellington, Kansas

Fred Angulo, PhD, DVM
Acting Associate Director for Science, NCEH/ATSDR
Centers for Disease Control and Prevention
Atlanta, Georgia

Philip W. Askenase, MD
Section of Allergy and Clinical Immunology
Department of Medicine
Yale University School of Medicine
New Haven, Connecticut

Paul Auerbach, MD
Professor of Surgery—Emergency Medicine
Stanford University School of Medicine
Stanford, California

Connie C. Austin, DVM, MPH, PhD
State Public Health Veterinarian
Division of Infectious Disease
Illinois Department of Public Health
Springfield, Illinois

Nili Avni-Magen, DVM
Head Veterinarian
Tisch Family Zoological Gardens
Jerusalem, Israel

Sarah L. Babcock, DVM, JD
Animal & Veterinary Legal Services
Harrison Township, Michigan

Michele Barry, MD, FACP
Senior Associate Dean of Global Health
Health Consultant Overseas Program, Ford
    Foundation;
Director of Global Health Programs in Medicine
Director, Yale/Stanford Johnson & Johnson Global Health
    Scholars Program, Stanford University Site
Professor, Department of Medicine
Stanford University School of Medicine
Stanford, California

Emily Beeler, DVM
Los Angeles County Department of Public Health
Veterinary Public Health and Rabies Control Program
Downey, California;
College of Veterinary Medicine
Western University of Health Sciences
Pomona, California

Jeff B. Bender, DVM, MS, DACVPM
Veterinary Public Health
Center for Animal Health and Food Safety
College of Veterinary Medicine
University of Minnesota
St. Paul, Minnesota

Tegan K. Boehmer, PhD, MPH
LCDR U.S. Public Health Service
Epidemiologist
Air Pollution and Respiratory Health Branch
National Center for Environmental Health
Centers for Disease Control and Prevention
Atlanta, Georgia

Jonathan Borak, MD, DABT, FACP, FACOEM
Clinical Professor of Epidemiology & Public Health
Clinical Professor of Medicine
Yale University School of Medicine
New Haven, Connecticut

Edward B. Breitschwerdt, DVM
Professor of Medicine and Infectious Diseases
College of Veterinary Medicine
North Carolina State University
Raleigh, North Carolina

Anne Brewer, MD
Associate Director
Family Medicine Residency Program
The Stamford Hospital
Stamford, Connecticut

Victoria E. Bridges, DVM, MS
Veterinary Epidemiologist
U.S. Department of Agriculture
Fort Collins, Colorado

Sondra Brown, DVM, MS
Northwood Animal Hospital and
The Animal Hospital & Pet Resort at Southwood
Tallahassee, Florida

Stanley D. Bruntz, DVM, MPH
MAHRS Coordinator
National Surveillance Unit
Centers for Epidemiology and Animal Health
U.S. Department of Agriculture, Animal and Plant Health
    Inspection Service Veterinary Service
Fort Collins, Colorado

Arlene Buchholz, DVM, MPH, DACVPM
Veterinary Medical Officer
Hawaii State Department of Health
Honolulu, Hawaii

Danielle Buttke, DVM, PhD Candidate
The Baker Institute for Animal Health
College of Veterinary Medicine
Cornell University
Ithaca, New York

Bryan Cherry, VMD, PhD
State Public Health Veterinarian
New York State Department of Health
Albany, New York

James E. Childs, ScD
Senior Research Scientist/Scholar
Department of Epidemiology and Public Health
Yale University School of Medicine
New Haven, Connecticut

Kerry L. Clark, MPH, PhD
Associate Professor and MPH Program Director
Epidemiology & Environmental Health
Department of Public Health
Brooks College of Health
University of North Florida
Jacksonville, Florida

Mark R. Cullen, MD
Chief, Division of General Internal Medicine
Stanford University School of Medicine
Stanford, California

Radford Davis, DVM, MPH, DACVPM
Associate Professor of Public Health
Department of Veterinary Microbiology and Preventive
    Medicine
College of Veterinary Medicine
Iowa State University
Ames, Iowa

F. Joshua Dein, VMD, MS
Veterinary Medical Officer
USGS National Wildlife Health Center
Madison, Wisconsin

Millicent Eidson, MA, DVM, DACVPM (Epidemiology)
State Public Health Veterinarian and Director, Zoonoses
    Program
New York State Department of Health;
Associate Professor
Department of Epidemiology and Biostatistics
School of Public Health
State University of New York
Albany, New York

Paul Ettestad, DVM, MS
State Public Health Veterinarian
Epidemiology and Response Division
New Mexico Department of Health
Santa Fe, New Mexico

Durland Fish, PhD
Professor of Epidemiology and Public Health
Professor of Forestry and Environmental Studies
School of Public Health;
Director
Yale Institute for Biospheric Studies Center for
    EcoEpidemiology
Yale University
New Haven, Connecticut

Renée Funk, DVM, MPH & TM, DACVPM
LCDR, United States Public Health Service
Emergency Preparedness and Response Office NIOSH
Centers for Disease Control and Prevention
Atlanta, Georgia

Paul Garbe, DVM, MPH
Chief, Air Pollution and Respiratory Health Branch
Division of Environmental Hazards and Health Effects
National Center for Environmental Health
Centers for Disease Control and Prevention
Atlanta, Georgia

Gary Ginsberg, PhD
Division of Environmental and Occupational Health
Connecticut Department of Public Health
Hartford, Connecticut

Carol Glaser, DVM, MPVM, MD
Viral and Rickettsial Disease Laboratory
California Department of Health Services
Richmond, California

Larry Glickman, VMD, DrPH
Professor of Epidemiology
Department of Emergency Medicine
University of North Carolina;
Senior Epidemiologist
OneEpi Consulting
Pittsboro, North Carolina

Jerome Goddard, PhD
State Medical Entomologist
Mississippi State Department of Health
Jackson, Mississippi

Robert P. Gordon, DVM
Owner and Director
Oakland Animal Hospital
Oakland, New Jersey

Zimra J. Gordon, DVM, MPH
Private Practice
Stamford, Connecticut

Marilyn Goss Haskell, DVM, MPH
NCDHHS Public Health Veterinarian
Epidemiology, CD Medical Unit
Raleigh, North Carolina

Ellis C. Greiner, PhD
Professor, Parasitology
Department of Infectious Diseases and Pathology
College of Veterinary Medicine
University of Florida
Gainesville, Florida

Sharon Gwaltney-Brant, DVM, PhD, DABVT, DABT
Vice President & Medical Director
ASPCA Animal Poison Control Center
Urbana, Illinois

Steven A. Hale, MD
Senior Physician
Orange County Health Department
Orlando, Florida

Michael L. Haney, PhD, NCC, LMHC
Division Director for Prevention and Intervention
Children's Medical Services
Florida Department of Health
Tallahassee, Florida

Frederick G. Hayden, MD, FACP
Professor of Medicine, Infectious Disease and International
    Health
University of Virginia School of Medicine
Charlottesville, Virginia

Robert Hood, PhD, CIP
Ethics and Human Research Protections Program Assistant
    Director
Office of Public Health Research
Florida Department of Health
Tallahassee, Florida

Martin E. Hugh-Jones, Vet MB, MA, MPH, PhD
Coordinator of the World Health Organization Working
    Group on Anthrax Research and Control
Geneva, Switzerland;
Professor Emeritus
Department of Environmental Sciences
School of the Coast and Environment
Louisiana State University
Baton Rouge, Louisiana

Suzanne R. Jenkins, VMD, MPH, ACVPM
State Public Health Veterinarian (Retired)
Virginia Department of Health
Richmond, Virginia

Anne E. Justice-Allen, DVM
Wildlife Health Specialist
Arizona Game and Fish Department
Phoenix, Arizona

Bruce Kaplan, DVM, DAVES (Hon)
Sarasota, Florida

Jeffrey D. Kravetz, MD
Veterans Affairs Healthcare System
West Haven, Connecticut;
Yale University School of Medicine
New Haven, Connecticut

Charlotte A. Lacroix, DVM, JD
Owner and CEO
Veterinary Business Advisors, Inc.
Whitehouse Station, New Jersey

Mira J. Leslie, DVM, MPH
Public Health Veterinarian
Ministry of Agriculture and Lands
Abbotsford, British Columbia
Canada

Joann M. Lindenmayer, DVM, MPH
Associate Professor of Public Health
Department of Environmental
    and Population Health
Cummings School of Veterinary Medicine
Tufts University
North Grafton, Massachusetts

Jean Malecki, MD, MPH, FACPM
Director
Palm Beach County Health Department
West Palm Beach, Florida

Leonard C. Marcus, VMD, MD
Travelers' Health and Immunization Services
Newton, Massachusetts

Rosanna Marsella, DVM, DACVD
Professor
Department of Small Animal Clinical Sciences
College of Veterinary Medicine
University of Florida
Gainesville, Florida

Catherine McManus, VMD, MPH, DACVPM
Veterinary Epidemiologist
Division of Environmental Epidemiology
Virginia Department of Health
Richmond, Virginia

CDR David McMillan, MD, MPH, ACOEM
Head, Navy Occupational Medicine Programs and Policy
Navy Surgeon General's Office
Washington, DC

Kathleen A. Smith, DVM, MPH
State Public Health Veterinarian
Ohio Department of Health
Reynoldsburg, Ohio

Andre N. Sofair, MD, MPH
Associate Professor of Medicine, Epidemiology, and Public
    Health
Yale University School of Medicine
New Haven, Connecticut

Daniel L. Sudakin, MD, MPH, FACMT, FACOEM
Associate Professor
Department of Environmental and Molecular
    Toxicology
College of Veterinary Medicine
Oregon State University
Corvallis, Oregon

David E. Swayne, DVM, PhD, DACPV
Laboratory Director
Southeast Poultry Research Laboratory
USDA/Agricultural Research Service
Athens, Georgia

Wendy T. Thanassi, MA, MD
Chief, Occupational Health Services
Palo Alto VA Health Care System;
Clinical Assistant Professor of Surgery (Emergency
    Medicine)
Stanford Hospitals and Clinics and Lucile Packard
    Children's Hospital
Stanford University School of Medicine
Stanford, California

Greg Troll, MD
Associate Dean
Faculty & Curriculum Development
Touro University College of Osteopathic Medicine
Sebastopol, California

†Jeff W. Tyler, DVM, MPVM, PhD, DACVIM
Professor
Director of Strategic Program Initiatives
Director of Clinical Research
Department of Veterinary Medicine and Surgery
College of Veterinary Medicine
University of Missouri
Columbia, Missouri

Mark Jerome Walters, DVM
Associate Professor
Department of Journalism & Media Studies
University of South Florida
St. Petersburg, Florida

Kalman L. Watsky, MD
Clinical Professor of Dermatology
Yale University School of Medicine;
Section Chief of Dermatology
Hospital of Saint Raphael
New Haven, Connecticut

J. Scott Weese, DVM, DVSc, DACVIM
Department of Pathobiology
Ontario Veterinary College
University of Guelph
Guelph, Ontario
Canada

Sara C. Wilson, RN/CNS, MSN, APHN-BC
Registered Nursing Consultant
Office of Public Health Nursing
Tallahassee, Florida

James C. Wright, DVM, PhD, DACVPM
Associate Professor
Veterinary Public Health
Department of Pathobiology
College of Veterinary Medicine
Auburn University
Auburn, Alabama

---

†Deceased.

Preface

INTRODUCTION AND HOW TO USE THIS BOOK

This book is designed to help clinicians and public health professionals manage a wide range of clinical problems at the intersection of human and animal health. It presents a "One Health" approach to such problems, in recognition that the health of human beings, animals, and their environments is interrelated.

BACKGROUND AND CONCEPTUAL APPROACH

The relevance of nonhuman animals to human health takes at least three basic forms. First, a number of health risks are related to animal contact, including zoonotic infectious diseases transmitted from animals to human beings; animal allergens that cause allergic disease in human beings; and animal bites, stings, and other direct trauma. Second, important psychosocial effects of the human-animal bond may have physical benefits as well. Third, animals may serve as "sentinels" for toxic or infectious health hazards in the environment that are also a risk for human beings.

Despite the fact that the majority of American households include at least one animal, communication between the veterinarian caring for the family pets and the human health care providers treating the human household members is currently limited. Similarly, there may be limited contact between public health professionals and their animal health counterparts. The growing recognition of the links among human health, animal health, and the environment requires new tools for cooperation and communication between professionals working in these sectors. Such intersectoral cooperation demands further development of a common body of knowledge (what we call *human-animal medicine*) and a common scientific and clinical vocabulary for understanding diseases affecting both human beings and animals that often are related to environmental factors. This book is an attempt to outline this body of knowledge and suggests practical steps for implementing the concept of "One Health" in the daily practice of human and animal medicine and public health.

Emerging infectious diseases such as SARS, West Nile Virus infection, and avian/swine influenza have focused attention on infectious diseases that cross between animals and human beings; we believe that many of these diseases are manifestations of important environmental changes related to land use, climate change, intensification of food production, and other factors. Therefore preventing such diseases must involve creating and maintaining healthy environments. Other environmental health risks that may be shared by human beings and animals include toxicants, allergens, and psychosocial issues. Working to improve such environments is a complex process that involves both professionals and communities.

We believe that human and animal health clinicians have an important role to play in identifying specific factors affecting the health of their patients. Public health professionals can look at factors affecting both animals and human beings in their communities and take steps to ameliorate conditions. Informed communities can work on a policy and practical level to implement a variety of solutions.

In the future, we envision the need for an expanded cadre of veterinarian "specialists" in human-animal medicine concepts who can function as part of integrated clinical care and prevention teams for human health. We also see the possibility for human health clinicians who receive special veterinary medical training to better deliver services such as occupational health care to persons with animal contact and evaluation of environmental hazards affecting both human beings and other animals. The escalating role of veterinarians in public health over the last several years is just the first step in a necessary and ongoing process that is detailed in several sections of this book.

We hope this book can provide additional impetus to this evolution.

WHO WILL BENEFIT FROM THIS BOOK

- For human health clinicians, including primary care providers, home health care providers, and specialists in infectious disease, allergy, dermatology, and psychiatry, this book provides a core body of knowledge regarding the role of animals in human infectious and allergic disease, the psychosocial aspects of human-animal contact, and the potential for animals to serve as sentinels for toxic and other environmental health risks to human beings. Armed with such knowledge, human health clinicians can more effectively screen for human-animal health problems and make appropriate referrals to both veterinarians and public health departments.
- For physicians and other clinicians providing occupational health services to persons with animal contact, including farmers, veterinarians, zookeepers, pet store employees, and laboratory animal workers, this book details the special risks of injury, allergy, infection, and psychosocial stress that these workers may experience. It provides guidelines for designing and implementing appropriate preventive services for these occupational risk groups.
- For veterinarians in community-based practice, this book outlines the human health implications of zoonotic diseases, animal allergy, and human-animal interaction. It provides guidelines for communication with clients and human health care providers about reducing animal-related disease risk, and how to recognize when animals may be serving as potential sentinels of environmental health risks. It also details some of the legal and ethical

ramifications of veterinarians playing a greater role in human health care.

- For public health professionals in environmental health, the book explains how specific hazards in the home and environment can affect the health of human beings and animals in the community, and how animals can serve as sentinels for human health risks, and vice versa.
- For public health officials engaged in disease surveillance, the book provides examples of how outbreaks in animal populations can provide information about human disease risk and how to investigate the human health implications of such outbreaks, in cooperation with agricultural and other animal health agencies.

ORGANIZATION

To address these needs, this book attempts to outline clinically important areas where human and animal health are linked and some key similarities and differences in the ways that human and animal health is affected by environmental factors. For each area, we have enumerated specific roles for human health, veterinary health, and public health professionals in the detection, management, and prevention of disease.

Chapter 1 outlines the factors driving the convergence of human, animal, and environmental health as well as the "One Health" concept that has been proposed to encourage greater cross-specialty interaction on vital issues of emerging diseases and environmental change. Chapter 2 provides some cautionary guidance regarding potential legal and ethical pitfalls that must be faced and avoided during this process of increasing intersectoral collaboration. Chapter 3 provides a guide to the history that both human and animal health clinicians can incorporate into their daily care of patients to identify important human-animal health links. Chapter 4 provides charts of important sentinel signs in human beings and animals that could indicate human-animal health risks. Chapter 5 outlines the different facets of the psychosocial bonds between human beings and animals and how human-animal interaction can be a therapeutic tool as well as an important factor to consider in a wide range of clinical situations. Chapter 6 highlights the need to consider health effects from indoor and other built environments. Chapter 7 deals with allergens related to human-animal contact and clinical manifestations of allergic disease in human beings and animals. Chapter 8 provides an overview of important clinical syndromes in human beings and animals related to acute and chronic exposure to toxic hazards in the environment, the ability of animals to serve as sentinels for human environmental health hazards from toxicants, and preventive steps for toxicant avoidance. Chapter 9 reviews selected zoonotic diseases of importance, and Chapter 10 presents particular infectious disease risk scenarios, including travel and immunocompromised individuals. Chapter 11 provides an overview of common issues regarding foodborne illness.

Chapter 12 outlines the occupational hazards facing workers who handle animals on a regular basis and provides guidelines for preventive health care services for such individuals. Chapter 13 discusses the special role that public health agencies play in the prevention and management of disease risk facing human and animal populations. Chapter 14 concludes the book with practical suggestions for integrated primary, secondary, and tertiary disease prevention activities among the human health, animal health, and public health sectors as well as templates for communication between professionals working in these sectors.

We have endeavored to make this book as evidence based as possible by referencing, when available, original studies in the biomedical literature in support of specific recommendations. At the same time, we acknowledge that for many human-animal health issues there are important gaps in knowledge, and much of the available evidence is anecdotal in nature. A notable exception is the recommendations of the U.S. Public Health Service in "Guidelines for Preventing Opportunistic Infections Among HIV-Infected Persons" (see Chapter 10).[1] It is our hope that such evidence-based recommendations can serve as a model for future guidelines on other human-animal medicine issues.

DISTINCTIVE FEATURES

For each clinical problem covered, the book presents:

- Comparative charts of the presentation and treatment of the disease in human beings and nonhuman animals.
- Specific steps for human health, animal health, and public health professionals to take to prevent and manage the particular condition.
- The role of environmental factors in the causation of the clinical problem.

Other features include:

- Treatment of emerging disease issues, including emerging zoonoses, harmful algae blooms, and animal-related pesticides.
- Legal and ethical aspects of greater interaction between human and animal health professionals.
- Sample protocols for professional communication between veterinarians, human health clinicians, and public health professionals.

REFERENCE

1. Mofenson LM, Brady MT, Danner SP et al: Guidelines for the prevention and treatment of opportunistic infections among HIV-exposed and HIV-infected children: recommendations from the CDC, the National Institutes of Health, the HIV Medicine Association of the Infectious Diseases Society of America, the Pediatric Infectious Diseases Society, and the American Academy of Pediatrics, *MMWR Recomm Rep* 58 (RR-11):1-66, 2009.

Acknowledgments

Because this is a book about partnerships, it could not have been created without the help of many individuals and organizations to whom we would like to express our deep appreciation.

The concept for the book grew out of discussions over a number of years with some wonderfully original thinkers, including Zimra Gordon, Joshua Dein, Thomas Chase, Augustus Ben David II, Jakob Zinsstag, Juan Lubroth, Elizabeth Mumford, Alonzo Aguirre, Peter Daszak, William Karesh, Lonnie King, Don Levy, Mark Pokras, Stephan Delaroque, Katinka deBalough, Michael Perdue, and Craig Stephens.

Bruce Kaplan drew on his many professional contacts to introduce the authors to each other and to encourage the development of the book throughout its many stages. His partners in the One Health initiative, Laura Kahn and Thomas Monath, have tirelessly worked to explore many of the themes that appear in the book.

Katherine Quesenberry helped introduce the idea of the book to Elsevier, where editor Anthony Winkel took it under his wing. Catherine Bowers helped with organization of early drafts. Maureen Slaten, our developmental editor, used unimaginable patience and perseverance to help us mold the many different sections into a consistent format and a recognizable whole, aided by Brandi Graham, Brian Dennison, and many others. Publisher Penny Rudolph assumed responsibility for the project in its later stages and helped finalize the many remaining decisions.

The work on the book drew us away from other professional responsibilities, and we are indebted to the supportive colleagues who helped make this possible. At Yale, some of those who generously helped provide coverage during Peter's sabbatical included Patrick O'Connor, Mark Cullen, Carrie Redlich, Oyebode Taiwo, Mark Russi, Martin Slade, Sharon Kirsche, Deron Galusha, Lynda Odofin, Frank Nusdeu, and Judy Sparer.

Any acknowledgments are inadequate to the large team of coauthors and chapter reviewers whose names appear elsewhere in the book. A special thanks is due to the members of the National Association of Public Health Veterinarians who consistently responded to requests for assistance in reviewing chapters. These individuals took time away from other duties to provide text and unsparing but always constructive critiques for the section drafts. We are incredibly fortunate to have been able to tap some of their vast funds of knowledge. Responsibility for any errors in the final version rests, however, with us, not them.

Although it may be a cliché to mention long-suffering family members, there are no words to describe the support, understanding, and insight provided by Peter's wife Nelly, who lived and breathed every step of the book's creation; children Aaron and Natasha, who waited patiently for the end of writing sessions; stepsons Sasha and Eliosha, who provided long-distance encouragement; and parents Alan and Andrea, who always had useful advice. Lisa's husband Tommy offered empathy, strength, and encouragement during the process; son Dane allowed his mom nights and weekends to attend to the project; and Aunt Mary brightened any day with her sanguine disposition.

We hope that this book does justice to the efforts and inspiration provided by these wonderful friends, family, and colleagues.

Foreword: Clinical Perspective

Ronald Davis, MD, MPH, and Roger Mahr, DVM

Serving as presidents of our respective national associations, the American Medical Association (AMA) and the American Veterinary Medical Association (AVMA), and representing our professions around the world, was, for us, the honor of a lifetime.

As each of us prepared to assume our presidencies, we focused on our respective Association missions and contemplated the following question: What are the values and responsibilities of our professions to global society?

We believe that animal and human health are at a crossroads. The convergence of animal, human, and environmental health dictates that the "One Health" concept be embraced and that the health science professions assume major leadership roles to translate that concept from a vision to reality.

It was on that basis of value to global society, and that sense of responsibility to the future, that we articulated our collective vision for a One Health Initiative. We have traveled the world, meeting and talking with veterinarians, physicians, public health professionals, academicians, students, government officials, legislators, and other stakeholders about the interrelationships among health science professions.

Through our respective leadership roles, we were able to achieve a collaborative relationship between the AVMA and AMA. In April 2007, the AVMA Executive Board took official action to establish the AVMA One Health Initiative Task Force. The charge to the Task Force was to study the feasibility of a One Health Initiative that would facilitate collaboration and cooperation among health science professions, academic institutions, governmental agencies, and industries and that would help with the assessment, treatment, and prevention of cross-species disease transmission and mutually prevalent, but nontransmitted, human and animal diseases and medical conditions. In June 2007, the AMA House of Delegates approved a resolution calling for the AMA to support the One Health Initiative and to engage in a dialogue with the AVMA to discuss means of enhancing collaboration between the two professions in medical education, clinical care, public health, and biomedical research.

We were privileged to serve as liaisons to the One Health Initiative Task Force and are proud of the dedicated efforts of its visionary members. We are enthusiastic about the potential impact of this initiative throughout the world. One Health has been defined as the collaborative efforts of multiple disciplines—working locally, nationally, and globally—to attain optimal health for people, animals, and our environment.

Certainly the One Health concept is not new. The pioneering efforts of many health science professionals in the past, including Sir William Osler, Rudolph Virchow, and Louis Pasteur in the nineteenth century, and Assistant Surgeon General James Steele and Dr. Calvin Schwabe in the twentieth century, have significantly influenced the development of comparative medicine and biomedical research and advanced the prevention and control of zoonotic diseases internationally.

As we face the challenges of the twenty-first century, it is imperative that One Health become a central focus within each health science profession. While the AVMA and AMA will continue to be key advocates for this effort, the success of the One Health Initiative will depend on the collaboration of various health science professional associations, academic institutions, governmental agencies, nongovernmental organizations, and industries.

It is most fitting and timely that *Human-Animal Medicine: Clinical Approaches to Zoonoses, Toxicants, and Other Shared Health Risks* be written collaboratively by a physician, Dr. Peter Rabinowitz, and a veterinarian, Dr. Lisa Conti. This book promises to be a valuable contribution to the One Health Initiative and will serve to demonstrate the significant benefit of interdisciplinary collaboration. In addition, it will further underscore the importance of coordination, communication, and cooperation among multiple disciplines, professions, and organizations.

This clinical guide is well designed and written for human health, animal health, public health, environmental health, and wildlife professionals. Through our individual careers as a clinical veterinary practitioner and a public health and preventive medicine physician, we appreciate the value this book will offer to students, practitioners, educators, researchers, and other professional disciplines. It can also be used as a resource to help the general public develop an awareness and understanding of One Health.

It is our fervent hope that professionals engaged in the health sciences will work to bring our disciplines into closer harmony, which will surely demonstrate that an integrated One Health enterprise is stronger and more valuable than the sum of its parts. Drs. Rabinowitz and Conti have provided evidence of that synergy through their collaboration in the publication of this extraordinary book.

[†]*Ronald Davis, MD, MPH*
Past President
American Medical Association

Roger Mahr, DVM
Past President
American Veterinary Medical Association

[†]Deceased.

Foreword: Public Health Perspective

James H. Steele, DVM, MPH, and Lonnie King, DVM, MS, MPA

While the foundation for the One Health concept as a convergence of human and animal health has been well articulated by key champions in the past, we are now entering a new era of awareness among public health professionals, clinicians, and the public about the inextricable links of human, animal, and environmental health. This era is making the One Health concept more expansive, accepted, global, and evidence based rather than characterized by single events. Understanding the One Health paradigm and our ability to effectively work at the human-animal interface is now a new dictum for health professionals. The publication of this book is further evidence of this transformation.

In the nineteenth century, Louis Pasteur confirmed that disease transmitted by microbes could affect both human beings and animals. This laid the groundwork for cross-disciplinary cooperation in public health research and practice, with veterinarians and physicians working side by side. It was a veterinary student named Daniel Salmon who isolated the enteric organism that now carries his name—*Salmonella*. One of the first activities of the Veterinary Public Health program at the then Centers for Disease Control (CDC, now Centers for Disease Control and Prevention) was to investigate the possibility that *Salmonella* was an important human pathogen. At that time, poultry and meat producers argued that *Salmonella* did not cause infection in human beings. CDC investigators, however, were able to confirm that the bacteria were indeed an important cause of human enteric disease. Today, we have more sophisticated diagnostic tools and growing technological capacities that enable us to gain more insights into the complex dynamics and full dimensions of human-animal health links. Over a decade ago, the CDC introduced a new DNA fingerprinting diagnostic system termed PulseNet. Working with state public health laboratories, PulseNet has enabled us to better diagnose multistate foodborne outbreaks and better understand the ecology and epidemiology of these outbreaks. *Salmonella* in peanut butter, peppers, and pot pies and *Escherichia coli* in spinach are just a few examples of discovering new vehicles for foodborne pathogens and helping reveal the importance of understanding how microbes are transmitted and maintained in the environment and readily move across species lines. The use of microarrays and new molecular diagnostics has also helped us elucidate the science of infectious disease ecology. We now appreciate that bats may harbor Ebola, Hendra, Nipah, and Marburg viruses and that H5N1 avian influenza is found in multiple wild bird and domestic poultry species and populations worldwide. Technological advances have given us new tools and insights into the convergence of human, animal, and environmental health and have reinforced a growing scientific foundation that further undergirds the principles of One Health. The scope, scale, and global implications of emerging infectious diseases and other contemporary public health challenges demand that scientists, researchers, health care workers, and practitioners move beyond the confines of their own disciplines and explore new models of team science as well as establish new working relationships among human, animal, and environmental professionals, especially between veterinary practitioners and physicians. Thus a One Health construct is now essential for us to target earlier interventions and new prevention strategies.

There is every indication that the driving forces that have dramatically resulted in a new and profound era of emerging infections will continue to grow even more complex, challenging, and important to our work and lives. Thus this book is especially timely and relevant. We now live in a world where we must prepare for an H5N1 pandemic, appreciate our rapidly growing and expanding global food system, understand the importance of emerging zoonoses, grow increasingly concerned about antimicrobial resistance, and acknowledge new threats from the expansion of vector-borne, foodborne, and water-borne diseases both domestically and globally.

This book is especially beneficial to raise the awareness and appreciation of private practitioners, both veterinary and human, to envision themselves and their clinical work as key to putting One Health into practice. At the same time, the book is enormously helpful in building momentum toward a more universal acceptance of One Health and encourages us to work across disciplines, professions, and organizations. Just as important, the book is instructive to help us shift from the concept of One Health to actually implement daily actions and strategies that bring the nexus of human, animal, and environmental health into better focus to ensure positive and real health impact.

Furthermore, this book serves as a wonderful contribution for educating public and animal health professionals and practitioners about working together at the human-animal interface. Yet much more needs to be done to ensure that our researchers, diagnosticians, laboratory scientists, and practitioners take a more holistic view of health and realize the many overlaps between human and animal medicine and health. We appreciate that the authors have demonstrated the benefits of working together and have encouraged us to be part of a larger community with mutual respect and new tools and thinking that will continue to improve human, animal, and environmental health. We are grateful for both the intellectual and practical contributions of this book and will use the examples and ideas contained in it to better prepare us to address the threats and challenges of the future. Lastly, this book will also be enormously helpful to stimulate us to continue our pioneering efforts and leadership in public and animal health to create a more integrated worldview of One Health.

James H. Steele, DVM, MPH
Chief Veterinary Officer
Assistant Surgeon General
U.S. Public Health Service

Lonnie King, DVM, MS, MPA
Director of National Center for Zoonotic, Vector-Borne
  and Enteric Diseases
Centers for Disease Control and Prevention
Atlanta, Georgia

Contents

The Convergence of Human and Animal Medicine

Laura H. Kahn, Bruce Kaplan, and Thomas P. Monath

1

HOW HUMAN AND ANIMAL HEALTH CONVERGE

The relationship between human and animal health is becoming increasingly complex and includes biological, chemical, physical, and social factors (Figure 1-1). Both endemic and newly emerging infectious diseases have grabbed headlines and heightened awareness of the role of wild and domestic animal populations in transmitting diseases to human beings. Although the importance of zoonotic disease is not new—approximately 60% of all infectious pathogens of human beings are zoonotic in origin—an even higher percentage of newly emerging diseases over the past 2 decades are zoonoses, many originating from wildlife (Figure 1-2).[1] All but one of the bioterrorism agents considered to have the highest potential for use as a weapon of biological warfare are zoonotic pathogens.

Pets and Wildlife

More than half of households in the United States own a dog, cat, or both. In addition, millions of exotic wild animals, birds, and reptiles are kept in U.S. households as pets, and the worldwide trade in such animals is accelerating (see Chapter 10).[2] Therefore the average patient visiting his or her health care provider is likely to share his or her living space with a pet, and the health of the pet (which may have originated in a wildlife population across the globe) may hold clues to health or disease issues that the patient is experiencing. Furthermore, as suburban developments encroach on wildlife habitat (see Chapter 6), contact with domestic animals, wildlife, and insect vectors may be frequent, allowing pathogens to pass in both directions and bringing human beings into the mix. At the same time, veterinarians in small animal practice have understood for years that pets contribute to improved human mental health and well-being and that the benefits of companion animals usually far exceed the risks of zoonotic disease. A growing body of research now supports the concept of this "human-animal bond phenomenon"; avenues for physician-veterinarian cooperation to maximize these benefits are detailed in Chapter 5.

Food Animals

On a global scale, the growing human population has led to a rapid and unprecedented increase in the numbers and density of animals raised for food production in many parts of the world and the United States (see Chapter 11). The rearing, transportation, marketing, and processing of these animals have significant implications for the occupational health of the human beings working with the animals (Figure 1-3); wildlife that may have contact with such animals; as well as the air, soil, and water quality of agricultural areas (see Chapter 12). The widespread outbreaks of avian influenza among domestic poultry and the threat of the emergence of new strains with pandemic potential are a reminder of these connections. In addition, the increasing reliance on bush meat consumption in many developing countries affects wildlife populations and species diversity and exposes human beings to zoonotic disease threats.[3]

THE IMPORTANCE OF ENVIRONMENTAL HEALTH TO HUMAN BEINGS AND OTHER ANIMALS

Zoonotic disease represents just one of the ways that the health of companion animals, livestock, and wildlife is inextricably linked with human health. The global environment is rapidly changing, and animals and human beings are exposed to shared environmental health risks. Environmental disasters such as Hurricane Katrina wreak havoc on both human and animal populations. Many zoonotic diseases are emerging as a result of environmental factors, including climate change, deforestation, alterations of wildlife habitat, and other land use change[4]; human population growth; movement of human beings and animals across borders; and increased production of food animals. The built environment may contribute to a sedentary lifestyle and manifest as an obesity epidemic in both human beings[5] and their pets (Figure 1-4). Animals and human beings often share exposure risks from noninfectious disease threats, such as air and water quality problems, pesticides, lead, and carbon

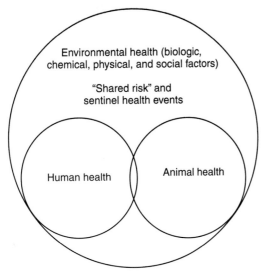

Figure 1-1 ■ Relationships among environmental, human, and animal health.

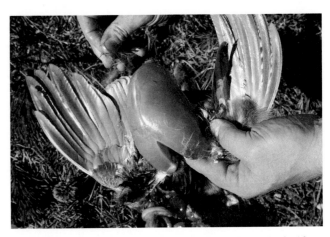

Figure 1-3 ■ Removing the breast and leg meat from a bird without using gloves. (Courtesy Melissa Anderson. From Auerbach PS: *Wilderness medicine*, ed 5, Philadelphia, 2007, Mosby Elsevier.)

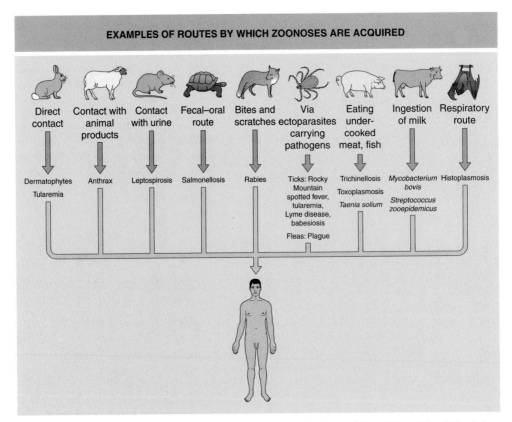

Figure 1-2 ■ Examples of routes by which zoonoses are acquired by human beings. (From Cohen J, Powderly WG: *Infectious diseases*, ed 2, London, 2003, Mosby Elsevier.)

monoxide. Just as canaries once warned coal miners of the presence of deadly gases and dead songbirds sent a message to human beings about the risks of pesticides in Rachel Carson's *Silent Spring*, a disease occurrence in an animal can be a "sentinel event" warning human beings of an environmental threat.[6] Alternatively, at times a human being has a diagnosed disease that provides information about an environmental risk to animals living nearby. Chapter 4 in this book, as well as the disease-specific chapters, provide many examples of sentinel events and how clinicians and public health professionals can detect them and act on such information to prevent further cases.

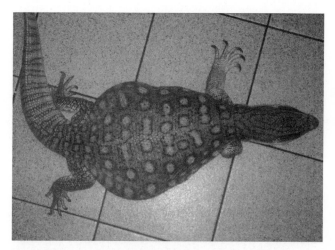

Figure 1-4 ■ Obese Savannah monitor *(Varanus exanthematicus).* (Courtesy S.J. Hernandez Divers. From Mader DR: *Reptile medicine and surgery,* ed 2, St Louis, 2005, Saunders Elsevier.)

SIMILARITIES AND DIFFERENCES AMONG THE TRAINING AND PRACTICE OF HUMAN HEALTH, ANIMAL HEALTH, AND PUBLIC HEALTH PROFESSIONALS

The training and practice patterns of human health care providers, veterinarians, and public health professionals differ in important ways. Table 1-1 outlines some of the key points differentiating the groups.

Despite many curricular similarities between human medical and veterinary medical schools, veterinarians receive more training in zoonotic diseases, whereas medical students learn virtually nothing about animal health issues. Both groups receive only limited training in public health theory and practice.

After completing their training, physicians in practice rarely make home or worksite visits to directly see the environments where their patients live and work, whereas large animal veterinarians frequently visit farms. Public health professionals may be more likely to visit locations where environmental health threats have been identified. The rate at which veterinarians perform necropsies on animals that have died may be higher than the rate at which physicians perform autopsies. As a result of these training and practice differences, the approaches to detecting and preventing problems related to interactions among human beings, animals, and the environment may differ greatly among these groups.

Role of Veterinarians in Human Health

Many physicians may not be aware of the routine contributions made by practicing veterinarians to human health. Veterinarians regularly educate pet owners and farmers

Table 1-1 ■ Training and Practice Statistics: Veterinary Medicine, Human Medicine, and Public Health

Category	Veterinary Medicine (DVM/VMD)[7]	Human Health (MD, DO)[7]	Public Health (MPH, DrPH)
Minimum years of professional school	4 Approximately 2 years basic sciences + 2 years clinical studies Curricula comparable to medical schools	4 Approximately 2 years basic sciences + 2 years clinical studies Curricula comparable to veterinary medical schools	2-4 Studies include epidemiology, biostatistics, and public health administration
Amount of training in zoonotic diseases	Moderate	Minimal	Varies
Amount of training in animal health issues	High[8]	None	Varies (e.g., there are combined DVM/MPH programs)
Curriculum hours in public health	Minimal	Minimal	High
Number of practitioners in the United States	Approximately 69,170 (active)[8]*	633,000	†
Specialties	70% of private practice veterinarians focus on small animal medicine/surgery (dogs, cats, etc.) Board certifications in various specialties	Primary care professions Specialists	Includes environmental health, occupational health, maternal and child health, infectious diseases, biostatistics
Practice organization	Prevailing model solo or small group practices with some evolving large group practices	Increasing role of health maintenance organizations	Public health agency
House calls/site visits	Large animal DVMs/VMDs visit farms; rare for small animal practitioners (via mobile veterinary clinics)	MDs rarely make house calls Home health care nurses provide many services in homes	Some public health professionals perform site visits
Licensing agency in states	Departments of consumer affairs, professional regulation, or departments of public health (usually the same department in state)		

*As of October 31, 2007.
†Data not available.

about the risks of acquiring zoonotic diseases. They reduce transmission risks to human beings by vaccinating large numbers of pets and livestock against zoonotic diseases. Many are involved in caring for wildlife and exotic animals.

The expanding role of veterinarians at the U.S. Centers for Disease Control and Prevention (CDC, http://www.cdc.gov) reflects a growing trend to create joint teams of veterinarians and human health professionals to deal with human-animal health issues. The team approach has proved synergistic; more rapid and precise evaluations enhance more efficacious control. At the time of this writing, approximately 90 veterinarians work at the CDC.[9] The CDC's National Center for Zoonotic, Vector-Borne, and Enteric Diseases (NCZVED) provides leadership, expertise, and service in laboratory and epidemiological science, bioterrorism preparedness, applied research, disease surveillance, and outbreak response for infectious diseases. Its ecological framework includes human beings, animals, and plants interacting in the complex, changing natural environment. Until September 1, 2009, NCZVED was directed and administered by a veterinarian with previous experience as administrator of the U.S. Department of Agriculture's (USDA) Animal and Plant Health Inspection Service (APHIS).

From 1953 through 2008, more than 228 veterinarians have completed the Epidemic Intelligence Service (EIS) training at the CDC (Figure 1-5). The EIS represents the U.S's critical unit for investigating the causes of major epidemics. Over the past 50 years, EIS officers have played crucial roles in combating the root causes of epidemics of major consequence. The EIS has served as a model for similar services in about 25 other countries worldwide.

The Special Pathogens Unit at the CDC concerns itself with the investigation of the highly pathogenic, zoonotic viral hemorrhagic fevers, such as Ebola virus, Marburg hemorrhagic fever, and Lassa fever. The unit is currently directed by a veterinarian and includes a number of physicians who collaborate on laboratory and field research aimed at elucidating the reservoirs of infection in nature, transmission of viruses to human beings, the control of outbreaks, and groundbreaking research on diagnostic methods and vaccines.

Outside the CDC, state public health veterinarians (http://www.nasphv.org) are involved in a wide range of public health issues. They often interact with their federal colleagues at the CDC and other professionals in state and federal departments of agriculture on issues related to food safety, importation of animal diseases, bioterrorism preparedness, pandemic preparedness, environmental health, and many areas of shared concern (see Chapter 13).

Other Professionals Critically Involved With Human-Animal Medicine Issues

In addition to physicians, veterinarians, and public health professionals, many other professionals play key roles in human and animal health and should be considered in any discussion of how these fields converge. A significant percentage of health care services in the United States is provided by advanced practice registered nurses (APRNs) or physician assistants (PAs), and hospital-based and home health nurses perform frequent health assessments and contribute to the development of care plans. On the veterinary side, veterinary technicians and other veterinary staff provide many animal health care services, as do wildlife rehabilitators. Public health efforts to manage zoonotic disease risk and other environmental health issues require the expertise of vector ecologists, wildlife biologists, disease ecologists, environmental health professionals, industrial hygienists, toxicologists, anthropologists, farmers, and agricultural extension officers, among others. Although human health and animal health clinicians may detect sentinel cases of disease related to environmental factors, the actual intervention to improve such environments requires a team approach of diverse professionals, as is described in other sections of this book.

EFFORTS TO BRIDGE THE GAPS BETWEEN HUMAN AND ANIMAL HEALTH

Communication Between Human and Animal Health Care Providers

The convergence of these health issues involving human beings and other animals would seem to demand ongoing

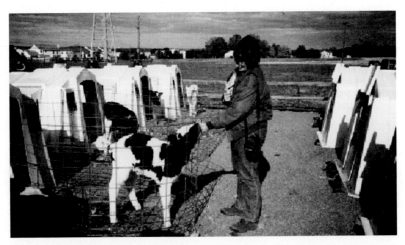

Figure 1-5 ■ A CDC investigator examines a calf as part of an outbreak investigation. (Courtesy Centers for Disease Control and Prevention, Atlanta, Ga.)

and substantive interactions between human health care providers and veterinarians, as well as a shared body of knowledge regarding health links between human beings and animals. Yet professional interaction of this type is often limited. Research indicates that many physicians and other health care providers may be uncomfortable discussing animal health issues with their patients.[10] Veterinary medical health care providers may be cautious about discussing human health issues with their clients, in some circumstances because of caution to not overstep professional boundaries and possibly because of concerns about malpractice liability or privacy issues (see Chapter 2). Both human health and veterinary clinicians may be unfamiliar with public health and environmental health concepts and their relevance to their practices.

Some of the key differences among the professions, as well as the One Health Initiative aimed at overcoming professional barriers to communication and collaboration, are described below.

Collaborations Between Animal and Human Health Care Providers

Historical precedents do exist for productive collaboration between animal and human health care providers. The nineteenth-century physician pathologist Dr. Rudolf Virchow (who coined the term *zoonosis*) emphasized the need for medical scientists to learn from comparative medicine approaches to research. Sir William Osler (called the "Father of Modern Medicine"), a physician who studied with Virchow, helped establish the first departments of veterinary pathology in North America in the late nineteenth century. Drs. Theobald Smith, a physician, and F. L. Kilborne, a veterinarian, discovered that *Babesia bigemina,* the cause of cattle fever, was transmitted by ticks. Their work set the stage for Walter Reed's discovery of yellow fever transmission via mosquitoes.[11] More recently, Rolf Zinkernagel, a physician, and Peter C. Doherty, a veterinarian, shared the 1996 Nobel Prize for their discoveries of how the body's immune system distinguishes normal cells from virus-infected cells.

One Health Initiative

In the 1960s, veterinarian Dr. Calvin W. Schwabe, a parasitologist and veterinary epidemiologist, coined the term *One Medicine* in his textbook, *Veterinary Medicine and Human Health.*[12] Schwabe proposed a collaborative effort between veterinary and human health professionals to combat zoonotic diseases. In recent years, a number of organizations and collaborations have sought to build on and further expand this model, producing concepts such as conservation medicine,[13] Ecohealth,[14] and "One World, One Health."[15] The common theme of these diverse efforts is that the health of human beings, wildlife, domestic animals, and the environment is vitally interconnected and future efforts to improve global health must take these interrelationships into account.

Recently the American Medical Association (AMA) and American Veterinary Medical Association (AVMA) began collaborative efforts on a One Health Initiative (also referred to as *One Medicine, One Medicine-One Health*, and *One World One Medicine One Health*). The One Health Initiative promotes the model of physicians, veterinarians, and allied medical and environmental scientists in clinical, public health, and biomedical research settings working more closely together than in the past to better understand, manage, and prevent health risks involving animals, human beings, and their environments (Figure 1-6).[11,16]

A joint One Health Task Force created by the AMA and AVMA was formed to study ways to facilitate collaboration and cooperation among human health and animal health professions, educational institutions, and agencies to improve assessment, treatment, and prevention of cross-species disease transmission and mutually prevalent noninfectious human and animal diseases and medical conditions. The recommendations of the One Health Task Force were published in 2008 (available online at http://www.avma.org/onehealth).[17] Key recommendations of the task force included a call for a national research agenda for One Health and outreach efforts to involve medical, veterinary medical, and public health students and their respective organizations in One Health concepts.

Similarly, a consultation document, "Contributing to One World, One Health: Strategic Framework for Reducing Risks of Infectious Diseases at the Animal-Human-Ecosystems Interface," was produced by the Food and Agriculture Organizations of the United Nations (FAO), World Organization for Animal Health (OIE), World Health Organization (WHO), United Nations System Influenza Coordination, United Nations Children's Emergency Funds (UNICEF), and the World Bank (see http://www.oie.int/downld/AVIAN%20INFLUENZA/OWOH/OWOH_14Oct08.pdf).

The six specific objectives suggested for prioritization by national authorities are as follows:

1. Develop international, regional, and national capacity in surveillance, making use of international standards, tools, and monitoring processes
2. Ensure adequate international, regional, and national capacity in public and animal health—including communication strategies—to prevent, detect, and respond to disease outbreaks

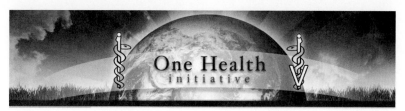

Figure 1-6 ■ The One Health Initiative logo. (From B. Kaplan, http://www.onehealthinitiative.com.)

3. Ensure functioning national emergency response capacity as well as a global rapid response support capacity
4. Promote interagency and cross-sectoral collaboration and partnership
5. Control highly pathogenic avian influenza and other existing and potentially re-emerging infectious diseases
6. Conduct strategic research

Research approaches linking human and animal health in a One Health model hold great promise. Improved vaccine development and delivery for animal diseases such as brucellosis and avian influenza may reduce human risk from these diseases. Conversely, the conservation of great apes in Africa, currently affected by outbreaks of Ebola virus, could benefit if a human vaccine were developed. Similarly, pharmaceutical developments and sustainable environmental health practices often have benefits across species.

The Human Genome Project has resulted in the availability of sequencing the genomes of multiple animal species and an understanding of epigenetics. These molecular tools are helping define the similarities and differences between species with regard to host-environment interactions as well as drug pharmacodynamics and pharmacokinetics.

Disease surveillance represents another area of improved collaboration between human and animal health. Improved early warning systems for disease risk that use both human and animal data could help highlight environmental factors driving disease outbreaks in wildlife, domestic animals, and human beings, leading to better disease prevention.

A better understanding of disease ecology and the impact of environmental change on disease risk for both animals and human beings is essential to the One Health approach. As clinicians become increasingly aware that the diseases observed in their human and animal patients are related to shared environmental health risks, this can create synergy in collaboration with environmental health and disease ecology experts to reduce such risks.

In the midst of such developments, human and animal health professionals working on the front lines of clinical and public health practice will play an important role in the recognition and management of a wide range of health issues involving overlaps between human and animal health. This book provides numerous practical suggestions for helping such professionals retool and implement One Health concepts into their daily practice routines, which could enhance the preventive and therapeutic care they provide and lead to further convergence between the disciplines.

References

1. Woolhouse ME, Gowtage-Sequeria S. Host range and emerging and reemerging pathogens. *Emerg Infect Dis.* 2005;11(12):1842–1847.
2. Chomel BB, Belotto A, Meslin FX. Wildlife, exotic pets, and emerging zoonoses. *Emerg Infect Dis.* 2007;13(1):6–11.
3. Wolfe ND, Daszak P, Kilpatrick AM, et al. Bushmeat hunting, deforestation, and prediction of zoonoses emergence. *Emerg Infect Dis.* 2005;11(12):1822–1827.
4. Patz JA, Daszak P, Tabor GM, et al. Unhealthy landscapes: policy recommendations on land use change and infectious disease emergence. *Environ Health Perspect.* 2004;112(10):1092–1098.
5. Wakefield J. Fighting obesity through the built environment. *Environ Health Perspect.* 2004;112(11):A616–A618.
6. Carson R. *Silent spring.* Boston: Houghton Mifflin; 1962.
7. Bureau of Labor Statistics, U.S. Department of Labor. *Occupational outlook handbook,* 2008-09 edition. http://www.bl.gov/oco/ocos076.htm. Accessed August 26, 2008.
8. National Research Council, Committee on the National Needs for Research in Veterinary Science. *Critical needs for research in veterinary science.* Washington, DC: National Academies Press; 2005.
9. King LJ. Personal communication. 2008.
10. Grant S, Olsen LW. Preventing zoonotic diseases in immunocompromised persons: the role of physicians and veterinarians. *EID.* 1999;5(1):159–163.
11. Kahn LH, Kaplan B, Steele JH. Confronting zoonoses through closer collaboration between medicine and veterinary medicine (as "one medicine"). *Veterinaria Italiana.* 2007;43(1):5–19.
12. Schwabe CW. *Veterinary medicine and human health,* ed. 3. Baltimore: Williams & Wilkins; 1984.
13. Aguirre AA, Ostfeld RS, Tabor GM, et al. *Conservation medicine: ecological health in practice.* New York: Oxford University Press; 2002.
14. Wilcox B, Kueffer C. Transdisciplinarity in EcoHealth: status and future prospects. *EcoHealth.* 2008;5(1):1–3.
15. Wildlife Conservation Society. *The Manhattan principles on "One World-One Health."* http://www.oneworldonehealth.org/index.html. Accessed August 11, 2008.
16. Kahn LH, Kaplan B, Monath TP, et al. Teaching "one medicine, one health." *Am J Med.* 2008;121(3):169–170.
17. King LJ, Anderson LR, Blackmore CG, et al. Executive summary of the AVMA one health initiative task force report. *J Am Vet Med Assoc.* 2008;233(2):259–261.

Legal and Ethical Issues in Human-Animal Medicine

2

Peter M. Rabinowitz and Lisa A. Conti

The concept of increasing communication and collaboration among public health, human health, and animal health professionals in a One Health model has numerous advantages. Important legal and ethical issues apply to such professional interactions. Clinicians and public health professionals need to be aware that such issues can be complex and are continuing to evolve. This chapter outlines some of these issues. Health care providers should query local authorities such as health department attorneys, risk managers, and their professional associations about state and local regulations. Although some international disease reporting requirements apply to animal and human health in the United States, professionals in other countries also will need to be informed about country and region-specific regulations.

Key Points for Clinicians and Public Health Professionals

Public Health Professionals

- Educate human health and veterinary clinicians about requirements for reporting certain diseases to public health authorities.
- Facilitate communication between animal and human health professionals while protecting patient confidentiality.

Human Health Clinicians

- Report notifiable diseases to public health authorities.
- Become knowledgeable about zoonotic and other animal-related disease risks. Competently assess such risks during the care of patients.
- Provide written information on zoonotic and other animal-related disease risks (such as the CDC's Pets-Scription: http://www.cdc.gov/healthypets/health_prof.htm#petscription) to patients with animal contact. Information if include advice about seeking medical care if symptoms develop.
- Respect patient confidentiality when communicating with veterinary professionals and abide by applicable laws and professional guidelines.

- Do not treat animals or give veterinary medical advice because these activities fall outside the scope of practice for human medical licensure.
- Provide medical services that promote public health, such as preventive care for zoonotic disease.

Veterinary Clinicians

- Comply with the state's scope of veterinary practice.
- Counsel clients about zoonotic disease risks and how to reduce such risks. Document in the veterinary medical record all public health advice given to clients.
- Provide clients with written information on zoonotic and other animal-related disease risks (such as the CDC Pets-Scription), including advice about seeking medical care if clinical signs develop.
- Provide competent preventive care for zoonotic disease prevention.
- If clients decline preventive, diagnostic, or treatment services for their animals for zoonotic disease, request that they sign a waiver documenting refusal of these services.
- Avoid giving human medical advice but offer to assist in communication with physicians or other human health care providers regarding zoonotic or other animal-related health risks.
- Request permission of client before discussing the client's animals with human health care providers.
- Respect the confidentiality of client medical information and do not include protected health information (PHI) about clients and their families in a veterinary medical record.
- Report suspected animal abuse to appropriate authorities.
- Provide veterinary medical services that promote public health, such as strategic deworming and vaccination against zoonotic diseases.

LEGAL CONSIDERATIONS

The convergence of animal health and human health described in Chapter 1 raises a number of potentially important legal issues of which human health and veterinary providers should be aware.

Scope of Practice

In some instances, physicians have been asked to treat animals belonging to their patients. Likewise, veterinarians have been asked to treat people or provide medical advice and/or medications that could be used for human beings as well as other animals, especially when dealing with zoonotic diseases. Both human and veterinary health professionals need to be aware of the concept of professional scope of practice and the need not to overstep professional bounds in such situations.

Physicians and other human health care providers, including nurse practitioners and physician assistants, are licensed to evaluate and treat diseases in human beings. Individuals without such licenses who provide medical treatment (such as administration of prescription medication or performing a surgical procedure such as suturing a wound) are "practicing medicine without a license," which is a violation of state professional licensing (and possibly criminal) statutes. The justification for licensing professionals is in part to ensure they are appropriately qualified and can provide necessary care. The exact scope of practice of physicians and other medical professionals is determined by medical examining boards of individual states and therefore can vary among states. For example, licensed psychologists have the authority to prescribe medications in some states but not in many others.[1] Obviously, the scope of practice for medical care providers does not include providing veterinary care for animals.

Similarly, veterinarians are licensed to evaluate and treat animals other than human beings. Veterinary practice acts in different states define the practice of veterinary medicine and the scope of practice for veterinary professionals in that state, including veterinarians and associated providers such as veterinary technicians. Someone who diagnoses and treats an animal (other than one he or she owns) without such licensing is at risk of being charged with "practicing veterinary medicine without a license." The American Veterinary Medical Association (AVMA) publishes a Model Veterinary Practice Act (MVPA) that has been used by some states in drafting scope of practice legislation.[2] Veterinary providers should be aware of their state's current definition of veterinary medicine and scope of veterinary practice. The definition of veterinary practice in the MVPA is shown in Box 2-1.

Veterinary Practice Act

As shown in Box 2-1, the "rendering of advice or recommendation" about animal diseases is part of the practice of veterinary medicine, and this should be kept in mind by human health care providers who are discussing animal health issues with their patients. The MVPA does not include any provisions for veterinarians offering medical advice to their clients regarding human diseases. However, in addition, the oath of practice that veterinarians take when entering the profession (Box 2-2) includes a commitment to "the promotion of public health, and the advancement of medical knowledge." Therefore counseling clients about reducing zoonotic disease risk, providing preventive care to reduce such risk, and notifying public health departments in a timely manner about human health risks would appear to be an intrinsic part of good preventive veterinary care. Failure on the part

---

of a veterinarian to perform such activities could potentially lead to legal liability (see below). Veterinarians consequently must carefully consider ways to fulfill their public health obligations while not exceeding their professional scope of practice.[3]

Malpractice Liability

Both physicians and veterinarians are liable for malpractice (damages awarded for professional negligence). Many human health and veterinary providers carry malpractice insurance, but such insurance covers only activities within the scope of practice for that professional.

There is a growing realization of particular risks to both human and veterinary medical providers related to zoonotic diseases in terms of malpractice liability related to human-animal medicine issues, although legal precedent in this area remains sparse. There is potential malpractice liability for physicians and other human health care providers who fail to correctly diagnose an animal-related disease such as a zoonosis in their patients because they failed to take an adequate history of animal exposures or otherwise consider the diagnosis. For example, a physician who fails to obtain a history of bird contact in the household and consequently fails to correctly diagnose a disease such as psittacosis in a person who shares the household with the bird could be at risk of being sued for negligence (see Chapter 9). Management of this liability can include training for physicians and other medical providers in the recognition of zoonotic disease risk and other animal-related risks.

Veterinarians are in a knowledgeable position to warn clients about the risks of zoonoses and control the risk to human beings by competently managing disease in the animal population. Consequently, there appear to be a number of areas of potential malpractice liability for veterinarians related to negligence in the management of zoonotic disease.

The first area of potential negligence is the failure to correctly diagnose a zoonotic disease in an animal. For example, if a veterinarian fails to detect dermatophytosis in a cat used for animal therapy (see Chapter 5) and an immunocompromised person who is in contact with the cat becomes infected with *Microsporum* as a result (see Chapter 9), the veterinarian could be blamed for failing to diagnose the zoonotic risk. In the past, it may have been more difficult to definitively link an animal infection to a subsequent infection in a human, but the use of molecular techniques to characterize particular strains of an organism crossing from animals to human beings now allows such causative linkages to be made. Such evidence could surface in a medicolegal setting.[3]

Another area of malpractice liability for veterinarians related to zoonotic disease is the failure to recommend preventive measures for common zoonotic diseases. This situation could occur if a veterinarian failed to isolate an unvaccinated stray cat with bite wounds with the subsequent need for rabies postexposure prophylaxis among human contacts if the cat develops rabies (see Chapter 9). In such a case, the veterinarian could be held liable for not taking steps to control the zoonotic risk. Another example would be if a veterinarian diagnosed leptospirosis in a dog, failed to adequately warn the owner regarding the zoonotic risk of disease, and leptospirosis that could be traced back to the strain that infected the dog later develops in the owner.

In the case of exotic and wildlife pets that could harbor unusual zoonotic diseases (such as monkeypox) or pose envenomation risks (such as venomous reptiles), a veterinarian could be held liable for not warning clients about the dangers of keeping such animals. Even in the case of rare and unusual zoonoses and other disease risks related to exotic pets with which a veterinarian may be less familiar, it could be argued that the veterinarian should have referred the owner to a specialist for diagnosis or treatment of a species or condition that was not within the practitioner's expertise (see Chapter 10). [3]

An additional potential area of veterinarian malpractice liability involves a failure to advise a client to seek care from a physician for diagnosis and treatment of a zoonotic disease. This could occur if a client reports certain symptoms such as fever or diarrhea to a veterinarian after an exposure to a sick animal and the veterinarian fails to counsel that person to seek medical care.

Management techniques to avoid these malpractice liabilities include the following:

1. Educating clients about the risks of zoonotic disease and methods to reduce such risks, and documenting such education. To supplement such teaching, handouts about zoonotic disease risks can be given to clients by veterinarians to educate them. An example of such a handout is the "Pet-Scription" and "Pet-Scription for Reptile Owners" available from the CDC Healthy Pets Healthy People website. Discussions about zoonotic disease risk should be documented in the veterinary medical record.
2. Asking clients who decline preventive treatment (such as routine deworming) for their animals to sign a waiver documenting the refusal of such treatment. Examples of such legal consent forms are available, but veterinarians should seek advice from a local attorney about such documentation because local statutes may vary.[3]
3. Increasing direct professional communication between human health care providers and veterinarians. Direct physician-veterinarian contact offers several advantages, including ensuring that diagnostic and therapeutic information is accurately conveyed, learning of other animal-human interaction health concerns, and increasing dual awareness on the part of both types of practitioners about the health issues related to animal-human contacts. Many sections of this book contain specific suggestions for the content of direct communication between human and animal professionals. Such communications, however, need to consider concerns about patient confidentiality (see below).

Workers' Compensation Liability

Employers of animal workers, including owners of veterinary practices, zoos, and animal care facilities, are liable for work-related diseases in employees as a result of human-animal contact. Examples of potentially compensable diseases in animal workers include skin rashes, asthma or other allergy, animal bites, and zoonotic infections as well as diseases resulting from exposure to anesthetic gases, cleaning agents, and workplace noise. Incidents of work-related injury and illness are compensable under state workers' compensation statutes, with the employee being potentially eligible for reimbursement of medical expenses, lost work time, and other awards related to the illness or injury. Veterinarians and other employers of animal workers can manage liability for work-related illness and injury by taking steps to reduce risks in the workplace through engineering and work practice controls for biological, chemical, physical, and psychosocial hazards and by ensuring the provision of adequate occupational health services for such workers (see Chapter 12).

Other Liability

Veterinarians may be liable for physical injury to a human (such as a dog bite) if it could be shown that the veterinarian failed to properly counsel owners about ways to reduce the risk of such injury and failed to intervene appropriately in the care of a potentially dangerous animal. Again, educating owners about warning signs of behavioral problems in dogs and other animals and steps to take to reduce risks of aggressive animals, and documentation of such education, is one way to manage liability.

Confidentiality and the Health Insurance Portability and Accountability Act

The Health Insurance Portability and Accountability Act (HIPAA, known as the Privacy Rule) has tightened the rules regarding the release and sharing of personal health information (PHI) by medical providers treating patients. This rule also applies to health plans and health care clearinghouses.[4] PHI refers to health information that can be linked to an identifiable individual and that relates to the following:

1. Past, present, or future physical or mental health or condition of the individual
2. Provision of health care to the individual
3. Payment for the provision of health care to the individual

"Covered entities" under HIPAA include persons, businesses, or agencies that furnish, bill, or receive payment for health care in the normal course of business.[5] The Privacy Rule does not directly address confidentiality in veterinary practices. Provisions of the Privacy Rule allow PHI to be released to public health authorities for the purpose of surveillance and disease control. However, public health authorities must take steps to preserve the confidentiality of such information.[6]

Veterinarians also have laws that govern the confidentiality of veterinarian-client interactions.[7] In some states, veterinarians are forbidden to release details regarding the treatment of an animal without the written permission of the animal's owner. Although exceptions allow for communications between veterinarians or between veterinarians and human health professionals or animal control officers, in general veterinarians should obtain the permission of their clients before releasing information about an animal's diagnosis and treatment.[7] HIPAA legislation does not specifically mention veterinarians, but some communications of health information between veterinarians and human health care providers could involve HIPAA-defined PHI (see Chapter 3). For example, if a client mentions to the veterinarian that he or she has a medical condition that could predispose others to zoonotic infection (see Chapter 10), such information could be considered PHI.

Guidelines for practice in this environment for veterinarians include the following:

- Excluding identifiable health information about clients or other persons in the household that could be considered PHI from the veterinary record (see Chapter 3)
- Refusing to provide medical advice to human beings (see also the scope of practice discussion above)
- Offering assistance to speak with the person's physician, with the person's permission
- Educating the physician or other human health care provider on questions he or she may have regarding pets, zoonoses, and pet care

Notification and Reporting

Both human health care and veterinary providers are required by state and federal regulations to report certain diseases and conditions to the appropriate health agencies, although the lists of reportable human and animal diseases have areas of overlap and some differences (see Chapter 13 for a listing of nationally notifiable human and animal diseases). Whereas human health providers must report notifiable diseases to public health authorities, veterinarians may need to report animal and other diseases to agriculture departments, public health departments, or both (see Chapter 13).

In addition to reportable diseases, other medical conditions require notification by health professionals. Human health care providers are required to report cases of suspected child abuse. Similarly, in some states veterinarians are required to report suspected animal abuse (see Chapter 5).[8]

If human health care providers, veterinary providers, or their employees incur an occupational injury or illness, including animal bites and zoonotic or allergic disease among workers in an animal hospital or other animal care facility, such incidents need to be recorded on the Occupational Safety and Health Administration (OSHA) reporting log of work-related injuries and illnesses for that facility (see Chapter 12). Instructions regarding OSHA reporting can be found at http://www.osha.gov/doc/outreachtraining/htmlfiles/cfr1904.html.

ETHICAL ISSUES

Professionalism

One set of ethical issues concerns professionalism and expectations of practitioners. For example, patients have an expectation that health care providers are honest and truthful, are knowledgeable and current in their field, and act in the best interests of their patients. The idea that professionals act in the best interests of their patients is both a legal and ethical obligation known as a *fiduciary duty*. This duty refers to the relationship of trust or confidence between professionals and their patients or clients. Professionals are expected to be loyal, not put personal interests above those of the patient or client, and not profit from the relationship unless the patient or client consents. An implication of this last point is the expectation that professionals minimize and disclose conflicts of interests.

Ethical Principles in Human Health

Another set of issues concerns ethical principles regarding the conduct of human medical and veterinary practice. These can be characterized in ethical codes, in general principles, or by reference to cases (cases of good behavior and cases of nonoptimal behavior). Because a profession may have more than one code of ethics (for example, there are a number of codes in medicine, some tailored to the particular practice specialty), one broad approach to ethics is to identify and analyze practice using general ethical principles. In medicine there is widespread agreement on three principles: respect for persons (autonomy), beneficence, and justice.[9]

Respect for persons means that health care professionals recognize the ability of patients to make their own choices and exercise personal autonomy. Even when patients are not able to exercise autonomy (for example, in cognitively impaired populations), clinicians have an obligation to involve patients as much as their abilities permit and to pay particular attention to dissent. *Beneficence* means that the benefits of medical treatments should outweigh the harms. *Justice* means that patients are treated fairly and receive equal moral consideration, and that nonmedical criteria such as financial ability to pay for care do not influence treatment decisions by the clinician. In addition, there is a recognition that additional principles may apply to certain areas, such as public health. In public health an additional principle is the idea of *proportionalism*, which means that public health officials should use the least-intrusive means to achieve a public health goal. Another principle important in public health is the idea of *transparency* and *public disclosure* about public health interventions.

Ethical Principles in Animal Health

General ethical principles also can be applied to the care of animals.[10] The concept of respect for animals involves consideration of their general welfare. The principles of animal welfare have been summarized as "five freedoms," which were developed as goals for farm animal husbandry but are applicable to the care of other animals.[11] These freedoms are listed in Box 2-3.

The ethical concept of beneficence may be applied to the treatment of animals and human beings. As with medical treatment of human beings, veterinary treatments for individual animals should be grounded in the idea that benefits should outweigh harms. However, in addition to treating particular animals, veterinarians also may be called on to address the welfare of populations of animals as part of public health. Control of zoonotic diseases may require interventions to separate infected populations from uninfected populations and may require various control measures of infected populations. When dealing with populations of animals, the principle of proportionality is important to animal ethics, just as it is relevant to public health ethics focusing on the health of people. For example, if intrusive control measures, such as culling, are necessary, the requirement would

be to use the least-intrusive methods out of concern to minimize suffering and to exercise respect for animals.

Applying the principle of justice with regard to animal welfare ethics presents several challenges. The idea that all people deserve equal moral consideration (which may result in different treatment to serve the people's different needs) is generally accepted. However, there is no general consensus that animals deserve equal consideration, either with people or with respect to other kinds of animals. For example, in many states, agricultural animals are exempt from animal cruelty laws. At the same time, agricultural animals may be viewed by some to have greater moral importance than indigenous predatory animals such as wolves. One way of thinking about the idea of justice in veterinary medicine is that interventions should minimize unfair treatment of both people and animals. For example, as a matter of justice it may be the right thing for a government to compensate those who own animals if there is a need to cull such animals for public health purposes, such as in an outbreak of avian influenza.

Overarching ethical principles for public health and clinical considerations include eliminating environmental pollution and addressing habitat restoration. Focusing on environmental health is beneficial for human and other animal populations.

References

1. American Psychology Association. *Louisiana becomes second state to enact prescription privileges law for psychologists.* http://www.apa.org/releases/louisianarx. Accessed September 23, 2008.
2. American Veterinary Medical Association. *Model veterinary practice act.* http://www.avma.org/issues/policy/mvpa.asp. Accessed September 23, 2008.
3. Babcock S, Marsh AE, Lin J, et al. Legal implications of zoonoses for clinical veterinarians. *J Am Vet Med Assoc.* 2008;233(10):1556–1562.
4. US Department of Health and Human Services. *Health information privacy.* http://www.hhs.gov/ocr/hipaa/. Accessed September 23, 2008.
5. US Department of Health and Human Services. *Covered entity charts.* http://www.cms.hhs.gov/HIPAAGenInfo/Downloads/CoveredEntity-charts.pdf. Accessed September 23, 2008.
6. Centers for Disease Control and Prevention. HIPAA privacy rule and public health. Guidance from CDC and the U.S. Department of Health and Human Services. *MMWR Morb Mortal Wkly Rep.* 2003;52(suppl 1–17):19–20.
7. Babcock SL, Pfieffer C. Laws and regulations concerning the confidentiality of veterinarian-client communication. *J Am Vet Med Assoc.* 2006;229(3):365–369.
8. Babcock SL, Neihsl A. Requirements for mandatory reporting of animal cruelty. *J Am Vet Med Assoc.* 2006;228(5):685–689.
9. American Medical Association. *Principles of medical ethics.* http://www.ama-assn.org/ama/pub/category/2512.html. Accessed June 19, 2008.
10. American Veterinary Medical Association. *Principles of veterinary medical ethics of the AVMA.* http://www.avma.org/issues/policy/ethics.asp. Accessed June 19, 2008.
11. Webster AJ. Farm animal welfare: the five freedoms and the free market. *Vet J.* 2001;161(3):229–237.

BOX 2-3 *THE "FIVE FREEDOMS" OF ANIMAL WELFARE*

The Five Freedoms and Provisions

1. Freedom from thirst, hunger and malnutrition—by ready access to fresh water and a diet to maintain full health and vigor.
2. Freedom from discomfort—by providing a suitable environment including shelter and a comfortable resting area.
3. Freedom from pain, injury, and disease—by prevention or rapid diagnosis and treatment.
4. Freedom to express normal behavior—by providing sufficient space, proper facilities, and company of the animal's own kind.
5. Freedom from fear and distress—by ensuring conditions which avoid mental suffering.

From Webster AJ: Farm animal welfare: the five freedoms and the free market, *Vet J.* 161(3):229-37, 2001.

Establishing a New Approach to Clinical Health History

3

Peter M. Rabinowitz and Lisa A. Conti

Despite the growing sophistication of medical technologies for imaging and chemical diagnosis of disease states in both human and veterinary patients, the clinical history remains a critical part of medical decision making in human and animal health care. In an era when human health care providers and veterinarians rarely visit the homes, neighborhoods, and workplaces of their clients, the process of history taking remains the principal method of gathering information about environmental factors that could be relevant to the health status of the patient.

Despite a growing realization of connections between the health of human beings and other animals living in close proximity, the idea of a human health care provider including in the evaluation of a patient any directed questions about the contact with companion and other animals may seem foreign to many clinicians. Animal exposures are often overlooked during medical evaluations. A study of primary care physicians found that the majority of the time they failed to take a history of animal exposures when evaluating patients with presumed infectious gastroenteritis and diarrhea.[1] Possible exposures to pet shops, exotic and domestic pets, farm animals/environments, and zoos and other wildlife centers, although apparently clinically relevant, were routinely omitted in the medical history. As a result, the study authors concluded that a significant number of zoonotic disease events are missed. As explained in Chapter 2, potential exists for both missed diagnoses[2] and medicolegal liability in overlooking the importance of animal exposures when taking a medical history. For the veterinary clinician as well, there is some potential legal liability for overlooking a zoonotic or other human-animal–related health risk.

This chapter outlines essential elements of human-animal health concerns that should be (1) included in the clinical history taken by human health care providers and (2) asked of animal owners by veterinary health professionals.

ANIMAL HEALTH INFORMATION IN THE HUMAN MEDICAL HISTORY

Human health care providers should routinely ask questions about animal contacts as part of the medical history for four major reasons:

1. To identify possible zoonotic disease risks, thereby facilitating the diagnosis and prevention of disease transmission from animals to the patient.
2. To determine whether animals nearby could be a source of allergen exposure (see Chapter 7).
3. To understand the patient's psychosocial issues, including the emotional bond between a patient and one or more companion animals, the effect of animal care and feeding on daily routines, and the warning signs of neglect or abuse of an animal. Animals may be more significant in a patient's life than other social support networks that are routinely asked about in the social history (see Chapter 5).
4. Asking about the health of animals living nearby could provide information about toxic and infectious exposures in the environment as well as whether animal medications are stored in the house and could pose a risk to human beings.

In addition, asking about animal contacts may increase the rapport between clinician and patient, allow a better understanding of family relationships and health beliefs, and provide additional information about the patient's daily routine and environment.

Animal Contact History as Part of the Acute Care Visit

During an acute care visit, time available for history taking can be limited and priority must be given to the most important medical information gathering. At the same time, failure to gather important information about animal contacts, especially if no baseline data exist in the chart, can increase the risk of missing important clues to the correct diagnosis and treatment of the acute condition. Therefore it may be appropriate to ask several brief screening questions about animal contacts as part of the history of a patient with an acute illness.

Some patients may be surprised by their health care provider asking questions about family pets or other animals. The health care provider can begin these questions with an explanatory statement, such as:

These days, we are discovering that several diseases may pass between people and pets or other animals. I'm going to ask you some routine questions about pets in the house

Table 3-1 ▪ Screening and Follow-Up Questions for the Acute Care Visit	
Screening and Follow-Up Questions About Animal Contacts	
If the following screening questions are answered "yes,"	**Ask these follow-up questions:**
1. Do you have pets or other contact with animals?	*If yes, go to #2.*
2. Are the pets or other animals showing signs of illness?	*Please describe specific signs and any diagnoses and current treatment.*
3. Do you think that your illness is related to your pet or other animals?	*What exactly is your concern?*
4. Do your animals need vaccinations or deworming to be up to date?	*Do you know which vaccinations are not up to date?*
5. Has your veterinarian mentioned any human health care concerns?	*Name and telephone number of veterinarian, exact concern mentioned, and recommended course of action.*

and any other animal contacts that you may have, and whether your pets have had any health problems. This information can help me know whether there could be any connection between the health of animals that you live with and your health concerns.

Table 3-1 lists screening and follow-up questions for the acute care visit. The general screening questions can be modified for the particular situation, and examples of modified screening questions appear throughout this book (see, for example, Chapter 10). If the response to any of the screening questions is "yes," additional follow-up questions are indicated. Specific follow-up questions are mentioned in other sections of this book.

Baseline Information for the Medical Chart

An important setting for incorporating animal health information into the human health medical record is baseline medical information gathered for the patient's inpatient or outpatient chart. Because time is often limited for health care professionals to take an extensive inventory of animal contacts, one way to gather such information may be through a self-administered checklist completed by the patient (Figure 3-1). This can be completed while other baseline medical information is being gathered and incorporated later into an electronic or paper medical record.

In addition to asking about pets, the primary care assessment of zoonotic and other animal contact disease risks should include asking about wildlife and farm animal contacts for both human beings and pets living with them. This type of questioning has particular importance if a person's home is situated near wildlife habitat, on or near a farm, and/or when pets living in the house are allowed to roam free outdoors where they might come in contact with wildlife or livestock.

Home Health Assessment of Companion Animals and Human Health

A home visit, such as during the delivery of visiting nurse or other home health care services, provides an important opportunity to identify health risks and other issues relating to pets in the house. As before, these include zoonotic, allergic, psychosocial, and toxic risks. Figure 3-2 provides a form for home health care workers to complete as part of a home health risk assessment. A key aspect of such an assessment is whether there is a "mismatch" between the patient and animals in the house in terms of an animal that poses a direct health risk to the patient or indicates that the patient is becoming unable to care for and handle.

HUMAN-ANIMAL CONTACT INFORMATION IN THE VETERINARY HISTORY

For veterinary health care providers, the important categories of human-animal contact information that should be included in the veterinary history are similar to those for human health providers. If a known zoonotic disease is diagnosed in an animal with close human contact, the veterinarian should inform the client of common human symptoms of the disease and direct the animal owner to his or her physician if such symptoms have been noted in the human beings sharing the animal's environment or if any persons in the home are at increased risk for the disease. The veterinarian can stress preventive steps to reduce exposure risks. Similarly, if the animal's disease is likely from an environmental exposure, the veterinarian can recommend that persons in the household be screened and/or help eliminate the household exposure. For the well-being of the pet or other animal, it is also important for the veterinarian to know information about human-animal bonding and potential for abuse and neglect.

Baseline Human Health History for Veterinarians

Just as with the primary care medical visit and the animal health history, having baseline information in the veterinary medical chart regarding medical issues in persons living in proximity of a particular animal can be useful. Certain individuals, including infants, young children, and persons with impaired immune function, can be at increased risk of zoonotic diseases. Conversely, human beings with communicable diseases can pose a risk to nearby animals. Allergy in a human household member may be related to the presence of an animal in the house. Smokers in the house may put the animals at risk of health complications. Numerous other examples can be found throughout this book. However, any discussion of which aspects of human health history can be obtained by veterinarians and recorded in a veterinary medical record leads rapidly to a consideration of patient medical record privacy rules and regulations, in particular the Health Insurance Portability and Accountability Act (HIPAA) (see Chapter 2). To date, the extent to which HIPAA applies to the veterinary health care setting is unclear because it was written to focus on health care settings such as hospitals and outpatient medical offices where patients are often covered

Baseline Animal Health History Checklist (to be completed by the patient)

Date: _____ Name and telephone number of veterinarian: _____

_____

Animal contacts:

Please list all the different pets that live in your home and indicate whether they have had any health problems.

	Type of pet (cat, dog, bird, rabbit, reptile, etc.)	Approximate age (years)	Roams free outside? (yes/no)	In the past year, has the pet been treated for any infections or had any other health problems? If so, please list.	Currently taking medication? If so, please list (prescription and nonprescription).
1.					
2.					
3.					
4.					
5.					
6.					

Does your work involve contact with animals? ☐ Y ☐ N

If yes, please describe. _____

Do you frequently visit any of the following and have direct contact with animals (check all that apply)?

Farms where animals are kept ☐ Y ☐ N

Pet stores ☐ Y ☐ N

Petting zoos ☐ Y ☐ N

Animal markets ☐ Y ☐ N

Residential contact with wildlife:

Dwelling (check one): ☐ House ☐ Apartment ☐ Other

Size of property: _____ acres

Property is: ☐ Urban ☐ Suburban ☐ Rural

Please note which of the following are within 100 yards of your house:

☐ Lawn ☐ Woods ☐ Pond or other wetlands

Is property fenced? ☐ Y ☐ N

Have you noticed ticks around your yard? ☐ Y ☐ N

Do you have a bird feeder? ☐ Y ☐ N If yes, how far from your home? _____

Have you noticed mice or rats near your home? ☐ Y ☐ N

Figure 3-1 ▪ Self-administered checklist for a patient's animal contact history.

Please state which wildlife species can be found either on your property or in a half-mile vicinity:

☐ Deer ☐ Coyotes ☐ Foxes ☐ Canada geese

Other (please specify): _____

Farm animals:

On property or immediate vicinity, please state whether the following exist, and how many:

☐ Chickens ☐ Ducks ☐ Other poultry ☐ Horses ☐ Goats ☐ Sheep ☐ Domestic rabbits ☐ Pigs

Other (please specify): _____

Number: _____

Hunting and other wild game exposures:

Please check which of the following apply.

I or another household member regularly hunt for:

☐ Deer ☐ Waterfowl ☐ Other gamebirds ☐ Rabbits ☐ Feral hogs

Other (please specify): _____

Such hunting involves:

☐ Skinning carcasses without gloves or other protection ☐ Eating wild meat

Other (please specify): _____

Figure 3-1 ▪ Cont'd

by health insurance. In such settings, HIPAA sets clear guidelines for the protection of personal health information (PHI) that includes identifiable information about the health of individuals. Detailed information can be found at http://www.hhs.gov/ocr/hipaa/. For example, even if no names are recorded in a written record at a veterinary office, noting that a 29-year-old woman in the house has diabetes constitutes PHI because the person is potentially identifiable by address, age, and gender. In general, therefore, it is best that the veterinarian not record confidential human medical information in a veterinary medical record.

Figure 3-3 is an example of a human health questionnaire that can be completed by a client without revealing confidential medical information about individuals. This baseline information is potentially useful if the client agrees to complete the form. For a single household, it may be useful to record the names and contact information of health care providers, such as pediatrician, family physician, physician assistant, nurse practitioner, obstetric health provider, and so on. This information can be recorded in the chart in an anonymous manner as shown in Figure 3-3.

Health Assessment During the Sick Animal Visit

As with human health care, the acute care animal visit takes place in a time-limited environment, and any attempt to gather information about the health of human beings in the household must be streamlined. This can be accomplished by using screening questions listed in Table 3-2.

More detailed screening and follow-up questions can be found in the sections of the book relating to particular conditions.

Animal Health Risk Assessment Form

1. **Inventory of animals in the home:**

_____ # Cats _____ # Dogs _____ # Birds

Other pets (please specify): _____

☐ Animals share living space with persons in house

☐ Pets allowed to roam outside

2. **Zoonotic risks:** Is there evidence of a high-risk animal or high-risk situation for zoonotic disease transmission (such as poor hygiene around puppies or kittens)? Check all that apply:

☐ Exposure to animal feces

☐ Pets share dishes with persons

☐ High-risk animal (reptile, puppy or kitten, duckling, sick animal)

3. **Allergic issues:** Are there animals that could be causing allergy?

☐ Visible accumulation of pet hair, dander, or feathers

4. **Psychosocial:** Significant bonding between patient and animals, or evidence of abuse or neglect?

☐ Patient appears attached to particular animal (please specify):_____

☐ Evidence of neglected or abused animals

5. **Toxic issues:** Are there veterinary medications unsecured that could be confused with human medications, or other toxic exposures?

☐ List veterinary medications in the home_____

6. **Other mismatch between animal(s) and patient:**

☐ Patient increasingly unable to care for pets

☐ Type of pet inappropriate for patient (example: dog too active or large, animal in need of great deal of care)

Other (please specify): _____

Figure 3-2 ■ Animal health risk assessment form for home health nurses and other home health care providers.

Human-Animal Disease Risk Survey

The following questions will help indicate whether people in your household are at increased risk of animal-related disease. Please answer the following questions. All information will be kept confidential.

Type of pet or other animal: _____

Name of family health care provider and contact information:_____

_____

Number of persons in the household: _____

Dwelling: ☐ House ☐ Apartment ☐ Other _____

In the household are there:

Any children under 5 years of age? ☐ Y ☐ N

Any people with immune problems or chronic health problems? ☐ Y ☐ N

Any woman who may be or is planning to become pregnant? ☐ Y ☐ N

Any smokers? ☐ Y ☐ N

Any person(s) with allergies to animals? ☐ Y ☐ N

If yes, list animals known to be source of allergy for person: _____

Would you like more information about pet-related health issues? ☐ Y ☐ N

If yes, please specify: _____

Figure 3-3 ▪ Human health risk survey completed by animal owner to include in the veterinary chart.

Table 3-2 ▪ Human Health Risk Screening Questions for the Sick Animal Visit

Screening and Follow-Up Questions About Health Problems in Pet Owners and Other Household Members

If the following screening questions are answered "yes,"	Ask these follow-up questions:
1. Are any persons in the household sick?	If yes, go to #2.
2. Has this animal had contact with household members or other people?	Please describe specific types of contact, including frequency.
3. Do you have any concerns about human health problems related to your animal's illness?	What exactly is your concern?
4. Has your health care provider mentioned any concerns regarding the animals in the household?	Name and telephone number of health care provider, exact concern mentioned.

References

1. Warwick C. Gastrointestinal disorders: are health care professionals missing zoonotic causes? *J R Soc Health.* 2004;124:137–142.
2. Mohapatra PR, Janmeja AK, Kaur R. The answer you get depends on the question you ask. *Am J Med.* 2006;119(3):e19.

Sentinel Disease Signs and Symptoms

4

Peter M. Rabinowitz and Lisa A. Conti

Key Points for Clinicians and Public Health Professionals

Public Health Professionals

- Investigate human cases of zoonotic disease when animal zoonoses are reported.
- Consider potential for biological or chemical threat.

Human Health Clinicians

- Consider information about clinical disease in animals as potentially relevant to human disease (do not diagnose disease in animals or discuss specific animal treatments).
- Report diseases of public health significance to local or state public health authorities.*
- Consider contacting a veterinarian to coordinate disease control efforts.

Veterinary Clinicians

- Pursue etiologic diagnosis of disease in animals for appropriate treatment and determination of public health risk.
- Provide pet owners information concerning public health aspects of zoonoses and document this information in the medical record (do not diagnose diseases in human beings or discuss specific human treatments).
- Report diseases of public health significance to local or state public health authorities.

---

*Each state has a listing of reportable conditions. Contact your state epidemiologist for more information; http://www.cste.org/dnn/StateEpidemiologists/tabid/80/Default.aspx.

SIGNS OF ILLNESS IN ANIMALS THAT MAY BE RELEVANT TO HUMAN HEALTH

As mentioned in Chapter 3, in providing their medical histories, human patients may spontaneously mention particular health problems that have developed in their pets or other animals, perhaps thinking their own condition may be associated in some way with an ill animal. They may also provide information about the health of their animals in response to the directed questions listed in Chapter 3. Although a human health care provider should not attempt to offer advice about veterinary treatment (see Chapter 2), there are fundamental steps that he or she can take that may enhance the opportunities for early detection and prevention of human disease. In the case of the release of biological or chemical agents, either intentional or accidental, it is possible that sudden animal mortality or morbidity clusters could be an early warning sentinel event that would need to be recognized and acted on as soon as possible to reduce human health risks (see Chapter 13). The following section provides an overview of common clinical signs in animals, potential etiological agents, clinical and public health implications, and the next steps that human and animal health care providers should take if they learn of such conditions.

Types of Animal Diseases That May Be Important to Human Health Care Providers

In general, the human health consequences of a particular animal illness fall into two main categories (Figure 4-1). The first category is direct infection risk. The clinical sign is related to an infectious agent that could pass from the animal to the person, with the animal serving as a source for the zoonotic infection risk. An example may be the direct infection of a person tending a calf with cryptosporidial diarrhea after fecal material splashes directly into the person's mouth. The second is as an environmental sentinel event. The clinical signs of the animal disease provide an indication of an environmental hazard, either infectious or toxic, to which human beings may also be exposed. For example, identification of

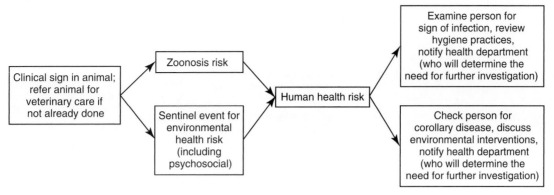

Figure 4-1 ▪ Relationship between clinical signs in animals and human health risks.

Rocky Mountain spotted fever in dogs has led to the discovery and treatment of disease in a human patient.[1] Similarly, a dog that becomes ill after ingesting toxic berries on an ornamental plant signals a potential danger for children who could inadvertently ingest the berries. Elevated blood lead levels in pets are an indicator of lead exposure risk in children living nearby.

Specific Signs in Animals and Appropriate Follow-up Steps for Human Health Professionals

Table 4-1 includes selected animal disease conditions for which a heightened index of suspicion for human disease risk is warranted, potential etiological agents and public health implications, and next steps for the human health care provider in protecting public health. A diagnosis in the animal should be pursued and human case findings similarly investigated while considering a common source of exposure.

HUMAN DISEASE SYMPTOMS THAT MAY BE RELEVANT FOR ANIMAL HEALTH

Just as animals can serve as sentinels of human health risk, it is conceivable that disease symptoms in the owner of an animal being treated or in human beings in the community could have important ramifications for veterinarians and animal health. It is possible that clients will spontaneously volunteer information about a medical condition they or household members are experiencing, and they may provide information in response to the directed questions listed in Chapter 3. Veterinarians should not provide medical advice or otherwise attempt to diagnose disease in a person based

on reported signs, but reports of certain symptom complexes in human beings should trigger steps, such as advising the client to contact a human health care provider for follow-up, as well as possibly affect the type of animal health care required.

Types of Human Disease Symptoms That May Be Important to Veterinarians

Table 4-2 includes human diseases for which a veterinarian may take appropriate action. The relevance to animal health professionals of a particular disease or symptom in human beings can be classified into several categories:

- *Zoonotic disease acquired from an animal.* This may necessitate referral of a person to a health care provider, evaluation of suspect animal(s), and a review of hygienic and biosafety practices and other preventive measures. Immunocompromised persons (e.g., from chemotherapy, chronic debilitation) are at increased risk of severe complications from a zoonotic disease, and there is consequently a need for increased vigilance to prevent zoonotic transmission from a pet-related infection such as diagnosing and treating any animal infections and reviewing infection hygienic practices.
- *Reverse zoonoses (disease passing from the human to the animal).* This could require screening the animal for infection as well as ensuring that the human being receives appropriate treatment and review of infection control practices and prevention measures.
- *Potential environmental sentinel event.* Signaling a risk of biological, chemical, or physical hazards in the environment to which animals or other people may also be exposed and

Table 4-1 ■ Clinical Signs in Animals That Patients May Report and Possible Human Health Care Provider Responses

Sign in Animal	Animal Species	Possible Causes (Differential Diagnosis) With Human Health Implications	Appropriate Actions for Human Health Care Providers*
Diarrhea	Dogs, cats, livestock	Bacterial: *Campylobacter, Escherichia coli, Salmonella, Yersinia*	Counsel about hygiene with excretions, avoid close contact; hand hygiene; consider common food source (see Chapter 11)
		Parasitic: *Ancylostoma, Cryptosporidium, Giardia*	
		Toxic: Pesticides, human medications	Ensure children are not at risk for ingesting toxins
Vomiting	Dogs, cats	Lead poisoning, ingestion of toxic substances such as human medications or poisonous plants	Check lead level and report to public health department if elevated; provide guidance for identification and removal of substances that can put children at risk
Upper respiratory signs (coughing, nasal or sinus congestion, sneezing)	Cats	*Chlamydophila felis,* SARS (Coronavirus), *Francisella tularensis, Yersinia pestis*	Counsel about hygiene with secretions, avoid close contact; hand hygiene; ask about respiratory symptoms in human beings; consider increased zoonotic potential in immunocompromised persons
	Ferrets, chickens/ducks	Influenza	
	Birds	*Chlamydophila*	
	Dogs	*Bordetella*	
Labored breathing, wheezing	Cats, dogs, horses, cattle	Environmental sentinel (not well documented): environmental allergens, irritants	Ask about respiratory problems in human beings sharing living space; eliminate possible irritants from the household or barn; eliminate indoor tobacco smoke
Nonhealing wounds	Dogs, cats	Methicillin-resistant *Staphylococcus aureus,* mycobacteriosis	Zoonotic and reverse zoonotic risks; hand hygiene; disinfection of or exposure reduction to contaminated environment
Hemorrhage	Dogs, cats	Toxin: coumarin derivatives, arsenic, lead, zinc	Ensure children are not at risk of ingesting rodent poison or heavy metals
		Infection: *Leptospira*	Consider zoonotic risks
		Trauma	Consider risk of violence
Neuropathology (ataxia, somnolence)	Cats, raccoons, skunks, bats, foxes, coyotes, dogs, bobcats	Rabies	Evaluate possible human exposures; contact public health officials
	Cattle	BSE	
	Horses	Equine encephalitis	
	Dogs, cats, birds	Carbon monoxide, lead	
	Dogs, cats, cattle, horses, sheep, pigs, rabbits, geese	Cyanobacteria (in stagnant fresh water)	
Skin rashes, crusting	Dogs, cats, rodent pets, hedgehogs, horses	Dermatophytes (Figure 4-2), *Leishmania,* allergies	Ask about lesions in human contacts, contact veterinarian for coordinated household treatment; counsel about handwashing and other methods of transmission risk
Sudden death	Pet birds	Teflon fumes	Eliminate exposure, immediately assess risk to human beings; ask about breathing problems in human beings; contact public health officials
	Wild birds	West Nile virus	
	Cattle, sheep, goats	*Bacillus anthracis*	
	Horses	Venezuelan equine encephalitis virus	
Neoplasia (weight loss, weakness, fatigue)	Dogs	Indoor air carcinogens (sinonasal cancer), asbestos (mesothelioma), pesticides (lymphomas)	Consider obtaining an environmental assessment, screening for disease in human beings
Fetal losses	Cattle, goats, sheep, dogs	*Brucella, Coxiella*	Assess associated disease symptoms in human beings
Signs of trauma, neglect, or abnormal behavior	Dogs, cats, other animals	Domestic violence, family dysfunction, neglect	Screen for domestic violence or other psychosocial problems

*These actions should also include recommending that patients consult their veterinarians.
BSE, Bovine spongiform encephalopathy; *SARS,* severe acute respiratory syndrome.

Table 4-2 ■ Human Disease Signs and Symptoms and Appropriate Actions for Veterinarians

Human Symptom or Sign Reported by Client or Other Human Beings in Household	Possible Causes (Differential Diagnosis)	Steps for Veterinary Professionals to Consider*
Diarrhea	Bacterial: *Salmonella, Campylobacter, Yersinia, Giardia*	Request examination and treatment of animals with clinical signs; review biosafety practices (hand hygiene); consider food safety issues
Vomiting	Staphylococcal food poisoning	Inquire about any shared food, vomiting in animals
Upper respiratory symptoms (nasal congestion, sore throat)	Influenza	If in risk area for zoonotic influenza, ensure human being is receiving care, look for evidence of infection in animals; may be a reverse zoonosis for pet ferrets
	Hypersensitivity reaction: air quality, brevitoxins, animal allergy, pneumonitis	Ask about indoor air quality and other environmental conditions; consider consulting health department; evaluate signs in animals; consider allergy to pet and methods to reduce allergens; eliminate tobacco smoke
Acute lower respiratory tract symptoms (cough, shortness of breath, fever)	*Chlamydophila, Francisella, Yersinia pestis,* Hantavirus	Review zoonotic disease risks
Chronic lower respiratory tract symptoms (chronic cough, weight loss)	*Mycobacterium tuberculosis*	Ensure person is receiving follow-up and is aware of reverse zoonosis risk
Nonhealing wound	Methicillin-resistant *Staphylococcus aureus* Mycobacteriosis	Consider culture of companion animals if this is a recurring issue in the person and other household members have had cultures. Consider a common source of exposure for companion animal
Hematochezia, hemoptysis	Poisoning with coumarin derivatives	Consider whether companion animals could have ingested poison as well
Skin rash Excoriations Serpiginous rash, especially on feet Papules Eschar	Rocky Mountain spotted fever (maculopapular [Figure 4-4]), *Borrelia burgdorferi* (ECM rash [Figure 4-5]), dermatophytes Ectoparasites (scabies, other mites) Cutaneous larva migrans Flea (Figure 4-6), ant/mosquito bites Anthrax (Figure 4-7)	Ectoparasite and endoparasite control and prevention; counsel about zoonotic risks; examine animal; consider presumptive treatment
Trauma (broken bones, bruises, bruises in unusual places or not consistent with history of trauma) Behavior problems in children or adults	Accidents, domestic violence Psychosocial dysfunction in household	Look for signs of physical or behavioral trauma in pet or signs of neglect; referral for social services
Pregnancy	Agents that could complicate pregnancy (*Toxoplasma, Salmonella, Coxiella, Listeria*)	Review hygiene/biosafety practices, particularly of food preparation and avoidance of handling animal waste, and appropriate pet selection
Weight loss, weakness, fatigue	Cancer, HIV, other immunosuppression	Review hygiene/biosafety; ensure pets are adequately treated for infection
Arthritis	*Borrelia burgdorferi*	Tick control for pets, environment around house

*In all cases, recommend that the client consult a human health care provider.
HIV, Human immunodeficiency virus; *ECM,* erythema chronicum migrans.

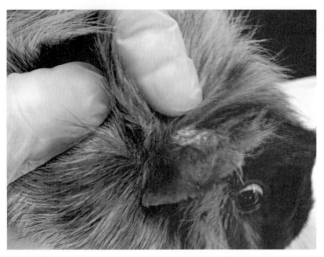

Figure 4-2 ■ A guinea pig with a crusted area on the dorsal pinna consistent with dermatophytosis. A *Trichophyton* organism was cultured from the site. (From Mitchell M, Tully TN Jr: *Manual of exotic pet practice*, St Louis, 2008, Saunders Elsevier.)

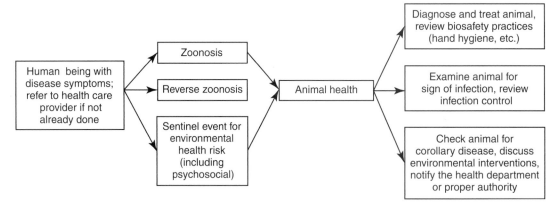

Figure 4-3 ■ Human disease symptoms, according to animal health ramifications.

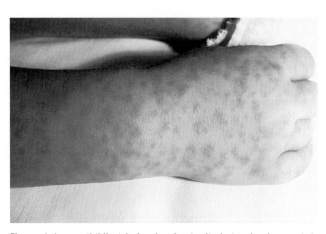

Figure 4-4 ■ Child's right hand and wrist displaying the characteristic spotted rash of Rocky Mountain spotted fever. (From Centers for Disease Control and Prevention Public Health Image Library, Atlanta, Ga.)

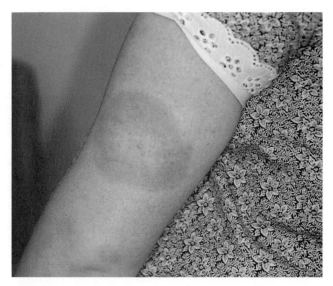

Figure 4-5 ■ Lyme disease rash. (From Cohen J, Powderly WG: *Infectious diseases*, ed 2, Philadelphia, 2003, Mosby.)

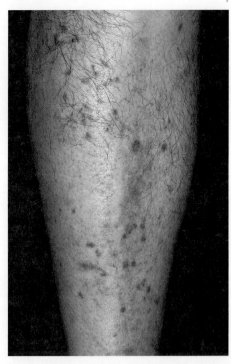

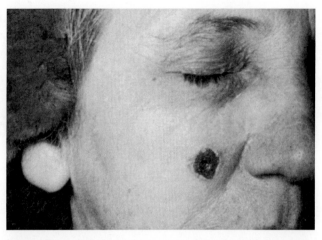

Figure 4-7   ■   Cutaneous anthrax on an employee of a goat-hair processing mill spinning department. (From Centers for Disease Control and Prevention Public Health Image Library Atlanta, Ga.)

Figure 4-6   ■   Flea bites in human. (From Habif TP: *Clinical dermatology: a color guide to diagnosis and therapy,* ed 4, St Louis, 2003, Mosby.)

at risk. This should initiate a search for the environmental hazard, examination of the animal(s) to see whether corollary disease is present, notification of the health department and/or state veterinarian's office, if indicated, and consideration of ways to reduce the environmental risk. This category includes allergic disease, neglect, and domestic violence. These possibilities are summarized in Figure 4-3.

Reference

1. Paddock CD, Brenner O, Vaid C, et al. Short report: concurrent Rocky Mountain spotted fever in a dog and its owner. *Am J Trop Med Hyg.* 2002;66(2):197–199.

Psychosocial and Therapeutic Aspects of Human-Animal Interaction

5

Rebecca A. Johnson

People derive physiological and psychological benefits from interactions with animals. Animals can play a therapeutic and health-promoting role in a wide variety of human health conditions and in settings ranging from the community to primary, inpatient, and long-term health care. Human and veterinary health care providers need to be aware of the potential health benefits of human-animal interaction (HAI) and the important role that the human-animal bond may play in the health status of patients. This chapter outlines some of the therapeutic uses of animals and other psychosocial issues related to the human-animal bond (Figure 5-1).

Key Points for Clinicians and Public Health Professionals

- Educate human health and veterinary clinicians about ways to maximize public health benefits of HAI.
- Support policies that encourage appropriate infection control and other safeguards for animal assisted-therapy and other forms of HAI.
- Support developed environment enhancements that encourage physical activity for people and companion animals (e.g., parks, sidewalks, landscaping, traffic calming).

Human Health Clinicians

- Be aware of indications and precautions for the therapeutic use of animal-assisted activity (AAA), animal-assisted therapy (AAT), and pet ownership for patients.
- Coordinate AAA, AAT, and pet ownership referrals with social workers, physical or occupational therapists, and veterinarians.
- Ensure that animals used in therapy have been screened by veterinarians and are used by certified AAT professionals.
- Consider human-animal bond issues when dealing with acute illness or disaster response involving separation of patients from pets.
- Consider the psychological impact of the death or loss of a pet on the owner and family.

Veterinary Clinicians

- Encourage routine animal wellness examinations and zoonotic disease screening for animals used in therapeutic settings.
- Become familiar with the American Veterinary Medical Association (AVMA) *Guidelines for Animal-Assisted Activity, Animal-Assisted Therapy and Resident Animal Programs.*[1]
- Provide training to veterinary staff in the provision of pet loss support services.
- Report animal abuse to appropriate authorities and consider signs of abuse in pets as a possible warning of domestic violence risk to human beings in the household (see also Chapter 2).
- Keep current on zoonoses prevention, such as for methicillin-resistant *Staphylococcus aureus* (MRSA) (e.g., http://www.avma. org/reference/backgrounders/ mrsa_bgnd.pdf).

HUMAN-ANIMAL INTERACTION: ANIMAL-ASSISTED ACTIVITY, ANIMAL-ASSISTED THERAPY, AND SERVICE DOGS DEFINED

Human-animal interaction (HAI) is the term used to encompass the human-animal bonds developing from pet ownership, uses of animals for recreation (such as horseback riding), animal husbandry, and therapeutic settings. Perhaps the first therapeutic use of animals was Florence Nightingale's introduction of birds as distractions for hospital patients in the mid-1800s. The practice of facilitating HAI for therapeutic purposes has expanded in recent years, in advance of consistent research-based evidence supporting the health benefits of HAI. Today, HAI is used in countless clinical settings and is generally believed to improve patient outcomes.

Animal-assisted activity (AAA) refers to relatively brief visits (usually lasting up to 1 hour) occurring in a variety of settings in which people talk to, pet, groom, offer treats to, and/or play with companion animals with the animal's human handler present.

Animal-assisted therapy (AAT) refers to structured encounters in which the animal with its handler becomes part of a treatment plan for a particular patient. In this instance, the

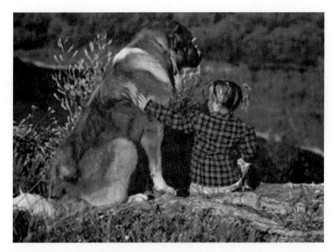

Figure 5-1 ■ A child interacting with her dog. (From Centers for Disease Control and Prevention: *Healthy pets, healthy people: infants and young children.* http://www.cdc.gov/healthypets/child.htm.)

patient may walk with, reach out to, groom, or engage in various games with the animal, with all such activities designed to address particular functional deficits in the person. These activities may be included as goals in the patient's plan of care. Thus the animal becomes an instrument through which a patient's progress may be measured (e.g., a patient goal may be to daily increase the number of strokes brushing the dog using an impaired hand or arm). The most common situations in which AAT is used are in cerebrovascular accident or traumatic brain injury rehabilitation or in various behavioral and other psychotherapy contexts, such as with depressed

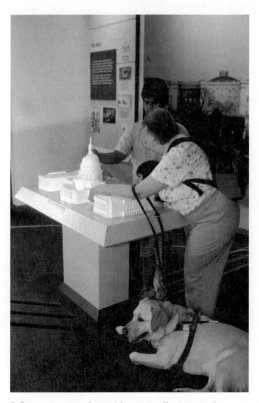

Figure 5-2 ■ Service dog with a visually impaired person. (From Centers for Disease Control and Prevention Public Health Image Library, Atlanta, Ga.)

| BOX 5-1 *USES OF AAA, AAT, AND SERVICE DOGS* |

Current Uses of AAA

Social interaction
- Instructional purposes in school classrooms
- Social purposes in nursing homes, retirement facilities, hospitals, prisons
- Instructional purposes with social and service organizations

Companionship purposes with shut-ins

Current Uses of AAT

Rehabilitation
- Cerebrovascular accident or traumatic brain injury
- Behavioral and other psychotherapy contexts, including depression
- Child abuse
- Autism spectrum disorder

Current Uses of Service Dogs

Leading a person who has a visual impairment around obstacles to destinations (e.g., seating, across street, to/through door, to/into elevator)

Sound discrimination to alert a person with a hearing impairment to the presence of specific sounds, such as the following:
- Smoke/fire/clock alarms
- Telephone
- Baby crying
- Sirens
- Another person
- Timers buzzing
- Knocks at door
- Unusual sounds (things that go bump in the night, mice in the cabinet, etc.)

General Assistance, Including

- Mobility (helping person balance for transfer/ambulation, pulling wheelchair, helping person rise from sitting or fallen position)
- Retrieval (getting items that are dropped or otherwise out of reach, carrying items by mouth)
- Miscellaneous (e.g., open/close doors and drawers, help person undress/dress, carry items in backpack, act as physical buffer to jostling by others, put clothes in washer/remove from dryer, bark to alert for help)

Sense and alert owners to oncoming seizures. It is currently unknown why or how some dogs are able to do this, but a number of dogs have demonstrated the ability to warn their owners of oncoming seizures, enabling the owners to position themselves safely.

From the Delta Society, Bellevue, Wa.

adults, children who have been abused, or those with autism spectrum disorder.

As Box 5-1 demonstrates, service dogs (Figure 5-2) are currently used in long-term patient-animal relationships for a variety of health care settings, both in institutional and home-based care.

HEALTH BENEFITS OF HUMAN-ANIMAL INTERACTION

Research into the health benefits of HAI began in the late 1970s with a study of nursing staff perceptions of psychosocial benefits of older adults interacting with a cat mascot in long-term care.[2] Subsequently, despite a growing number and wide range of studies that have been conducted with varying populations, there remain methodological issues associated with small samples, nonexperimental designs, nonrandomized treatment groups, and the influence of confounding variables.[3]

One problem commonly seen in literature discussing benefits of HAI is the assumption that similar health effects are found in pet ownership (or with service animals) and more casual pet interaction contexts, such as AAA or AAT. It is important to identify the distinction and to clarify these terms because pet/service animal ownership implies a longer, more committed relationship than what can be relatively brief encounters in other pet interactions. In many cultures, companion animals are viewed as family members, occupying homes, sleeping on human beings' beds, and sharing food and recreational activities—they are treated almost as children.[4,5] The distinction is made between this long-term relationship and more casual encounters in which people interact with companion animals in public or in therapeutic contexts, such as schools, clinics, or a range of health care facilities (AAA and AAT).

Several physiological benefits of HAI have been found in AAA, AAT, and pet ownership contexts (Table 5-1). The strong bond that human beings can develop with animals may stem from an innate human affinity with nature, including animals (termed *biophilia*, the love of living things[6]), predicated on the dependence of human beings on animals for food throughout history.[7] This natural tendency may help to provide an understanding of some of the effects of HAI.

AAA and AAT: Psychological and Psychosocial Effects

Clinical evidence indicates that even in therapeutic settings, in relatively short encounters with varying degrees of frequency, an intense attachment can rapidly develop between people and pets. In a laboratory setting serum cortisol levels were found to decrease when people interacted quietly with a dog.[9] During this interaction, additional beneficial changes in neurohormones were found (phenylethylamine, prolactin, oxytocin, dopamine, and endorphin levels increased significantly), as was a significant decrease in blood pressure. A parallel result was found in the dogs during the interaction, suggesting that they also benefited. Similarly, investigators found significantly smaller increases in blood pressure and heart rate when a dog was present during challenging mathematical tasks than when either a friend or an investigator was present.[10]

In a therapeutic horsemanship context, a relaxation response was observed in children with spastic cerebral palsy who experienced 8 minutes of riding. Electromyogram readings showed improved symmetry in muscle activity both during and for some time after the riding episodes.[11] Improved walking and muscle coordination also has been found in disabled children after therapeutic horseback riding.[12] Generally, children have been an understudied population in the HAI literature. Preliminary findings seem promising but additional data are needed to clarify the most beneficial contexts for AAT and AAT in children.

Table 5-1 ■ Research Evidence Showing Physiological Benefits of HAI

Benefit	Population	Pet Ownership (O), AAA, or AAT
Decreased cortisol levels	Adults with own or unfamiliar pet	O
Decreased blood pressure and heart rate/cardiovascular reactivity	Adults	O, AAA
Increased parasympathetic nervous system activity	Adults	O, AAA
Increased phenylethylamine, prolactin, oxytocin, serotonin	Adults with own or unfamiliar pet	O, AAA
Decreased pain, analgesia use, anxiety, and epinephrine levels	Adults	AAA
Decreased cholesterol and triglyceride levels	Adults	O
Better 1-year survival after myocardial infarction	Adults	O
Buffered blood pressure response to stress in hypertensive patients treated with lisinopril	Adults	O
Fewer patient-initiated physician visits	Elderly	O
Improved self-perceived health	Elderly	O
Increased physical activity levels and weight loss with dog walking	Adults and elderly	O, AAA
Increased longevity	Elderly	O
Increased food intake (with aquarium watching)	Elderly	AAA
Decreased muscle spasticity	Children with cerebral palsy	AAA, AAT

In clinical settings, hospitalized patients reported less pain and used fewer analgesics during and after an animal visit,[13] and patients with heart failure had decreased anxiety and epinephrine levels during and after an animal visit.[14] For older adults with dementia in long-term care settings, watching fish swim in an aquarium at mealtimes was associated with longer periods sitting to eat and greater nutritional intake (Figure 5-3).[15] Newly admitted nursing home residents exposed to a series of dog visits were found to have lower cortisol levels than those who had human visitors.[16]

Among community-dwelling older adults, walking with a "loaner" dog was associated with significantly greater parasympathetic nervous system activity (high-frequency heart rate variability) than walking without a dog.[17] When

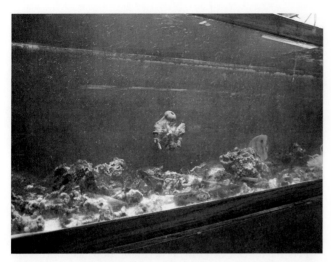

Figure 5-3 ▪ Watching fish swim in an aquarium has a relaxing effect on human beings. (From Mitchell M, Tully TN Jr: *Manual of exotic pet practice*, St Louis, 2008, Saunders Elsevier. Photo courtesy Trevor Zachariah.)

Table 5-2 ▪ **Psychosocial Benefits of HAI**		
Benefit	**Population**	**Pet Ownership (O), AAA, or AAT**
Decreased depression	Elderly, patients with AIDS	O, AAA, AAT
Decreased anxiety	Adults and patients with psychiatric disorders	O, AAA, AAT
Decreased loneliness	Adults, elderly	O
Improved morale	Elderly	O
Fun, relaxation	Elderly	O
Unconditional love and support	Elderly, cancer patients	O
Pets perceived as family members	Adults	O
Improved "prosocial" behaviors in nursing home	Elderly	AAA, AAT
Increased social interaction (pets as catalysts)	Adults	O, AAA, AAT
Increased interaction between staff and nursing home residents	Adults	AAA
Facilitators of attachment	Children	O

AIDS, Acquired immunodeficiency syndrome.

participants interacted quietly with the dog while it visited them in their own home, this activity increased by 1.87 times over their levels while at home without the dog. In overweight residents of public housing, an adherence rate of 72% and average weight loss of 14 pounds in a "loaner" dog-walking program was demonstrated because the participants believed that "the dogs need us to walk them." Participants in a community shelter dog-walking program were motivated to increase their exercise outside the walking program. Investigators found a significant increase in exercise and physical activity stage of change (participants went from vigorous exercise less than three times per week or moderate exercise less than five times per week to 30 minutes a day of moderate exercise five or more days per week for 1 to 5 months).[18]

A variety of psychosocial benefits have been reported by investigators studying outcomes of AAA and AAT (Table 5-2).[19] These benefits include increased social contact, reduced loneliness and depression in hospitalized patients and homeless persons,[20,21] and decreased anxiety in psychiatric patients.[22] The most commonly studied context is long-term care. For example, one study found nursing home residents' prosocial behavior (e.g., smiles, looks, leaning in, and touching) toward the animal and toward others benefited from the presence of a visitor dog or a resident dog.[23] Nursing home staff interacted more and in more positive ways with each other and with residents when a dog was present. However, another study found that nursing home residents enjoyed a visit from a "happy" human visitor as much as one from a dog and its handler.[24] Similarly, in a small study, investigators found that human visits were as favorable as dog/handler visits on nursing home residents' daily hassles, daily uplifts, mood, and social support.[25] Patients with cancer showed no significant differences in mood and social support when they received a series of dog/handler visits, human visits, or participated in quiet reading.[26] Interaction with animals in AAA has been associated with prosocial behaviors and decreased agitation among older adults with dementia.[27,28] Clinical evidence has shown that they are more likely to verbalize (even appropriately) in response to visiting with an animal.

Among children with autism spectrum disorder, investigators found that children were more attentive to and likely to respond appropriately in therapy sessions involving a live dog than with either a stuffed toy dog or a ball.[29] Given the difficulty of children with autism attending to faces, one fruitful area of inquiry in this topic might be to investigate the extent to which an animal face is more likely than a human face to receive the children's attention.

Generally, clinical evidence supports that people receiving AAA or AAT benefit from the following:

- Distraction from their own circumstances by interacting with the pet
- Feelings of being accepted by the animal
- Feeling happy, less lonely, and more included
- Having something pleasant to look forward to in anticipating subsequent visits by the animal and its handler

Pet owners experiencing AAA commonly engage in reminiscence about a previous pet or in comparison with a current pet. Stimulation of this activity may be beneficial in itself and could benefit from scientific scrutiny.

Pet Ownership: Physiological and Psychosocial Effects

It may seem commonsense that the mutual attachment between a pet and its human family would be stronger and thus more powerful in promoting beneficial outcomes than in short-term interactions common in AAA and AAT. Research has shown significant benefits in several parameters indicative of health. Early research findings showed lowering of blood pressure and a relaxation response when people interacted with pets.[30-32] For example, physiological arousal decreased in response to the presence of one's dog even while the human being was engaged in a stressful situation such as completing a difficult mathematical task.[33] Beneficial responses in neurohormonal changes were similar in direction (and even stronger) when people interacted with their own dogs.[9] Other investigators found pet ownership associated with lower triglyceride and cholesterol levels, particularly among women.[34] The 1-year survival rate was positively associated with dog ownership among patients discharged from a coronary care unit irrespective of age, severity of illness, or comorbid conditions.[35] Data on 4435 adults showed that the relative risk of death from heart attack was 40% higher for those who had never owned a cat.[36] The findings may have significant implications for health care expenditures. Older adult pet owners were found to have fewer patient-initiated physician visits and better health. Pet owners were healthier and made fewer physician visits, accounting for an estimated savings of $988 million in health care expenditures in Australia over a 1-year period.[37] The finding was similar in an analysis of German data, in which people who continuously owned pets were found to be the healthiest and to have 15% fewer physician visits.[38] The investigators controlled for previous health and a wide range of other potentially confounding variables to address directional causality or the criticism of HAI research that healthier people are more likely to acquire pets.

Older adult pet owners walked longer and had lower triglyceride and cholesterol levels than non–pet owners.[39] Commitment to dogs involves exercising them and thus may lead to healthier physical activity patterns. Dog walking may be one factor motivating increased physical activity. In Australia, dog owners walked 18 minutes per week more than non–dog owners and were more likely to meet physical activity recommendations of 150 min/wk.[40] A study in the United Kingdom found that dog owners accumulated significantly more exercise than either cat owners or adults without pets.[41] Findings from the National Household Travel Survey in the United States revealed that nearly half of adults who walked dogs in 2001 accumulated at least 30 minutes of walking in bouts of at least 10 minutes daily.[42] An intervention trial in the United States found that obese pet owners increased their moderate physical activity over that of non–pet owners and that the majority of this increase resulted from dog-related activities. The study concluded that companion dogs can serve as social support for weight loss and 1-year weight maintenance.[43] These patterns may differ across ethnic groups, which is a topic that has received little study. For example, although Latino elders expressed a very strong bond with their pet dogs, they did not necessarily exercise with them.[44] The implications for maintaining function among older adults who exercise with pets are being tested.[45] Dog walking may have a role in preventing disability and functionally limiting effects of chronic illnesses.

Older pet owners have been found to function better in activities of daily living than nonowners when studied over a 1-year period[46] and to have fewer patient-initiated physician appointments than non–pet owners, irrespective of the number and type of stressful life events they experienced during the study period.[47]

Pet attachment was related to decreased depression (particularly in older adult pet owners,[48] people with acquired immunodeficiency syndrome [AIDS][49]) and in another study to improved morale. When people have a positive affect and morale, they are more likely to engage with others socially, to participate in recreational activities, and to avoid sedentary, isolated situations.[50] This mind-body connection has been well established in research and can be a factor in maintaining older adults' health and thus preventing or minimizing disability.

Pets have been extensively written about as sources of unconditional love and support[51] and facilitators of attachment in children[52] and were viewed as fun, dependent, and relaxing.[53] Other authors reported on the multiple health benefits of pet ownership, many of which involved lessened anxiety, depression, and social isolation and increased physical activity.[54] Dogs were found to be catalysts for social interactions (Figure 5-4).[55] People walking their dogs in a park had significantly more chance conversations with other park users than when they walked the same route alone.[56] A person's perceived likeability by others was increased by the presence of a dog.[57] These findings were extended more recently when investigators in Australia identified that pet owners scored higher than non–pet owners on social capital (defined as social engagement, social reciprocity or doing favors for each other, trusting others, a sense of community, and civic engagement). The findings are relevant for health care professionals advising clients about how to become more physically and socially active because pet owners indicated that they had met and had varying levels of interaction with other pet owners, but also that they

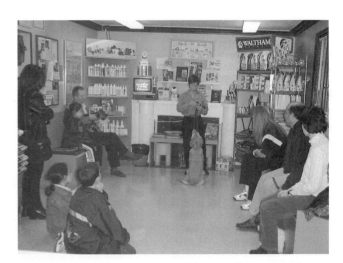

Figure 5-4 ■ A puppy party can combine an open house with an entertaining and informative session about puppy socialization, play, and training. The trainer demonstrates the power of positive reinforcement at a puppy party at the Doncaster Animal Clinic. (From Landsberg GM: *Handbook of behavior problems of the dog and cat*, ed 2, Oxford, 2008, Saunders Elsevier.)

had met others because of their dogs. Pet owners were 57% more likely to engage in volunteer work, school-related activities, or sports and recreational clubs and activities than were non–pet owners. Pet ownership was significantly and positively related to reciprocity (giving and receiving favors from others). Pet owners attributed feeling safe in their homes and when out walking their dogs. Further, sense of community was significantly higher in pet owners, who reported it less difficult than non–pet owners to generally get to know others.[58] Similar findings held in disabled persons accompanied by a service dog; the dog was found to facilitate social interaction.[59-61]

FACILITATING HUMAN-ANIMAL INTERACTION

Referral for AAA or AAT

Applying the extant research and clinical evidence on beneficial effects of HAI, it is possible to make some guarded recommendations for facilitating AAA and AAT with particular patient populations and situations (Table 5-3). Patients may benefit from AAA if they are experiencing anxiety-inducing disease states or treatment protocols, such as patients with cancer undergoing chemotherapy or radiation treatments. In this population, AAA may provide support and distraction.[41] In populations needing companionship, AAA or pet ownership may be beneficial to increase social interaction and decrease loneliness, anxiety, and depression.[26] In obese patients, AAA or pet ownership can provide motivation for increasing physical activity.[18,59]

However, AAA or AAT may not be appropriate for various patient populations, or special precautions may need to be taken. In particular, if a patient is significantly immunocompromised, introduction of animals may not be appropriate or special precautions may be needed.

The most common way to make a referral for AAA or AAT is through a social worker or department of social work. In some inpatient facilities, the department of physical or occupational therapy may be the correct conduit through which to prescribe AAA or AAT. It is incumbent on health care professionals who are in a position to recommend or prescribe

AAA or AAT to identify the proper mechanism for this in their own institution. If no existing AAA or AAT program operates in the facility, referral can result in an affiliation of the facility with the nearest animal visitation group. There are many such groups throughout North America. If health care professionals in the facility are interested in starting an AAA/AAT program by affiliating with an animal visitation group, the resources identified in this chapter provide a starting point for developing policies and procedures to guide such a program.

As a discipline, the field of social work has a growing affiliation with AAA/AAT groups and facilitating the human-animal bond and education of veterinary medical students about the bond through their practice in teaching hospitals of veterinary medicine. For example, the Denver University Graduate School of Social Work offers an animal-assisted intervention certification program preparing social workers to use animals in their practice. The program is sought by students seeking a master's degree in social work and by those seeking a post-master's certification or doctorate.

Medical Recommendations for Pet Ownership

All human health histories should include questions about patients' pets given the beneficial findings about pet ownership and health as well as the possible health risks (see Chapter 3). Care must be taken when health care professionals recommend pet ownership to patients. In particular, it is important to ascertain to what extent the patient is physically and cognitively able or has sufficient support systems (e.g., home helpers or family) to enable the proper care of the animal. When a patient's disability is significant and support is minimal, a dog, cat, or bird may not be an appropriate recommendation; a self-cleaning aquarium may be a better option. Similarly, the costs of providing proper veterinary care, feeding, grooming, and training must be considered. To date, little financial assistance is available for low-income pet owners to offset the costs of keeping pets. Clinical evidence of pet owners withholding food themselves to provide care for their pet has been reported. Finally, during impending hurricanes, some pet owners have elected to stay in harm's way rather than leave their pets when no pet-friendly shelter options were available.

Physical and cognitive disability must be considered in recommending pet ownership. When patients are immunocompromised, certain pets—such as reptiles—are off-limits due to the risk of *Salmonella* infection (see Chapters 9 and 10). However, when precautions are taken, such as keeping cats indoors, good handwashing after handling pets, wearing gloves when cleaning cat litter boxes, and regular screening of the cat or dog for pathogens by a licensed veterinarian, risk of infection may be minimized.[62]

When a patient needs increased physical activity, exercising a dog may be recommended with or without recommending pet ownership. If pet ownership is desirable, breed recommendations must be made carefully. It may seem intuitive to recommend a breed requiring considerable exercise or of great athleticism. However, matching the breed characteristics

Table 5-3 ■ Guidelines for Recommending AAA, AAT, or Pet Ownership	
Clinical Indication	**AAA, AAT, or Pet Ownership (O)***
Anxiety-inducing disease states or treatment protocols for distraction	AAA and/or O (cat, bird, dog, or self-contained aquarium if dementia is present)
Settings or populations needing social interaction (animals to facilitate)	AAA and/or O (cat, bird, or dog)
Situations where companionship is needed	AAA and/or O (cat, bird, or dog)
Obesity/sedentary lifestyle	AAA and/or O (dog)

*If patient is physically able to care for a pet.

with the expectations of the prospective owner may be a more effective approach than trying to make the animal fit the maximum therapeutic level of physical activity desired. Most reputable animal shelters have surveys that attempt to identify an owner-breed match (http://www.hsus.org/pets/pet_adoption_information/choosing_the_right_dog.html). Given that the most common reasons for pet relinquishment to animal shelters are behavior problems that often have not been approached with proper owner training, ensuring that prospective owners are aware of likely breed-specific behavior is a must. When the health care professional is unsure of the patient's motivation to increase physical activity, it may be beneficial to recommend that the person volunteer to walk dogs at a local animal shelter as an intermediate step to owning a dog that needs regular exercise. This may serve two important purposes. First, the person can have regular exposure to a variety of breeds and possibly can learn what breed might be preferred. Second, the person can begin a regimen of increased physical activity gradually without putting an animal's health at risk if he or she does not follow through with the prescribed exercise regimen.

Clearly a team approach is needed involving physicians, nurses, physical therapists, social workers, and veterinarians (Table 5-4) to help assess the factors that may impede or facilitate pet ownership. This approach to recommending pet ownership will have greater likelihood of success for both the patient and the pet.

Credentialing for AAA and AAT Programs

In both AAA and AAT, the animal and handler are trained to engage in the activities. The handler commonly joins an

Table 5-4 ▪ Types of Behavioral Services Offered by the Veterinary Practice

Approach	Considerations
Preselection consultation	Consult with prospective pet owners to help them select an appropriate pet for their circumstances. Advise the owner about the health, behavior, and nutritional requirements of their new pet so that the home and family can be prepared in advance.
Preventive counseling	Counsel owners to raise their pet to minimize behavioral problems. Use handouts, pamphlets, books, and videos. Take full advantage of puppy and kitten vaccination visits to educate the family.
Puppy parties/training	Encourage owners to participate in puppy programs to enhance early socialization and provide training advice. If you have the space and expertise, consider offering classes in the clinic.
Behavior management products	Recommend and supply appropriate training devices (leashes, halters, chew toys, motion-activated alarms, etc.) to prevent or correct undesirable behaviors. If you do not recommend the right products, the owners may make improper decisions.
Surgery	Neutering can prevent estrous cycles in females and in males may reduce behavior problems associated with the effects of androgens, such as sexual attraction to females, roaming, marking, masturbation, mounting, and some forms of aggression.
Basic behavior counseling	As puppies and kittens mature, undesirable behaviors may develop. Intervene early and dedicate sufficient time to counseling for each specific behavior problem. If managed unsuccessfully, consider an anesthesiologist referral before the behavior becomes even more ingrained and the family becomes more frustrated.
Behavioral screening	Diseases of any organ or body system can cause or contribute to changes in behavior. Therefore screening for behavior problems and any behavioral changes is an important component of each health care visit and can aid in the early identification and diagnosis of medical conditions.
Medical history and diagnostics	Practice good-quality medicine and complete medical assessment on all patients routinely. Perform a medical workup on every patient that requires a behavioral assessment. Run appropriate diagnostics to rule out all possible medical problems for the presenting behavioral signs.
Behavioral history and diagnostics	Once medical problems for behavioral signs have been ruled out (or resolved), the behavioral diagnosis requires some knowledge and expertise in history-taking and familiarity with the differential diagnoses for the presenting signs. A videotape, interactive discussion with the owner, observation of the pet and owner, and a written history might all be used.
Advanced behavioral consultations	Make sure you feel competent in performing behavior counseling for advanced problems, such as aggression or phobic behaviors. If in doubt, contact a behavior referral center for advice or refer the case. Inappropriate counseling benefits neither the patient nor the veterinary practice.
Pharmacological management	Drug therapy (as well as alternative therapies such as nutritional management and supplements) can be an important component or even a necessity for the successful resolution of many behavior problems. This might be the case if there are medical conditions causing or contributing to the signs (e.g., pain management, interstitial cystitis, seizure focus). Psychotropic drugs may be a useful therapeutic option or an integral part of the treatment program for some problems.

From Landsberg GM: *Handbook of behavior problems of the dog and cat*, ed 2, 2004, Oxford, Saunders.

established animal visitation group that has affiliations with health care facilities and may provide some assistance with liability insurance. Most importantly, the visitation groups have health screening, certification, and AAA/AAT implementation guidance and standards. Persons who want to become registered as a pet-visitor team typically ensure that their animals are in good health (based on recent examination by a licensed veterinarian, including screening for internal and external parasites and administration of needed vaccinations; see below). The animal and handler must complete obedience training (in the case of dogs), and the dog must pass the American Kennel Club's Canine Good Citizen test. This test is offered by certified testers throughout the United States and identifies the dog's basic level of obedience mastery. Next, the pair must complete a training and testing protocol to ensure readiness to make visits in health care facilities. A commonly used training and registration protocol in the United States is the Delta Society's Pet Partners Program (http://www.deltasociety.org/) in which the handler and dog must complete course materials and training exercises and the dog must undergo a temperament and behavior examination. The purpose of this examination is to identify the dog's suitability to behave reliably and under control of the handler, accept awkward handling, loud noises, and rapidly changing situations. Cats are similarly tested. Upon completion of the Pet Partners Program, in accordance with the rules of their animal visitation group, the handler and dog or cat may begin making visits in facilities either already affiliated with or making a new affiliation with the animal visitation group. Many animal visitation groups in the United States follow the standards manual (based on compilation of existing research evidence and consensus of health care professionals) created by the Delta Society. The book *Standards of Practice for Animal-Assisted Activities and Therapy*[63] provides a guide for animal visitation groups and health care facilities in developing policies and procedures for AAA and AAT. The standards include topics such as animal grooming standards, areas within facilities appropriate for accessibility to AAA and AAT teams, selection of the most (and least) applicable patient situations, successful implementation of visits, and lines of accountability.

No national service animal certification currently exists, although several groups can assist with specific instruction and training. The Americans with Disabilities Act requires businesses to permit people to be accompanied by their service animals "regardless of whether [their animals] have been licensed or certified by a state or local government."[64]

Minimizing Infectious Disease and Other Risks in AAA and AAT

The use of animals for therapy of persons with underlying medical problems involves a certain risk of zoonotic disease transmission. There is also a risk of animals becoming infected from human beings. For example, a human epidemic strain of *Clostridium difficile*, an emerging pathogen in health care settings, has been found in a visitation dog.[65] Other pathogens reported in visitation dogs include antibiotic-resistant *Escherichia coli*, *Salmonella*, *Giardia*, *Toxocara*, *Ancylostoma*,

---

BOX 5-2   COMPONENTS OF A HEALTH CLEARANCE EXAMINATION FOR SERVICE ANIMALS

- Thorough physical examination, including nutritional and oral health assessment, screening for selected infectious and parasitic diseases, and an evaluation for congenital diseases and/or conditions. NOTE: Disabilities should not necessarily eliminate an animal from participation. For example, amputees or deaf animals, if otherwise healthy, can have a positive impact on special populations. Disabled animals must be monitored closely by the responsible person and the attending veterinarian to ensure that the animal's participation does not exacerbate an existing medical condition or adversely affect its ability to provide needed services.
- Current rabies and other vaccinations as appropriate.
- Internal and external parasite prevention and control.
- Interactions of animals with immunocompromised individuals may justify use of certain screening tests that would not be necessary if those animals were interacting only with immunocompetent populations.
- The animal's hair coat and nail quality should be maintained. NOTE: Excessive grooming or bathing (including the use of harsh products) in preparation for AAA or AAT or as part of a maintenance protocol for a resident animal may be deleterious.
- Recommendations for health maintenance should include behavior management, daily exercise, play, diet, preventive dental care, and the potential advantages of spaying/neutering in selected species.
- Medications administered to participating animals should be reviewed for their appropriateness (e.g., animals treated with immunosuppressive medications may be at greater risk of contracting infectious agents).

Adapted from AAA/AAT guidelines; http://www.avma.org/issues/policy/animal_assisted_activity.asp.

---

and *Pasteurella*.[66] It is important that animals used for AAA or AAT receive an appropriate veterinary health assessment (Box 5-2). This assessment also should include a behavioral evaluation to ensure that the animal is suitable for working with a variety of human encounter situations (Figure 5-5). An interdisciplinary working group of health care professionals (in veterinary medicine, AAA/AAT, infection control, and public health) developed standards for AAA and AAT in health care facilities.[62] The AAA/AAT standards recommend exclusion of reptiles, amphibians, nonhuman primates, recently domesticated species, and other animals that cannot be litter trained (Table 5-5). The standards also recommend exclusion of animals receiving a raw meat diet (due to the risk of shedding *E. coli* and other pathogens), those coming directly from animal shelters, dogs and cats younger than 1 year, or animals not in a permanent home for at least 6 months. Detailed recommendations are made about handwashing and other components of the AAA and AAT patient-animal encounters. Adherence to such standards helps to ensure that AAA or AAT do not occur thoughtlessly or without significant commitment and contribution on the part of animal handlers and animal visitation groups. This helps to reassure those working in health care facilities regarding the likely safety of patients receiving AAA or AAT and maximizes the probability that patients will receive the benefits of this human–companion animal interaction.

Initial observations:

Animal friendly? ☐Y ☐N

Animal appears responsive? ☐Y ☐N

Any sign of aggression or fear when approached? ☐Y ☐N

Overactive or highstrung? ☐Y ☐N

Behavioral examination: Any adverse reactions with the following:

Door slamming? ☐Y ☐N

Pulling of hair or ears or tail? ☐Y ☐N

Being petted aggressively? ☐Y ☐N

Being hugged? ☐Y ☐N

When someone approaches animal's owner? ☐Y ☐N

Figure 5-5　■　Example of behavioral evaluation for therapy dog.

Table 5-5 ■ Exclusion Criteria for AAA and AAT animals	
Criterion	**Exclusion**
Species	Reptiles, amphibians, nonhuman primates; recently domesticated species; other animals that cannot be litter trained
Age	Dogs and cats younger than 1 year
Origin	Directly from animal shelters Permanent home for less than 6 months
Health issues	Being fed a raw-meat diet Immunocompromised Lack of complete vaccinations certified by a licensed veterinarian
Affiliation	Not affiliated with a visitation group Not registered by an AAA or AAT training program
Behavior	Any aggressive incident in a health care facility

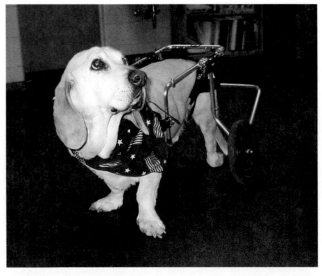

Figure 5-6　■　A paretic patient acclimated to a wheelchair or cart. The cart can be used as a therapy tool in the absence of aquatic therapy or as an ambulation aid at home if improvement is not expected. (From Fossum TW: *Small animal surgery*, ed 3, St Louis, 2007, Mosby Elsevier.)

HEALTH EFFECTS OF LOSS OF OR SEPARATION FROM A PET

As with human health care, improvements in veterinary care have increased the longevity of companion animals (Figure 5-6). Nevertheless, both human health care professionals and veterinary professionals may need to assist patients in ultimately dealing with pet loss. Pet owners who have lost a beloved pet often indicate that they feel ashamed to mention their feelings of loss because they fear they will be treated insensitively.

Human health care providers need to understand the magnitude of the loss of a pet on psychosocial and physiological functioning.

Despite the rapidly growing popularity of pet ownership, many health care providers may not recognize that pet loss can be as traumatic as or even more traumatic than losing a human family member. One study showed that nearly 30% of owners recently bereaved of a pet experienced severe grief. The most apparent risk factors for grief were level of attachment, euthanasia, societal attitudes toward pet death, and professional support from the veterinary team.[67] In addition to grief, patients may feel guilt at not providing better care or making the determination to euthanize the pet, denial that the pet is actually gone, and anger. These emotions may lead to sleep disturbances, depression, or anxiety.

During acute illness episodes requiring hospitalization, patients may experience significant psychosocial stress related to separation from the pet. Sources of stress may include concerns over the pet's welfare and loss of companionship. This is one justification for inquiring about pet ownership in the evaluation of a hospitalized patient (see Chapter 3).

During natural disasters such as hurricanes and earthquakes, separation from pets and other animals can be associated with similar stress reactions (see Chapter 13).

Sensitivity of human health and veterinary care providers during the process of pet euthanasia or other events leading to the death of a pet is crucial. If the euthanasia occurs in the veterinary clinic, the owner may want to bring the animal's favorite bedding, toy, or treat to provide comfort during the process. It is important that the owner not feel rushed and that the veterinary staff are kind and respectful of the pet and the owner's need to be present if that is his or her preference.

Encouraging owners to express their feelings of loss and reassuring them that it is normal to feel such loss will help them to progress through the grief process. Listening while they reminisce about their pet and acknowledging the pet's importance to them may be of further help. The veterinarian may be the only health care professional with whom the owner talks about this loss. This conversation may stimulate memories and discussion of previous losses of both pet and human family members. A follow-up phone call to the owner a few days to a week later is important to express care and concern and to rule out signs of extreme grief (owner unable to leave home, eat, dress, or do usual daily activities; extreme crying; statements about life being not worth living or about thoughts of suicide). If the owner identifies suicidal intentions, asking the name of the owner's physician, and contacting the physician to share this information or calling 911 may save the owner's life. If nonsuicidal extreme grief is identified, the veterinarian may encourage the owner to contact his or her physician for an appointment and may call a second time a few days later to check on the owner.

PETS AS INDICATORS OF HUMAN BEHAVIOR AND DOMESTIC VIOLENCE

There is little doubt that violence toward animals and other forms of domestic violence occur in tandem. In a recent study, investigators found that 54% of women participants who were staying in domestic violence shelters reported pet abuse in their households. The animal abuse included injury, torture, permanent loss of function, or death. In 87% of the women, the animal was identified as very close to them.[68] Animal abuse also presents serious problems for children who witness this violent and manipulative behavior in adult role models and may learn to imitate what they see. Experts in the field of animal and domestic violence and abuse agree that children exposed to domestic violence are more likely to be cruel to animals and that battered women and children may be more likely to stay in abusive homes to protect their pets, thereby exposing themselves to further abuse.[69]

Health care professionals who encounter such abuse have significant responsibilities. Human health care professionals are mandated to report child and elder abuse to law enforcement agencies. Veterinarians have an ethical responsibility to report suspected child and elder abuse but may not be mandatory reporters. More than 42 states have delineated various forms of animal abuse as felonies.[70] However, animal cruelty laws are inconsistent across states, and such crimes are commonly prosecuted only in extreme cases. Some states have mandated that veterinarians report animal abuse (termed *nonaccidental injury*) to authorities designated in their respective statutes. The rules vary considerably so it is incumbent on veterinary health care professionals to know the expectations in their particular state. The issues associated with veterinarians reporting animal abuse are similar to those encountered as child protection laws were being created. The role of the veterinarian in diagnosing the abuse is undisputed, but the process of diagnosis is not so clear-cut. The Tufts Animal Care and Condition Scales help to provide consistent, objective criteria for the diagnosis.[71] However, veterinarians may not feel sufficiently trained to identify, intervene, and report such cases. A recent study indicated that veterinarians in Australia believed that they should intervene in animal and child abuse cases but felt ill-equipped to do so.[72] Along with diagnosis, the issues for veterinarians reporting animal abuse parallel those encountered when health care providers in human medicine report child, domestic partner, or elder abuse. Specifically, the issues reflect concern about making a valid diagnosis, confidentiality with clients, liability of reporting suspected cases, the ethical duty to report, involvement of the veterinarian in the investigative and court process after reporting occurs, and the practical implications of all of these issues on the veterinary practice and business.[73] However, the AMVA's position is that veterinarians have the responsibility to report cases of animal abuse or neglect.[73]

The Humane Society of the United States developed the "First Strike" campaign in 1997 to increase awareness about animal abuse and neglect and the connection between this type of abuse and domestic violence. A variety of materials are available on their Web site to help health care professionals who need information about this connection, how to report such violence, and what steps can be taken in communities to prevent it. The following URL may be of assistance: http://www.hsus.org/hsus_field/first_strike_the_connection_between_animal_cruelty_and_human_violence/. Box 5-3 lists warning signs associated with possible abuse and domestic violence related to animals.

BOX 5-3   *POSSIBLE WARNING SIGNS OF ANIMAL ABUSE AND DOMESTIC VIOLENCE*

- Unexplained death of an animal
- Unusual fractures
- Unexplained weight loss
- Anxiety symptoms
- Incontinence in an animal that was formerly housebroken
- Animal hoarding (accumulating large numbers of cats or other domestic animals)

RESEARCH NEEDS

Although the body of evidence continues to grow, clearly more research about the health benefits of HAI is needed with robust designs and larger samples. But many areas about which we know relatively little—from either a clinical or empirical evidence point of view—need to be investigated. For example, research is needed to investigate the extent to which one species may be more effective than another in particular clinical settings for AAA and AAT. Interaction with a dog or cat is significantly different than what can be accomplished with a bird or fish in an aquarium. However, beneficial outcomes have been shown with all of these species. It is unclear to what extent individual preference may play a role in the efficacy of AAA and AAT. If we believe in the placebo effect in setting the stage for any intervention to be effective (as any nurse can attest to the importance of introducing a "take as needed" analgesic as "a very powerful drug that I think will help you," in predicting the efficacy of the drug), then individual preferences may be important in clinical prescriptions of AAA and AAT.

Clearly for people who are fearful of or dislike animals, AAA and AAT are not applicable interventions, just as we would not attempt a drug or other intervention to which a patient had an allergy or an aversion. Additionally, increased rather than decreased stress may be present in households where there is little or no capacity to properly care for a companion animal.

Presently we know nothing about effective "dosage" of AAA or AAT. Is a 15-minute session of petting a dog sufficient to produce the desired effects in anxiety reduction, depression alleviation, or pain relief? Does the session need to occur every day, or will three times per week suffice? Is it beneficial if the AAA or AAT session involves more active movement than just petting? Clinical evidence suggests that dogs provide comfort to patients during the dying process. In many settings, dogs are present on the patient's bed during this process. To date, there has been no clinical trial showing to what extent this experience provides comfort to the patient or the patient's family. Yet clinical reports show that dying patients request pet visits—either from their own pet or an AAA pet, and that these provide a loving, comforting environment.

Even less investigated have been the effects on animals of AAA and AAT work. One study showed that dogs who visited patients with cancer had no significant increases in urinary cortisol in response to the work, yet behavioral assessments revealed that the dogs commonly abstained from food and slept for an additional 2 to 3 hours after a day of visiting patients with cancer.[26] Yet clinical reports indicate that dogs sometimes have aversive responses to dying patients. The extent to which an animal may seek out or avoid particular patients has not been studied, nor has the mechanism through which this selection/aversion process occurs. Areas in need of investigation in the case of service dogs relate to their responses to their work and measures taken to minimize work-related stresses. For example, in service dogs working with children with autism, lack of rest and recreation, aggressive behavior toward the dog, and lack of predictability of daily routines have been identified as factors contributing to the dog's behavior, welfare, and performance, as well as parental satisfaction with the dog.[74] These areas have not been addressed in the AAA/AAT context and would enhance our understanding of the AAA/AAT experience for the dog.

The field of HAI continues to grow rapidly in a clinical sense (more programs for AAA and AAT emerge almost daily), but the research evidence base is growing slowly. Many aspects of the complex interactions between human beings and animals are still unknown (a 1987 National Institutes of Health expert panel called for animal-related variables in every major health study in the United States). The research is growing such that it is possible to begin to guide practice relying on this evidence. The ultimate goal of evidence-based study—clinical observations and practical application—is to optimize health through human animal interactions.

References

1. American Veterinary Medical Association. *Guidelines for animal assisted activity, animal-assisted therapy and resident animal programs.* http://www.avma.org/issues/policy/animal_assisted_guidelines.asp. Accessed August 27, 2008.
2. Brickel C. The therapeutic roles of cat mascots with a hospital-based geriatric population: a staff survey. *Gerontologist.* 1979;19:368–372.
3. Johnson RA, Odendaal JS, Meadows RL. Animal assisted intervention research: issues and answers. *West J Nurs Res.* 2002;24:422–440.
4. Cohen SP. Can pets function as family members? *West J Nurs Res.* 2002;24:621–638.
5. Cusack O. *Pets and mental health.* New York: Haworth Press; 1988.
6. Wilson E. *Biophilia.* Cambridge, MA: Harvard University Press; 1986.
7. Beck AM, Katcher AH. Future directions in human-animal bond research. *Am Behav Scientist.* 2003;47:79–93.
8. Reference deleted in proofs.
9. Odendaal JS. Animal assisted therapy—magic or medicine? *J Psychosom Res.* 2000;49:275–280.
10. Allen K, Blascovich J, Mendes WB. Cardiovascular reactivity and the presence of pets, friends, and spouses: the truth about cats and dogs. *Psychosom Med.* 2002;64:727–739.
11. Benda W, McGibbon N, Grant K. Improvements in muscle symmetry in children with cerebral palsy after equine-assisted therapy (hippotherapy). *J Altern Complement Med.* 1998;9:817–825.
12. McGibbon NH, Andrade CK, Widener G, et al. Effect of an equine movement therapy program on gait, energy expenditure, and motor function in children with spastic cerebral palsy: a pilot study. *Dev Med Child Neurol.* 1998;40:754–762.
13. Stoffel JM, Braun CA. Animal-assisted therapy: analysis of patient testimonials. *J Undergrad Nurs Schol.* 2006;8. Available at http://juns.nursing.arizona.edu.

14. Gawlinski A, Steers N, Kotlerman J. Animal-assisted therapy in patients hospitalized with heart failure. *Am J Crit Care*. 2007;16:575–588.
15. Edwards NE, Beck AM. Animal assisted therapy and nutrition in Alzheimer's disease. *West J Nurs Res*. 2002;24:697–712.
16. Banks MR, Banks WA. The effects of group and individual animal-assisted therapy on loneliness in residents of long-term care facilities. *Anthrozoos*. 2005;18:396–408.
17. Motooka M, Koike H, Yokoyama T, et al. Effect of dog-walking on autonomic nervous activity in senior citizens. *Med J Aust*. 2006;184:60–63.
18. Johnson RA, McKenney C, Cline K. Walk a hound, lose a pound: a walking program using shelter dogs as motivators. Unpublished manuscript. 2008.
19. Beck A. The use of animals to benefit humans, animal-assisted therapy. In: Fine AH, ed. *The handbook on animal assisted therapy: theoretical foundations and guidelines for practice*. San Diego, CA: Academic Press; 2000.
20. Cole K, Gawlinski A. Animal assisted therapy in the intensive care unit. *Res Util*. 1995;30:529–536.
21. Kidd A, Kidd R. Benefits and liabilities of pets for the homeless. *Psychol Rep*. 1994;74:715–722.
22. Barker SB, Dawson KS. The effects of animal-assisted therapy on anxiety ratings of hospitalized psychiatric patients. *Psychiatr Serv*. 1998;49:797–801.
23. Kongable L, Buckwalter K, Stolley J. The effects of pet therapy on the social behavior of institutionalized Alzheimer's clients. *Arch of Psychiatr Nurs*. 1989;3:191–198.
24. Kaiser L, Spence L, McGavin L, et al. A dog and a "happy person" visit nursing home residents. *West J Nurs Res*. 2002;24:671–683.
25. Johnson RA, McKenney C, Cline K. Pet pals pilot study: testing a dog visit protocol with newly admitted nursing home residents. Unpublished manuscript. 2008.
26. Johnson RA, Meadows R, Haubner J, et al. Animal assisted activity with cancer patients: effects on mood, fatigue, self-perceived health and sense of coherence. *Oncol Nurs Forum*. 2008;35:1–8.
27. Batson K, McCabe BW, Baun MM, et al. The effect of a therapy dog on socialization and physiological indicators of stress in persons diagnosed with Alzheimer's disease. In: Wilson CC, Turner DC, eds. *Companion animals in health*. Thousand Oaks, CA: Sage Publications; 1997.
28. Beyersdorfer P, Birkenhauer D. The therapeutic use of pets on an Alzheimer's unit. *Am J Alzheimer's Care Related Disord Res*. 1990;5:13–17.
29. Martin F, Farnum J. Animal-assisted therapy for children with pervasive developmental disorders. *West J Nurs Res*. 2002;24:657–670.
30. Katcher AH, Friedmann E, Beck AM, et al. Looking, talking and blood pressure: the physiological consequences of interaction with the living environment. In: Katcher AH, Beck AM, eds. *New perspectives on our lives with companion animals*. Philadelphia: University of Pennsylvania Press; 1983, p. 351–359.
31. Baun MM, Bergstrom N, Langston N, et al. Physiological effects of human/companion animal bonding. *Nurs Res*. 1984;33:126–129.
32. Baun MM, Oetting K, Bergstrom N. Health benefits of companion animals in relation to the physiological indices of relaxation. *Holistic Nurs Pract*. 1991;5:16–23.
33. Allen K, Blascovich J, Tomaka J, et al. Presence of human friend and pet dogs as moderators of autonomic responses to stress in women. *J Pers Soc Psychol*. 61:582–589.
34. Anderson W, Reid C, Jennings G. Pet ownership and risk factors for cardiovascular disease. *Med J Aust*. 1992;157:298–301.
35. Friedmann E, Thomas S. Pet ownership, social support, and one-year survival after acute myocardial infarction in the cardiac arrhythmia suppression trial (CAST). *Am J Cardiol*. 1995;76:1213–1217.
36. Morrison D. A feline lifeline? Owning a cat is linked to a lower risk of heart attack. *University of Minnesota News*. http://www1.umn.edu/umnnews/Feature_Stories/A_feline_lifeline3F.html. Accessed June 2, 2008.
37. Headey B. Health benefits and health cost savings due to pets: preliminary estimates from an Australian national survey. *Soc Indicators Res*. 1999;47:233–243.
38. Headey B, Grabka M. Pets and human health in Germany and Australia: national longitudinal results. *Soc Indicators Res*. 2007;80:297–311.
39. Dembicki D, Anderson J. Pet ownership may be a factor in improved health of the elderly. *J Nutr Elder*. 1996;15:15–31.
40. Baumann AE, Russell SJ, Furber SE, et al. The epidemiology of dog walking: an unmet need for human and canine health. *Med J Aust*. 2000;175:632–634.
41. Serpell JA. Beneficial effects of pet ownership on some aspects of human health and behaviour. *J Royal Soc Med*. 1991;84:717–720.
42. Ham SA, Epping J. Dog walking and physical activity in the United States. *Prev Chronic Dis*. 2006;3:A47.
43. Kushner RF, Blatner DJ, Jewell DE, et al. The PPET study: people and pets exercising together. *Obesity*. 2006;14:1762–1770.
44. Johnson RA, Meadows RL. Older Latinos, pets and health. *West J Nurs Res*. 2002;24:609–620.
45. Johnson R. *Walk a hound, lose a pound, and stay fit for older adults, funded grant proposal*. St. Petersburg, FL: Waltham Foundation & American Association of Human Animal Bond Veterinarians; 2007.
46. Raina P, Waltner-Toews D, Bonnett B, et al. Influence of companion animals on the physical and psychological health of older people: an analysis of a one-year longitudinal study. *J Am Geriatr Soc*. 1999;47:323–329.
47. Siegel J. Stressful life events and use of physician services among the elderly: the moderating role of pet ownership. *J Pers Soc Psychol*. 1990;58:1081–1086.
48. Garrity T, Stallones L, Marx M, et al. Pet ownership and attachment as supportive factors in the health of the elderly. *Anthrozoos*. 1989;3:35–44.
49. Siegel J, Angulo F, Detels R, et al. AIDS diagnosis and depression in the multicenter AIDS cohort study: the ameliorating impact of pet ownership. *AIDS Care*. 1999;11:157–170.
50. Lago D, Delaney M, Miller M, et al. Companion animals, attitudes toward pets, and health outcomes among the elderly: a long-term follow-up. *Anthrozoos*. 1989;3:25–34.
51. Beck AM, Katcher AH. *Between pets and people: the importance of animal companionship*. West Lafayette, IN: Purdue University Press; 1996.
52. Melson G, Schwarz R, Beck AM. Importance of companion animals in children's lives—implications for veterinary practice. *J Am Vet Med Assoc*. 1997;211:1512–1518.
53. Berryman J, Howells K, Lloyd-Evans M. Pet owner attitudes to pets and people: a psychological study. *Vet Rec*. 1985;17:659–661.
54. Beck AM, Meyers N. Health enhancement and companion animal ownership. *Ann Rev Health*. 1996;17:247–257.
55. McNicholas J, Collis G. Dogs as catalysts for social interactions: robustness of the effect. *Brit J Psychol*. 2000;91:61–70.
56. Messent P. Social facilitation of contact with other people by pet dogs. In: Katcher AH, Beck AM, eds. *New perspectives on our lives with companion animals*. Philadelphia: University of Pennsylvania Press; 1983.
57. Rossbach KA, Wilson JP. Does a dog's presence make a person appear more likable? Two studies. *Anthrozoos*. 1992;5:40–51.
58. Wood L, Giles-Corti B, Bulsara M. The pet connection: pets as a conduit for social capital? *Soc Sci Med*. 2005;61:1159–1173.
59. Eddy J, Hart LA, Boltz RP. The effects of service dogs on social acknowledgements of people in wheelchairs. *J Psychol*. 1988;122:39–44.
60. Hart LA, Hart BL, Bergin B. Socializing effects of service dogs for people with disabilities. *Anthrozoos*. 1987;1:41–44.
61. Mader B, Hart LA, Bergin B. Social acknowledgements for children with disabilities: effects of service dogs. *Child Dev*. 1989;60:1529–1534.
62. Lefebvre SL, Golab GC, Christensen E, et al. Guidelines for animal-assisted interventions in health care facilities. *Am J Infect Control*. 2008;36:78–85.
63. Delta Society. *Standards of practice for animal-assisted activities and therapy*. Renton, WA: Delta Society; 1996.
64. U.S. Department of Justice. *Commonly asked questions about service animals in places of business*. http://www.ada.gov/qasrvc.htm. Accessed August 27, 2008.
65. Lefebvre SL, Arroyo LG, Weese JS. Epidemic *Clostridium difficile* strain in hospital visitation dog. *Emerg Infect Dis*. 2006;12(6):1036–1037.
66. Lefebvre SL, Waltner-Toews D, Peregrine AS, et al. Prevalence of zoonotic agents in dogs visiting hospitalized people in Ontario: implications for infection control. *J Hosp Infect*. 2006;62(4):458–466.
67. Adams CL, Bonnett BN, Meek AH. Predictors of owner response to companion animal death in 177 clients from 14 practices in Ontario. *J Am Vet Med Assoc*. 2000;217:1303–1309.
68. Ascione FR, Weber CV, Thompson TM, et al. Battered pets and domestic violence: animal abuse reported by women experiencing intimate violence and by nonabused women. *Violence Against Women*. 2007;13:354–373.

69. Arkow P. Animal maltreatment in the ecology of abused children: compelling research and responses for prevention, assessment, and intervention. *Protecting Children.* 2007;22:66–79.

70. Arkow P. *The veterinarian's roles in preventing family violence: the experience of the human medical profession.* http://www.animaltherapy.net/Vets-abuse.html. Accessed June 1, 2008.

71. Patronek G. Issues and guidelines for veterinarians in recognizing, reporting and assessing animal neglect and abuse. *Society and Animals.* 1997;5(3):267–280.

72. Green P, Gullone E. Knowledge and attitudes of Australian veterinarians to animal abuse and human interpersonal violence. *Aust Vet J.* 2005;83:619–625.

73. Babcock S, Neihsl A. Requirements for mandatory reporting of animal cruelty. *J Am Vet Med Assoc.* 2005;228:685–689.

74. Burrows KE, Adams CL, Millman ST. Factors affecting behavior and welfare of service dogs for children with autism spectrum disorder. *J Appl Anim Welf Sci.* 2008;11:42–62.

The Built Environment and Indoor Air Quality

6

Clifford S. Mitchell, Carol Norris Reinero,
Peter M. Rabinowitz, Lisa A. Conti, and Judy Sparer

Our health is inextricably linked to both the natural and built environments. The *built environment* is defined as manmade surroundings ranging from individual buildings to developments and communities. The challenge is to design new, or retrofit existing, built environments to be sustainable and health promoting. *Indoor air quality* refers to gases and particulates or physical components of interior air that relate to building occupants' health and comfort. This chapter identifies certain links between clinical diseases in human beings and other animals relating to built environments and indoor air quality. Disease development in an animal or human being may be a sentinel sign of an environmental health hazard.

Key Points for Clinicians and Public Health Professionals

Public Health Professionals

- Monitor the health of the community and determine health associations with the built environment, including neighborhood and street planning and design of buildings.
- Work with urban planners, transportation engineers, environmental health specialists, and disease ecologists to implement improvements in neighborhoods and community design.[1] Resources are available at http://www.cdc.gov/healthyplaces, http://www.usgbc.org, http://www.smartgrowth.org, and http://www.epa.gov/dced.
- Provide technical advice to homeowners, contractors, and clinicians about ways to improve indoor air quality in homes and worksites.
- Provide information on energy conservation and sustainability such as Leadership for Energy and Environmental Design (LEED)-certified[2] status and LEED for Neighborhood Development (LEED-ND; see http://www.usgbc.org/DisplayPage.aspx?CMSPageID=148).

Human Health Clinicians

- Advocate for (re)development in the community that promotes healthy living, such as walking/biking and addition/maintenance of green spaces and parks.
- Encourage physical activity, including activities with healthy companion animals.
- Be alert to sentinel cases of disease in human beings related to the built environment or indoor air quality.
- Report possible cases of environmentally induced or exacerbated disease to the health department.
- If treating patients with diseases possibly related to the built environment or indoor air quality, inquire whether animals are also experiencing problems. This could help identify causative links.
- Consider building or retrofitting health care facilities to become certified.[2]

Veterinary Clinicians

- Advocate for (re)development in the community that promotes healthy living, such as walking/biking and addition/maintenance of green spaces and parks.
- Encourage physical activity with healthy companion animals.
- Be alert to sentinel cases of disease in animals related to the built environment and indoor air quality problems.
- Report possible cases of environmentally induced or exacerbated disease to the health department.
- If treating patients with problems possibly related to the built environment or buildings, inquire whether human beings in area are also experiencing problems. This could help identify causative links.

BUILT ENVIRONMENTS AND ACTIVE LIVING

On a large scale, habitat destruction affects species diversity; this results in loss of access to traditional medicines and novel pharmaceuticals as well as infectious disease emergence and spread.[3-5] Recent years have seen increasing realization that the design of neighborhoods and community environments has a profound impact on human health.[6] Moreover, issues such as traffic safety and injury risk, communities that sprawl (i.e., single-use development with design around the automobile), obesity,[7] and lack of exercise opportunities leading to inactivity have all been cited as important public health threats. These threats can eventually manifest as clinical problems, including

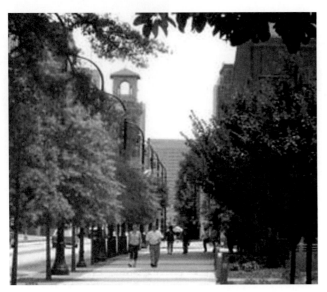

Figure 6-1 ■ Tree-lined, designated pedestrian paths increase the likelihood of walking. (From Centers for Disease Control and Prevention: *Healthy community design.* http://www.cdc.gov/healthyplaces/docs/Healthy%20Community%20Design.pdf.)

diabetes, asthma, hypertension, and stress-related illness.[8,9] Societal reductions of physical activity contributing to these poor health outcomes have been linked with designing our communities around motorized transportation and failing to design communities to promote neighborhood interaction. Active living is defined as participating in at least 30 minutes of physical activity on most days.[10] Research indicates that environmental factors, including accessibility (e.g., safe pedestrian and bike paths, parks, stores, churches, schools, libraries, and so on within safe walking distance), opportunities (e.g., sidewalks, a walkable neighborhood environment), and aesthetic attributes (e.g., tree-lined pedestrian paths, free of litter, with enjoyable scenery; Figure 6-1) all have a significant effect on the likelihood of engaging in physical activity,[11–13] "aging in place,"[*,14] and community resiliency.[15]

Less well considered is that companion animals and wildlife are also affected by changes in the built environment and, in turn, may contribute to human health issues. Human health care providers may not be aware that pet obesity is an increasing problem, presumably due to factors similar to those driving the rise in obesity prevalence in human beings, including lack of exercise related in part to neighborhood design and their owners' sedentary habits. The interactions between built environments with nearby wildlife areas can affect the risk of zoonotic disease transmission among wildlife, domestic animal, and human populations (Figure 6-2).

CLINICAL CONDITIONS IN HUMAN BEINGS AND OTHER ANIMALS RELATED TO BUILT ENVIRONMENTS

Table 6-1 lists conditions in human beings and other animals that could be related to problems with built environments

*Older adults continuing to live independently rather than moving to an institutional care setting.

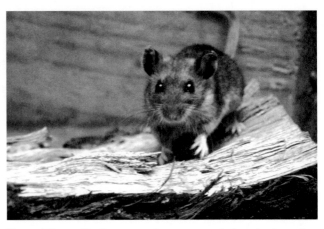

Figure 6-2 ■ The deer mouse, *Peromyscus maniculatus,* is a hantavirus carrier that becomes a threat when it enters human habitation in rural and suburban areas. (From Centers for Disease Control and Prevention Public Health Image Library, Atlanta, Ga. Photo courtesy James Gathany.)

and that should make clinicians consider this possibility. Similar clinical conditions can arise in both human beings and companion animals.

The impact of the built environment on health is complex. Nevertheless, identifying individuals with medical problems apparently related to the built environment can contribute to raising awareness in the community about specific environmental health issues.

BUILDING HEALTHY COMMUNITIES

Public health and health care involvement in community design is critical to addressing and improving population health. Activity-promoting environments are those with pedestrian-centric design and aesthetic appeal, and are joined with historic core public health issues such as water, soil, and air quality concerns.[19] Urban designers and planners, with their roots in public health protection, can be advocates in concert with public health professionals and clinicians to alter zoning codes to encourage working, shopping, and attending school within neighborhoods and to provide green space with its attendant violence prevention and mental health improvements.[20] Veterinarians, wildlife biologists, and other animal health professionals can play key roles in this effort by working with planners, land use experts, and developers to help design and build environments that encourage healthy pet ownership, including adequate sidewalks and paths for pet walking (Figure 6-3), parks that encourage pet sanitation, and approaches to limit forest fragmentation and problems such as peridomestic rodent infestation and disease vector abundance. Specific guidelines for reducing rodent infestation and tick control are found in Chapter 9.

INDOOR ENVIRONMENTS

Americans spend the majority of each day indoors[21] both at home and at work, and the indoor environment is becoming recognized as an important factor in respiratory, allergic, and other health issues.[22,23] Many companion animals are kept

Table 6-1 ■ Health Hazards and Clinical Conditions Related to the Built Environment

Health Hazard Associated With Built Environment	Sentinel Health Event in Human or Companion Animal	Mitigation
Lack of safe pedestrian areas	Pedestrian, bicyclist, or animal injured by motorist	Provide safe walking paths for people and pets (Figure 6-3); (re)design communities for pedestrians rather than automobiles, mixed-use and higher-density zoning and design (for sprawl); protection and creation of green spaces
Lack of exercise areas and opportunities	Obesity and chronic disease[16,17]	
Lack of green space or other aesthetic attributes	Reduction in physical activity[11,18]	
Suburban encroachment on wildlife habitat	Tick-borne disease (such as Lyme disease or Rocky Mountain spotted fever)	Management of open space and wildlife habitat near housing, integrated pest management techniques
Rodent infestation in and around buildings	Rodent-associated illness (such as hantavirus)	
Inadequate policies on pet sanitation in playgrounds and public areas	Hookworm disease, toxoplasmosis	Policies addressing pets in public areas (e.g., picking up after pets to keep areas free of feces)

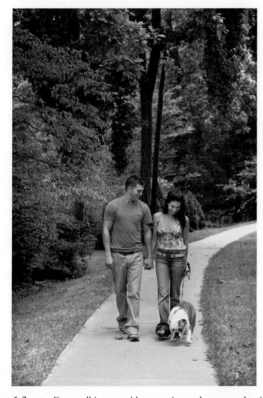

Figure 6-3 ■ Dog-walking provides exercise and stress reduction for both people and their pets.

Table 6-2 ■ Common Contaminants in Indoor Air

Class of Hazard	Hazard Sources
Volatile organic compounds (formaldehyde and others)	Plywoods, particle board; new vinyl flooring, rubber-backed nylon carpeting; adhesives, paints, resins, solvents; printed materials, printer and photocopier emissions; cleaning chemicals, personal products, fragrances, pesticides, cooking fumes
Dust	Dirt, house dust, construction, paper dust, paint dust (lead)
Fibers	Insulation (asbestos, fiberglass)
Bioaerosols	Bacteria, fungi/molds, dust mites, viruses, pollen, human skin particles, animal and insect dander and excreta
Entrapped outdoor sources	Vehicle exhaust (including carbon monoxide, ozone, and particulate matter), industrial exhaust
Physical factors	Temperature, humidity, noise, lighting
Other chemicals	Cooking odors, combustion products, radon, pesticides, cleaning agents, environmental tobacco smoke, building materials

Adapted from Hodgson M, Addorisio MR. Exposures in indoor environments. In: Rosenstock L, Cullen MR, Redlich C, et al, eds: *Textbook of clinical occupational and environmental medicine*, ed 2, Philadelphia, 2004, Saunders.

indoors because of lifestyle (apartment living), to avoid injury (from automobiles or other animals), or to minimize contact with zoonotic disease threats from wildlife and arthropod vectors (as recommended in some sections of this book). As a result of these changes in the Western lifestyle, human beings and other animals share indoor environments to a significant extent and are exposed to many similar indoor air health hazards. These hazards include chemicals from cleaning, renovation, pesticides, personal care products, and even cooking; allergens; and infectious pathogens (Table 6-2). Specific infectious diseases are discussed in Chapter 9, and the shared exposures of animals and human beings to specific toxic

chemicals are described in Chapter 8. In most living areas, the total loading of chemicals is not high compared with an industrial environment, but low levels of chemicals without good ventilation have an effect on health. In addition, as described in Chapter 7, animals and people are exposed to each other's allergens. Animal dander has been linked to an increasing prevalence of asthma and other allergic conditions in human beings in developed countries.[24] In a similar manner, human dander has been associated with feline asthma[25] and canine eosinophilic bronchopneumopathy.[26]

As Table 6-2 shows, indoor air environments can contain complex mixes of contaminants, often caused by inadequate ventilation. Persistent water intrusion from leaks or condensate can lead to mold growth (Color Plate 6-1). Sources of potential contaminants include renovation and remodeling materials, cleaning compounds, pesticides, paint, carpet or flooring, improperly stored volatile material, glue, copy machines, printers, and perfumes. Any water leaks are also of concern because molds can find hospitable growth conditions in damp carpet, ceiling tile, or even wallboard. The resulting exposures can produce certain nonspecific clinical syndromes.

Clinical Conditions in Human Beings and Other Animals Related to Indoor Air Quality

Not surprisingly, human beings and other animals exposed to indoor air contaminants can develop a number of health conditions (Figure 6-4). In human beings, the nonspecific cluster of symptoms known as "sick building syndrome" or nonspecific building-related illness (NSBRI) can include itching, watery eyes, nasal congestion, headaches, fatigue, and pruritus.[27] The causes of NSBRI appear to be multifactorial, including low-level exposure to airborne irritants and temperature and humidity fluctuations. Symptoms often improve with increased fresh air ventilation. A key factor in improving conditions is the opinion of the health care professional about the relationship between reported illness and the indoor air environment. Box 6-1 provides suggested intake questions to assist with this determination.

Less is known about diseases in other animals related to indoor air environments, but it appears that some conditions experienced by human beings may have corollaries in pets (Table 6-3). Importantly, pets tend to spend a greater portion of each day inside the home compared with human beings and consequently experience greater exposure to many

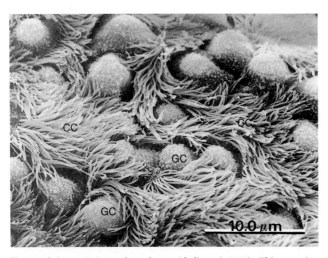

Figure 6-4 ■ Primary bronchus epithelium (×2000). This scanning electron micrograph illustrates the surface of a primary bronchus; the film of surface mucus has been removed. The ciliated epithelial cells (CC) have numerous surface cilia, each several microns long, that move in a coordinated fashion to sweep mucus up the bronchus. Scattered goblet cells (GC) are recognizable by their bulbous surface outline, lack of cilia, and the presence of small surface projections associated with mucus secretion. The fragile cilia are particularly vulnerable to damage and destruction by inhaled toxic chemicals (cigarette smoke, car exhaust fumes) and by bacterial and viral infections. (From Young B, Lowe JS, Stevens A, et al: *Wheater's functional histology: a text and colour atlas*, ed 5, Edinburgh, 2006, Churchill Livingstone Elsevier.)

BOX 6-1   DIAGNOSTIC CHECKLIST FOR ASSESSING POTENTIAL HUMAN ILLNESS ASSOCIATED WITH INDOOR AIR QUALITY

- When did the [symptom or complaint] begin?
- Does the [symptom or complaint] exist all the time, or does it come and go? That is, is it associated with times of day, days of the week, or seasons of the year?
- If so, are you usually in a particular place at those times?
- Does the problem abate or cease, either immediately or gradually, when you leave that location? Does it recur when you return?
- What is your work? Have you recently changed employers or assignments, or has your employer recently changed location?
- If not, has the place where you work been redecorated or refurnished, or have you recently started working with new or different materials or equipment? (These may include pesticides, cleaning products, craft supplies, and so on.)
- What is the smoking policy at your workplace? Are you exposed to environmental tobacco smoke at work, school, home, or other places?
- Describe your work area.
- Have you recently changed your place of residence?
- If not, have you made any recent changes in, or additions to, your home?
- Have you or anyone else in your family recently started a new hobby or other activity?
- Have you recently acquired a new pet?
- Does anyone else [or any pets] in your home have a similar problem? How about anyone with whom you work? (An affirmative reply may suggest either a common source or a communicable condition.)

From Environmental Protection Agency: *Indoor air pollution: an introduction for health professionals*. http://www.epa.gov/iaq/pubs/hpguide.html.

indoor air contaminants. Therefore signs of ill health in animals may be an indication of a health risk to the human beings, and vice versa, making diagnosis in one species relevant to the health of the other.

Building-related illness associated with indoor air quality tends to improve when human beings and animals are away from the building and recur after returning to the building.

Evaluation and Improvement of Indoor Air Quality

The health of occupants in indoor environments—whether human or other animal—depends on the same factors: the creation of an environment that is well ventilated and relatively free of agents that are harmful to the biological organism. The goal is not to create a sterile environment but one that promotes comfort and health. The U.S. Green Building Council has established the LEED rating system, a set of standards based primarily on energy conservation and sustainable construction, although it offers some encouragement to improve air quality. New or renovated buildings may apply for LEED certification that its standards have been met.[38]

EVALUATING INDOOR AIR PROBLEMS

Indoor air quality evaluations, which can be performed by an industrial hygienist, usually focus on two aspects of a building. The first is the identification and evaluation of potential

Table 6-3 ▪ Conditions in Human Beings and Other Animals Related to Indoor Air Quality Problems		
Indoor Air Quality Problem	**Sentinel Event in Human Beings**	**Sentinel Event in Other Animals**
Allergens (see Chapter 7), including those to chemicals in personal and pet care products	Asthma, rhinitis, atopic dermatitis	Allergic skin disease,[28] feline asthma (possible), canine eosinophilic bronchopneumopathy, equine hypersensitivity pneumonitis due to mold, dermatitis
Environmental tobacco smoke, a major source of indoor air contamination	Bronchitis, rhinitis, pharyngitis, asthma, lung cancer, conjunctival irritation, headache	Nasal neoplasia[29] and possible chronic bronchitis[30] in dogs; oral squamous cell carcinoma[31] and malignant lymphoma in cats[32]; pneumotoxicity in birds[33]; possible chronic respiratory conditions in captive reptiles[34]
Radon	Lung cancer	Lung cancer in rats[35]
Inadequate ventilation, VOCs, temperature and humidity fluctuation	"Sick building syndrome" (nonspecific building-related illness)	Calves grouped indoors are at increased risk for exposure to ammonia fumes and subsequent *Pasteurella multocida* colonization of the lungs[36]; increased mastitis rates in cattle[37]

sources of contaminants in the air (see Table 6-2). The other important aspect affecting indoor air quality is the ventilation system. To achieve good air quality, the system must be able to supply sufficient fresh air to all occupied spaces and remove the contaminants. An evaluation includes determination of how much fresh air is being provided, the quality of that fresh air, and how well the distribution system functions. The air system must be balanced, delivering enough air to each room, and must ensure mixing of new and old air within each space for proper cleaning and temperature equilibrium.

Sometimes measurements of carbon dioxide, total airborne hydrocarbons, or airborne molds are taken to help determine ventilation effectiveness. The carbon dioxide measurement is used as a marker. If the air circulation is poor and the fresh air insufficient, carbon dioxide, derived primarily from occupants' breathing, builds up (carbon dioxide is not a good marker of air quality if there are few people or animals present and breathing in the space). Carbon dioxide serves as an easily measured marker for poor ventilation, which is often associated with complaints of fatigue, dry or irritated eyes, scratchy throat, or headache. (Although the Occupational Safety and Health Administration [OSHA] standard for carbon dioxide is 5000 parts per million [ppm], when indoor levels rise above 700 to 800 ppm, building occupants report discomfort. For reference, carbon dioxide levels outdoors are usually between 250 and 450 ppm, depending on traffic or other sources of combustion.)

Particulates (airborne dust particles) are a common problem in indoor air environments. If the ductwork or unit ventilators have become dirty, the filters overloaded or breached, or some part of the structure (sometimes the insulation of the ductwork) has deteriorated, the ventilation system itself can become a source of contamination. It is not unusual for construction dust to enter the ventilation system. Systems designed with an open return plenum are especially susceptible. Poorly maintained fuel-burning heating systems can be a source of carbon monoxide. Systems should have annual maintenance.

Excessive dryness (relative humidity below 30%) adds to winter discomfort from respiratory complaints. Excessive humidity (above 60%) encourages the growth of mold. Levels of airborne mold are sometimes measured but levels are not yet sufficiently understood to predict illness. Mold is always present in both indoor and outdoor air and varies tremendously from season to season and place to place. A history of water damage is generally more helpful in identifying a mold problem than measuring mold levels. Therefore mold measurements are not recommended. Any porous materials that have become damp with water for any reason should be dried immediately. If they have been wet for a prolonged period, they should be removed and replaced because effective mold removal from porous materials is extremely difficult.

The American Society of Heating, Ventilating, Refrigerating and Air Conditioning Engineers (ASHRAE) recommends that a minimum of 20 cubic feet per minute (cfm) of fresh outdoor air per occupant be provided in business offices and 15 cfm per occupant in reception areas. Any additional sources of air contaminants increase the demand for fresh air. There is no specific recommendation for physicians' or veterinarians' offices, but hospitals and nursing homes are recommended to provide 25 cfm per occupant for patients' rooms, 15 cfm for medical procedure rooms, 30 cfm for operating rooms, and 15 cfm for recovery rooms, intensive care units, and autopsy rooms. Many homes, especially older ones and stand-alone homes, do not have a regular source of fresh air but depend on leakage, open windows, or the opening and closing of doors to provide adequate ventilation.

In many situations the principles of good practice listed in Box 6-2 can prevent the indoor environment from causing health problems for human beings and companion animals.

Clinicians may often feel ill-equipped to make recommendations or initiate interventions to improve indoor air quality. The environmental health division of the local health department may be able to offer technical advice to homeowners, contractors, and clinicians about improving indoor air quality. The Environmental Protection Agency (EPA) also has useful educational materials on its Web site (http://www.epa.gov/iaq/pubs). Human health clinicians and veterinarians may be able to collaborate to work toward improvement of a particular building where both human beings and animals are affected.

BOX 6-2   *INTERVENTIONS TO IMPROVE INDOOR AIR ENVIRONMENTS*

Reduce or Eliminate Sources of Indoor Air Pollution

- Perform regular maintenance on home heating systems to reduce potential carbon monoxide exposure.
- Minimize the use of products that become airborne, such as cleaning chemicals with VOCs, personal products and perfumes, air fresheners, and pesticides. Renovation and decorating materials may also "off-gas" VOCs for some time.
- Prohibit smoking in buildings and away from entrances and air intakes.
- Keep the home as free as dust and allergens as possible by:
  - Frequent cleaning
  - Putting walk-off mats by entrances, wiping pets' feet when returning from walks
  - Using vacuums with HEPA filters rather than regular vacuum cleaners or brooms
  - Using microfiber dust cloths rather than traditional dusters
  - Furnishing with items that are easily cleaned and do not become reservoirs for dust and allergens
- Develop an integrated pest management program to effectively control pests while minimizing the use of toxic pesticides.
- Prevent mold by promptly fixing water leaks and drying spills. Any absorbent material that has been damp for longer than 48 hours can become an indoor source of mold.
- Test and mitigate for radon.

Ensure Proper Ventilation

- Good ventilation is essential to removing contaminant-laden air and bringing in fresh outdoor air.

VOC, Volatile organic compound; *HEPA,* high-efficiency particulate air.

References

1. Jacobs DE, Kelly T, Sobolewski J. Linking public health, housing, and indoor environmental policy: successes and challenges at local and federal agencies in the United States. *Environ Health Perspect.* 2007;115(6):976–982.
2. US Green Building Counsel. *LEED for healthcare.* http://www.usgbc.org/DisplayPage.aspx?CMSPageID=1765.
3. Cassis G. Biodiversity loss: a human health issue. *MJA.* 1998;169:568–569.
4. Grifo F, Rosenthal J, eds. *Biodiversity and human health.* Washington DC: Island Press; 1997.
5. Swaddle J, Calos S. Increased avian diversity is associated with lower incidence of human West Nile infection: observation of the dilution effect. *PLoS ONE.* 2008;3(6):e2488.
6. Jackson RJ. The impact of the built environment on health: an emerging field. *Am J Public Health.* 2003;93(9):1382–1384.
7. Frances L, Gordenard B, Jalaludin B. Impact of urban sprawl on overweight, obesity, and physical activity in Sydney, Australia. *J Urb Health.* 2008;186(1):19–30.
8. Rutt C, Dannenberg AL, Kochtitzky C. Using policy and built environment interventions to improve public health. *J Public Health Manag Pract.* 2008;14(3):221–223.
9. University of Colorado Denver. *Children, youth, and environments center for research and design.* http://www.cudenver.edu/Academics/Colleges/ArchitecturePlanning/discover/centers/CYE/Pages/index.aspx.
10. Active Living by Design. http://www.activelivingbydesign.org.
11. Sallis J, Cervera R, Archer W, et al. An ecological approach to creating active living communities. *Ann Rev Pub Health.* 2006;27:297–332.
12. Gauvin L, Riva M, Barnett T, et al. Association between neighborhood active living potential and walking. *Am J Epidemiol.* 2008;167(8):944–953.
13. Wells NM, Ashdown P, Davies EHS, et al. Environment, design, and obesity. *Environ Behav.* 2007;39(1):6–33.
14. Michael YL, Green MK, Farquhar SA. Neighborhood design and active aging. *Health Place.* 2006;12(4):734–740.
15. Campanella TJ. Planning for postdisaster resiliency. *Ann Am Acad Pol Soc Sci.* 2006;604(1):192–207.
16. McCann BA, Ewing R. *Measuring the health effects of sprawl: a national analysis of physical activity, obesity and chronic disease.* Smart Growth America Surface Transportation Project; 1993. http://www.smartgrowthamerica.org/report/HealthSprawl8.03.pdf.
17. German AJ. The growing problem of obesity in dogs and cats. *J Nutr.* 2006;136(suppl 7):1940S–1946S.
18. Farley TA. *Prescription for a healthy nation: a new approach to living our lives by fixing our everyday world.* Boston: Beacon Press; 2005.
19. Prevention Institute. *The built environment and health: 11 profiles of neighborhood transformation.* http://www.preventioninstitute.org/builtenv.html.
20. Jackson RJ, Kochtitzky C. *Creating a healthy environment: the impact of the built environment on public health.* Washington DC: Sprawl Watch. http://www.cdc.gov/healthyplaces/articles/Creating%20A%20Healthy%20Environment.pdf.
21. Leech JA, Nelson WC, Burnett RT, et al. It's about time: a comparison of Canadian and American time-activity patterns. *J Expo Anal Environ Epidemiol.* 2002;12(6):427–432.
22. Wu F, Jacobs D, Mitchell C. Improving indoor environmental quality for public health: impediments and policy recommendations. *Environ Health Perspect.* 2007;115(6):953–957.
23. National Institute for Occupational Health and Safety. *Indoor environmental quality.* http://www.cdc.gov/niosh/topics/indoorenv.
24. Liccardi G, Cazzola M, D'Amato M, et al. Pets and cockroaches: two increasing causes of respiratory allergy in indoor environments. Characteristics of airways sensitization and prevention strategies. *Respir Med.* 2000;94(11):1109–1118.
25. Corcoran BM, Foster DJ, Fuentes VL. Feline asthma syndrome: a retrospective study of the clinical presentation in 29 cats. *J Small Anim Pract.* 1995;36(11):481–488.
26. Clercx C, Peeters D, German AJ, et al. An immunologic investigation of canine eosinophilic bronchopneumopathy. *J Vet Intern Med.* 2002;16(3):229–237.
27. Burge PS. Sick building syndrome. *Occup Environ Med.* 2004;61(2):185–190.
28. August JR. *Consultation in feline internal medicine.* 5th ed. St. Louis: Saunders; 2006.
29. Ford RB, Mazzalferro E. *Kirk and Bistner's handbook of veterinary procedures and emergency treatment.* 8th ed. St Louis: Saunders; 2006.
30. Birchard SJ, Sherding RG. *Saunders manual of small animal practice.* 3rd ed. St Louis: Saunders; 2006.
31. Bertone ER, Snyder LA, Moore AS. Environmental and lifestyle risk factors for oral squamous cell carcinoma in domestic cats. *J Vet Intern Med.* 2003;17:557–562.
32. Bertone ER, Snyder LA, Moore AS. Environmental tobacco smoke and risk of malignant lymphoma in pet cats. *Am J Epidemiol.* 2002;156:268–273.
33. Plumlee K. *Clinical veterinary toxicology.* St Louis: Mosby; 2004.
34. Mader DR. *Reptile medicine and surgery.* 2nd ed. St Louis: Saunders; 2006.
35. Collier CG, Strong JC, Humphreys JA, et al. Carcinogenicity of radon/radon decay product inhalation in rats—effect of dose, dose rate and unattached fraction. *Int J Radiat Biol.* 2005;81(9):631–647.
36. Divers TJ, Peek SF. *Rebhun's diseases of dairy cattle.* 2nd ed. St Louis: Saunders; 2008.
37. Radostits OM, Gay CC, Hinchcliff KW, eds. *Veterinary medicine: a textbook of the diseases of cattle, horses, sheep, pigs and goats.* 10th ed. Oxford: Saunders Elsevier Ltd.; 2007.
38. US Green Building Council. *LEED.* http://www.usgbc.org/DisplayPage.aspx?CategoryID=19.

Allergic Conditions

7

Carol Norris Reinero, Clifford S. Mitchell, and Peter M. Rabinowitz

Although concern is ongoing about the risks of zoonotic disease transmission from animal exposure, allergic diseases caused by animal allergens may be a greater public health and clinical problem because of the prevalence of disease and potential for mortality. Diagnosing and managing animal allergy can be challenging in part because many people are reluctant to give up their pets.

Pets and other animals can develop allergic conditions that may be triggered by the allergens that cause problems in people. In addition, because of the similarity of animal and human disease, animals serve as research models for human beings. Therefore increased communication among public health, human health, and veterinary clinicians may lead to improved management and prevention of allergic conditions.

Key Points for Clinicians and Public Health Professionals

Public Health Professionals

- Educate the public that exposure to allergens can be a significant contributor to rates of asthma and other allergic conditions in the community.[1]
- Support surveillance and analysis of asthma data (for case definition, see http://www.cste.org/ps/1998/1998-eh-cd-01.htm).

Human Health Clinicians

- Allergen exposure reduction is a part of a comprehensive management program for asthma and allergies. Pets may be an important source of allergens, but elimination of the pet may not be the only therapeutic option and should be considered in light of a comprehensive treatment and prevention approach. Clinicians may wish to discuss options with the family veterinarian. (NOTE: Cat allergens can persist in the environment years after the elimination of the pet.) Other animals such as rats and mice also can contribute to indoor air allergen load.
- When evaluating a patient with allergic symptoms, inquire also about contacts with animals and the health of the animals. Animals may also manifest clinical reactions to environmental allergens.

Veterinary Clinicians

- Communication with human health clinicians can help explore alternatives to removing a pet from the household of an allergic person.
- Allergic conditions in an animal may suggest an indoor air contaminant with human health relevance. Veterinarians treating an animal with an allergic condition can inquire about human beings with problems related to allergies or airborne contaminant exposures and whether causative agents have been identified. Contact with the treating health care provider may help coordinate household allergen management.

ANIMAL ALLERGY IN HUMAN BEINGS

Human beings can become sensitized to a wide range of animal allergens (Table 7-1). As much as 10% of the general population and 50% of persons with atopy (allergic predisposition) may be sensitized to dogs and cats. Other animals causing significant allergy in human beings include rodents, horses, insects, and birds.[5]

Much symptomatic animal allergy is associated with pet ownership, but allergy can also be a significant occupational problem for individuals working with animals, including laboratory animal workers[3] and veterinarians (see Chapter 12). Occupational allergens include rodent urine, cat dander, and horse dander. Because animal allergens may persist in the environment long after elimination of a pet and can be carried distances in dust, cat and dog allergens may be present in homes where no pets are present and in schools.

Allergy to Cats and Dogs

A common misconception is that human beings are allergic to cat and dog hair and that short-haired breeds of cats and dogs are less allergenic than long-haired breeds. In fact, human allergy to cat and dogs is related to specific protein allergens, such as Fel d 1 and Can f 1, respectively, rather than

Table 7-1 ■ Sources of Animal Allergens Associated with Human Allergy

Animal Species	Source of Allergen
Rats and mice	Urine, hair, saliva
Guinea pigs	Urine, dander, saliva, hair
Rabbits	Urine, saliva, hair
Cats	Dander, saliva
Dogs	Dander
Birds	Feathers, serum
Horses	Serum, dander
Cattle	Hair, dander
Reptiles	Scales[3]
Nonhuman primates	Hair
Cockroaches	Feces, saliva, debris from dead animals[4]
Mites	Feces

hair per se. For this reason, despite advertising claims to the contrary, there are currently no "nonallergenic" breeds of cats and dogs. However, some species appear to provoke allergies in certain individuals and efforts are under way to develop breeds with lower allergenic potential. Cats produce a number of proteins that can act as human allergens. The one considered the most important, Fel d 1, is produced by sebaceous and salivary glands, basal squamous epithelial skin cells, and anal glands of cats.[6] It can be carried on particles less than 5 microns in diameter that can remain airborne for long periods of time.[7] A naturally selected line of cats with deficient Fel d 1 is being developed.[2] Dog breed, gender, and seborrhea appear to influence the levels of Can f 1 allergen detected on fur.[8] Cat and dog allergens may persist for extended periods in a house even after a pet has left, and both Fel d 1 and Can f 1 have been detected in homes without pets.[9]

Risk Factors for Pet Allergy

Despite the prevalence of pet allergy, it is not clear whether having a pet in the house increases the overall risk of allergy. Host factors play an important role, especially the presence of atopy, defined as "the genetic propensity to develop immunoglobulin E [IgE] antibodies in response to exposure to allergen."[10] Studies have shown that children born into families that already own dogs (where there is no history of atopy) have a lower risk of allergic disease by 2 years of age compared with families that did not have a dog.[11] The genetic basis of allergic predisposition is a subject of active scientific investigation. The timing of allergen exposure also appears to play a role. Although it has been reported that early exposure to cats can increase the risk of early sensitization and development of an immune response to cat allergens, other studies have shown a protective effect for pet ownership early in life, and still others have demonstrated inconsistent results regarding the development of early clinical allergic disease (particularly asthma).[12,13] Farm exposure in early life is also associated with an allergy-protective effect in human beings.[14]

CLINICAL CONDITIONS RELATED TO ANIMAL ALLERGY

Rhinitis and Upper Airway Symptoms

Rhinitis and upper airway symptoms are among the most common complaints in outpatient medical practice. The prevalence in the general population is as high as 20%, but in patients with asthma the prevalence is generally much higher. Symptoms include sneezing, nasal passage obstruction, lacrimation, and itching of the nasopharynx. The diagnosis is generally made by history and physical examination. One of the most important distinctions to make in chronic rhinitis and sinusitis is whether it is allergic or nonallergic. Nonallergic rhinitis and rhinosinusitis can occur in the context of exposure to airborne irritants in the environment. Especially if these irritant exposures continue, this condition is less amenable to treatment with pharmacotherapy.

Diagnostic testing for rhinitis and other allergic conditions related to indoor air exposure can include skin prick or blood testing for IgE antibodies to specific antigens. Skin prick testing involves noting the immediate wheal-and-flare reaction to antigens introduced under the skin. Blood testing using radioallergosorbent testing (RAST) can screen for a wide number of IgE antibodies to specific antigens. Both skin testing and RAST testing are associated with false-positive and false-negative results, and this possibility must be considered in reviewing the results of such testing.

Management of upper airway disorders is generally a combination of exposure reduction and pharmacotherapy. Exposure reduction typically involves multiple measures, such as eliminating irritating chemicals, cleaning more frequently and/or adopting changes in cleaning techniques, and (if relevant) removing or isolating pets from the bedroom and removing fabrics that retain dander and allergens. These measures have been effective in reducing allergen exposure and improving symptoms in the aggregate but not necessarily in the individual patient. Pharmacotherapy includes nasal steroid sprays and antihistamines to control allergic symptoms.

Asthma

Human asthma is characterized by bronchoconstriction and inflammation with airway secretions, leading to obstruction of the airways. Clinically, the hallmark symptoms of asthma are wheeze, cough, and dyspnea. The pathogenesis of asthma involves reversible airway obstruction, and treatment with both short- and long-acting medications can reverse or prevent the symptoms. A variety of allergens can lead to sensitization and new onset of asthma, or exacerbation of underlying asthma in previously sensitized individuals, including animal-related allergens such as dander, cockroach excreta, and dust mites. The role of domestic animals in asthma causation and prevention is complex. Some studies show that possession of pet dogs and cats may be associated with a lower incidence of early childhood asthma, whereas other studies suggest that pet possession may lead to an increased risk of asthma. These differences may be due in part to the nature of the population in question. The effect seems to vary with the age of the children, whether they are in environments with high or low prevalence of pet ownership, and whether there is a family history of allergic disorders.[15] At this time, therefore, it is not possible to offer general recommendations regarding ownership of pets for young families if there is no current asthma or atopy in the family.

In evaluating a patient with suspected asthma, it is important to confirm that reversible airway disease is present. If a patient has spirometry showing obstruction, reversibility can be demonstrated by improvement in spirometry flow rates after bronchodilator administration. If spirometry is normal at baseline, a methacholine challenge test can document abnormal bronchial reactivity.

As with rhinitis, allergic asthma must be distinguished from nonallergic asthma. Nonallergic asthma may be due to exposure to chemical irritants. Diagnostic testing often involves skin prick or RAST testing. A variety of agents are available for asthma treatment, including inhaled corticosteroids, bronchodilators, leukotriene inhibitors, and mast cell stabilizers.

Anaphylaxis

Anaphylaxis is an acute, severe, IgE-mediated reaction to environmental allergens that can occur in sensitized individuals. The clinical presentation of anaphylaxis can involve swelling of the lips and throat with progressive airway edema leading to obstruction and respiratory collapse and death if not treated.

Anaphylaxis can occur as a result of exposure to insect stings (see Chapter 8) but can also occur with exposure to other animal allergens. Anaphylactic reactions can also occur when the immediate precipitating factor is unknown. The diagnosis is typically made by clinical history; laboratory testing is of limited value. Although tryptase or histamine levels may be elevated acutely after an anaphylactic episode, they usually return to normal by the time of a clinical evaluation. The presence of elevated serum IgE to a specific antigen can be of benefit in a patient with a history of anaphylactic episodes, but it is of limited value in predicting whether an asymptomatic patient is at risk of future anaphylaxis because many people with elevated IgE levels do not have anaphylactic symptoms. Although the negative predictive value of IgE is relatively high, occasionally people with normal IgE levels can have anaphylactic reactions to an antigen.[16] The treatment of anaphylactic episodes may include epinephrine, antihistamines, and steroids.

Hypersensitivity Pneumonitis

Hypersensitivity pneumonitis (HP), also known as *extrinsic allergic alveolitis,* is an inflammatory reaction of the lower airways to a variety of environmental allergens. Also encountered in the occupational setting, HP can be caused by exposure to thermophilic bacteria in moldy hay ("farmer's lung"), mushrooms ("mushroom worker's lung"), and a large number of other animal and plant allergens, including wood dust. It can also be caused by certain chemicals such as isocyanates. Animal allergens that have been implicated in HP include pigeon antigens (pigeon breeder's lung) and feather dander from other birds, especially psittacine birds such as parakeets and parrots ("bird fancier's lung").

HP can have both an acute and insidious onset pattern. Acute symptoms may follow an exposure to antigen, such as cleaning an animal's cage, and can include cough, shortness of breath, and fever. Many cases are misdiagnosed and treated as pneumonia because chest radiographs may show fleeting infiltrates (Figure 7-1).[17] HP also can be mistaken for other forms of interstitial lung disease. Some exposed patients may not notice acute effects but instead have gradual onset of shortness of breath and progressive fatigue. If exposure continues, the pulmonary inflammation may lead to irreversible fibrosis and restrictive lung disease and even respiratory failure.

HP can be difficult to recognize and diagnose. The diagnosis of HP relies partly on a history of exposure to an antigen. Pulmonary function testing classically shows a restrictive pattern, although obstruction also can be seen, particularly with avian exposures. Like other interstitial disease, the diffusion capacity of carbon monoxide is reduced. Serum precipitins may be positive but have low sensitivity and depend on the laboratory and preparation of standards.[18] Bronchoalveolar lavage (BAL) shows a predominance of lymphocytes (30% to 90%) and macrophages. Computed tomographic scans may show a characteristic alveolitis pattern. Referral and co-management with a specialist in occupational pulmonary diseases are recommended.

The treatment of HP requires removal from exposure. Patients may be reluctant to give up their animals or otherwise take steps to reduce exposure and need to be counseled that they risk potentially fatal lung disease. Unlike some allergic conditions mentioned in this chapter, elimination of the exposure is generally required for patients with HP because of the risk of irreversible complications. Other adjuncts to treatment include oral steroids, although there is no supporting evidence that this affects the natural history of the disease.

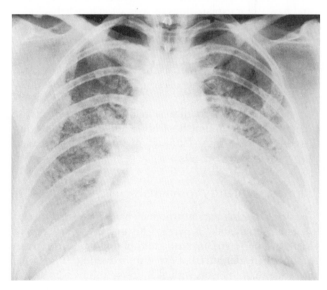

Figure 7-1 ▪ Chest radiograph of acute hypersensitivity pneumonitis. (From Adkinson NF Jr: *Middleton's allergy: principles and practice,* ed 6, St. Louis, 2003, Mosby.)

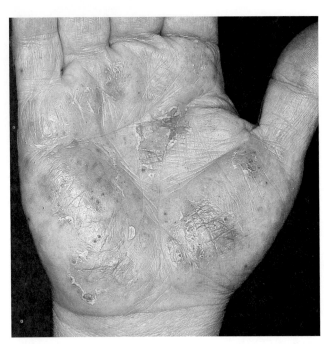

Figure 7-2 ■ Hand eczema. (From Habif TP: *Clinical dermatology: a color guide to diagnosis and therapy,* ed 4, St Louis, 2004, Mosby.)

Eczema/Dermatitis

Eczema, also known as *atopic dermatitis,* is a skin disorder (Figure 7-2) characterized by pruritus and scratching that often affects flexor surfaces and usually appears before the age of 5 years. Because it is associated with an atopic predisposition, in many children with eczema allergic rhinitis, asthma, or both eventually develop. The condition often persists into adulthood. The diagnosis is usually made by history and physical examination. As with other allergic disorders, it has been suggested that early exposure (indicated by ownership of a furry pet) may have a protective effect against the development of eczema, but this result is inconsistent and could have other explanations such as avoidance behavior.[19]

Management of eczema includes topical steroids and newer nonsteroidal antiinflammatory agents. Treatment may be required for secondary effects such as infection. Known triggers can be avoided but this is often not effective, and there are few data on either allergen reduction or removal of pets in eczema.

Other dermatitis conditions related to animal allergy include acute development of hives and itching following allergen exposure; such skin reactions may be accompanied by anaphylaxis (see below).

Diagnosing Allergy to Animals

When faced with a patient who may have an animal allergy, clinicians should take a detailed history of exposures and symptoms, perform diagnostic testing for response to antigens, and consider a trial of exposure reduction. It is simple to assume that a person with allergic symptoms who shares a house with an animal must be having allergic reactions to that animal, but this is not always the case. Another allergen exposure could be the causative agent instead.

An accurate history can reveal important details about the circumstances of exposure (see Chapter 3). The timing of symptom onset with the acquisition of a pet or contact with the pet or specific areas where the pet spends the most time can be helpful in making the association. It is also important to ask about occupation and possible association with occupational exposures. It is important to have a history of possible comorbid conditions and to establish which medications are already in use or have been tried. A family history and history of tobacco use are also essential.

It is important to inquire about any previous symptoms of anaphylactic reactions to animal contact or other allergens in taking the history of allergy.

Diagnostic testing for animal allergy can involve skin prick testing, RAST for animal-specific IgE, and/or a serum IgG panel for suspected HP. Chest radiographs often are useful for HP. Pulmonary function tests are helpful to establish baseline function and to distinguish obstructive disease from restrictive or mixed patterns but are not generally helpful in distinguishing allergic from other disorders.

If airway involvement is suspected (bronchial asthma), an adjunct to the patient history can be a peak flow diary, in which the patient records peak flow rates several times a day for 2 weeks to help determine whether decreases in peak flows are related to times of animal exposure.[20]

Trials of avoidance for animal allergy can be both diagnostic and therapeutic. In the home setting, they involve either removing the animal from the house for a period to see whether symptoms improve or having the person spend time in another house or other environment free from the presumptive allergen. Removal of the animal for a few days or weeks may not be sufficient because 20 weeks or longer may be required for levels of animal antigen to fall to background levels, and allergens may be highly transportable.[21]

MANAGEMENT OPTIONS FOR ALLERGY TO ANIMALS

Once it is clear that an individual has allergies and is sensitized to a pet in the house, there are three basic management options: (1) removal of the animal or person, (2) reduction of the allergen load without removal of the animal or person, and (3) desensitization therapy. Robust evaluation of the differential effectiveness of these measures is lacking.[22]

Removal of the Animal or Person

The National Asthma Education and Prevention Program Expert Panel Report 3 recommends animal removal as the treatment of choice for those with known animal dander sensitization. If removal is not acceptable to the patient, then exposure should be minimized by keeping the pet out of the patient's room, keeping the bedroom door closed, removing upholstered furniture and carpeting, or keeping the pet from those items.[23] It is important to stress that this should be done as part of a comprehensive program of exposure reduction and effective medical management. Removal of the pet will reduce but may not eliminate an individual's total allergen exposure. This is especially important in cases of anaphylaxis, as well as HP and severe asthma, for which the outcomes can be irreversible or fatal.[24]

Allergen Reduction

The role of allergen load reduction in asthmatic patients with known sensitization to animal dander is well established. Studies of allergen reduction have generally demonstrated that multifaceted strategies are required to achieve significant reductions in allergen load. These strategies include thorough cleaning with high-efficiency particulate (HEPA) vacuum cleaners (to avoid resuspending particulates), removing carpeting and upholstered furniture from the bedroom, washing and covering bedding with impermeable covers, using HEPA air filtration, and keeping the pet out of the bedroom.[25] In one study, routinely washing cats resulted in only a short-lived (24-hour) reduction in Fel d 1 and was therefore not considered efficacious.[26] Although individually it is difficult to document how much each of these strategies adds to the total, the reductions in allergen loads are significant.

Desensitization

Allergen desensitization therapy has been used extensively to treat patients with more severe allergic conditions such as insect venom allergy. A recent innovation in immunotherapy is the use of sublingual administration in addition to the more traditional injections. Much of the data on the effectiveness of immunotherapy concerns allergens that pose significant risks to patients or cannot be easily avoided, such as dust mite, pollens, or bee stings. Some data show the effectiveness of immunotherapy for animal allergens, but this is not seen as a first-line therapy.[27] One question that remains unanswered is how long immunotherapy must be maintained.[28]

SELECTED ALLERGIC CONDITIONS IN ANIMALS

A number of conditions in companion animals may be related in part to allergens and could be corollaries of allergic conditions in human beings (Table 7-2). With more owners seeking veterinary medical care for their pets, the recognition of these diseases is increasing.

Feline Asthma

As in human beings, feline asthma is associated with eosinophilic airway inflammation, reversible airway obstruction, airway hyperreactivity, and airway remodeling. Aeroallergens are believed to drive the Th2 immune response leading to clinical signs of cough, wheeze, and episodic respiratory distress. Cats have tested positive to a variety of allergens (including weeds, trees, grasses, fungi, and house dust mites) using IgE serology and intradermal skin testing (Figure 7-3).[29-31] Cats may also develop clinical signs after exposure to nonallergen irritants such as cigarette or fireplace smoke, various sprays (e.g., hairspray, deodorant, flea spray, deodorizer), and dust from cat litter. Some cats have responded well to allergen avoidance.[32,33]

The diagnosis of feline asthma is usually made clinically. Thoracic radiographs may show signs of a bronchial or bronchointerstitial pattern with evidence of lung lobe collapse (due to mucus plugging of the major bronchus) or hyperinflation (due to air trapping secondary to bronchoconstriction). However, thoracic radiographs may also be unremarkable despite pronounced airway inflammation. Eosinophilic

Table 7-2 ▪ Common Allergic Diseases in Companion Animals

Species	Disease	Clinical Manifestations	Diagnosis	Treatment	Potential Causative Factors
Cats	Asthma	Cough, wheeze, respiratory distress	Thoracic radiographs, airway cytology, ancillary diagnostics	Bronchodilators, steroids	Aeroallergens (presumptive)
Dogs	Canine eosinophilic bronchopneumopathy (eosinophilic bronchitis/pneumonia)	Cough, respiratory distress, nasal discharge	Thoracic radiographs, airway cytology, exclusion of known causes of eosinophilic airway inflammation	Steroids (with or without antibiotics as indicated)	Aeroallergens (?)
Cats, dogs	Atopic dermatitis	Pruritus, redness, scaling, hyperpigmentation, hair loss	Intradermal skin testing (see Figure 7-3), RAST test	Steroids, allergen avoidance, allergen-specific immunotherapy, essential fatty acids, cyclosporine, antihistamines	Molds; tree, weed, and grass pollens; animal and human dander; fabrics (wool)
Horses	Recurrent airway obstruction (heaves)	Coughing, airway obstruction, exercise intolerance	History, physical examination, airway cytology	Environmental modification, bronchodilators, steroids	Molds, stable dusts
Cattle	Hypersensitivity pneumonitis	Weight loss, coughing, granulomatous inflammation, alveolitis, interstitial fibrosis	Tracheal wash, positive serology to *Micropolyspora faeni* suggestive, lung biopsy	Corticosteroids for acutely affected or severely recurrent cases, change in management (e.g., turning cattle outside)	Dusts from moldy hay (thermophilic actinomycetes spores)

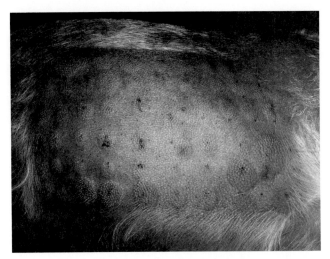

Figure 7-3 ■ Allergy skin testing in a cat. The positive reactions are well-demarcated erythematous wheals, which have the appearance of bee stings. (From Medleau L, Hnilica KA: *Small animal dermatology: a color atlas and therapeutic guide*, ed 2, St Louis, 2006, Saunders Elsevier.)

airway inflammation can be seen on lavage cytology. A positive response to a treatment trial of oral or inhaled glucocorticoids and bronchodilators is also helpful in the diagnosis of feline asthma. Unlike in human asthma, pulmonary function testing is not routinely performed in pet cats.

Canine Eosinophilic Bronchopneumopathy

Dogs are not known to develop asthma, although they do develop a syndrome more analogous to eosinophilic bronchitis in human beings that is characterized by eosinophilic airway inflammation without spontaneous airway obstruction or consistent hyperreactivity.[34] In contrast to what is seen in human beings, simultaneous bronchial and pulmonary parenchymal infiltration by eosinophils is usually present in dogs. Eosinophils and CD4+ T lymphocytes in bronchoalveolar lavage fluid support an allergic cause for this disorder. Intradermal skin testing in dogs with eosinophilic bronchopnemopathy has shown positive reactions against mites, human dander, and mixed feathers.[35]

Radiographic and bronchoalveolar lavage results support diagnosis. Thoracic radiographs show infiltrates centered around the airways and/or in the interstitium or alveolar spaces with bronchiectasis in many chronic cases. Lavage cytology demonstrates an increased eosinophil count. Other causes of airway eosinophilia (e.g., parasites) should be ruled out by blood or fecal testing or with a course of an appropriate antihelminthic.

Glucocorticoids are the mainstay of therapy of canine bronchopneumopathy. During clinical presentation, secondary infection may exacerbate disease, and a course of antibiotics based on culture results should be considered. Because it is suspected that aeroallergens may be responsible for eosinophilic bronchopnemopathy, hyposensitization/desensitization therapy based on intradermal skin testing results can be tried.[34]

Atopic Dermatitis

Dogs and cats commonly develop allergic skin disease associated with elevated IgE to a variety of indoor and outdoor environmental allergens. Along with elevations in allergen-specific IgE, other contributing factors thought to contribute to atopic dermatitis include increased susceptibility to bacterial and yeast infections (Figure 7-4), abnormal epidermal barrier function, T helper 2 cell polarity, and/or defective T-cell regulatory function.

The diagnosis of atopic dermatitis involves performing a careful clinical history and physical examination (Figure 7-5). It is necessary to exclude other disorders causing similar clinical signs, including ectoparasites, flea allergic dermatitis, adverse food reactions, and dermatophytosis. Intradermal skin testing and serum allergen-specific IgE testing are important aids to identifying specific allergens in making a diagnosis of atopic dermatitis in dogs and cats.

In dogs and cats, treatment for atopic dermatitis includes avoidance of identified allergens when possible, topical therapy (such as hypoallergenic and colloidal oatmeal–containing shampoos) to remove allergens from the skin and prevent dry skin, antiinflammatory drugs (steroids, fatty acids, cyclosporine), and allergen-specific immunotherapy.

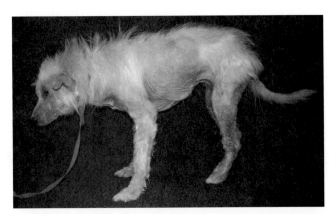

Figure 7-4 ■ Generalized alopecia in a dog secondary to atopy. (From Medleau L, Hnilica KA: *Small animal dermatology: a color atlas and therapeutic guide*, ed 2, St Louis, 2006, Saunders Elsevier.)

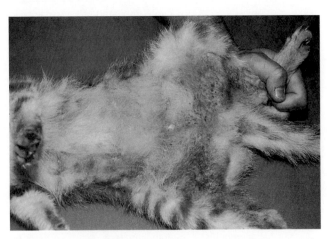

Figure 7-5 ■ Feline atopy. Alopecia and early eosinophilic plaques on the abdomen of an allergic cat. (From Medleau L, Hnilica KA: *Small animal dermatology: a color atlas and therapeutic guide*, ed 2, St Louis, 2006, Saunders Elsevier.)

Heaves in Horses

Heaves (also called *recurrent airway obstruction* and formerly called *equine chronic obstructive pulmonary disease*) appears to be a form of chronic allergic asthma or severe asthma that develops as a hypersensitivity reaction to mold and stable dusts. Unlike the case in cats and many human beings in which eosinophils are the predominant inflammatory cell, the neutrophil is the main cell type in equine heaves and eosinophils are rare.

Bovine Hypersensitivity Pneumonitis

Cattle can develop a respiratory condition that is similar to HP in human beings as a result of exposure to moldy hay. The presentation may be acute or chronic and includes cough, fever, and respiratory distress. The chronic form can involve anorexia and weight loss. Interstitial fibrosis of the lung may be found on necropsy. Treatment with steroids may lead to clinical improvement, but affected cattle can improve markedly when turned out to pasture in the spring.[36]

Resources

- National Institutes of Health, National Heart, Lung, and Blood Institute: Guidelines for the diagnosis and management of asthma (http://www.ncbi.nlm.nih.gov/bookshelf/picrender.fcgi?book=asthma&blobtype=pdf)
- Centers for Disease Control and Prevention: Asthma (http://www.cdc.gov/asthma)

References

1. Institute of Medicine. *Clearing the air: asthma and indoor air exposures.* Washington DC: National Academy Press. http://www.nap.edu/catalog.php?record_id=9610.
2. Ferguson BJ. Environmental controls of allergies. *Otolaryngol Clin North Am.* 2008;41(2):411–417, viii–ix.
3. San Miguel-Moncín MM, Pineda F, Río C, et al. Exotic pets are new allergenic sources: allergy to iguana. *J Invest Allerg Clin Immunol.* 2006;16(3):212–213.
4. Adkinson Jr NF. *Middleton's allergy: principles and practice.* 6th ed. St Louis: Mosby; 2003.
5. Elliott L, Heederik D, Marshall S, et al. Progression of self-reported symptoms in laboratory animal allergy. *J Allergy Clin Immunol.* 2005;116(1):127–132.
6. Liccardi G, Cazzola M, D'Amato M, et al. Pets and cockroaches: two increasing causes of respiratory allergy in indoor environments. Characteristics of airways sensitization and prevention strategies. *Respir Med.* 2000;94(11):1109–1118.
7. Bateman BJ, Dean TP. The Cheshire cat's grin—is cat allergy here to stay? *Clin Exp Allergy.* 1999;29(6):725–728.
8. Ramadour M, Guetat M, Guetat J, et al. Dog factor differences in Can f 1 allergen production. *Allergy.* 2005;60(8):1060–1064.
9. Arbes Jr SJ, Cohn RD, Yin M, et al. Dog allergen (Can f 1) and cat allergen (Fel d 1) in US homes: results from the National Survey of Lead and Allergens in Housing. *J Allergy Clin Immunol.* 2004;114(1):111–117.
10. Arshad SH, Tariq SM, Matthews S, et al. Sensitization to common allergens and its association with allergic disorders at age 4 years: a whole population birth cohort study. *Pediatrics.* 2001;108(2):E33.
11. Pohlabeln H, Jacobs S, Bohmann J. Exposure to pets and the risk of allergic symptoms during the first 2 years of life. *J Invest Allerg Clin Immunol.* 2007;17(5):302–308.
12. Perzanowski MS, Chew GL, Divjan A, et al. Cat ownership is a risk factor for the development of anti-cat IgE but not current wheeze at age 5 years in an inner-city cohort. *J Allergy Clin Immunol.* 2008;121(4):1047–1052.
13. Brussee JE, Smit HA, van Strien RT, et al. Allergen exposure in infancy and the development of sensitization, wheeze, and asthma at 4 years. *J Allergy Clin Immunol.* 2005;115(5):946–952.
14. Vogel K, Blümer N, Korthals M, et al. Animal shed *Bacillus licheniformis* spores possess allergy-protective as well as inflammatory properties. *J Allergy Clin Immunol.* 2008;122(2):307–312.
15. Chan-Yeung M, Becker A. Primary prevention of childhood asthma and allergic disorders. *Curr Opin Allergy Clin Immunol.* 2006;6(3):146–151.
16. Simons FE, Frew AJ, Ansotegui IJ, et al. Risk assessment in anaphylaxis: current and future approaches. *J Allergy Clin Immunol.* 2007;120 (suppl 1):S2–24.
17. Rosenstock L, Cullen MR, Redlich C, et al., eds. *Textbook of clinical occupational and environmental medicine.* 2nd ed. Philadelphia: Saunders; 2002.
18. Fenoglio CM, Reboux G, Sudre B, et al. Diagnostic value of serum precipitins to mould antigens in active hypersensitivity pneumonitis. *Eur Respir J.* 2007;29(4):706–712.
19. Langan SM, Flohr C, Williams HC. The role of furry pets in eczema: a systematic review. *Arch Dermatol.* 2007;143(12):1570–1577.
20. Plaschke P, Janson C, Balder B, et al. Adult asthmatics sensitized to cats and dogs: symptoms, severity, and bronchial hyperresponsiveness in patients with furred animals at home and patients without these animals. *Allergy.* 1999;54(8):843–850.
21. American Academy of Allergy, Asthma, and Immunology (ACAAI). Advice from your allergist…pet allergy. http://www.acaai.org/public/advice/pets.htm. Accessed August 20, 2008.
22. Morris A. ABC of allergology: aero-allergen avoidance measures—effective or futile? *Curr Allergy Clin Immunol.* 2008;21(2):101–102.
23. National Heart, Lung, and Blood Institute; National Asthma Education and Prevention Program. *Expert panel report 3: guidelines for the diagnosis and management of asthma.* http://www.nhlbi.nih.gov/guidelines/asthma/asthgdln.pdf. Accessed July 26, 2008.
24. Shirai T, Matsui T, Suzuki K, et al. Effect of pet removal on pet allergic asthma. *Chest.* 2005;127(5):1565–1571.
25. Eggleston PA. Improving indoor environments: reducing allergen exposures. *J Allergy Clin Immunol.* 2005;116(1):122–126.
26. Nageotte C, Park M, Havstad S, et al. Duration of airborne Fel d 1 reduction after cat washing. *J Allergy Clin Immunol.* 2006;118(2):521–522.
27. Alvarez-Cuesta E, Berges-Gimeno P, González-Mancebo E, et al. Sublingual immunotherapy with a standardized cat dander extract: evaluation of efficacy in a double blind placebo controlled study. *Allergy.* 2007;62(7):810–817.
28. Cox L, Cohn JR. Duration of allergen immunotherapy in respiratory allergy: when is enough, enough? *Ann Allergy Asthma Immunol.* 2007;98(5):416–426.
29. Halliwell RE. Efficacy of hyposensitization in feline allergic diseases based upon results of in vitro testing for allergen-specific immunoglobulin E. *J Am Anim Hosp Assoc.* 1997;33(3):282–288.
30. Moriello KA, Stepien RL, Henik RA, et al. Pilot study: prevalence of positive aeroallergen reactions in 10 cats with small-airway disease without concurrent skin disease. *Vet Derm.* 2007;18(2):94–100.
31. Norris Reinero CR, Decile KC, Berghaus RD, et al. An experimental model of allergic asthma in cats sensitized to house dust mite or bermuda grass allergen. *Int Arch Allergy Immunol.* 2004;135(2):117–131.
32. Prost C. Treatment of feline asthma with allergen avoidance and specific immunotherapy: experience with 20 cats. *Revue Française d'Allergologie et d'Immunologie Clinique.* 2008;48(5):409–413.
33. Corcoran BM, Foster DJ, Fuentes VL. Feline asthma syndrome: a retrospective study of the clinical presentation in 29 cats. *J Small Anim Pract.* 1995;36(11):481–488.
34. Clercx C, Peeters D. Canine eosinophilic bronchopneumopathy. *Vet Clin North Am Small Anim Pract.* 2007;37(5):917–935.
35. Clercx C, Peeters D, German AJ. An immunologic investigation of canine eosinophilic bronchopneumopathy. *J Vet Intern Med.* 2002;16(3):229–237.
36. Kahn CM, Line S. *The Merck veterinary manual.* 9th ed. Whitehouse Station, NJ: Merck; 2005.

Toxic Exposures

8

HEALTHY HOMES

Peter M. Rabinowitz and Lisa A. Conti

The concept of a "healthy home" as promoted by the U.S. Department of Housing and Urban Development (HUD) and other federal agencies involves not only aspects of the built environment (see Chapter 6), but also creating homes that are safe in terms of toxic hazards such as carbon monoxide and pesticides.[1] This concept is one in which human health care providers, public health professionals, and veterinarians can actively collaborate because it seems clear that what is good for the human beings in the household in terms of toxic hazard reduction is also good for animals living in the household.

In the early part of the twentieth century, miners in the United States and Great Britain brought caged canaries into mines to provide an early warning of the presence of deadly gases such as carbon monoxide and methane. Studies had shown that the canaries were more sensitive than other species to the effects of these gases,[2] and a canary becoming ill and falling from its perch was sufficiently recognizable to warn the miners of the hazard. In the same way, animals living in or near a household can serve as "sentinels" for human health hazards related to toxic exposures in the home and other environments. Much of what is known about the toxic properties of environmental chemicals is based on studies of laboratory animals such as rats and mice. However, pets, other domestic animals, and wildlife can provide both clinically important information to human health as well as useful "animal models" of cancer and other environmentally induced disease.[3]

At times it is the human being who first presents to medical care with a toxic syndrome that is relevant to animals in the household. Greater access to medical care and diagnostic services may result in diagnosis in the human case before related animal cases.

This chapter outlines acute poisoning and chronic toxic exposure situations for human beings and other animals and indicates certain scenarios in which a toxicant-related disease event in one species could be an indicator of risk for other species. This section provides an overview of acute and chronic toxic exposures in different species. Subsequent sections provide specific information on toxicity caused by carbon monoxide, lead, animal-related pesticides, envenomations, and harmful algae blooms (HABs).

Key Points for Clinicians and Public Health Professionals

Public Health Professionals

- Educate the public on principles for a safer, healthier home:
  - Eliminate tobacco smoking from the home.
  - Use safer substances for general cleaning (e.g., vinegar, lemon juice).
  - Store medications out of reach of children and pets.
  - Eliminate toxic substances from the home or store them out of reach of children and animals.
  - Use nontoxic plants in and around the home.
  - Use integrated pest management (IPM) techniques for rodent, weed, and insect control to reduce dependence on toxic substances. (See, for example, http://www.epa.gov/pesticides/factsheets/ipm.htm.) IPM is a commonsense and environmentally sensitive approach to pest management that uses current, comprehensive information on the life cycles of pests and their interaction with the environment.

Human Health Clinicians

- Consider toxic exposures in the differential diagnosis of both acute and chronic medical problems.
- If unusual health events are occurring in pets and/or other animals, consider whether this could be a sentinel event warning of human health risk from an environmental toxic hazard.
- An acute poisoning episode in a pet could be a warning of inappropriate access to hazardous substances and the need for steps to prevent exposures to children.
- Counsel smokers on the importance of smoking cessation to benefit their own health and the health of others in the household (including pets).

- Be aware of cultural and ritualistic use of toxic substances such as mercury, which may endanger household members and companion animals (see http://www.epa.gov/superfund/community/pdfs/merc_rep05.pdf).
- Judiciously prescribe medications and counsel patients to keep medications and other toxic hazards stored out of the reach of children and companion animals.

Veterinary Clinicians

- Consider toxic exposures in the differential diagnosis of both acute and chronic animal illness.
- If toxic exposures are identified in animal patients, consider whether human beings could also be at risk and contact public health authorities.
- An acute poisoning episode in a pet could be a warning of inappropriate access to hazardous substances and the need for steps to prevent exposures to children.
- If owners report toxic exposures diagnosed in human beings in the household, consider whether animals are also at risk.
- Judiciously prescribe medications and counsel owners to keep medications stored out of the reach of children and companion animals.
- Counsel owners not to use any medications in their animals unless prescribed by a veterinarian.
- Counsel owners about the least-toxic chemicals for pest control and the use of IPM techniques.

PRIMARY PREVENTION OF TOXIC EXPOSURE

Human health and veterinary health clinicians can recommend a number of preventive steps to their patients and clients, respectively, to reduce the risk of toxic exposures to human beings and other animals.

Pet Proofing and Child Proofing

Pets and children share the potential for accidentally ingesting toxic substances left around a house or yard. Keep toxic substances such as cleaning solutions, flea and tick preparations, other pesticides, and all medications out of reach of pets and children. Encourage smoking cessation to protect the health of the smoker and human beings and animals exposed to secondhand smoke (Figure 8-1).

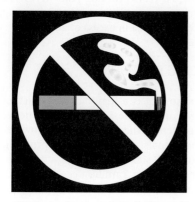

Figure 8-1 ▪ Eliminate tobacco smoke in the house. (From Centers for Disease Control and Prevention Public Health Image Library, Atlanta, Ga.)

Judiciously Prescribe Medications

Human and veterinary clinicians should weigh the relative value of prescribing medications by considering such issues as antibiotic resistance, drug interactions, entrance of pharmaceuticals into community drinking water, and assurance that drugs are taken only by the individuals for whom they are prescribed. Patient/owner education should be carefully reviewed such that judiciously prescribed medications should never be administered to other people, household pets, or other animals. In addition, over-the-counter medications should be administered only to a companion animal based on the veterinarian's treatment plan for that animal.

Substitution: "Green" Chemistry

One way to reduce the risk of acute and chronic poisoning is to consider less-toxic substitutes for many household uses. In general, keeping the residence uncluttered, food sources appropriately stored, and surfaces clean and dry will eliminate much of the need for more-toxic substances. In addition, "green" or "sustainable" chemistry encourages the design and use of products that ultimately eliminate the need for hazardous substances.

The public should use caution with herbal remedies in the belief that these substances as substitutes for conventional pharmacology. Adverse events may occur and antidotes may not be available.

ANIMALS AS SENTINELS FOR HUMAN TOXIC EXPOSURE RISK

Six years before the detection of Minamata disease, an outbreak of severe methyl mercury poisoning among families living near Minamata Harbor in Japan, strange clinical signs were seen in local cats that ate diets high in fish from the bay. This "dancing cat disease" included twitching, spasms, abnormal movements, and convulsions. Only later was the association made between the neurological signs in the cats and the devastating signs of mercury poisoning in children and adults (who also ate mercury-contaminated fish from the bay) that included mental retardation, seizures, and other neurological damage.[4]

The inappropriate use of melamine as a filler substance in pet foods has been blamed for thousands of animal deaths from renal failure.[5] Unfortunately, this scandal did not protect against the subsequent unscrupulous use of the "protein booster" in powdered baby formula in China, which led to illness and death in human infants the following year.[6]

A National Academy of Sciences panel has concluded that domestic animals and wildlife could serve as useful sentinels of human environmental health hazards because they may develop recognizable signs or biomarkers of toxicity in a timely way to provide a warning to human beings and to assist in human risk assessment.[7] Animals may function as sentinels when there are differences between animals and human beings regarding exposure, susceptibility, or latency to a particular hazard. At times, an unusual cluster of disease in an animal population may suffice to draw attention to a particular hazard. For example, when horses (and dogs) in Times Beach,

Missouri, began to die after their stable area was sprayed with oil to control dust, it was discovered that the oil was contaminated with dioxin.[8] The Times Beach incident was the largest community-wide exposure to dioxin in the United States.

Routes of Exposure

Perhaps the most likely opportunity for animals to serve as sentinels of household toxic exposures is by their greater exposure risk. Dogs are well known for their propensity to ingest a wide variety of substances, including lead-containing dusts and household cleaning agents, and therefore may be the first in a household to manifest signs. Household pets also spend more time in the home environment and thus could have a higher exposure risk to a number of substances present in the home. For example, cats and dogs may have increased exposure to dust compared with human beings because they live close to the floor level and often lick their fur during grooming (especially cats). Dust in a household may contain accumulations of chemicals, including flame retardants, lead, mercury, phthalates, and perfluorochemicals (used in nonstick cookware) and can lead to significant toxic exposures in human beings and other animals in the house. A recent study of levels of chemicals in the blood and urine of dogs and cats found levels of flame retardants in cats more than 20 times the average level in human populations, levels of mercury more than five times as high, and levels of perfluorochemicals in dogs more than double that found in the general human population.[9] These finding indicate that pets may have increased exposure to many toxicants found in household dust and fumes compared with human beings and therefore may be at risk of showing signs sooner or with greater severity.

Outdoors, dogs and cats may dig in the soil around a house or in adjacent neighborhoods, exposing themselves to lead, pesticides, arsenic, and other toxic chemicals that could be in soil. Some authorities have expressed concern that pets could then track such contaminated soil into a house on their paws and fur, potentially increasing the exposure risk for children and other inhabitants.[10] Wildlife and livestock often live continuously in outdoor environments near human beings and may be exposed to toxicants in water, air, soil, and food sources, including vegetation, at much higher levels than human beings.

Metabolic Fate/Susceptibility

Physiological differences in metabolism in some animals may make them more sensitive than human beings to certain toxicants. Canaries were found to be more sensitive than human beings to the toxic effects of carbon monoxide and methane gas in coal mines, allowing them to provide early warning to miners if they began to act sick (Figure 8-2). Dogs lack the metabolizing enzyme rhodanese and therefore may have effects of cyanide poisoning at lower doses than human beings. Birds appear to be more sensitive than human beings to inhalation of fumes from burning polytetrafluoroethylene (PTFE; Teflon [DuPont, Wilmington, Del.]).[11]

Susceptibility to acute and chronic exposure to toxicants may vary within species according to breed, sex, age, neutering status, or other differences. For example, the risk of nasal cancer in dogs (which has been linked to indoor air pollution; see below) may be higher in long-nosed dogs because of

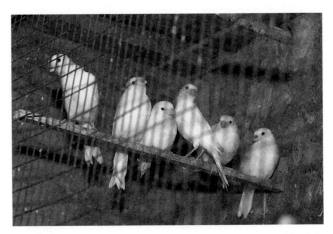

Figure 8-2 ■ Canaries are popular caged birds that are revered for their beauty and singing qualities. (From Tully TN Jr: Birds. In Mitchell MA, Tully TN Jr (eds): *Manual of exotic pet practice*, St Louis, 2008, Saunders Elsevier.)

anatomical differences that allow different degrees of contact between carcinogenic air pollutants such as polyaromatic hydrocarbons (PAHs) and the lining of their nasal passages compared with short-nosed dogs.[12] An increased risk of bladder cancer has been reported in obese female dogs; the reasons for this are not clear.[12]

An example of interspecies differences in susceptibility to toxic exposures can be seen in the list of human foods that are toxic to some companion animals (Table 8-1) and common human medications that may be highly toxic to pets at relatively low doses.

Latency

Another way in which animals may be a sentinel for human illness is if they develop signs in a shorter period of time (latency). This may be more important for chronic rather than acute toxic exposures. Most companion animals have a shorter average lifespan than human beings. Therefore chronic disease effects from environmental exposures tend to have a shorter latency. An example is the finding of mesothelioma in dogs whose owners had occupational or hobby exposure to asbestos (which resulted in secondary exposure of the household dog and other human beings in the household) (Color Plate 8-1). The average age of the dogs at time of diagnosis was 8 years (48 "dog years"), whereas mesothelioma in human asbestos exposure has a usual latency (time since asbestos exposure) in excess of 20 years.[14]

ACUTE TOXIC EXPOSURES

Accidental poisoning is a major cause of acute injury and death in the United States. The national network of poison control centers in the United States provides emergency advice to individuals and health care professionals about human poisonings (800–222–1222).[15]

Each year more than 2 million cases of acute toxic exposures are reported to regional poison control centers, and many others are treated in emergency departments without formal reporting.[16] The majority of human poisonings

Table 8-1 ▪ Partial List of Foods Toxic to Companion Animals

Food (Ingredient)	Toxic Effect in Dogs	Toxic Effect in Cats
Alcoholic beverages (ethanol)	Ataxia, respiratory depression, cardiac abnormalities, death (acute toxicity with 5-8 mL/kg; oral LD_{50} 5500 mg/kg in dogs)	Ataxia, respiratory depression, cardiac abnormalities, death (acute toxicity with 5-8 mL/kg)
Avocado (persin)	Vomiting, diarrhea	None known
Chocolate (theobromine)	Vomiting, diarrhea, tremors, seizures, death (250-500 mg/kg LD_{50} in dogs)	Vomiting, diarrhea, tremors, seizures, death (200 mg/kg LD_{50} in cats)
Coffee (all forms) (caffeine)	Vomiting, diarrhea, tremors, seizures, death (LD_{50} 140-150 mg/kg in dogs)	Vomiting, diarrhea, tremors, seizures, death (LD_{50} 100-150 mg/kg in cats)
Fatty foods	Steatorrhea, diarrhea, obesity, pancreatitis	Steatorrhea, diarrhea, obesity
Macadamia nuts	Vomiting, depression, ataxia (2.2 g/kg)[13]	None known
Moldy foods (tremorgenic mycotoxins)	Muscle tremors, seizures	Muscle tremors, seizures
Onions, onion powder, garlic, leeks, chives (propyl disulfide)[13]	Hemolysis (11 g raw onions/kg)	Hemolysis (28 g raw onion/kg)
Raisins and grapes	Acute renal failure (no apparent dose response)	None known
Yeast dough (ethanol)	Abdominal distention, ethanol toxicosis	Abdominal distention, ethanol toxicosis

LD_{50}, Median lethal dose.

Table 8-2 ▪ Top 25 Substances Involved in Human Exposures Reported to American Association of Poison Control Centers, 2006

Substance	No.	%*
Analgesics	284,906	11.9
Cosmetics/personal care products	214,780	8.9
Cleaning substances (household)	214,091	8.9
Sedative/hypnotics/ antipsychotics	141,150	5.9
Foreign bodies/toys/ miscellaneous	120,752	5.0
Cold and cough preparations	114,559	4.8
Topical preparations	108,308	4.5
Pesticides	96,811	4.0
Antidepressants	95,327	4.0
Bites and envenomations	82,133	3.4
Cardiovascular drugs	80,426	3.3
Alcohols	76,531	3.2
Antihistamines	75,070	3.1
Food products/food poisoning	66,115	2.8
Antimicrobials	66,017	2.7
Plants	64,236	2.7
Vitamins	63,331	2.6
Hormones and hormone antagonists	51,875	2.2
Gastrointestinal preparations	50,914	2.1
Hydrocarbons	49,526	2.1
Chemicals	47,557	2.0
Stimulants and street drugs	46,239	1.9
Anticonvulsants	40,476	1.7
Fumes/gases/vapors	39,586	1.6
Arts/crafts/office supplies	37,990	1.0

*Percentages are based on the total number of human exposures (2,403,539) rather than the total number of substances.
From Bronstein AC, Spyker DA, Cantilena LR Jr et al: 2006 annual report of the American Association of Poison Control Centers' National Poison Data System (NPDS), *Clin Toxicol (Phil)* 45(8):815-917, 2007.

involve young children, and the most common source of poisoning is from prescription medications. However, other common exposures include cleaning substances and pesticides. Table 8-2 shows the substances most commonly involved in human exposures reported to poison control centers.

Animals also experience acute poisoning episodes. In fact, a significant number of calls to human poison control centers involve nonhuman animals. As Table 8-3 shows, reported poisoning in dogs is much more frequent than in cats, and poisonings in other species, including livestock and wildlife, are much less likely to be reported.[11] In addition to animal reports to human poison control centers, acute poisoning episodes in animals are reported to veterinary practices and a network of animal poison control centers in the United States and other countries. The American Society for the Prevention of Cruelty to Animals (ASPCA) maintains the national Animal Poison Control Center, a 24-hour resource for practitioners managing acute toxic exposures in animals.[17] An online information system has been developed in Switzerland for the management of poisoning in large and small animals (http://www.clinitox.ch).[18] France also has a national service (http://www.vet-lyon.fr).[19]

Table 8-3 ■ Nonhuman Exposures by Animal Type Reported to American Association of Poison Control Centers

Animal	No.	%
Dog	114,599	89.3
Cat	12,002	9.4
Bird	482	0.4
Rodent/lagomorph	417	0.3
Horse	264	0.2
Sheep/goat	105	0.1
Cow	41	0
Aquatic	40	0
Other	403	0.3
Total	128,353	100

From Bronstein AC, Spyker DA, Cantilena LR Jr et al: 2006 annual report of the American Association of Poison Control Centers' National Poison Data System (NPDS), *Clin Toxicol (Phil)* 45(8):815-917, 2007.

Table 8-4 shows the distribution of substances accounting for toxic exposures in animals reported to poison control centers and veterinary practices in 2006. Chocolate ingestion, rodenticide exposure (also a hazard to children in a house), and medications (especially analgesics) account for the majority of animal poisoning reports. Animals can be exposed to pharmaceuticals from ingesting human medications that are left unsecured within a household and from inappropriate administration of human or veterinary medications by human beings. Inappropriate ingestion also accounts for much of exposure to rodenticides, pesticides (including slug bait), poisonous plants, and cleaning products.[20,21] An acute toxic poisoning in an animal can therefore be a warning sign of inappropriate access to hazardous products. This situation should alert human health and animal health care providers to take steps to avoid further pet or children's exposures.

Table 8-4 ■ Exposures of Animals to Various Toxic Agents Reported by Veterinary Clinics and Poison Control Centers

Agent	Relative Frequency (%)
Chocolate	26
Rodenticides	26
Pharmaceuticals	22
Pesticides	13
Plants	5
Miscellaneous	3
Glycols	1

Adapted from Gwaltney-Brandt SM: Epidemiology of animal poisonings. In Gupta RC (ed): *Veterinary toxicology: basic and clinical principles*, New York, 2007, Academic Press.

Clinical management of acute toxic exposures involves identification of the exposure, reduction of the exposure, administration of specific antidotes if available, and supportive care. In-depth discussion of treatment protocols for the complete range of specific chemical exposures is beyond the scope of this book, but a number of common toxic exposures found in homes are covered, in addition to those in the sections on carbon monoxide, lead poisoning, pesticides, envenomations, and HABs.

Common Medications and Their Toxicity in Human Beings and Animals

ACETAMINOPHEN

Acetaminophen, a principal component of a large number of analgesic medications, is an excellent example of differential interspecies susceptibility to toxic exposures. The drug is metabolized in the liver by uridine diphosphate (UDP)–glucuronyl transferase 1,6 to glucuronide and excreted via the kidneys. Another detoxification pathway is sulfation. Acetaminophen can also be oxidized through the cytochrome P450 (CP450) system to *N*-acetyl-*p*-benzoquinone imine, which is toxic to the liver. Cats have only one tenth of the glucuronyl transferase activity compared with dogs and are therefore highly susceptible to acetaminophen toxicity. The clinical signs of toxicity differ somewhat among human beings and dogs and cats; in human beings, the principal complication of overdose is liver toxicity, whereas in cats methemoglobinemia predominates. Both hepatocellular injury and methemoglobinemia develop in dogs.[11]

Treatment of acetaminophen poisoning is similar in human beings and other animals and involves decontamination with stomach evacuation and administration of activated charcoal to bind unabsorbed medication, as well as the use of the antidote: *N*-acetylcysteine, which prevents oxidative damage to the liver.

ASPIRIN

Aspirin (acetylsalicylic acid) is another common analgesic present in both over-the-counter and prescription analgesics. As with acetaminophen, cats are more susceptible than dogs or human beings, and fairly low doses can be fatal. The major complication of aspirin toxicity is gastrointestinal (GI) irritation and bleeding, but at higher doses it can cause metabolic acidosis and central nervous system (CNS) toxicity. Treatment involves gastric evacuation if a recent large ingestion is suspected, followed by activated charcoal, fluids, and alkalinization of urine.

NONSTEROIDAL ANTIINFLAMMATORY DRUGS

Nonsteroidal antiinflammatory drugs (NSAIDs), such as ibuprofen and naproxen, can cause GI irritation and bleeding in human beings, dogs, and cats. Dogs can be highly susceptible to the toxic effects of NSAIDs (Figure 8-3).[11] Table 8-5 lists the toxic effects in human beings and companion animals of several common analgesics.

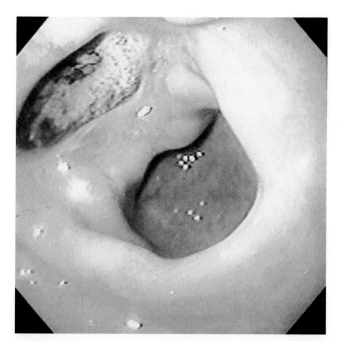

Figure 8-3 ▪ Gastric ulcer resulting from NSAID use in a dog. (From Peterson ME, Talcott PA: *Small animal toxicology*, ed 2, St Louis, 2006, Saunders Elsevier. Courtesy Dr. M. Kern.)

Other Household/Environmental Sources of Acute Toxic Exposures

ETHYLENE GLYCOL

Ethylene glycol (EG) toxicosis is relatively common in both human beings and domestic animals, especially dogs and cats. The most common source is antifreeze, which is approximately 95% EG. Its sweet taste is attractive, and EG can be found stored in many households. Exposure is usually by ingestion, although cutaneous exposure has been reported to cause toxicity in cats.[22]

Acute EG ingestion causes a toxicosis with CNS depression and gastric irritation. EG is metabolized in the liver by enzymes such as alcohol dehydrogenase to metabolites including glycoaldehyde and glyoxylate that can lead to further toxicity, including an anion gap metabolic acidosis, renal failure, and deposition of oxalic acid crystals in the kidney and other tissues.[23] Fomepizole (4-methylpyrazole) is an alcohol dehydrogenase inhibitor that is indicated for suspected or confirmed cases of EG (or methanol) toxicity in human beings.[24] It is also used in dogs. In cats, fomepizole is ineffective at the canine dosage and ethanol is used. Once renal failure develops in dogs and cats, the prognosis is poor. In contrast, the use of dialysis in human beings is one reason why renal insufficiency in EG poisoning has a relatively good prognosis.

CLEANING PRODUCTS (BLEACH, AMMONIA, OTHERS)

Cleaning products such as hypochlorite bleach and ammonia are toxic to animals and human beings through ingestion, inhalation of fumes, or skin contact. Ingestion by pets can occur through drinking from toilet bowls or other liquids treated with cleaners and can lead to GI distress, including vomiting and irritation. Respiratory exposure can result in irritation and difficulty breathing and the development or worsening of asthma symptoms. Dermal exposure leads to an irritative dermatitis. Treatment involves removal from exposure, substitution with less-irritating chemical cleaning agents, and symptomatic treatment of airway, skin, or GI irritation.

Table 8-5 ▪ Common Medications and Their Toxic Effects in Human Beings and Pets

Medication	Toxic Effect in Human Beings	Toxic Effect in Dogs	Toxic Effect in Cats	Treatment
Acetaminophen	Liver failure at high doses (acute intake of >150 mg/kg in children)	Toxic dose 100 mg/kg[22] Hepatocellular injury, methemoglobinemia, anorexia, abdominal pain, brown blood	Toxicity reported with doses of 10 mg/kg, most poisonings due to doses >50 mg/kg Methemoglobinemia at 60 mg/kg (brown blood, mucous membranes) Depression, weakness, hyperventilation, death, hepatic injury can also occur	Decontamination (emetics, gastric lavage, activated charcoal) *Antidote:* *N*-acetylcysteine
Aspirin	Potentially acute toxic dose 150 mg/kg/day[13] Anion gap Metabolic acidosis, respiratory alkalosis, GI bleeding	Gastric ulcers with doses of 75-105 mg/kg/day[11]	Doses between 100 and 110 mg/kg/day fatal[11] Depression, gastric ulceration, liver necrosis, fever, seizures, coma, death	Gastric evacuation for large recent ingestion, activated charcoal, fluids, alkalinize urine
NSAIDs	GI irritation, bleeding, renal toxicity	Dogs extremely susceptible to ibuprofen, naproxen toxicosis; toxicity with ibuprofen >5 mg/kg/day[11] Vomiting, diarrhea, nausea, abdominal pain, ulcers, anemia (see Figure 8-3)	GI irritation	Gastric evacuation for large recent ingestion, activated charcoal, fluids, H₂ blockers, sucralfate

H_2, Histamine; *NSAIDs*, nonsteroidal antiinflammtory drugs.

METALDEHYDE

Metaldehyde is a bait used to kill slugs, snails, and other garden pests. Baits in pellet form resemble dog food and are flavored with sweeteners such as molasses to attract snails. This can lead to poisoning in dogs, cats, birds, and other wildlife. Human poisoning can also occur, especially in children who accidentally ingest pellets, but such incidents are less common in human beings than in other animals. Human poisonings are usually not serious. Metaldehyde is a neurotoxin and exposure results in vomiting, tachycardia, tremors, seizures, and death.[11] Susceptibility varies slightly by species. Treatment involves removal of the agent from the GI tract, use of activated charcoal, and control of medical complications, including seizures and acidosis.

POISONOUS PLANTS

A wide variety of plants used as houseplants or in home landscaping are toxic to human beings and other animals if they are ingested. Exposures to leaves, stems, and berries of poisonous plants are a significant cause of poisoning in animals and can also pose a risk to children. Each year more than 100,000 calls to poison control centers involve plant exposures.[25] Table 8-6 shows the most common types of plant exposures involved in human poison center calls.

Most poisonous plant exposures to human beings are non–life-threatening because the quantities ingested by children are usually small. Certain plants, however, have high levels of toxins. An example is poisonous oleander (*Nerium oleander*) (Color Plate 8-2). The leaves of the oleander plant contain cardiac glycoside chemicals resembling digoxin. The toxicity of oleander in human beings and other animals resembles digoxin toxicity, with GI distress, nausea, and tachycardia and other arrhythmias. Treatment is with the digoxin-specific Fab antibody fragment.[25]

Ingestion of mushrooms and toadstools is another serious cause of plant poisonings in human beings and animals. The majority of human fatalities and serious dog poisonings as a result of mushroom poisoning involve mushrooms of the genus *Amanita* that contain *Amanita* toxin (Figure 8-4). Ingestion by human beings or animals leads to hepatocellular injury and liver and kidney failure. Puppies and children may be at increased risk. Treatment is supportive and involves gastric decontamination and activated charcoal for recent ingestion followed by management of medical complications.

RODENTICIDES

Rodenticides, used to control rats and mice around dwellings, represent another example of a potent toxic hazard to which animals are more often exposed than human beings. Rodenticides are often placed near places where rodent infestation exists but where pets and wildlife may also have access. The toxic elements in rodenticides are anticoagulants, including warfarin and related compounds, that kill rodents by causing internal bleeding. The symptoms of rodenticide ingestion are bleeding complications, including hematomas (Color Plate 8-3), GI bleeding, hematuria, anemia, and prolongation of the international normalized ratio. Treatment consists of administration of vitamin K to reverse the warfarin effect on the coagulation pathway.

Table 8-6 ■ Top 25 Poisonous Plant Exposures Reported to American Association of Poison Control Centers, 2006	
Botanical (Common) Name	**No.**
Spathiphyllum spp. (peace lily)	2133
Euphorbia pulcherrima (poinsettia)	1615
Ilex spp. (holly)	1572
Philodendron spp. (philodendron)	1514
Phytolacca americana (American pokeweed)	1358
Toxicodendron radicans (poison ivy)	1194
Schlumbergera bridgesii (Christmas cactus)	705
Ilex opaca (American holly)	608
Crassula argentea (jade plant)	604
Plants—cardiac glycosides	583
Malus spp. (crabapple)	582
Taraxacum officinale (dandelion)	581
Pepper mace	566
Epipremnum aureum (silver vine, money plant)	566
Plants—cyanogenic glycosides	555
Plants—pokeweed	543
Mold	538
Caladium spp. (elephant ear)	533
Nandina domestica	530
Narcissus pseudonarcissus (wild daffodil)	474
Spinacia oleracea (spinach)	467
Cactus (unknown type or name)	460
Rosa spp. (rose)	450
Quercus spp. (oak)	447
Hedera helix (common ivy)	446

From Bronstein AC, Spyker DA, Cantilena LR Jr et al: 2006 annual report of the American Association of Poison Control Centers' National Poison Data System (NPDS), *Clin Toxicol (Phil)* 45(8):815-917, 2007.

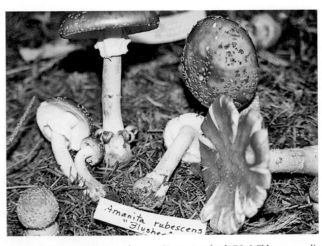

Figure 8-4 ■ *Amanita rubescens*. (From Auerbach PS: *Wilderness medicine*, ed 5, Philadelphia, 2007, Mosby Elsevier.)

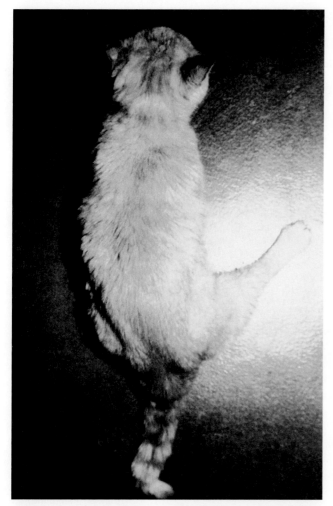

Figure 8-5 ▪ Hindlimb ataxia with decreased conscious proprioception in a cat 5 days after ingestion of bromethalin (found in rodenticides) (dose 0.45 mg/kg). (From Dorman DC: Emerging neurotoxicities. In August JR (ed): *Consultations in feline internal medicine,* vol 2, Philadelphia, 1994, WB Saunders.)

A newer rodenticide agent, bromethalin, is a neurotoxic agent that uncouples oxidative phosphorylation in the mitochondria of the CNS. Animals poisoned with bromethalin develop cerebral edema and neurological signs including ataxia and paralysis (Figure 8-5). Human cases are rare to date, but a fatality has been reported.[26] It is anticipated that treatment in human beings will be modeled after treatment in animals, including GI decontamination and treatment of cerebral edema.[26]

PTFE FUMES

Nonstick cooking pans containing PTFE (Teflon) release fumes (perfluorooctanoic acid [PFOA]) when overheated. These fumes are highly toxic to caged birds, and there are numerous reports of pulmonary hemorrhage and death. A syndrome known as *polymer fume fever* can develop in human beings exposed to fumes of burning PTFE and Teflon-containing sprays.[27,28] Flulike symptoms of fever, chills, and

cough have been reported. Treatment for inhalation of PTFE fumes is supportive.

Table 8-7 summarizes the comparative presentation and treatment of common toxic exposures in human beings and other animals. Consultation with a poison control center is recommended for serious acute poisoning exposures.

Identification of Exposure

Identification of the toxic exposure can involve checking product labels and searching online or through the distributing company for a copy of the material safety data sheet (MSDS) regarding the suspected chemical exposure (see the Resources section for Web site resources for MSDSs and other toxic hazards). During the medical evaluation of the exposure, specialized toxicologic testing may be indicated. Table 8-8 summarizes analytical toxicologic testing in animals. Similar testing can be performed in human beings.

In addition to eliminating the offending exposure and treating the patient, human health and veterinary clinicians can contact the environmental health officer in the local health department to report suspected environmental hazards to human beings or other animals.

A veterinarian who sees a pet animal with a toxic exposure that could also endanger the owner and family should consider directly contacting the human health care provider for the family to communicate this concern. Similarly, human health clinicians who identify environmental health hazards in the setting of pet ownership should counsel patients to contact their veterinarian or should contact the veterinarian directly.

CHRONIC TOXIC EXPOSURES AND HEALTH EFFECTS

Toxic exposures at levels below those associated with acute poisoning can produce long-term toxic effects in both human beings and other animals. Studies have linked certain low-dose household toxic exposures to chronic health effects in animals, suggesting that animals in a household could serve as sentinels for human beings exposed to the same substances.

Cancer

A number of studies have found associations between exposure to chemical and physical hazards and cancer in animals, especially in dogs. Table 8-9 lists some of these reported associations. Many of these associations are based on limited case-control studies or descriptive case reports and remain inconclusive. One obstacle to connecting animal cancers to environmental exposures is the existence of fewer tumor registries for domestic animals compared with human beings. Another is the lack of detailed data on environmental exposures; often data are not obtained for animals diagnosed with cancer. Much remains unknown regarding the linkages between animal risk and human risk of carcinogenesis, including reasons why the most common types and

Table 8-7 ■ Comparative Presentation and Treatment of Common Toxic Exposures in Human Beings and Other Animals

Toxic Exposure	Human Beings	Dogs	Cats	Birds[29]	Treatment*
Ethylene glycol (antifreeze)	Intoxication/ CNS depression, metabolic acidosis, oxalate crystals in urine, respiratory/ cardiac difficulty, renal failure, cerebral edema	(LD 4.4 cc/kg) *30 min-12 hr after ingestion:* polyuria, polydipsia, CNS depression, ataxia, vomiting, oxalate crystals in urine *36-72 hr after ingestion:* oliguria, lethargy, coma	(LD 1.4 cc/kg) *30 min-12 hr after ingestion:* CNS depression, ataxia, vomiting, polyuria, oxalate crystals in urine *12–24 hr after injection:* oliguria, lethargy, coma, swollen/ painful kidneys[23]	(poultry LD 7-8 cc/kg)[23] CNS depression, ataxia	Fluids, supportive care In human beings and dogs, fomepizole to inhibit ADH In cats, ethanol to inhibit ADH Dialysis effective for renal insufficiency in human beings
Household cleaners Chlorine bleach, ammonia, others	*Inhalation:* respiratory irritation (fumes): coughing, gagging, sneezing, asthma *Ingestion:* GI distress, vomiting *Dermal:* skin irritation	*Ingestion:* vomiting, hypersalivation, depression *Inhalation:* coughing, gagging, sneezing	Pulmonary irritation, retching, coughing Concentrated ammonia: seizures and death within 5 minutes[13]	Respiratory irritation, death[23]	Removal from exposure, substitution of less irritating cleaning agents, supportive care of irritation
Slug bait (metaldehyde)	Toxic level not known; most ingestions not serious Salivation, nausea, vomiting, abdominal pain, tachycardia can occur	*Immediate to 3 hr after ingestion:* Convulsions, tremors, hyperthermia, hyperpnea, vomiting, cyanosis, depression, ataxia, seizures, death LD$_{50}$ (ingestion) 100 mg/kg in dogs, 207 mg/kg cats[11]		LD$_{50}$ 500 mg/kg (chickens)	Remove from GI tract, activated charcoal; control seizures, spasms; treat acidosis
Plants	Many plants with low toxicity	Many plants toxic to animals, including lilies, azaleas, rhododendron			
Oleander (cardiac glycosides)	Dizziness, nausea, cardiac arrhythmias	Vomiting, diarrhea, cardiac toxicity (tachycardia, heart block)			GI decontamination, activated charcoal Cardiac monitoring, digoxin-specific Fab fragment
Mushrooms, toadstools (*Amanita* toxin; see Figure 8-4)	*Amanita:* Liver, kidney toxicity: vomiting, pain, jaundice				GI decontamination, activated charcoal
Rodenticides					
Warfarin and related compounds	Bleeding	Anemia, spontaneous bleeding, hematomas, melena (see Color Plate 8-3)			GI decontamination, charcoal, vitamin K
Bromethalin	Altered mental status, seizures[26]	Hindlimb ataxia (see Figure 8-5), tremors, hyperthermia, seizures, coma			GI decontamination, treatment of cerebral edema
Teflon fumes (PFOA)	Polymer fume fever (flulike symptoms)	None known		Respiratory distress, death[30]	Remove from exposure, supportive care

ADH, Antidiuretic hormone; *CNS*, central nervous system; *GI*, gastrointestinal; *LD*, lethal dose; *LD$_{50}$*, median lethal dose.
*Poison center consultation recommended.

sites of cancer may vary among species and differing biology of particular cancers across species.[12] Therefore linking the occurrence of animal cancers to either environmental exposures or human risks remains extremely difficult.

Nevertheless, considering the relationships between human and companion animal cancers may be of both clinical and scientific value. Dogs and human beings are the only animals that naturally develop lethal prostate cancers.

Breast cancer in female dogs spreads to bone, just as it does in women. The most frequent tumor in dogs, osteosarcoma, is an important tumor that affects young people. Such observations have led to the development of the field of "comparative oncology." A growing amount of research is studying similarities and differences between tumors of human beings and domestic animals, and new cancer registries for pet cancers are being established to better understand links between

Table 8-8 ▪ Samples That May Be Needed for Analytical Toxicology Testing*

Sample	Amount	Condition	Examples of Toxicoses
Antemortem			
Whole blood	1-3 mL	EDTA or heparin anticoagulant	Lead, arsenic, mercury, selenium, pesticides, anticoagulants
Urine	10-50 mL	Plastic screw-capped vial	Drugs, some metals, paraquat, alkaloids
Serum	5 mL	Remove from clot; element tubes	Trace metals (no rubber contact if testing for zinc), some drugs, ethylene glycol, electrolytes, botulinum, iohexol
Cerebrospinal fluid	1 mL	Clot tube	Sodium
GI contents	100 g	Obtain representative sample	Pesticides; plant-, metal-, and feed-related poisons
Body fluids	10-20 mL	Clot tubes	Anticoagulants
Hair	1-5 g	Rarely useful	Call laboratory; chronic selenosis
Postmortem			
Urine, serum, body fluids	1-50 mL	Same preparation and tests as for antemortem samples; get serum from heart clot	Drugs, arsenic
Liver	100 g	Plastic (foil for organics)	Pesticides, metals, botulinum
Kidney	100 g	Plastic (foil for organics)	Metals, compound 1080 (sodium monofluoroacetate), calcium, ethylene, glycol, cholecalciferol
Brain	50%	Cut sagittally; put half in plastic for analysis (fix other half for pathologic examination)	Organochlorines, sodium, bromethalin
Fat	100 g	Foil in plastic	Organochlorines
Lung	100 g	Plastic	Paraquat
Pancreas	100 g	Plastic	Metals (zinc)
GI contents	100 g	Obtain representative sample	Pesticides/baits; plant- metal-, or feed-related toxicants
Bone	100 g	One long bone	Fluoride
Miscellaneous		Injection sites, spleen	Some drugs (barbiturates in spleen)
Environmental			
Baits/sources	200 mL or g	Clean glass jar (liquid); plastic vial (write chemical name if available)	Unidentified chemicals, organics
Feed	1 kg	Plastic, box; must be representative	Mycotoxins, feed additives, plants, pesticides
Plants	Entire plant	Fresh or pressed, send all parts	Identification, chemical assay
Water	1 L	Clean mason jar; foil under lid for organics, plastic jar for metals	Metals, nitrates, pesticides, algae, salt, organics

EDTA, Ethylenediamine tetraacetic acid.
*Submit samples frozen except for blood or if very dry. Amounts given are optimum amounts; smaller samples may be accommodated (call laboratory about testing for smaller samples). Appropriate tissue samples should be fixed in formalin for histological analysis as well. Do not submit material in syringes.
Modified from Galey FD: Effective use of an analytical laboratory for toxicology problems. In Kirk RW, Bonagura JD, editors: *Current veterinary therapy, small animal practice,* vol XI, Philadelphia, 1992, WB Saunders. In Peterson ME, Talcott PA: *Small animal toxicology,* ed 2, St Louis, 2006, Saunders Elsevier.

environments and cancers.[37] Some studies have attempted to assess human environmental cancer risk by monitoring biomarkers such as lymphocyte micronucleus testing in dogs living near Environmental Protection Agency (EPA) Superfund sites to determine the extent of exposure to mixtures of chemicals that could be carcinogenic.[38]

When patients report a history of cancer in a pet, human health clinicians may wish to contact the veterinarian to determine whether a suspected environmental cause of a pet cancer exists. If there appears to be grounds for concern, the physician or veterinarian can contact the environmental health department of the local or state health department or one of the regional clinics in the Association of Occupational and Environmental Medicine Clinics (AOEC) to assess any possible human risk related to the exposures.

Table 8-9 ■ Reported Associations Between Cancer in Animals and Environmental Exposures

Species	Type of Neoplasia	Associated Environmental Exposure	Comments
Cats	Oral squamous cell carcinoma	Environmental tobacco smoke[31]	Tonsillar form is more common in urban cats than rural cats
Dogs	Bladder cancer	Pesticides	Higher risk in obese female dogs[32]
	Nasal carcinoma	Indoor coal or kerosene heaters[33]	Evidence stronger for long-nosed breeds
	Lymphoma	Lawn pesticide application,[34] electromagnetic fields[35]	Concern that such exposures cause cancer in human beings
Dogs (military)	Testicular cancer	Vietnam service	Exposed to variety of chemicals, infections, and medications during military service[36]

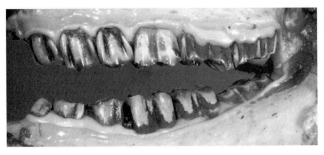

Figure 8-6   ■   Fluorosis in cheek teeth of a cow. The enamel is chalky and weak and the teeth are usually rapidly worn down. (From McGavin MD, Zachary JF: *Pathologic basis of veterinary disease*, ed 4, St Louis, 2007, Mosby Elsevier. Courtesy Dr. L. Krook, College of Veterinary Medicine, Cornell University.)

Table 8-10 ■ Noncancer Outcomes in Animals and Implicated Chronic Environmental Exposures

Species	Type of Disease	Exposure Implicated
Cat	Hyperthyroidism	Flame-retardant (PBDE) from carpet and furniture[43]
	Mercury poisoning	Fish consumption
Dog	Lung disease	Ambient air pollutants[42]
Cattle, horses, deer	Fluorosis of bones and teeth	Exposure to fluoride in pastures contaminated from nearby factories
Horses, dogs	Sudden death	Exposure to dioxin from contaminated oil used to spray roads, stables[8]
Cattle	Cadmium-induced renal disease	Cadmium in feed and pastures irrigated with sewage sludge

NONCANCER OUTCOMES

Just as with cancer, a number of other diseases in animals have been attributed to chronic exposures to toxicants, and there is evidence that animals can serve as sentinels for human beings. Recently an association has been reported between hyperthyroidism in cats and high levels of the flame retardant polybrominated diphenyl ether (PBDE) related to house dust and diet exposures.[39] This association is an example of the current scientific controversy regarding the potential of chemicals in the environment to cause alterations in endocrine function ("endocrine disruption") in animals and possibly human beings.

As previously described, cats were sentinels of methyl mercury poisoning in Minamata, Japan, and the deaths of dogs and horses provided warning of a human health risk from dioxin in oil sprayed for dust control in Times Beach, Missouri. Other examples of animals providing sentinel information about chronic toxic exposures in homes and outdoor environments include horses and deer that develop fluorosis of their bones and teeth while grazing near areas of fluoride-contaminated soil in the vicinity of aluminum smelters and other industrial sources (Figure 8-6).[40] In a similar fashion, livestock can develop signs of cadmium toxicity when grazing on cadmium-contaminated soils.[41] Dogs have been used to monitor the effects of air pollution on lungs and cardiac function.[42] Table 8-10 lists some of these reported associations between environmental toxic exposures and noncancer outcomes in animals that have potential sentinel value for human health.

WEB RESOURCES

- **National Healthy Homes Training Center and Network**
  http://www.healthyhomestraining.org/
- **Environmental Protection Agency**
  Using Toxics and Pesticides Safely: http://www.epa.gov/epahome/home.htm#safe
- **TOXNET Toxicology Data Network**
  http://toxnet.nlm.nih.gov/
- **Agency for Toxic Substances Disease Registry (ATSDR) Toxicological Profiles**
  http://www.atsdr.cdc.gov/toxpro2.html
- **The Canary Database** (animals as sentinels of human environmental health hazards)
  http://canarydatabase.org
- **Tox Town** (consumer resource for information regarding environmental health concerns and toxic chemicals)
  http://toxtown.nlm.nih.gov/index.php
- **Material Safety Data Sheets**
  Available through University of Vermont SIRI MSDS database: http://siri.org/msds/

References

1. U.S. Department of Housing and Urban Development. *Healthy Homes Initiative.* http://www.hud.gov/offices/lead/hhi/index.cfm. Accessed April 5, 2009.

2. Burrell G, Seibert F. Experiments with small animals and carbon monoxide. *J Ind Eng Chem.* 1914;6(3):241–244.

3. Bukowski JA, Wartenberg D. An alternative approach for investigating the carcinogenicity of indoor air pollution: pets as sentinels of environmental cancer risk. *Environ Health Perspect.* 1997;105(12):1312–1319.

4. Eto K, Yasutake A, Nakano A, et al. Reappraisal of the historic 1959 cat experiment in Minamata by the Chisso Factory. *Tohoku J Exp Med.* 2001;194(4):197–203.

5. Thompson ME, Lewin-Smith MR, Kalasinsky VF, et al. Characterization of melamine-containing and calcium oxalate crystals in three dogs with suspected pet food-induced nephrotoxicosis. *Vet Pathol.* 2008;45(3):417–426.

6. Lattupalli R, Yee J, Kolluru A. Nephrotoxicity of mala fide melamine: modern era milk scandal. *Scientific World Journal.* 2008;8:949–950.

7. National Research Council. *Animals as sentinels of environmental health hazards.* Washington DC: National Academies Press; 1991.

8. EPA Superfund Record of Decision. *Shenandoah Stables.* http://www.epa.gov/superfund/sites/rods/fulltext/r0790042.pdf. Accessed October 28, 2008.

9. Environmental Working Group. *Polluted pets: high levels of toxic industrial chemicals contaminate cats and dogs.* http://www.ewg.org/book/export/html/26238.

10. Ginsberg G, Toal B. *What's toxic, what's not.* New York: Berkeley Books; 2006.

11. Gupta RC. *Veterinary toxicology: basic and clinical principles.* New York: Academic Press; 2007.

12. Kelsey JL, Moore AS, Glickman LT. Epidemiologic studies of risk factors for cancer in pet dogs. *Epidemiol Rev.* 1998;20(2):204–217.

13. Peterson ME, Talcott PA. *Small animal toxicology.* 2nd ed. St Louis: Saunders Elsevier; 2006.

14. Glickman LT, Domanski LM, MacGuire TG, et al. Mesothelioma in pet dogs with exposure of their owners to asbestos. *Environ Res.* 1983;32(2):305–313.

15. American Association of Poison Control Centers. *Poison Centers Can Help.* http://www.aapcc.org/dnn/Home/tabid/36/Default.aspx. Accessed April 5, 2009.

16. Bronstein AC, Spyker DA, Cantilena Jr LR, et al. 2006 Annual report of the American Association of Poison Control Centers' National Poison Data System (NPDS). *Clin Toxicol (Phila).* 2007;45(8):815–917.

17. Khan SA, Schell MM, Trammel HL, et al. Ethylene glycol exposures managed by the ASPCA National Animal Poison Control Center from July 1995 to December 1997. *Vet Hum Toxicol.* 1999;41(6):403–406.

18. Kupper J, Hellwig B, Demuth D, et al. Computer-based information system (clinitox) for the management of poisoning in small animals [in German]. *Schweiz Archiv Tierheilkd.* 2004;146(3):127–134.

19. Burgat V, Keck G, Guerre P, et al. Glyphosate toxicosis in domestic animals: a survey from the data of the Centre National d'Informations Toxicologiques Veterinaires (CNITV). *Vet Hum Toxicol.* 1998;40(6):363–367.

20. Cope RB, White KS, More E, et al. Exposure-to-treatment interval and clinical severity in canine poisoning: a retrospective analysis at a Portland veterinary emergency center. *J Vet Pharmacol Ther.* 2006;29(3):233–236.

21. Hornfeldt CS, Murphy MJ. American Association of Poison Control Centers report on poisonings of animals, 1993–1994. *J Am Vet Med Assoc.* 1998;212(3):358–361.

22. Kahn CM, Line S. ed. *The Merck veterinary manual.* 9th ed. Whitehouse Station, NJ: Merck; 2005.

23. Ford MD, Delaney KA, Ling L, et al. *Clinical toxicology.* Philadelphia: Saunders; 2001.

24. Holstege CP, Dobmeier SG, Bechtel LK. Critical care toxicology. *Emerg Med Clin North Am.* 2008;26(3):715–739, viii–ix.

25. Froberg B, Ibrahim D, Furbee RB. Plant poisoning. *Emerg Med Clin North Am.* 2007;25(2):375–433.

26. Pasquale-Styles MA, Sochaski MA, Dorman DC, et al. Fatal bromethalin poisoning. *J Forensic Sci.* 2006;51(5):1154–1157.

27. Patel MM, Miller MA, Chomchai S. Polymer fume fever after use of a household product. *Am J Emerg Med.* 2006;24(7):880–881.

28. Son M, Maruyama E, Shindo Y, et al. Case of polymer fume fever with interstitial pneumonia caused by inhalation of polytetrafluoroethylene (Teflon) [in Japanese]. *Chudoku Kenkyu.* 2006;19(3):279–282.

29. Animal Forum. *Animal poison control center offers pet poison safety tips for bird owners.* http://www.animalforum.com/birdpoison.htm. Accessed April 5 2009.

30. Stoltz JH, Galey F, Johnson B. Sudden death in ten psittacine birds associated with the operation of a self-cleaning oven. *Vet Hum Toxicol.* 1992;34(5):420–421.

31. Snyder LA, Bertone ER, Jakowski RM, et al. P53 expression and environmental tobacco smoke exposure in feline oral squamous cell carcinoma. *Vet Pathol.* 2004;41(3):209–214.

32. Glickman LT, Raghavan M, Knapp DW, et al. Herbicide exposure and the risk of transitional cell carcinoma of the urinary bladder in Scottish Terriers. *J Am Vet Med Assoc.* 2004;224(8):1290–1297.

33. Bukowski JA, Wartenberg D, Goldschmidt M. Environmental causes for sinonasal cancers in pet dogs, and their usefulness as sentinels of indoor cancer risk. *J Toxicol Environ Health A.* 1998;54(7):579–591.

34. Hayes HM, Tarone RE, Cantor KP, et al. Case control study of canine malignant lymphoma: positive association with dog owner's use of 2,4-dichlorophenoxyacetic acid herbicides. *J Natl Cancer Inst.* 1991;83(17):1226–1231.

35. Reif JS, Lower KS, Ogilvie GK. Residential exposure to magnetic fields and risk of canine lymphoma. *Am J Epidemiol.* 1995;141(4):352–359.

36. Hayes HM, Tyrone RE, Casey HW. Excess of seminoma observed in Vietnam service U.S. military working dogs. *J Natl Cancer Inst.* 1990;82(12):1042–1046.

37. Waters DJ, Wildasin K. Cancer clues from pet dogs. *Sci Am.* 2006;295(6):94–101.

38. Backer LC, Grindem CB, Corbett WT, et al. Pet dogs as sentinels for environmental contamination. *Sci Total Environ.* 2001;274(1–3):161–169.

39. Dye JA, Venier M, Zhu L, et al. Elevated PBDE levels in pet cats: sentinels for humans? *Environ Sci Technol.* 2007;41(18):6350–6356.

40. Vikoren T, Stuve G. Fluoride exposure in cervids inhabiting areas adjacent to aluminum smelters in Norway. II. Fluorosis. *J Wildl Dis.* 1996;32(2):181–189.

41. Kessels BG, Wensing T, Wentink GH, et al. Clinical, chemical, and hematological parameters in cattle kept in a cadmium-contaminated area. *Bull Environ Contam Toxicol.* 1990;44(2):339–344.

42. Calderon-Garciduenas L, Mora-Tiscareno A, Fordham LA, et al. Canines as sentinel species for assessing chronic exposures to air pollutants: part 1. Respiratory pathology. *Toxicol Sci.* 2001;61(2):342–355.

43. American Chemical Society. Cat disease linked to flame retardants in furniture and to pet food. *ScienceDaily.* http://www.sciencedaily.com/releases/2007/08/070815122354.htm. Accessed February 3, 2009.

CARBON MONOXIDE

Peter M. Rabinowitz and Lisa A. Conti

(ICD-10 T58.0 Toxic Effect of Carbon Monoxide)

Carbon monoxide (CO) is the most common cause of poisoning-related death.[1] Each year in the United States, several thousand individuals die or are hospitalized with CO poisoning related to smoke inhalation, and more than 400 deaths each year are attributed to non–fire-related accidental CO poisoning.[2] Because the gas has no warning odor or color and the symptoms are often subtle and nonspecific, the true incidence of CO poisoning in human beings may be much higher. In fact, CO has been termed the "unnoticed poison of the twenty-first century."[3] CO is an example of a toxicant for which companion animals could provide early warning of human exposure risk. However, it is likely that just as in human beings, the diagnosis is often overlooked. The classic animal sentinel for CO poisoning is the canary. Canaries were brought into mines in the United States and Great Britain in the first half of the twentieth century to provide early warning to miners of CO and other toxic gases. Canaries were chosen after experiments on this species, as well as guinea pigs, rabbits, chickens, dogs, mice, and pigeons, revealed that either canaries or mice were most suitable, with canaries more sensitive than mice to the effects of CO.[4] Canaries developed recognizable signs of toxicosis sufficiently early to allow the miners to take preventive steps to avoid further exposure. In the home setting as well, dogs and cats may sometimes serve as sentinels. Human cases of CO poisoning have been detected because the family dog and family members were displaying signs of intoxication.[5] Additionally, the 2007 ASPCA Cat of the Year award was given to a 2-year-old domestic short-hair cat that scratched at her sleeping owner's face to arouse her and save her from death from CO intoxication.[6]

Key Points for Clinicians and Public Health Professionals

Public Health Professionals

- Educate the public on preventive measures (Box 8-1).
- Maintain heightened alertness at the onset of the winter heating season as well as after natural disasters and emergencies such as power outages, hurricanes, and earthquakes.
- Consider CO exposure in unexplained deaths of animals or human beings.
- Monitor poison control data.
- Consider adding CO intoxication as a reportable condition if it is not already.

BOX 8-1   YOU CAN PREVENT CARBON MONOXIDE EXPOSURE

- **Do** have your heating system, water heater, and any other gas, oil, or coal-burning appliances serviced by a qualified technician every year.
- **Do** install a battery-operated CO detector in your home and check or replace the battery when you change the time on your clocks each spring and fall. (Some states have passed laws requiring their installation.[7]) If the detector sounds, leave your home immediately and call 911.
- **Do** seek prompt medical attention if you suspect CO poisoning and are feeling dizzy, lightheaded, or nauseated.
- **Don't** use a generator, charcoal grill, camp stove, or other gasoline- or charcoal-burning device inside your home, basement, or garage or near a window.
- **Don't** run a car or truck inside a garage attached to your house, even if you leave the door open.
- **Don't** burn anything in a stove or fireplace that is not vented.
- **Don't** heat your house with a gas oven.

Modified from Centers for Disease Control and Prevention: *Carbon monoxide poisoning: prevention guidelines.* http://www.cdc.gov/co/guidelines.htm.

Human Health Clinicians

- Provide the national or state poison control number to patients.
- In taking a history of a patient with suspected CO poisoning, ask about abnormal signs in household pets.
- Have a high index of suspicion in the autumn when home heating units are turned on, after storms when generators are used, or when gasoline-powered appliances are used.
- Encourage CO testing of pets as well as human beings.

Veterinary Clinicians

- In taking a history about an animal with suspected CO poisoning, ask about any similar symptoms (see Table 8-11) in people living in the household.
- Consider the diagnosis in unexplained sudden deaths of pets, and alert human beings living nearby as well as health professionals responsible for their care.
- Have a high index of suspicion for the diagnosis of CO intoxication in pets after storms, at the beginning of heating season, and for pets living in an economically depressed area.
- Encourage testing of human beings and animals when intoxication is suspected.
- Provide the national or state poison control number to clients.

AGENT

CO is an odorless, colorless, nonirritating gas that is produced by the incomplete combustion of fuels. Common sources include malfunctioning and improperly vented heating furnaces, automobile exhaust, and propane-powered equipment such as forklifts, generators, space heaters, and floor polishers (Figure 8-7).[8] CO is also a component of air pollution, leading to population-wide low-level exposures. CO is slightly lighter than air, so it tends to rise through a building.

ROUTES OF EXPOSURE AND METABOLIC FATE

The primary route of CO exposure is inhalation. Levels of CO in ambient air are usually less than 10 ppm but may be higher in urban areas. The Occupational Safety and Health Administration (OSHA)-permissible exposure level for CO exposures in the workplace is 50 ppm. After a gas stove is used for cooking, nearby air levels may exceed 100 ppm.[1] CO inhaled into the lungs binds tightly to hemoglobin in red blood cells (RBCs) to form carboxyhemoglobin (COHb). This process displaces oxygen from the hemoglobin-binding sites because it binds to hemoglobin more than 200 times more avidly than oxygen.[3] This reduces the oxygen-carrying capacity of the bloodstream, causing tissue hypoxia, particularly of the heart and brain. COHb is bright red in color, which is why tissues of a CO-poisoned individual may be "cherry red." The half-life of COHb in the human bloodstream is approximately 4 to 5 hours when the person is breathing room air. However, if 100% oxygen is administered, the half-life has been reported to shorten to 47 to 80 minutes[9] and is even shorter in a hyperbaric oxygen environment.

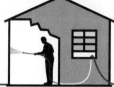

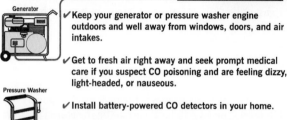

Say No to CO!

Keep generators and pressure washer engines OUTSIDE

Carbon monoxide (CO) is a poisonous gas that cannot be seen or smelled, but it can kill you or make you sick.

✔ NEVER use generators, pressure washers, or other gasoline-powered tools indoors or in a garage, carport, or basement. They all produce large amounts of CO that can build up to dangerous levels IN MINUTES.

✔ Keep your generator or pressure washer engine outdoors and well away from windows, doors, and air intakes.

✔ Get to fresh air right away and seek prompt medical care if you suspect CO poisoning and are feeling dizzy, light-headed, or nauseous.

✔ Install battery-powered CO detectors in your home.

✔ Read product directions for other important safety information.

Recommendations from the Centers for Disease Control and Prevention

Figure 8-7 ▪ CDC flyer on the proper use of generators and pressure washers. (From Centers for Disease Control and Prevention, Atlanta, Ga.

The level of COHb in the blood helps determine the degree of toxicity. Smokers may have chronically elevated levels around 7% to 12%. Normal levels in nonsmokers are generally less than 2%.[10]

GROUPS AT RISK

Individuals at high risk of CO poisoning include workers who use propane- or gasoline-powered equipment and individuals who improperly use propane- or gasoline-fired generators, space heaters, or other heating devices, including wood- and coal-burning stoves. Use of such equipment may increase in areas that have experienced natural disasters. Individuals with increased susceptibility include elderly people, individuals with cardiovascular disease, infants, and pregnant women (risk to the fetus).

Pets such as dogs may be at increased exposure risk relative to human beings because of their faster breathing rate and smaller volume of distribution. Birds have increased susceptibility relative to human beings because of their efficient gas exchange and higher mass-specific ventilation of tissues.[11] Pregnant animals and pets with underlying cardiac disease are at increased risk.

TOXICITY IN HUMAN BEINGS

CO can produce both acute and chronic effects (Figures 8-8 and 8-9).[3] Because of their high metabolic activity and oxygen demand, the brain and heart are the organs most affected by

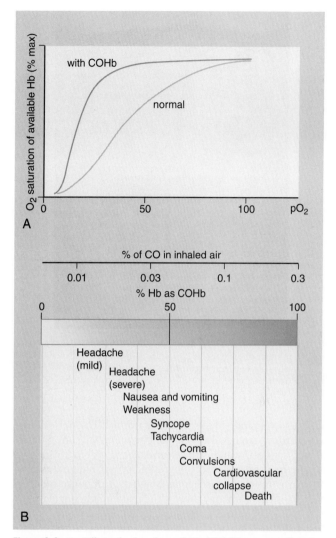

Figure 8-8 ▪ Effects of carboxyhemoglobin (COHb) on oxygen dissociation from hemoglobin *(A)*, and the symptoms associated with carbon monoxide *(CO)* poisoning *(B)*. The affinity of CO for hemoglobin *(Hb)* is 220 times higher than for oxygen, thereby decreasing the oxygen-carrying capacity of blood. In addition, COHb shifts the oxyhemoglobin–oxygen saturation curve to the left, making oxygen release during hypoxia more difficult. This is illustrated in the upper panel, which is normalized to 100% maximum. If the data were expressed as absolute oxygen content, the values in the presence of COHb would be decreased compared with normal. (From Page CP, Hoffman B, Curtis M et al: *Integrated pharmacology*, ed 3, Edinburgh, 2006, Mosby Elsevier.)

exposure. Low-level chronic exposure, as from a slowly leaking furnace, can cause headaches, fatigue, malaise, dizziness, chest pain, and abdominal pain. These nonspecific symptoms can easily be attributed to other causes, and the diagnosis may therefore be overlooked. Elevations in the COHb level to between 5% and 20% may be associated with subtle changes such as headache and behavioral changes. Chronic exposures are believed to predispose human beings to the development of cardiovascular disease and memory loss.

Acute, high-level exposure with COHb levels greater than 20% produces symptoms as described above, as well as ataxia, confusion, slurred speech, disturbances of visual or auditory function and, with increasing intoxication, eventual loss of consciousness. If exposure continues, death can result from respiratory arrest (Color Plate 8-4). The skin color of

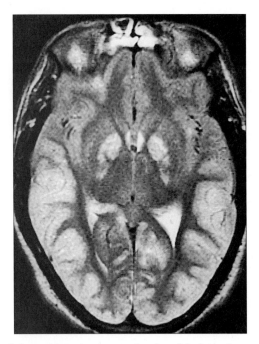

Figure 8-9 ■ Magnetic resonance imaging of the brain shows areas of infarction after carbon monoxide poisoning. This T2-weighted image shows abnormally high signal intensity in the basal ganglia, right frontal lobe, and cerebral cortex. (From Yanoff M, Duker J: *Ophthalmology*, ed 2, St Louis, 2004, Mosby.)

CO-poisoned individuals usually is normal. The pulse oximetry reading can be falsely elevated because conventional oximeters cannot distinguish between oxyhemoglobin and COHb. There may be electrocardiographic abnormalities including arrhythmias and ischemia. Magnetic resonance imaging (MRI) of the brain may show white matter high-signal intensities resulting from impaired diffusion.[3] Low-attenuation lesions in the globus pallidum have been reported.

Individuals who have recovered from acute episodes of intoxication may have long-term sequelae including chronic encephalopathy, parkinsonism, memory loss, and other signs of dementia.

TOXICITY IN ANIMALS

Dogs appear to be more resistant to COHb than human beings.[13] Acute signs include lethargy, incoordination, cherry-red mucous membranes, dyspnea, coma, and death. Tachycardia has been reported in dogs at levels of 15% COHb.[14] Chronic exposure in dogs and cats can manifest as decreased exercise tolerance and gait problems.

Birds exhibit drowsiness, difficulty breathing, weakness, ataxia, and seizures.[11] Chickens may become exposed in enclosed facilities and during transport in trucks. This can result in high mortality rates, with bright pink coloration of the viscera at necropsy.[15] Spontaneous abortion has been noted in sows that have experienced CO intoxication.[12] Table 8-11 shows key aspects of CO toxicity in human beings and other animals.

DIAGNOSIS

The cornerstone of diagnosis is the history of exposure and a COHb level. The COHb level should be measured as soon as the diagnosis is suspected because the half-life is 4 to 5 hours. A history of similar illness resembling CO intoxication in both animals and people is supportive of the diagnosis.

Measurement of air levels of CO in the area where the exposure occurred should also be done as soon as possible. Many fire departments or public health departments are able to obtain such measurements. Although CO standards have yet to be set for indoor air, the U.S. National Ambient Air Quality Standards are 9 ppm for 8 hours and 35 ppm for 1 hour for outdoor air.[18]

MANAGEMENT OF CO POISONING

Treatment in Human Beings

The principal approach to management of acute CO poisoning is to remove the patient from exposure, ensure adequate

Table 8-11 ■ Comparative Toxicity of Carbon Monoxide in Human Beings and Other Animals				
Species	**Risk Factors**	**Toxic Level**	**Clinical Manifestations**	**Diagnostic Findings**
Human beings	Inadequate ventilation when operating propane or gasoline appliances; pregnancy	COHb >10%	Lethargy, cherry-red mucous membranes, headaches, visual, auditory disturbances, confusion, ataxia, somnolence	Elevated COHb level, pulse O_2 usually normal, abnormal MRI, abnormal ECG
Dogs, cats[16]	Impaired cardiac or pulmonary function	>15% COHb	*Acute:* lethargy, incoordination, cherry-red mucous membranes, dyspnea, coma death *Chronic:* exercise intolerance, gait abnormalities	Elevated creatine kinase, whole blood COHb, blood pH lowered due to metabolic acidosis, ECG consistent with anoxia
Birds	Varying sensitivity in different species, canaries very sensitive[17]	20% COHb associated with motor impairment[11]	Drowsiness, respiratory difficulty, lethargy, seizures, sudden death	Bright pink viscera on necropsy
Pigs		Unknown	Spontaneous abortion	

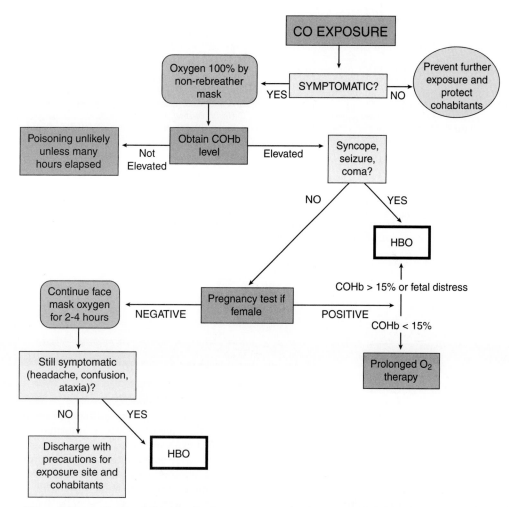

Figure 8-10 ▪ Suggested algorithm for the management of carbon monoxide poisoning. (From Ford MD, Delaney KA, Ling L et al: *Clinical toxicology*, Philadelphia, 2001, Saunders.) *HBO*, Hyperbaric oxygen.

oxygenation, and eliminate COHb from the body (Figure 8-10). All patients should receive 100% oxygen. Patients with significant symptoms (such as loss of consciousness with or without neurological deficits) levels of COHb greater than 25% and all pregnant patients are candidates for hyperbaric oxygen therapy, but hyperbaric oxygen therapy should be considered on a case-by case-basis in all patients in consultation with a bariatric medicine specialist.

Electrolytes should be monitored for the presence of lactic acidosis as a result of tissue hypoxia. Cardiac function should be monitored continuously during treatment. After the acute treatment, follow-up care should assess the impact on neuropsychiatric functioning. Follow-up MRI imaging of the brain and formal neuropsychiatric testing may be indicated.

TREATMENT IN ANIMALS

Treatment of CO poisoning in animals also depends on the COHb level and primarily involves restoration of oxygen to heart and brain tissue. Hyperbaric oxygen, when available,

promotes recovery. Treatment should also include elimination of exposure. Response to therapy should be evident within 4 hours of treatment. Physical activity should be limited for 2 weeks after exposure. After acute treatment, rehabilitation may be required for chronic neurological effects, which may become evident days to up to 6 weeks after exposure.

WEB RESOURCES

- **CDC: Carbon Monoxide Poisoning**
  http://www.cdc.gov/co/basics.htm
- **EPA: An Introduction to Indoor Air Quality: Carbon Monoxide (CO)**
  http://www.epa.gov/iaq/co.html
- **Consumer Product Safety Commission: Carbon Monoxide Detectors Can Save Lives**
  http://www.cpsc.gov/cpscpub/pubs/5010.html
- **U.S. Fire Administration (USFA): Exposing an Invisible Killer: The Dangers of Carbon Monoxide**
  http://www.usfa.dhs.gov/citizens/all_citizens/co/fswy17.shtm

References

1. Kao LW, Nanagas KA. Toxicity associated with carbon monoxide. *Clin Lab Med.* 2006;26(1):99–125.
2. Centers for Disease Control and Prevention (CDC). Carbon monoxide-related deaths, United States, 1999–2004. *MMWR.* 2007;56(50):1309–1312.
3. Prockop LD, Chichkova RI. Carbon monoxide intoxication: an updated review. *J Neurol Sci.* 262(1–2):122–130.
4. Burrell GA. *Relative effects of carbon monoxide on small animals.* United States Bureau of Mines; 1914.
5. The Boston Channel. Dog helps alert family to carbon monoxide poisoning. Viewed December 5, 2005.
6. Associated Press. *Life-saving dog, cat honored for heroic acts: pets feted by ASPCA after rescuing their masters.* http://www.msnbc.msn.com/id/21595558/. Accessed November 2, 2007.
7. Klein J. All clear: laws, codes expanding to help prevent carbon monoxide tragedies. *Occup Health Saf.* 2007;76(5):82–84.
8. Washington State Department of Labor and Industries. *Carbon monoxide.* http://www.lni.wa.gov/Safety/Topics/AtoZ/CarbonMonoxide/default.asp Accessed August 15, 2008.
9. Ford MD, Delaney KA, Ling L, et al. *Clinical toxicology.* Philadelphia: Saunders; 2001.
10. Rosenstock L, Cullen M, Brodkin C, et al. *Textbook of clinical occupational and environmental medicine.* 2nd ed. Edinburgh: Saunders; 2004.
11. Gupta RC. ed. *Veterinary toxicology: basic and clinical principles.* New York: Academic Press; 2007.
12. Pejsak Z, Zmudzki J, Wojnicki P. Abortion in sows associated with carbon monoxide intoxication. *Vet Rec.* 2008;162(13):417.
13. Penney DG. Hemodynamic response to carbon monoxide. *Environ Health Perspect.* 1988;77:121–130.
14. Farber JP, Schwartz PJ, Vanoli E, et al. Carbon monoxide and lethal arrhythmias. *Res Rep Health Eff Inst.* 1990;(36):1–17, discussion 19–27.
15. Kahn CM, Line S, eds. *The Merck veterinary manual.* 9th ed. Whitehouse Station, NJ: Merck; 2005.
16. Hipwell F. Suspected carbon monoxide poisoning in a dog. *Vet Rec.* 1995;136(11):275–276.
17. Brown RE, Brain JD, Wang N. The avian respiratory system: a unique model for studies of respiratory toxicosis and for monitoring air quality. *Environ Health Perspect.* 1997;105(2):188–200.
18. United States Environmental Protection Agency. *Carbon monoxide.* http://www.epa.gov/iaq/co.html. Accessed June 1, 2008.

LEAD

Peter M. Rabinowitz and Lisa A. Conti

(ICD-10 T56.0 Toxicity Due to Lead)

Other Names in Human Beings: Plumbism, Lead Colic

Other Names in Animals: Lead Poisoning

Lead is a common exposure in the environment. As a heavy metal, it has the ability to accumulate over time in bones and soft tissues, leading to a chronic body burden and a wide range of clinical effects in human beings and other animals. It is an example of toxicant for which there are numerous documented episodes of animals serving as sentinels providing warning of human exposure risk.

Key Points for Clinicians and Public Health Professionals

Public Health Professionals

- Ensure remediation for contaminated buildings and other sites in the health district.
- Perform follow-up investigations of cases identified in human beings and animals.
- Educate human health clinicians and veterinarians about the need to communicate about cases.
- Provide lead alerts for toys, candies, candles, and other product recalls.
- Educate human health clinicians and veterinarians about risks in the home or environment; see http://www.cdc.gov/nceh/lead/.

Human Health Clinicians

- Report cases to the health department.
- Gather medical history information about possible lead exposure risks, including older homes, dishes or glassware containing lead, and lead in toys or hobbies.
- Have a high index of suspicion in high-risk areas and with groups and individuals with occupational and environmental risk (painters, battery workers, old homes with peeling paint, etc.) and recent immigrants from countries with environmental exposure risk.
- When evaluating a suspected human case, inquire whether any animals are exposed and showing signs of illness.
- Encourage testing of pets as well as human beings.

Veterinary Health Clinicians

- Gather history information about lead exposure risks in indoor and outdoor environments.
- Have a high index of suspicion in pets that are younger than 1 year, live in an economically depressed area, or are in an old house or building that is being renovated.
- When treating an animal with lead poisoning, encourage the client to contact a health care provider to get children (and possibly adults) in the household tested.
- Contact the local health department to inform them of cases of lead poisoning diagnosed in animals.

AGENT

Lead is a toxic metal that is widely distributed in the environment. It the most common cause of heavy metal toxicity in human beings.[1] It is most commonly found in the inorganic form (Pb) but also can exist as an organic compound, such as the tetraethyl lead in leaded gasoline (phased out of use in the United States beginning in 1976 but still in use in many other countries). The most significant source of environmental exposure for children in the United States is lead-based paint. It is estimated that more than 27 million housing units built before 1950 still contain such paint.[2] Other sources in the environment include batteries; lead solder in plumbing joints; lubricating compounds; putty; tar paper; contaminated soil from paint, paint residues, or dusts, linoleum, solder, mining tailings, and industrial facility waste; and lead objects such as fishing sinkers. In households, plates, glassware, cans, and cooking vessels containing lead may contaminate food, water, and other beverages. Some folk remedies and herbal medicines may contain significant amounts of lead. Other household risks include drapery weights, stained glass, and the home use of lead for hobbies and home repair. Lead is a very stable compound and persists in the environment for a long time. It also tends to accumulate in the body of human beings or other animals, with a long half-life for elimination. As a result, even small exposures over a prolonged period can lead to significant body burdens.

ROUTES OF EXPOSURE AND METABOLIC FATE

The primary route of lead exposure in most cases is ingestion (Figure 8-11). Approximately 10% to 15% of ingested lead is absorbed from the GI tract by adults (absorption in children may be as high as 50%[1]) and is absorbed even faster in the presence of nutritional deficiencies. The second most important exposure pathway is inhalation of dust and vapors containing lead. Up to 100% of inhaled lead is taken up by the body. Dermal exposure plays a much smaller role, and inorganic lead is absorbed less through the skin than organic lead. Once lead enters the bloodstream, it binds to red blood cells. The half-life in the blood is approximately 30 to 60 days.[1] The body distributes lead among the blood, soft tissues (such as kidney and liver), and bone. Lead can pass the blood-brain barrier and affect the CNS. Once lead is taken up by bone, it remains as part of the bony matrix for many years. In growing bones, "lead lines" can be seen at the ends of long bones (Figure 8-12). Lead is eliminated from the body in the urine, but this is a slow process and, if exposure is ongoing, urinary excretion cannot keep pace with accumulation of the lead body burden.

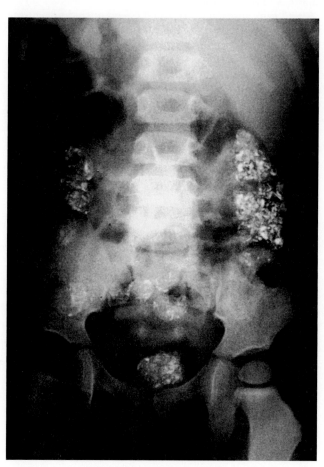

Figure 8-11 ▪ Abdominal radiograph shows lead in the intestines. (From Ford MD, Delaney KA, Ling L et al: *Clinical toxicology*, Philadelphia, 2001, Saunders.)

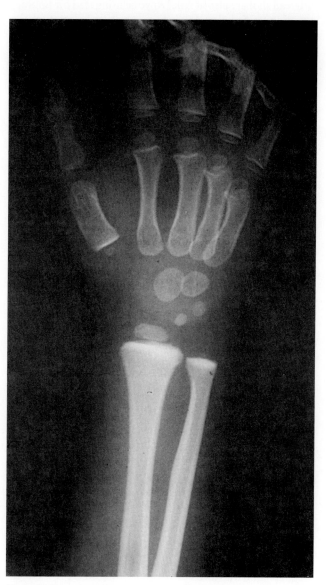

Figure 8-12 ▪ Lead lines in the distal radius. (From Ford MD, Delaney KA, Ling L et al: *Clinical toxicology*, Philadelphia, 2001, Saunders.)

GROUPS AT RISK

Among the general population, children have the highest risk of lead exposure and toxic effects of lead. It is estimated that more than 300,000 U.S. children have blood lead levels in excess of 10 mcg/dL.[3] Children living in houses with old peeling paint or dust or soil that contains lead are at risk because of their tendency to play on floors and on the ground and to ingest dirt and dust (especially if they have pica) through such activities. In addition, children are more susceptible than adults to the neurotoxic effects of lead exposure.

Among adults, certain occupations and hobbies place individuals at increased risk. Occupational hazards include sanding old paint from houses and other structures (Color Plates 8-5 and 8-6), making or recycling batteries, welding, or using solders that contain lead. Such workers can bring home lead dust on their clothes or shoes, posing a risk for other family members and family pets. Hunters who eat game with lead shot are also at risk.[4] Anyone using lead for hobbies including stained glass or the home melting of lead to make such items as fishing gear, hunting gear, or dive weights may be at risk.

Similarly, pets such as dogs may be at increased risk because of their tendency to also ingest dust and dirt around a house or yard. Dogs living in industrial areas have been found to have higher lead levels than those in rural areas.[5] Licking of contaminated fur, such as cats cleaning themselves, may be one source of ingestion of lead in dust and dirt. Lead intoxication in caged birds is well recognized.[6] Pet birds may ingest paint, lead in stained glass windows, and lead curtain weights. Pocket pets such as gerbils that gnaw on articles may also become lead poisoned.[6] Poultry living in areas of contaminated soil or old coops with lead paint can also become fatally intoxicated.[6]

There are a number of case reports of pets serving as early-warning sentinels of lead exposure risks to human beings living nearby. In one case, a dog developed persistent vomiting and weight loss 1 month after renovation of the home. After the dog was diagnosed with lead poisoning, the two young children living in the home were tested and found to have lead toxicity as well.[7] In another case, a pregnant woman was becoming overexposed to lead by removing paint from interior walls but realized this danger to herself and her fetus only after her two cats were hospitalized with lead poisoning.[8] Reported cattle deaths from lead poisoning related to contamination from mining have provided warning of the risk to children in the area.[9]

TOXICITY IN HUMAN BEINGS

Lead exposure produces toxic effects in a range of organs and a different spectrum of clinical effects in children and adults. Although acute toxicity can occur, chronic effects are more common. Importantly, many patients with lead poisoning may have nonspecific symptoms, and medical care providers can miss the condition if a careful exposure history is not taken.

In children, subclinical effects of lead neurotoxicity may occur at blood lead levels of 10 mcg/dL or lower. These effects include impaired school performance, attention problems, and aggressive behavior.[2] Therefore, although blood levels in excess of 10 mcg/dL in children are considered by the

Centers for Disease Control and Prevention (CDC) to represent overexposure, evidence suggests that the target level in children should be lowered further.[10,11] Even at higher lead levels requiring chelation therapy (see below), many children may have minor or only vague symptoms, reinforcing the importance of a high index of clinical suspicion. Rarely, children will present with extremely high lead levels and symptoms of severe toxicity, including mental confusion, weakness, abdominal pain, and vomiting and seizures.

In adults, subclinical neurological toxicity can manifest as depression, problems with memory and learning, headaches, fatigue, and abdominal discomfort. Peripheral nervous system effects include a motor neuropathy with weakness of the wrist and ankle extensor muscles. Encephalopathy and seizures can occur with severe cases of lead poisoning (blood levels generally in excess of 70 mcg/dL). A frequent toxic effect of lead is anemia, produced through a number of effects on the hematological system including impairment of hemoglobin synthesis and a destabilization of RBC membranes, thus leading to hemolysis. The toxic effect of lead on the bone marrow can result in coarse basophilic stippling of RBCs seen on the peripheral blood smear (Color Plate 8-7).

The kidney is another target of lead toxicity. In children, acute lead poisoning can lead to the development of Fanconi syndrome. In adults, chronic lead exposure can increase the risk of hyperuricemic gout, chronic lead nephropathy, renal failure, and hypertension.

Lead can cause a number of GI effects, including nausea, vomiting, constipation, and abdominal pain or "lead colic" as a result of the effects of lead on bowel smooth muscle.

At high exposure levels, lead may deposit along the gums producing a "lead line." Other reported manifestations of toxicity include infertility caused by the effects on sperm counts and the risk of spontaneous abortion, hearing loss, and thyroid dysfunction.

In children, lead toxicity may affect school performance and behavior. Acute significant toxicity can present with abdominal pain, irritability, and muscle cramps. Pregnant women can pass lead to their developing fetus, increasing the risks for premature birth, low birth weight, and neurological damage. After birth, lead can be passed from the mother to her newborn in breast milk.

TOXICITY IN ANIMALS

As in human beings, lead exposure can produce both acute and chronic signs, some of which may be nonspecific and easily missed by veterinarians. Companion animals such as cats and dogs can exhibit anorexia, abdominal discomfort, nausea and vomiting, seizures, and blindness. Cats can also manifest vestibular signs.

Large animals can develop lead poisoning; horses may be more sensitive than cattle. These animals can develop laryngeal paralysis, colic, abnormal bellowing, and seizures (Figure 8-13).[12]

In birds, signs can include emaciation, anorexia, tremors and leg weakness, loss of vision, wing drooping, reproductive failure, and death. Anemia and renal dysfunction may occur. Such signs can be seen in caged birds and wild and domestic waterfowl that ingest lead in fishing sinkers and lead shot from hunting.

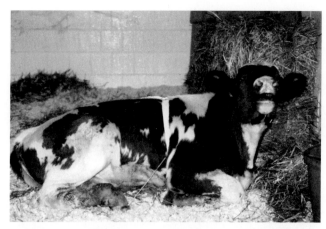

Figure 8-13 ▪ Lead poisoning causing recumbency, blindness, and bellowing. This 16-month-old heifer also showed uncontrolled, jerky movements. (From Divers TJ, Peek SF: *Rebhun's diseases of dairy cattle*, ed 2, St. Louis, 2008, Saunders Elsevier.)

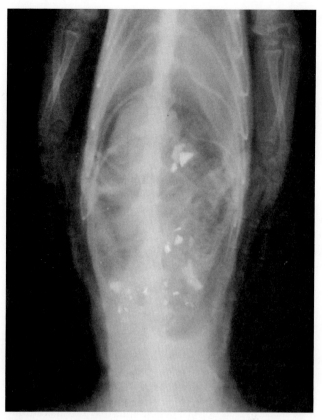

Figure 8-14 ▪ Radiograph shows metallic densities in a green iguana (*Iguana iguana*) with lead poisoning. Blood lead levels were measured at 600 mcg/dL The source of lead was never determined. (From Mader DR: *Reptile medicine and surgery*, ed 2, St Louis, 2006, Saunders Elsevier.)

Reported cases of lead poisoning in reptiles are rare, but captive iguanas have been found to have toxic levels of lead (Figure 8-14). Wild snapping turtles that ingested lead sinkers have been observed to have weakness, difficulty walking, and CNS dysfunction.[13] Table 8-12 shows the comparative clinical presentations of lead toxicity in human beings and other animals.

Table 8-12 ▪ Comparative Toxicity of Lead in Human Beings and Other Animals

Species	Risk Factors	Toxic Level	Clinical Manifestations	Laboratory Findings
Human beings	*Children:* lead paint (in U.S. houses built before 1950), soil, lead objects, water *Adults:* lead paint, water, occupational or hobby exposure, folk medicines	25-40 mcg/dL (adults) 10 mcg/dL or below (children)	*Children:* learning problems, confusion, seizures, renal dysfunction *Adults:* lethargy, depression, abdominal pain, anorexia, CNS effects, weakness, renal toxicity	Elevated blood lead level, ZPP, anemia, basophilic stippling of RBCs, abnormal liver and renal function tests, "lead lines" in radiographs of long bones, elevated bone lead by x-ray fluorescence
Dogs, cats	Exposure to old paint in buildings or soil	>40 mcg/dL	Anorexia, colic, emesis, diarrhea, constipation, CNS depression or excitation, ataxia, nystagmus, convulsions[14,15]	Basophilic stippling of RBCs, nucleated RBCs, hepatocyte intranuclear inclusion bodies, abnormal liver function tests (elevated AST and ALT), elevated blood lead levels
Birds	*Caged:* lead around windows, curtains, pet toys *Wild:* ingestion of lead sinkers, lead shot by waterfowl	Varies with species: 20-40 mcg/dL	Regurgitation, depression, weakness, excitability, seizures, wasting, death	Hemoglobinuria, anemia, elevated liver and kidney function tests
Cattle, horses	Forage contaminated with lead from agriculture, calves at increased risk, ingestion of lead from batteries or shot in soil	35 ppm	Anorexia, colic, constipation, ataxia, muscle tremors, convulsions	Anemia, basophilic stippling of RBCs
Reptiles	Lead fishing sinkers, other lead ingestion	Insufficient evidence	Abnormal behavior, weakness, gait difficulties	Elevated blood lead level

ALT, Alanine aminotransferase; *AST,* aspartate aminotransferase; *CNS,* central nervous system; *PPM,* parts per million; *RBCs,* red blood cells; *ZPP,* zinc protoporphyrin.

DIAGNOSIS

The cornerstone of diagnosis of lead poisoning in human beings and other animals is obtaining an accurate exposure history and documenting elevated blood lead levels. The two principal tests are the venous lead level and the zinc protoporphyrin (ZPP) level. The ZPP level is a measure of the impact of lead on RBC synthesis and reflects exposures over a period of several months. Therefore the finding of an elevated level of venous lead but a normal ZPP test result suggests acute rather than chronic exposure. Normal values of ZPP are usually below 35 mcg/dL. Other conditions that elevate ZPP levels are iron deficiency anemia and hereditary porphyria. Urine lead is sometimes measured but is considered to be variable and does not accurately reflect the body lead burden. Similarly, analysis of lead in hair and nails is considered unreliable.

For individuals with long-term exposure, it is sometimes useful to assess the body lead burden. Chelation challenge with ethylenediamine tetraacetic acid (EDTA) is the most common method. This test measures the urinary excretion of lead after administration of the chelating agent EDTA. EDTA challenge appears especially useful for assessing the burden of lead in soft tissues.

Another method to assess body lead burden is K-shell x-ray fluorescence (XRF) measurement of lead in bone. This test is not widely available. In birds and other animals that have ingested lead objects, radiographs may reveal accumulation of lead in the digestive system. However, many birds and wild animals have lead toxicosis without radiographically visible metallic objects.

MANAGEMENT OF LEAD TOXICITY

Treatment in Human Beings

The fundamentals of management of lead poisoning in human beings are elimination of further exposure, removal of any metallic lead from the GI tract, and chelation therapy, which is generally reserved for children and acute severe toxicity in adults.

Removing an individual from exposure allows the body to slowly eliminate the body's accumulation of lead through the urine over time. It is therefore imperative to identify and eliminate exposure sources by removal of the individual from the environment and/or environmental decontamination. Even if the source of exposure is clear, a complete history should be obtained to rule out other concurrent exposures (Box 8-2).

The health department should be contacted for assistance in identifying and eliminating the exposure. Table 8-13 provides guidelines for ongoing management of lead poisoning in human beings based on the venous lead level and the clinical status of the patient.

Chelation is never a substitute for aggressive environmental intervention to eliminate all further exposure. Chelation should not be given if there is persistent lead exposure or residual lead in the GI tract. In addition, periodic monitoring is necessary to ensure that blood lead levels are declining. Table 8-14 lists guidelines for chelation therapy in human beings and animals.

For high-level exposure and/or significant symptoms, treatment with a chelating agent may be indicated. Possible indications for chelation in adults include blood lead level

---

> **BOX 8-2   QUESTIONS FOR THE MEDICAL HISTORY REGARDING LEAD EXPOSURE RISKS**
>
> The following are some issues a physician might discuss with the patient and/or family:
> - Condition of household pets
> - Drinking water source and type of pipes
> - Family history, including possibility of maternal/family exposure and potential use of unusual medicines or home remedies
> - Hobbies of all family members
> - Home-remodeling activities
> - Location, age, physical condition of current residence, school, and day-care center, and so on (to identify potential for lead paint, as well as proximity to industrial facilities, hazardous waste sites, and other potential lead sources)
> - Nutritional status
> - Occupational history of all home occupants
> - Past living conditions (international background is important)
> - Siblings or playmates in whom a diagnosis of lead poisoning has been made
> - Use of imported or glazed ceramics

From Agency for Toxic Substances and Disease Registry: *Lead toxicity: how should patients exposed to lead be evaluated?* http://www.atsdr.cdc.gov/csem/lead/pbpatient_evaluation2.html. Accessed February 15, 2008.

Table 8-13 ■ Guidance for Treatment Actions According to Blood Lead Level

Blood Lead Level (BLL) (mcg/dL)	Treatment Actions
10-19	Provide lead education and referrals Provide diagnostic testing within 3 months and follow-up testing within 2 to 3 months Proceed according to guidelines in 20-44 mcg/dL range if BLLs persist in 15-19 mcg/dL range (The presence of a large proportion of children in the 10-14 mcg/dL range should trigger community-wide lead poisoning prevention)
20-44	Provide lead education and referrals Provide coordination of care (case management) Perform clinical evaluation and management Provide diagnostic testing (from within 1 month to within 1 week) and follow-up testing (every 1 to 2 months) Perform aggressive environmental intervention
45-69	Provide lead education and referrals Provide coordination of care (case management) *within 48 hr* Perform clinical evaluation and management *within 48 hr* Provide diagnostic testing *within 24-48 hr* and follow-up testing (in accordance with chelation therapy, at least once a month) Perform aggressive environmental intervention Provide appropriate chelation therapy
≥70 (or in case of encephalopathy)	*This is a medical emergency* Perform diagnostic testing immediately as an emergency lab test Hospitalize and begin immediate chelation therapy Begin other activities as above

BLL, Blood lead level.
From Agency for Toxic Substances and Disease Registry: *Lead toxicity: how should patients exposed to lead be treated and managed?* http://www.atsdr.cdc.gov/csem/lead/pbmanage_therapy2.html. Accessed March 2, 2008.

greater than 70 mcg/dL, ongoing hemolysis, and encephalopathy. In children, oral chelation with dimercaptosuccinic acid (DMSA) is indicated for blood levels in excess of 45 mcg/dL. For extremely high lead levels, intravenous chelation with CaNa2EDTA is recommended.[2] Na$_2$EDTA (disodium ethylenediamine tetraacetic acid or edetate disodium) should *not* be used for chelation in children because it can cause fatal hypocalcemia.[17] Other risks of chelation include worsening of lead toxicity and hepatic effects of DMSA. Before initiating chelation therapy, consultation with a regional poison center or pediatric or adult toxicology unit should be obtained.

Treatment in Animals

Treatment in animals depends on the blood lead level. Treatment must involve elimination of exposure. Lead objects in the GI tract should be removed and, in a haired animal such as a dog or cat, it is necessary to remove possible lead contamination from the coat. Cathartics such as magnesium sulfate (400 mg/kg orally) can remove lead from the GI tract if acute ingestion is suspected in cattle.[6] Balanced electrolyte solutions to replace hydration deficit, gastric lavage, and seizure control may be necessary. Chelation therapy should be considered for severe animal toxicity cases.

WEB RESOURCES

- **CDC: Lead Poisoning Prevention Program**
  http://www.cdc.gov/nceh/lead/
- **EPA: Lead Awareness Program**
  http://www.epa.gov/opptintr/lead/index.html
- **HUD: Office of Healthy Homes and Lead Hazard Control**
  http://www.hud.gov/offices/lead/

References

1. Ford MD, Delaney KA, Ling L, et al. *Clinical toxicology*. Philadelphia: Saunders; 2001.
2. Moline JM, Landrigan PJ. Lead. In: Rosenstock L, Cullen MR, Brodkin CA, et al., eds. *Textbook of clinical and occupational environmental medicine*. 2nd ed. Edinburgh: Saunders; 2005.
3. Centers for Disease Control and Prevention. *Lead: topic home*. http://www.cdc.gov/lead/. Accessed December 12, 2008.
4. Guitart R, Serratosa J, Thomas VG. Lead-poisoned wildfowl in Spain: a significant threat for human consumers. *Int J Environ Health Res.* 2002;12(4):301–309.
5. Ghisleni G, Spagnolo V, Roccabianca P, et al. Blood lead levels, clinicopathological findings and erythrocyte metabolism in dogs from different habitats. *Vet Hum Toxicol.* 2004;46(2):57–61.
6. Kahn CM, Line S. *The Merck veterinary manual*. 9th ed. Whitehouse Station, NJ: Merck; 2005.
7. Dowsett R, Shannon M. Childhood plumbism identified after lead poisoning in household pets. *N Engl J Med.* 1994;331(24):1661–1662.
8. Doumouchtsis SK, Martin NS, Robins JB. Veterinary diagnosis of lead poisoning in pregnancy. *BMJ.* 2006;333(7582):1302–1303.
9. Feely E, Garavan C, Kelleher K. Dead cattle, lead and child health. *Ir Med J.* 2003;96(8):232–234.
10. Agency for Toxic Substances and Disease Registry. *Lead toxicity: what are the physiological effects of lead exposure?* http://www.atsdr.cdc.gov/csem/lead/pbphysiologic_effects2.html. Accessed February 15, 2008.
11. Centers for Disease Control and Prevention. *Preventing lead poisoning in young children*. http://www.cdc.gov/nceh/lead/publications/PrevLeadPoisoning.pdf. Accessed December 12, 2008.
12. Gupta RC, ed. *Veterinary toxicology: basic and clinical principles*. New York: Academic Press; 2007.

Table 8-14 ▪ Chelation Guidelines for Lead Toxicity in Human Beings and Other Animals

Species	Blood Level or Signs	Primary	Alternative
Adult human beings	Consider chelation for markedly elevated blood lead level (>80 mcg/dL)[1], ongoing hemolysis, encephalopathy	Succimer (DMSA) 10 to 30 mg/kg/day for 5 days	Ca-EDTA chelation
Children	>45 mcg/dL (see Table 8-12)	Succimer (DMSA) safety and effectiveness in pediatric patients younger than 12 months have not been established *Dose:* 10 mg/kg or 350 mg/m² q8h for 5 days, then 10 mg/kg or 350 mg/m² q12h for 14 days	
Dogs	>40 mcg/dL or >20 mcg/dL with evidence of clinical signs and exposure	Ca-EDTA 25 mg/kg diluted in D$_5$W q6h for 5 days *Or* succimer 10 mg/kg PO tid × 10 days[16]	D-Penicillamine 10-15 mg/kg PO q12h × 2 weeks (do not give if there is lead in the GI tract)
Cats		Ca-EDTA 25 mg/kg diluted in D$_5$W SC, IM, IV q6h for 5 days	
Cattle		Ca-EDTA 110 mg/kg/day IV/SC divided and diluted in D$_5$W bid × 3 days, repeat after 2 days,[6] thiamine 2-4 mg/kg/day SC	
Birds		Ca-EDTA 30-50 mg/kg diluted in D$_5$W IM or SQ, bid, or tid 5-7 days After a 5- to 7-day rest, repeat treatment may be warranted[6]	D-Penicillamine 30-50 mg/kg bid

D$_5$W, 5% dextrose in water.

13. Wellehan JFX, Gunkel CI. Emergent diseases in reptiles. *Seminars in Avian and Exotic Pet Medicine.* 2004;13(3):160–174.
14. De Francisco N, Ruiz Troya JD, Agüera EI. Lead and lead toxicity in domestic and free living birds. *Avian Pathol.* 2003;32(1):3–13.
15. Knight TE, Kumar MS. Lead toxicosis in cats—a review. *J Feline Med Surg.* 2003;5(5):249–255.

16. Ramsey DT, Casteel SW, Faggella AM, et al. Use of orally administered succimer (meso-2,3-dimercaptosuccinic acid) for treatment of lead poisoning in dogs. *J Am Vet Med Assoc.* 1996;208(3):371–375.
17. Brown MJ, Willis T, Omalu B, et al. Deaths resulting from hypocalcemia after administration of edetate disodium: 2003–2005. *Pediatrics.* 2006;118(2):e534–e536.

PESTICIDES

Lisa A. Conti and Peter M. Rabinowitz

> ### Pesticides (ICD-10: T60.0 Toxic Effect of Organophosphate and Carbamate Insecticides; T60.2 Toxic Effect of Other Insecticides; T60.8 Toxic Effect of Other Pesticides; T60.9 Toxic Effect of Pesticide, Unspecified)

Pesticides are chemicals, biologicals, antimicrobials, or disinfectants used to control insects, weeds, mollusks, mammals, fish, birds, nematodes, plant pathogens, and microbes. Historically, pesticides have been a common cause of poisoning in human beings and other animals. In recent years the number of serious poisonings reported to U.S. poison control centers appears to be declining,[1] related in part to phasing out of several toxic organophosphate insecticides (including chlorpyrifos) for residential use and an increased interest in using "green" products. Yet pesticide poisoning remains an important clinical problem in the United States and worldwide. Although pesticides are usually developed and marketed for specific purposes, their toxic effects may cross many species. In addition, trace amounts may find their way into drinking water with as yet unknown effects from chronic exposure. Differences in toxicokinetics (and toxicodynamics) between human beings and other animals can result in differential susceptibility (a pesticide may be more or less toxic, depending on the species that has been exposed).

This section focuses on toxic hazards associated with animal-related pesticides. Some of the zoonotic diseases discussed in this book are controlled through the use of pesticides applied directly to animals or their bedding or by the use of insect repellents applied to human skin or clothing. Such uses can involve a risk of toxicity to both human beings and animals. In recent years the U.S. EPA has taken steps to phase out of commercial use a number of pet-related pesticides, especially organophosphate compounds such as chlorpyrifos, because of concerns about the short- and long-term health effects in human beings and other animals (Figure 8-15). Other groups, such as the Humane Society of the United States, have recommended that newer, apparently less-toxic pesticides be used for animal care.[2] Perhaps in part as a result of such actions, in 2006 fewer than 200 human exposures to veterinary insect repellents were reported to U.S. poison control centers.[3] In addition, animals may become sickened through inappropriate use of a human insect repellent on a pet, although this appears to be a rare occurrence.

Although there are several major classes of pesticides (and some of the newer pesticides are in entirely new chemical classes) with markedly different chemical composition and

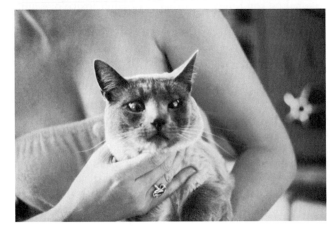

Figure 8-15 ■ An ideal flea and tick control is one that is specific to target the organism and safe for nontarget species such as human beings and companion animals. (From Centers for Disease Control and Prevention Public Health Image Library, Atlanta, Ga.)

spectra of toxic effects, many commercial formulations contain mixtures of different compounds, resulting in complex clinical syndromes. In addition, symptoms of pesticide toxicity are often nonspecific, and it is likely that many cases of mild toxicity are never reported.

Key Points for Clinicians and Public Health Professionals

Public Health Professionals

- Ensure that local animal care facilities and exterminators are using only approved pesticides for flea and tick control and are storing and using them with strict adherence to the product labeling instructions.
- Educate human health clinicians to communicate about cases and veterinarians to contact public health if there is a possibility of human exposure from these products.
- Educate the public about the judicious use of products. See "Using Pesticides Safely" (http://www.epa.gov/opp00001/health/safely.htm), which includes links to documents on protecting pets, children, and so forth with an emphasis on the importance of compliance with labeling instructions for pesticide products in human beings and other animals.
  - Always store pesticides and other household chemicals away from children and animals.
  - Read the label.
  - Before applying pesticides or other household chemicals remove children, pets, and toys from the area.

- ◦ Never transfer pesticides to another container.
- Report incidents to the EPA via the National Pesticide Information Center; see http://oregonstate.edu/npmmp/contact.php (general information: http://npic.orst.edu/).

Human Health Clinicians

- Encourage the use of cleanliness and sanitation around the home in lieu of the use of pesticides. Integrated pest management emphasizes using a combination of approaches toward taking care of pest problems (not just using pesticides). See http://www.epa.gov/opp00001/factsheets/ipm.htm.
- For patients who own pets or farm animals, inquire about pesticide use practices and storage and counsel about symptoms of toxicity.
- Have a high index of suspicion in persons occupationally exposed or otherwise exposed to pet pesticides.
- Counsel pet owners not to use *N,N*-diethyl-meta-toluamide (DEET)-containing products on pets.
- Report incidents to state or local public health officials and the EPA via the National Pesticide Information Center; see http://oregonstate.edu/npmmp/contact.php (for general information, see http://npic.orst.edu/). The EPA's *Recognition and Management of Pesticide Poisonings* is a good resource for information about the clinical toxicology of pesticides and is available online at http://npic.orst.edu/rmpp.htm.

Veterinary Clinicians

- Encourage pet owners to use appropriate alternatives to pesticides or lower toxicity pesticides to control fleas and ticks and to keep cats indoors.
- Discourage the use of organophosphate or carbamate pesticides for animals.
- Ensure that veterinary workers applying flea or mite dips and other treatments are adequately protected and trained in the proper handling and storage of these products. Consider use of less-toxic compounds for such purposes.
- Report incidents to the EPA via the National Pesticide Information Center; see http://oregonstate.edu/npmmp/contact.php (general information: http://npic.orst.edu/).

INSECT REPELLENTS USED ON HUMAN BEINGS

Table 8-15 lists agents for prevention of insect bites for human beings (Figures 8-16 and 8-17). The EPA reviews the use of particular compounds as insect repellents.[4] Most of these repellents do not work on lice or fleas (Figure 8-18).

DEET

DEET was developed for use by the U.S. Army in 1946 and approved for use by the general public in 1957. It is one of the insect repellents judged by the EPA to provide longer-lasting protection than some others. It is considered safe for use by both adults and children 2 years and older when used as directed (Figure 8-19). Each year, approximately one third

of the U.S. population uses some quantity of DEET.[5] In 2006, more than 8000 exposures to DEET were reported to U.S. poison control centers.[3] Although residues of DEET have been identified in environmental water samples, the impact on the ecosystem is considered to be minimal.[8] The EPA recommendations for safe use of DEET products are listed in Box 8-3.

Picaridin

Picaridin (2-(2-hydroxyethyl)-1-piperidinecarboxylic acid 1-methylpropyl ester) was registered as an insect repellent with the EPA in 2001 and is thus a much newer agent than DEET. It is believed to have comparable efficacy, have very low toxicity, and be safe for human use as directed.[9] Advantages over DEET include the fact that it is odorless, less greasy, and does not damage clothing.

Pyrethroids/Permethrin

Permethrin is a synthetic chemical compound, along with other pyrethroids, similar to that produced by pyrethrum flowers (*Chrysanthemum cinerariifolium* and *C. coccineum*). These chemicals are poorly absorbed by the skin but can cause hypersensitivity reactions. These chemicals are neurotoxic to insects by maintaining patency in sodium channels in neuronal membranes.

Oil of Lemon Eucalyptus

Oil of lemon eucalyptus is a plant-based repellent that the CDC considers to be an alternative to DEET as an insect repellent. The active ingredient is *p*-methane 3,8-diol (PMD). The mechanism of action is unclear, and aside from eye irritation no significant toxicity has been reported.[7] However, according to the product labeling, products containing oil of lemon eucalyptus *should not be used on children younger than 3 years.*[10]

Other products are being developed with regard to safety and efficacy.[11,12]

PESTICIDES USED ON ANIMALS

In addition to being nuisances, fleas, ticks, and mosquitoes are carriers of disease agents such as plague (fleas), Rocky Mountain spotted fever (ticks; Figure 8-20), and arboviral disease (mosquitoes). Table 8-16 provides information about the pesticides used on companion animals to control these arthropods.

Pesticides With Low Relative Mammalian Toxicity

Fipronil is an *N*-phenylpyrazole compound that was introduced in 1996. When applied to a dog or cat, it spreads over the skin and accumulates in sweat glands, where it is slowly released over time. Skin absorption is thought to be minimal. It acts by blocking gamma-aminobutyric acid (GABA) receptors in insects, disrupting nervous system function. It appears to have less affinity for mammalian

Table 8-15 ■ Agents for Prevention of Insect Bites for Human Beings

Compound	Use	Insects	Comment
DEET (e.g., Off, Cutter, Repel, many other products, some combined with sunscreen)[5]	Apply to clothing or exposed skin NOTE: DEET (along with the other repellents) should not be applied under clothing (on unexposed areas); applying underneath clothing can increase the extent of absorption and is more likely to result in irritant reactions	Flies, mosquitoes, ticks	Combined sunscreen/DEET products not recommended[6,7] DEET products should not be used on animals Not to be used on children <2 years
Picaridin (e.g., Cutter Advanced)	Apply to clothing and skin	Biting flies, mosquitoes, chiggers, ticks, fleas	
Pyrethroids/permethrin	Apply to clothing and gear but not skin	Mosquitoes, ticks, other arthropods	
Oil of lemon eucalyptus (e.g., Repel Lemon Eucalyptus Insect Repellent)	Apply to skin and clothing	Mosquitoes, ticks (not yet studied in malaria mosquitoes)	Not to be used in children younger than 3 years old

DEET, *N,N*-diethyl-m-toluamide.

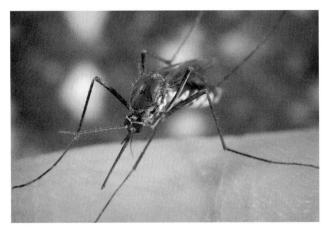

Figure 8-16 ■ Mosquito about to take a blood meal. (From Centers for Disease Control and Prevention Public Health Image Library, Atlanta, Ga. Courtesy James D. Gathany.)

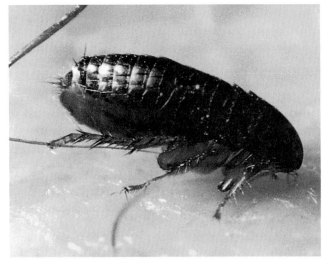

Figure 8-18 ■ Flea. Thin wingless insects with very hard bodies and large hind legs adapted for jumping. (From Habif TP: *Clinical dermatology: a color guide to diagnosis and therapy*, ed 4, St Louis, 2004, Mosby. Courtesy Ken Gray, Oregon State University Extension Services.)

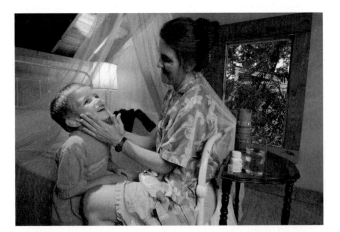

Figure 8-17 ■ A mother applying mosquito repellent to her child's skin to prevent mosquitoes from biting, thereby, preventing many arboviral infections such as West Nile virus. (From Centers for Disease Control and Prevention Public Health Image Library, Atlanta, Ga. Courtesy James D. Gathany.)

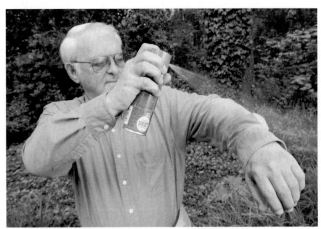

Figure 8-19 ■ Applying DEET repellent to clothing. (From Centers for Disease Control and Prevention Public Health Image Library, Atlanta, Ga. Courtesy James D. Gathany.)

EPA GUIDELINES FOR SAFE USE OF DEET-CONTAINING PRODUCTS

Consumers can reduce their own risks when using DEET by reading and following product labels. All DEET product labels include the following directions:

- Read and follow all directions and precautions on the product label.
- Do not apply over cuts, wounds, or irritated skin.
- Do not apply to hands or near eyes and mouth of young children.
- Do not allow young children to apply this product.
- Use just enough repellent to cover exposed skin and/or clothing.
- Do not use under clothing.
- Avoid overapplication of this product.
- After returning indoors, wash treated skin with soap and water.
- Wash treated clothing before wearing it again.
- Use of this product may cause skin reactions in rare cases. The following additional statements appear on the labels of all aerosol and pump spray formulation labels:
- Do not spray in enclosed areas.
- To apply to face, spray on hands first and then rub on face. Do not spray directly onto face.

From Environmental Protection Agency: *The insect repellent DEET.* http://www.epa.gov/pesticides/factsheets/chemicals/deet.htm. Accessed April 14, 2008.

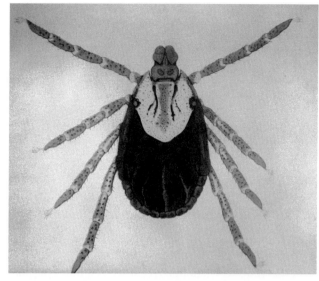

Figure 8-20 ▪ This illustration depicts a dorsal view of a female "hard" or *Ixodidae*, "American dog tick" (wood tick), *Dermacentor variabilis*. (From Centers for Disease Control and Prevention Public Health Image Library, Atlanta, Ga.)

Table 8-16 ▪ Pesticides Used on Animals

Compound	Uses	Dogs	Cats	Other	LD$_{50}$
Fipronil (e.g., Frontline, Top Spot)	Flea and tick control	X	X		*Dermal dose:* >5000 mg/kg in rats *Orally:* 750 mg/kg in rats
Imidacloprid (e.g., Advantage, Advantix [which also includes permethrin])	Flea control	X	X		*Dermal dose:* >5000 mg/kg in rats *Orally:* 450 mg/kg in rats
Spinosad (e.g., Comfortis)	Flea control	X			*Orally:* >3000 mg/kg in rats; >2000 mg/kg in rabbits (translates to over 30 times recommended oral dose)
Metaflumizone (with Amitraz) (e.g., ProMeris)	Flea control Tick control	X X	X		*Metaflumizone:* >5000 mg/kg dermally in rats *Amitraz:* 515-938 mg/kg orally in rats; 100 mg/kg orally for dogs
Selamectin (e.g., Revolution)	Endoparasites and ectoparasites (heartworm, roundworm, hookworm, mites)	X	X		*Dermal dose:* >1600 mg/kg in rats
Nitenpyram (e.g., Capstar)	Fleas	X	X		*Orally:* 1575 mg/kg in rats
Lufenuron (e.g., Program, Sentinel [and milbemycin for additional parasites])	Fleas (sterilization)	X	X		*Orally:* >2000 mg/kg in rats
Pyrethrins/pyrethroids (e.g., permethrin, phenothrin, cyphenothrin)	Tick and flea control, mite and lice (birds)	X		X	*Orally:* 430-4000 mg/kg in rats
Organophosphates (e.g., low toxicity: tetrachlorvinphos; moderately toxic: diazinon, chlorpyrifos; extremely toxic: coumaphos)	Tick and flea control	X	X		*Orally:* 22 to >1000 mg/kg in rats
Carbamates (e.g., low toxicity: propoxur, carbaryl; extreme toxicity: carbofuran)	Tick and flea control	X	X		*Orally:* 4-850 mg/kg in rats

LD$_{50}$, Median lethal dose.

GABA receptors and is considered to have low acute toxicity. The major acute sign appears to be skin and eye irritation. In young rabbits, however, there have been anecdotal reports of anorexia, lethargy, seizures, and death. Fipronil is classified as a possible human carcinogen based on studies in rats showing an increase in thyroid tumors.[13]

Imidacloprid is a chloronicotinyl nitroguanidine compound. It acts by blocking nicotinic acetylcholine receptors in the insect nervous system and, like fipronil, appears to have less affinity for mammalian receptors. It is capable of being absorbed through the skin but appears to have low acute toxicity. Animals fed significant amounts of imidacloprid over time have developed thyroid disturbances. It is classified as having evidence of noncarcinogenicity in human beings.[13]

Spinosad is a macrolide insecticide derived from a naturally occurring actinomycete bacterium that activates nicotinic acetylcholine receptors by a novel mechanism. It also has effects on GABA receptor function that may contribute further to its insecticidal activity. It has a low mammalian toxicity. It requires topical application and spreads in the skin oils (requiring a day or two for distribution).

Metaflumizone is a semicarbazone insecticide derived from the pyrazolone sodium channel blocker insecticides discovered in the early 1970s. Metaflumizone has greatly improved mammalian safety over its ancestors.

Nitenpyram is a neonicotinoid chemical, interfering with nerve transmission in the flea but not the pet.

Luferuron is an insect growth regulator through chitin inhibition. Therefore lufenuron does not kill adult fleas.

Selamectin is a semisynthetic avermectin developed for use in dogs and cats. It treats a wide range of ectoparasites and endoparasites. It affects chloride channels in the nervous system of insects, producing paralysis, and has less effect on mammalian nerves. It is applied topically and absorbed systemically, where it acts in both the intestine and the skin glands to eliminate parasites. It is considered to have low toxicity in human beings, cats, and dogs. The major side effect is skin irritation.

Pesticides With Moderate Relative Mammalian Toxicity

Beginning in 2000, the EPA acted to phase out the use of organophosphate insecticides in residential environments. As a result, the number of pyrethrin- and pyrethroid-related exposures reported to poison control centers has increased in recent years.[14] Pyrethrins are derived from the chrysanthemum plant. They have a quick onset of paralytic action on insects and are often used in household settings. However, they break down quickly in sunlight. Synthetic pyrethrins (pyrethroids) are more stable and have wider use in agricultural applications and mosquito control. Pyrethrins are poorly absorbed across the skin and are rapidly broken down in the mammalian digestive system.[15] Pyrethrins are often used with potentiating agents such as piperonyl butoxide, which inhibit breakdown of the compound by inhibiting mixed function oxidase action in insects.

Pesticides With High Relative Mammalian Toxicity

Organophosphate compounds phosphorylate and inactivate acetylcholinesterase and pseudocholinesterase enzymes that are responsible for breaking down acetylcholine (ACh) in nerve endings, RBCs, and muscle. As a result, ACh accumulates, resulting in disruption of normal nerve stimulus control and excess stimulation of both central and peripheral nerve junctions, including muscarinic and nicotinic receptors. (NOTE: Cats have most of their cholinesterases in their plasma rather than RBCs like most other species. Measuring RBCs for cholinesterase activity in cats detects only the pseudocholinesterase activity, which can drop to zero by exposure to subtoxic doses of ACh inhibitors. Plasma ACh activity, not RBC ACh, should therefore be measured in cats to reduce false-positive findings due to the inhibition of RBC pseudocholinesterases.)

N-methyl carbamates cause reversible carbamylation of acetylcholinesterase (AChE) and therefore cause clinical syndromes similar to organophosphates, with muscarinic, nicotinic, and CNS effects. However, inhibition of AChE is more reversible than organophosphate poisoning, resulting in shorter duration of signs and somewhat easier treatment.

GROUPS AT RISK

Children, the elderly, and pregnant women may be at particularly high risk for toxicity from pesticides and insect repellents. Individuals at increased risk of exposure to pet pesticides include pet groomers and handlers, pet parlors, pet store employees, veterinary workers, agricultural workers, and children who pet animals that have been topically treated with pesticide.

Pet groomers and veterinary workers have become poisoned after skin contact with flea dips containing phosmet (organophosphate). In one case the dog being bathed shook his coat and showered the worker with fluid from the dip.[16] Symptoms included skin irritation, shortness of breath, abdominal cramping, and nausea. In another case, a pet store employee sprayed her face with a solution containing pyrethrins while spraying a flea-infested house. She developed eye irritation and wheezing.

Certain animals have increased susceptibility to particular pesticides. For example, cats are particularly sensitive to carbamates and permethrins. The pyrethroids are also very toxic to aquatic species, which is important to mention to people who have aquariums or fish ponds at home. In addition, animals may be susceptible to toxicity from insect repellents used on human beings. Therefore such compounds should never be used on animals unless specifically labeled for such use.

TOXICITY IN HUMAN BEINGS

Table 8-17 compares clinical manifestations of acute pesticide poisoning in human beings and other animals. Acute organophosphate poisoning in human beings manifests as

Table 8-17 ■ Clinical Manifestations of Acute Pesticide Poisoning in Human Beings and Other Animals

Type of Pesticide	Human Beings	Dogs	Cats	Birds
Organophosphates	Hypersalivation, lacrimation, urination, miosis, bradycardia, blurred vision, mental status changes, depressed cholinesterase levels	Hypersalivation, miosis, diarrhea, vomiting, colic, bradycardia, dyspnea, ataxia, hyperthermia, excessive bronchial secretions (thick, ropy mucus blocking the respiratory tract is one of the more common causes of death in dogs and cats), CNS stimulation progressing to seizures followed by onset of weakness and paralysis, respiratory depression, depressed cholinesterase levels[22]		Diarrhea, ataxia, tremors, seizures, dyspnea, respiratory failure, increased secretions, paralysis
Carbamate	Resembles organophosphate poisoning but shorter lived; seizures; bradycardia less frequent			
Pyrethrin/pyrethroids	Allergic symptoms (crude pyrethrum), respiratory irritation, paresthesias, seizures (rare)	*Mild:* hypersalivation, fasciculation *Moderate:* vomiting, diarrhea, depression, ataxia, tremors *Severe:* seizures or death (cats are more sensitive than dogs)		Depression, weakness; possible tremors, seizures[23]

signs of cholinergic overstimulation, including salivation, sweating, lacrimation, urination, diarrhea, bradycardia, muscle twitching, and nausea. CNS effects include headache and agitation. In severe cases, there can be respiratory depression, seizures, and loss of consciousness. Miosis may occur. Cholinesterase levels are depressed.

Carbamate toxicity resembles organophosphate poisoning but tends to be shorter lived. Bradycardia and seizures are less frequent. Cholinesterase levels may be "falsely normal" in the setting of carbamate toxicity because of the presence of a carbamylated enzyme that can be reactivated in vitro.

Crude pyrethrum and, to a lesser extent, purified pyrethrin preparations and pyrethroids may cause allergic reactions including skin and eye irritation and asthma.[17] The chief effect of pyrethroids appears to be on the nervous system. In mild cases, nausea and paresthesia can occur (at the site of contact, which generally resolve within 24 hours after exposure). Seizures have been reported in more severe exposures.

There are case reports of DEET toxicity in human beings, including CNS effects such as slurred speech and seizures; these have generally been the result of ingestion of large doses,[18] and the anecdotal nature of these reports requires caution in interpretation. Dermal application has been reported to rarely cause rashes, itching, and mucosal irritation; eye and skin irritation are considered the major possible side effects of conventional DEET use.[7]

No major toxic effects of picaridin or lemon eucalyptus oil have been reported to date. Both are believed to cause less skin and eye irritation than DEET. However, long-term toxicity studies are lacking.

TOXICITY IN ANIMALS

Organophosphates and carbamates have higher toxicity in animals with lower cholinesterase activity. Cats are more sensitive to these products than dogs. Young and leaner animals are more susceptible. Signs include predominantly parasympathetic stimulation. Toxicity occurs with inappropriate application: overuse or use of yard products as topical insecticides or dog products used on cats, and with accidental ingestion of lawn products (typically out of containers by dogs) or cats walking through wet, recently treated areas and grooming the product off their coats.

Cats are quite sensitive to the effects of concentrated pyrethroids such as permethrin (e.g., >10% permethrin; dog products are 20% to 85% permethrin). Despite label warnings, cats are poisoned by permethrin spot-on treatments for ticks and fleas that were intended for use on dogs. Young, old, or debilitated animals are also more likely to suffer ill effects. Signs result from idiosyncratic and neurotoxic reactions and include twitching, muscle spasms and fasciculations, and seizures.[19] Hypothermic patients are more likely to show signs.

DEET at very high oral doses (400 mg/kg/day) has been reported to cause vomiting, ataxia, tremors, and convulsions in dogs,[20] and a DEET/fenvalerate topical product for dogs has resulted in seizures. However, the ASPCA Animal Poison Control Center has issued a press release that recommends not using DEET on companion animals because of the risk of neurologic effects in dogs and cats.[21]

DIAGNOSIS

Diagnosis of pesticide poisoning is often a clinical diagnosis made when typical symptoms or signs develop after exposure. Organophosphate pesticides depress serum and RBC cholinesterase levels (<25%). Any patient with organophosphate toxicosis should have blood levels determined immediately because the administration of pralidoxime hydrochloride can normalize test results. As stated previously, cholinesterase levels may be spuriously normal in carbamate intoxication. Cholinesterase levels are also useful in the diagnosis of animal intoxication. (Care must be used when interpreting cholinesterase activity results between species. Use toxicologist and laboratory normal values for comparison.)

Table 8-18 ▪ Treatment of Acute Pesticide Poisoning in Human Beings and Other Animals

Type of Pesticide	Human Beings	Dogs	Birds
Organophosphate	Moderately severe *Adult:* Atropine sulfate 2-4 mg IV q15min until decreased secretions, pulse 140. *Children <12 years:* 0.05-0.1 mg/kg body weight, minimum dose 0.1 mg *Severe poisoning:* *Adults:* Pralidoxime 1-2 mg IV slowly *Children <12 years:* 20-50 mg/kg body weight (depending on severity of poisoning) IV, in 100 mL of normal saline infused over 30 min[15]	Atropine sulfate 0.2 mg/kg (¼ given IV and the remainder SC) q3-6h *should be given only to relieve excessive bronchial secretions or severe bradycardia.* (Over-atropinization is a common cause of serious illness and death in dogs and cats when atropine is given without regard for the condition of the animal. Unfortunately, over-atropinzied animals may display CNS signs that resemble some of the CNS effects of the OP/carbamate, which may result in yet more atropine being administered.) Pralidoxime chloride 10-15 mg/kg IM or slow IV (over 5-10 min) q8-12h until recovery If seizures, diazepam (0.05-1 mg/kg IV) or phenobarbital (3-30 mg/kg IV) to effect	Atropine sulfate 0.01-0.02 mg/kg SC, IM (most species, ranges up to 0.5 mg/kg) or pralidoxime 10-100 mg/kg IM q24-48h or repeat once in 6 hr (use lower dose in combination with atropine)[24]
Carbamates	Atropine, anticonvulsants, as with organophosphates		
Pyrethrin/pyrethroids	Antihistamines for allergic reactions	Bathe with a mild detergent If tremors or seizures, methocarbamol 55-220 mg/kg IV not to exceed 330 mg/kg/day, diazepam to control seizures	Bathe with mild detergent, diazepam 0.5-1.0 mg/kg IM, IV q8-12h as anticonvulsant[24]

OP, Organophosphate; *IV,* intravenous; *SC,* subcutaneous; *IM,* intramuscular.

MANAGEMENT OF ANIMAL-RELATED PESTICIDE POISONING

Management of acute pesticide exposures involves assessment of exposure amount and route, decontamination (removal of clothing, washing, etc.), supportive measures, and consideration of specific antidotes. Contact the poison control center at 800-222-1222 or the Animal Poison Control Center at 888-426-4435 (a fee may apply to the latter call). Table 8-18 presents treatment options of acute pesticide poisoning in human beings and other animals.

WEB RESOURCES

- **National Pesticide Information Center**
  http://npic.orst.edu
- **CDC: Insect Repellent Use and Safety** (including duration of effectiveness)
  http://www.cdc.gov/ncidod/dvbid/westnile/qa/insect_repellent.htm
- **EPA: Ten Tips to Protect Children from Pesticide and Lead Poisonings**
  http://www.epa.gov/pesticides/factsheets/child-ten-tips.htm

References

1. Blondell JM. Decline in pesticide poisonings in the United States from 1995 to 2004. *Clin Toxicol (Phila).* 2007;45(5):589–592.
2. Humane Society of the US. *What you should know about flea and tick products.* http://www.hsus.org/pets/pet_care/what_you_should_know_about_flea_and_tick_products/. Accessed February 20.
3. Bronstein AC, Spyker DA, Cantilena Jr LR, et al. 2006 Annual Report of the American Association of Poison Control Centers' National Poison Data System (NPDS). *Clin Toxicol (Phila).* 2007;45(8):815–917.
4. Environmental Protection Agency. *How to use insect repellent safely.* http://www.epa.gov/pesticides/health/mosquitoes/insectrp.htm. Accessed April 14, 2008.
5. Environmental Protection Agency. *The insect repellent DEET.* http://www.epa.gov/pesticides/factsheets/chemicals/deet.htm. Accessed April 14, 2008.
6. Centers for Disease Control and Prevention. *Insect repellent use and safety: using repellents properly.* http://www.cdc.gov/ncidod/dvbid/westnile/qa/insect_repellent.htm#proper. Accessed April 14, 2008.
7. Kendrick DB. Mosquito repellents and superwarfarin rodenticides—are they really toxic in children? *Curr Opin Pediatr.* 2006;18(2):180–183.
8. Costanzo SD, Watkinson AJ, Murby EJ, et al. Is there a risk associated with the insect repellent DEET (N,N-diethyl-m-toluamide) commonly found in aquatic environments? *Sci Total Environ.* 2007;384(1-3):214–220.
9. Environmental Protection Agency. *New pesticide fact sheet: Picaridin.* http://www.epa.gov/opprd001/factsheets/picaridin.pdf. Accessed April 14, 2008.
10. Centers for Disease Control and Prevention. *Insect repellent use and safety.* http://www.cdc.gov/ncidod/dvbid/westnile/qa/insect_repellent.htm. Accessed September 15, 2008.
11. Schwantes U, Dautel H, Jung G. Prevention of infectious tick-borne diseases in humans: comparative studies of the repellency of different dodecanoic acid-formulations against *Ixodes ricinus* ticks (Acari: Ixodidae). *Parasit Vectors.* 2008;1(1):8.
12. Thorsell W, Mikiver A, Tunón H. Repelling properties of some plant materials on the tick *Ixodes ricinus* L. *Phytomedicine.* 2006;13(1–2):132–134.
13. Hovda LR, Hooser SB. Toxicology of newer pesticides for use in dogs and cats. *Vet Clin North Am Small Anim Pract.* 2002;32(2):455–467.
14. Power LE, Sudakin DL. Pyrethrin and pyrethroid exposures in the United States: a longitudinal analysis of incidents reported to poison centers. *J Med Toxicol.* 2007;3(3):94–99.

15. Reigart JR, Roberts JR. *Recognition and management of pesticide poisoning.* 5th ed. Washington DC: U.S. Environmental Protection Agency; 1999.

16. Centers for Disease Control and Prevention. Illnesses associated with occupational use of flea-control products—California, Texas, and Washington, 1989–1997. *MMWR.* 1999;48(21):443–447.

17. Franzosa JA, Osimitz TG, Maibach HI. Cutaneous contact urticaria to pyrethrum—real? common? or not documented? An evidence-based approach. *Cutan Ocul Toxicol.* 2007;26(1):57–72.

18. Koren G, Matsui D, Bailey B. DEET-based insect repellents: safety implications for children and pregnant and lactating women. *CMAJ.* 2003;169(3):209–212.

19. Sutton NM, Bates N, Campbell A. Clinical effects and outcome of feline permethrin spot-on poisonings reported to the Veterinary Poisons Information Service (VPIS), London. *J Feline Med Surg.* 2007;9(4):335–339.

20. Schoenig GP, Osimitz TG, Gabriel KL, et al. Evaluation of the chronic toxicity and oncogenicity of N,N-diethyl-m-toluamide (DEET). *Toxicol Sci.* 1999;47(1):99–109.

21. The American Society for the Prevention of Cruelty to Animals (ASPCA). *Press release: the ASPCA Animal Poison Control Center Alerts Dog Owners to Important Information Regarding West Nile Virus.* http://www2.aspca.org/site/News2?page=NewsArticle&id=10900&news_iv_ctrl=1101. Accessed April 14, 2008.

22. Kahn CM, Line S. eds. *The Merck veterinary manual.* 9th ed. Whitehouse Station, NJ: Merck; 2005.

23. Willis GA. *Hamilton & District Budgerigar Society, Inc: Avian poisoning.* http://www3.sympatico.ca/davehansen/avpoison.html. Accessed April 14, 2008.

24. Carpenter JW. *Exotic animal formulary.* 3rd ed. St Louis: Saunders; 2005.

ENVENOMATIONS

Peter M. Rabinowitz and Lisa A. Conti

(ICD-10 T63.0 Toxic Effect of Contact With Venomous Animals)

A wide variety of animals are equipped with venom of different types for protective and sometimes feeding purposes. Human beings and other animals may be exposed to such venoms through bites, stings, and ingestion.[1] Envenomation may be a complication to consider in evaluating a patient who seeks emergency care after an animal bite (see Chapter 10).

Envenomation scenarios often illustrate the overlap between human and veterinary medicine. For a number of hazards, such as snakebite, poisoning episodes are much more common in dogs than in human beings because of greater exposure to snakes in the wild. For example, several thousand human beings are bitten by poisonous snakes each year in the United States, but the number of dogs and cats that sustain snakebites annually may be as high as 150,000.[2] Pets can therefore serve as sentinels about the environmental risk of venomous animals. For marine envenomations, documented cases in companion animals or wildlife are uncommon. When cases of poisoning do occur in animals, they often closely resemble the clinical picture in human beings. In terms of treatment, moreover, veterinarians must sometimes rely on the use of antivenin developed for human beings when treating poisoned animals. A significant issue for both human health and veterinary clinicians is the risk of poisoning from exotic pets (see Chapter 10), such as reptiles,[3] amphibians, and invertebrates such as scorpions.[4] Many owners are unaware that these pets pose an envenomation risk to human beings and other animals living in the house.[5] Another issue is the potential for animal envenomation during foreign travel from bites, stings, and even exotic foods such as toad soup.[6]

Key Points for Clinicians and Public Health Professionals

Public Health Professionals

- Describe the public health risk in the community from venomous animals, both wild and captive, including pet swap meets and private collectors.

- When appropriate, help coordinate with regional poison control centers and emergency medical providers to ensure access to antivenin and other information necessary to treat possible envenomations that may occur locally.[7]
- Increase the public's awareness of the risks of venomous animals kept as pets and in the wild.

Human Health Clinicians

- When taking a history of animal exposures (see Chapter 3), ask about any venomous pets. If patients report such a history, ensure they are aware of emergency procedures if envenomation should occur. If patients have questions about a particular animal, consult the patient's veterinarian.
- In evaluating a patient with an animal bite, determine the species responsible and the possibility for envenomation. Consult a regional poison control center.
- Counsel travelers about the risk of animal envenomation (including in exotic foods) and necessary steps to take in case of envenomation in countries that the patient plans to visit.

Veterinary Clinicians

- Recognize the envenomation potential of particular species kept as pets. Discuss with clients the risk to companion animals in the house, and counsel clients to discuss human health risks with their medical provider.
- Only highly trained individuals should handle venomous animals.
- Counsel pet owners with venomous animals on envenomation risks and methods to reduce them (bite prevention; see Chapter 10 on animal bites), as well as the need to seek immediate medical care if envenomation occurs.
- Ensure that the local emergency departments and regional poison control centers are aware of certain venomous animals being housed in the community, as well as venomous wildlife species, and that steps are being taken to prepare for an envenomation incident (such as availability of appropriate antivenin).

- When treating a dog or other animal for envenomation from a snake or other venomous animal, consider the risk to human beings as well and counsel owners on risk reduction.
- If a pet is traveling to another country or region, counsel the owner about local envenomation risks and steps to take in an emergency.

HYMENOPTERAN ENVENOMATION

Stings from insects of the order Hymenoptera (bees, yellow jackets, wasps, and ants) can cause reactions ranging from mild local discomfort to life-threatening systemic reactions in human beings and other animals. They are the most frequent arthropod-associated envenomation seen in U.S. poison control centers, with more than 4000 reported cases in 2005.[8] Honeybees have a barbed stinger that is left in the skin, eviscerating the insect. Honeybees are attracted to carbon dioxide, bright colors, and sweet odors but are usually docile unless provoked.[9] Africanized bees, in contrast, may be aggressive and cause mass envenomations. Yellow jackets and hornets may be more aggressive than honeybees and have nonbarbed stingers that can sting repeatedly and deliver more venom than a bee sting (Figure 8-21). Hymenoptera stings usually result in local redness, pain, and swelling. A small number of persons have Hymenoptera allergy and are at risk of severe allergic reactions that can include anaphylaxis (see Chapter 7 on allergic conditions). Even without allergy, systemic reactions can occur including nausea, dizziness, and vomiting, especially after multiple stings.

Treatment involves local measures, including ice and topical steroids or oral antihistamines. Anaphylaxis needs to be treated promptly with epinephrine and steroids. Honeybee stingers should be removed using a credit card or fine tweezers to remove the apparatus without expressing additional venom into the wound.[9]

Other hymenopterans capable of significant envenomations include fire ants, which can give painful stings producing a ring of small pustules (Color Plate 8-8). Mass envenomation can occur when a child or animal disturbs a large ant colony. Treatment is supportive with cool compresses, antihistamines, and topical steroids if necessary.

Individuals with Hymenoptera allergy should carry epinephrine in an injectable form (Epi-Pen, DEY L.P., Napa, Calif.) (Figure 8-22) whenever there is potential for stings to occur.

In animals, anaphylactic reactions to hymenopteran stings have been reported in dogs but not in livestock.[10] Local reactions (pain and swelling) from stings in dogs, cats, and other mammals resemble those in human beings (Figure 8-23), and systemic reactions can occur with multiple stings. Treatment is similar to that in human beings and involves antihistamines, corticosteroids, and fluids (see Table 8-20). Epinephrine is used for suspected anaphylactic reactions.

LEPIDOPTERISM

Certain species of caterpillars are capable of producing minor envenomations (lepidopterism) on direct skin contact. Symptoms include local redness and irritative dermatitis (Color Plate 8-9). Other caterpillars can inflict painful stings (Color Plate 8-10).

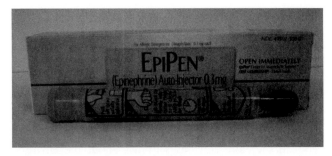

Figure 8-22 ■ EpiPen preloaded delivery system for injection of aqueous epinephrine.

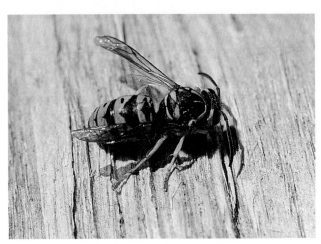

Figure 8-21 ■ Yellow jacket, *Vespula maculiforma*. (From Auerbach PS: *Wilderness medicine*, ed 5, Philadelphia, 2007, Mosby.)

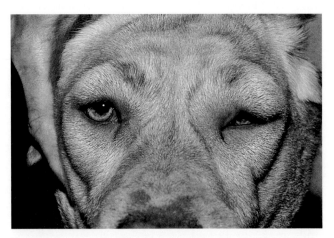

Figure 8-23 ■ Angioedema. Severe swelling of the face and periocular tissue developed after a venomous insect sting. (From Medleau L, Hnilica KA: *Small animal dermatology: a color atlas and therapeutic guide*, ed 2, St. Louis, 2006, Saunders Elsevier.)

SPIDER BITES

More than 34,000 species of spiders exist worldwide, but only a small percentage can penetrate the skin of a large mammal and cause envenomation.[11] Antivenin has been developed for three of the most dangerous spiders: the brown recluse, the black widow, and the funnel-web spider. However, such antivenin may not be widely available.

Tarantulas are found in parts of the United States and are frequently sold as pets. Tarantula bites usually do not cause significant envenomations but may cause local tissue swelling. Another hazard of tarantulas is that contact with the hairs of the back, which are released when the tarantula is distressed, can cause local skin reactions as well as a granulomatous reaction of the cornea and conjunctiva of the eye (ophthalmia nodosa) that requires urgent ophthalmologic attention.[9] Dogs or cats that attempt to eat tarantulas may gag or vomit.[10]

Bites of the brown recluse spider (*Loxosceles reclusa*, also known as the *fiddleback spider* because of the violin-shaped dark band on its cephalothorax; Figure 8-24) are initially painless but later cause local tissue necrosis. Systemic reactions (loxoscelism) can include fever, jaundice, vomiting, convulsions, rash, and intravascular hemolysis.[11] The bite typically first appears as an erythematous bull's-eye lesion that then progresses over days and weeks to a necrotic ulcer.[11] The wound margin and necrosis may take weeks to fully develop, and follow-up with a plastic surgeon is advisable for wound care.[9]

Brown recluse bites to companion animals produce similar pathology and are treated in a similar manner with local wound care and pain control.[10]

Bites of the female black widow spider and related widow spiders (*Latrodectus* spp.; Figure 8-25) result in a neurotoxic envenomation caused by α-latrotoxin. α-Latrotoxin is a polypeptide that binds to nerve receptors at the neuromuscular junction and in the autonomic nervous system, producing excess acetylcholine at the synapse. Clinical manifestations include abdominal pain and rigidity, headache, hypertension, and nausea, vomiting, and diaphoresis that can be mistaken for appendicitis or other acute medical problems.[9]

Most widow spider envenomations are not life threatening. Supportive measures can include pain control and muscle relaxants (benzodiazepines). However, for serious cases, the Food and Drug Administration (FDA) has approved an equine-derived antivenin for black widow spider envenomation. Indications for the use of the antivenin include predisposing conditions (cardiovascular disease, pregnancy, chronic obstructive pulmonary disease, elderly or very young patients) as well as failure of supportive treatment.[11] In

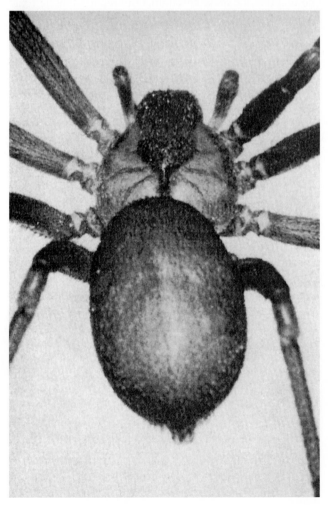

Figure 8-24 ■ The brown recluse spider is 10 to 15 mm long, light to dark brown, and has a species-specific dorsal, dark, violin-shaped band. (From Dillaha CJ, Jansen GT, Honeycutt WM et al: North American loxoscelism. Necrotic bite of the brown recluse spider, *JAMA* 188:33–36, 1964.)

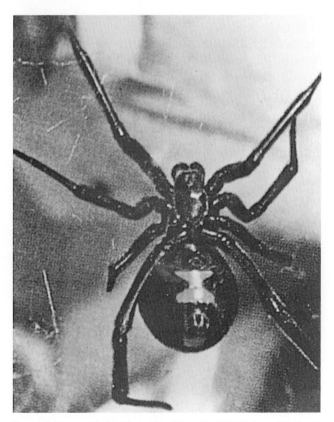

Figure 8-25 ■ Black widow spider. (From Ford MD, Delaney KA, Ling L et al: *Clinical toxicology*, Philadelphia, 2001, Saunders.)

patients with known horse allergy, the risks of allergic reaction versus the benefits of the antivenin must be weighed,[9] and resuscitation equipment and medications should be available to handle a severe allergic reaction.[1]

Cats are very sensitive to black widow envenomation and have a high fatality rate. There are case reports of cats being successfully treated with antivenin.[10]

Funnel-web spiders are found in Australia and produce a neurotoxic venom. Symptoms of a funnel-web spider bite include painful lymphadenopathy, headache, nausea, sweating, and muscle spasms of the legs and abdomen. Renal failure, hypertension, and cardiovascular collapse can occur. The bite can be fatal within 2 hours, and elderly and very young victims are at increased risk. An antivenin has been developed but is not commercially available in the United States.[11] Susceptibility to funnel-web spider bites appears to vary among species, with human beings very sensitive, whereas dogs and cats experience only mild and transient effects. In animals, the bite of the male spider appears to be more potent than that of the female.[10]

SCORPION STINGS

Most scorpion stings cause only local pain and swelling and respond to local measures such as cold compresses and wound care. A number of species, however, possess potent venom and can cause significant envenomations. These species include the bark scorpion (*Centruroides* spp.) found in the Southwestern United States (Figure 8-26 and Color Plate 8-11), scorpions of the genus *Tityus* in the Caribbean, and members of the genera *Androctonus*, *Buthus*, and *Parabuthus* in Africa. Such scorpion stings can result in excess cholinergic activity with symptoms of delirium, nausea, bradycardia, salivation, and sweating. With some species, adrenergic toxicity and tissue necrosis can also occur. Treatment is supportive. An antivenin has been developed for *Centruroides* stings but is not often used because of the frequency of allergic hypersensitivity reactions.[7]

There is a lack of evidence that scorpion envenomation in dogs and cats is a significant concern.[10]

REPTILE EVENOMATIONS

It has been estimated that worldwide each year more than 5 million individuals are bitten by snakes, resulting in more than 2.5 million cases of envenomation and as many as 125,000 deaths.[12] A large number of snakes worldwide possess significant venom and their bites can lead to serious complications and mortality. As stated previously, many more dogs and cats than human beings are bitten by venomous snakes each year in the United States. In many parts of the world, venomous snake bites are an occupational hazard. Examples of groups at risk include rice farmers and plantation workers in Asia, farmers in West Africa, herdspeople, persons catching snakes in China for human consumption, fishermen in Asia encountering sea snakes, wildlife biologists, forestry workers, zoo workers, and pet store workers. Snakebites can occur during recreational activities, including wilderness travel to many regions (see Chapter 10 on travel and animal contact). The increasing number of reptile enthusiasts who keep venomous snakes as exotic pets in their homes has created new risk groups in the United States (see Chapter 10).[11] Table 8-19 shows the number of indigenous and exotic snake envenomations reported to the Toxic Exposure Surveillance System (TESS), a database of poison center calls.

Venomous snakes are members of four families: Viperidae, Elapidae, Colubridae, and Atractaspididae.[7] In North America, indigenous venomous snakes include pit vipers of the family Viperidae (subfamily Crotalinae) and coral snakes (of the family Elapidae, which also includes cobras, sea snakes, and others). The clinical manifestations and treatment of their bites vary by species. Antivenin is a key part of treatment of snakebite, but in the United States only antivenin for Crotaline and coral snake envenomations are approved by the FDA for commercial use. However, the FDA allows zoos to keep stocks of antivenin for exotic species in case of occupational exposure. The Association of Zoos

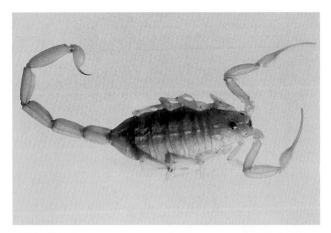

Figure 8-26 ■ *Centruroides exilicauda (C. sculpturatus)*, the bark scorpion of Arizona. (From Auerbach PS: *Wilderness medicine*, ed 5, Philadelphia, 2007, Mosby Elsevier.)

Table 8-19 ■ Snakebites Reported to Toxic Exposure System in United States (2003–2005)			
Snake	**2003**	**2004**	**2005**
Copperhead	997	1098	1051
Coral	97	99	58
Cottonmouth	175	192	194
Crotaline: unknown	397	431	413
Rattlesnake	1245	1178	1255
Venomous exotic snake	126	131	98
Nonvenomous exotic snake	138	131	42
Unknown exotic	9	2	6
Nonvenomous snake	1818	1803	1552
Unknown snake	1887	2147	1972

From McNally J, Boesen K, Boyer L: Toxicologic information resources for reptile envenomations, *Vet Clin North Am Exot Anim Pract* 11(2):389–401, viii, 2008.

and Aquariums (AZA) maintains an electronic database of these stockpiles known as the Antivenom Index that is available to regional poison control centers.[7]

Pit Vipers

The Crotalinae subfamily of pit vipers includes venomous snakes such as copperheads, water moccasins, and rattlesnakes. The name *pit vipers* comes from heat-sensing glands (pits) located on either side of the triangle-shaped head (Figure 8-27).

The fangs of pit vipers are hollow and can deliver a dose of venom deep into tissues. Pit viper venom is a highly complex mix of toxins, including metalloproteinases that cause local tissue destruction and thrombin-like proteins that cause a coagulopathy. Some species have venom with significant amounts of neurotoxins such as a phospholipase A_2 that blocks nerve transmission. The Mojave rattlesnake, *Crotalus scutulatus,* produces a potent neurotoxin that is a compound of phospholipase A_2 and an acidic subunit (Mojave toxin). As a result, victims of pit viper bites can have complicated clinical syndromes involving local pain, tissue swelling, edema, and necrosis (Figures 8-28, 8-29, and Color Plate 8-12) as well as hemorrhage, shock, and signs of neurotoxicity, including paresthesias and respiratory failure. Renal failure as a result of rhabdomyolysis can occur. Other complications can include allergy to components of the toxin and bacterial wound infection. Laboratory findings include leukocytosis and elevated creatine phosphokinase.

Although controlled studies are few, it is not clear whether first-aid measures for snake bites are beneficial. Such measures include incising and suctioning of the wound or the

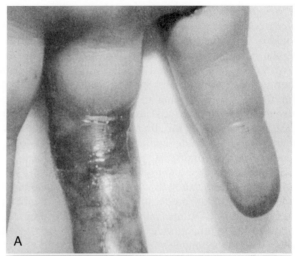

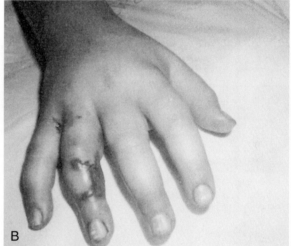

Figure 8-28 ▪ Crotalid envenomation. **A,** Photograph taken 60 minutes after bite. Marked swelling and ecchymosis are apparent. Fang marks are barely visible. **B,** In the same patient, the back of the hand shows extensive swelling. (From Wolf MD: Envenomation. In Halbrook PR, editor: *Textbook of pediatric critical care*, Philadelphia, 1993, WB Saunders.)

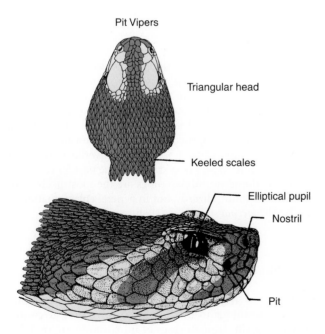

Figure 8-27 ▪ Pit viper's head. Note the elliptical pupil and the heat-sensing pit for which these reptiles are named. Viewed from above, the head has a distinctly triangular shape. Many nonvenomous snakes also possess triangular heads; therefore this is not a reliable means of differentiation. (From Auerbach PS: *Wilderness medicine*, ed 5, Philadelphia, 2007, Mosby Elsevier. Courtesy Marlin Sawyer.)

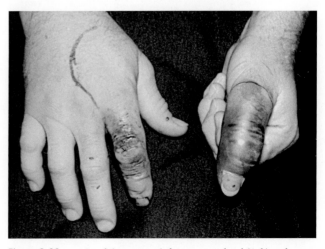

Figure 8-29 ▪ Local tissue necrosis from a copperhead (*Agkistrodon contortrix*) envenomation. (From Ford MD, Delaney KA, Ling L et al: *Clinical toxicology*, Philadelphia, 2001, Saunders.)

use of a tourniquet. In fact, such measures could worsen outcomes.[11] Most bites are to extremities, and the extremity should be immobilized in the field and the victim taken to a hospital. Hospital care includes wound treatment, supportive care to prevent shock, and management of swelling and other medical complications. Specific treatment involves the administration of Crotaline antivenin. The FDA-approved antivenin is an ovine-derived Fab immunoglobulin fragment (CroFab; Protherics US Inc., Brentwood, Tenn.).[1] Indications for antivenin use include significant progression of swelling, coagulopathy, neuromuscular paralysis, and cardiovascular collapse.[1]

Among domestic animals, dogs are most frequently bitten by pit vipers. Dogs are commonly bitten on the front legs and head (Figure 8-30 and Color Plate 8-13), horses are bitten most often on the muzzle (Figure 8-31), and cattle tend to be bitten on the tongue or muzzle. Cats are believed to be

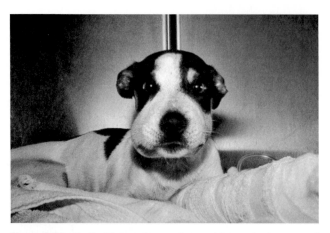

Figure 8-30 ■ Swelling on the muzzle resembling angioedema caused by a snakebite. (From Medleau L, Hnilica KA: *Small animal dermatology: a color atlas and therapeutic guide*, ed 2, St Louis, 2006, Saunders Elsevier.)

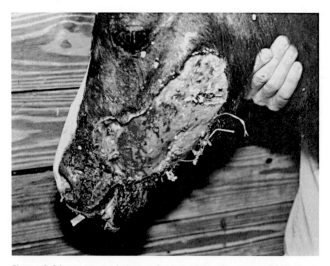

Figure 8-31 ■ Face of a horse after being bitten by an Eastern diamondback rattlesnake. (From Reed S, Bayly WM, Sellon DC: *Equine internal medicine*, ed 2, St Louis, 2004, Saunders.)

less sensitive than other species to Crotaline venom but are more likely to be bitten on the abdomen, with severe consequences. Cats also tend to run and hide after a bite, delaying veterinary treatment. The local and systemic effects of pit viper bites in animals resemble those in people (Table 8-20 and Figure 8-32). Treatment of Crotaline bites in animals is similar to that in human beings (see Table 8-20). A rattlesnake vaccine has recently been developed for dogs (*Crotalus atrox* toxoid; Hygeia Biological Laboratories, Woodland, Calif.), and twice-yearly vaccination is recommended for dogs that have potential for rattlesnake exposure.[10]

Elapids

The family Elapidae includes cobras, mambas, and sea snakes (see Marine Envenomations). In North America, the family is represented by the coral snake *Micrurus* spp. (Color Plate 8-14). The venom of many members of the elapid family is predominantly neurotoxic. The bite of an elapid such as a coral snake can produce local pain (but usually not swelling), headache, nausea, paresthesias, cranial nerve involvement, altered mental status, and respiratory failure. As with pit viper bites, medical care should be sought immediately. Treatment involves administration of a *Micrurus*-specific antivenin as soon as possible. Some evidence suggests that pressure and immobilization of the wound area until antivenin can be administered is beneficial for the outcome of elapid bites. This treatment method is shown in Figure 8-33.

Coral snake bites also cause significant morbidity and mortality in cats and dogs. As with human beings, neurotoxic effects predominate and treatment is based on the use of antivenin.[10]

Poisonous Lizards

North America is home to the only poisonous lizards: the Gila monster *(Heloderma suspectum)* and the Mexican beaded lizard *(Heloderma horridum)*. Their bite is often complicated by local tissue trauma owing to the chewing action of their powerful jaws. The venom is similar to pit viper venom in causing local tissue destruction and swelling. Treatment is supportive; no specific antivenin is available. Human fatalities have not occurred in the past 50 years.

Among domestic animals, dogs are the most likely to be bitten by poisonous lizards, but in general envenomation of pets by *Heloderma* spp. is rare (Figure 8-34).[10]

AMPHIBIAN INTOXICATIONS

Toads (genus *Bufo*) produce a potent toxin (bufotoxin) in their parotid gland that is similar to cardiac glycosides such as digoxin. Human cases of intoxication are rare, but in Asia ingestion of toad egg soup has led to significant toxicity. Treatment involves gastric decontamination and management of arrhythmias. In serious human poisonings a digoxin antidote (digoxin-specific Fab fragment) has been used.

Table 8-20 ■ Terrestrial Envenomations in Human Beings and Companion Animals

Venomous Animal	Particular Species and Geographic Location	Symptoms and Treatment in Human Beings	Clinical Signs and Treatment in Other Animals
Arthropods			
Hymenopterans (wasps, bees, ants)	Worldwide	Local pain, redness, swelling, anaphylaxis in allergic individuals *Treatment:* Antihistamines, steroids For treatment of severe allergy: 0.1% adrenaline (0.5-1.0 mL for adults, 0.01 mL/kg for children)[13]	Urticaria, peripheral edema, anaphylaxis in sensitized animals *Treatment:* Antihistamines, steroids *Anaphylactic shock:* epinephrine (1-5 mL of 1:10,000 SC)
Spiders	Brown recluse spiders, widow spiders, funnel-web spiders, wandering spiders (South America)	Local tissue necrosis, anaphylaxis, systemic conditions, including muscle spasms and abdominal pain, hypertension, cardiovascular collapse *Treatment:* Supportive treatment, tetanus prophylaxis, antivenin (widow spider)	Tissue necrosis Systemic signs may develop after 3-4 days *Treatment:* Early application of cold packs, steroids to prevent necrosis; consider dapsone (4,4'-diaminodiphenylsulfone), a leukocyte inhibitor, 1 mg/kg q8h for 10 days (dogs),[14] antibiotics to animals not treated with dapsone Restlessness, muscle rigidity, severe cramping *Treatment:* Black widow antivenin given slowly IV diluted in crystalloid solution. Monitor the inner pinna for evidence of hyperemia as an indicator for allergic response to antivenin (envenomation in cats is usually fatal without antivenin), treat intractable hypertension with sodium nitroprusside, methocarbamol for spasms, analgesia, diazepam, tetanus prophylaxis[14]
Scorpions	North and South America, Africa, Middle East, South Asia	*Local:* pain, swelling, redness *Systemic:* cholinergic phase (vomiting, sweating, salivation, bradycardia, hypotension) followed by adrenergic phase (hypertension, tachycardia, cardiac failure) *Treatment:* Pain control, tetanus prophylaxis, control blood pressure; in United States, consider antivenin[13]	Pain, swelling *Treatment:* Antihistamine
Reptiles			
Crotalids (pit vipers) Responsible for most human snakebites in United States; approx. 6000 cases annually,[1] and 150,000 dog or cat cases annually in United States	*In United States:* rattlesnakes, water moccasin, and copperhead	Local pain, swelling, tissue destruction, some neurotoxicity with certain species *Treatment:* Immobilization in field, followed by antivenin (consult with poison control on urgent basis for specific antivenin by species)	*Dogs and cats:* Pain, weakness, dizziness, nausea, severe hypotension, thrombocytopenia; clinical signs can last up to 1½ weeks; may be fatal *Treatment:* Crystalloid fluids IV, 1 vial of antivenin[2] mixed with 200 mL crystalloid fluids and given slowly IV, monitoring the patient for hypersensitivity to the antivenin; vaccine available for dogs *Horses:* Pain, swelling, systemic signs, rarely fatal unless bite to head/neck *Treatment:* Supportive measures, antivenin if available[15]

Continued

Table 8-20 ■ Terrestrial Envenomations in Human Beings and Companion Animals—cont'd

Venomous Animal	Particular Species and Geographical Location	Symptoms and Treatment in Human Beings	Clinical Signs and Treatment in Other Animals
Reptiles—cont'd			
Elapidae	Coral snakes (United States), cobras (Asia)	Neurotoxicity *Treatment:* Antivenin (check with poison control for specific species), supportive care	Neurotoxicity, bites often occur on the lip, clinical signs can last for up to 1½ weeks, bulbar paralysis with respiratory collapse as primary cause of fatality *Treatment:* Administer 1-2 vials of antivenin. If no antivenin available, provide ventilator support for several days in a critical care facility, broad-spectrum antibiotics for 7-10 days
Lizards (Heloderma)	The only two poisonous lizards in the world are in southwest United States and Mexico: Gila monster and Mexican beaded lizard	Venom effect similar to many rattlesnakes: local pain, swelling, tissue destruction; bite can be tenacious with chewing and tissue destruction; dislodge lizard with hot water or instrument; wound cleansing and irrigation important; no commercially available antivenin, no human fatalities in past 50 years[11]	Bleeding from the site of the bite, ptyalism, hypotension *Treatment:* Flush bite site with lidocaine and probe for tooth fragments, soak bitten area with Burrow's solution; pain control, broad-spectrum antibiotics
Amphibians			
Toads (especially *Bufo marinus* and *Bufo alvarius*)	U.S. marine toad and Colorado River toad produce defensive toxin from the parotid glands: indole alkyl amines (similar to LSD), cardiac glycosides, and noncardiac sterols	Toxic ingestion of toad eggs reported, may resemble digitoxin overdose: nausea, tachycardia, arrhythmias, hyperkalemia *Treatment:* Emesis/gastric decontamination, cardiac monitoring, electrolyte monitoring and correction; consider digoxin-specific Fab fragment antidote if syndrome of digoxin toxicity[6]	Profuse hypersalivation after an exposure, brick-red buccal membranes Marine toad contact is a medical emergency with a high fatality rate, whereas Colorado River toad fatalities are uncommon after decontamination *Treatment:* Flush mouth with copious amounts of water for 10 min, monitor temperature (cool bath for hyperthermic animal >105 °F), atropine (0.04 mg/kg IM, SC), cardiac monitoring

LSD, Lysergic acid diethylamide; *IV,* intravenous; *SC,* subcutaneous; *IM,* intramuscular.

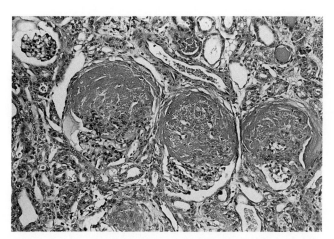

Figure 8-32 ▪ Photomicrograph of canine renal tissue after exposure to snake venom. Three glomeruli have varying degrees of hemorrhage and necrosis (mesangiolysis) (×10). (From Plumlee K: *Clinical veterinary toxicology*, St. Louis, 2004, Mosby.)

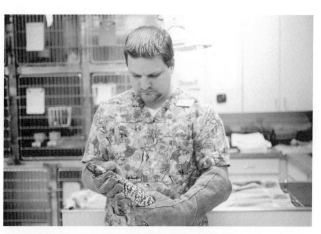

Figure 8-34 ▪ Training technicians to handle reptiles and provide for their daily needs is critical to successful treatment. This experienced technician is handling a venomous Gila monster (*Heloderma suspectum*) for treatment. (From Mader DR: *Reptile medicine and surgery*, ed 2, St Louis, 2006, Saunders Elsevier.)

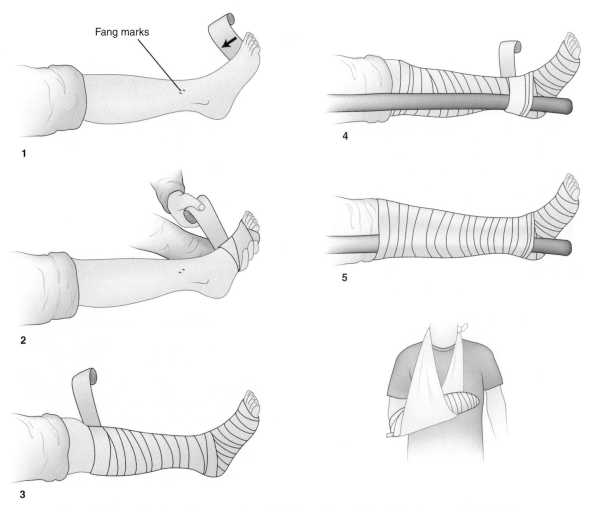

Figure 8-33 ▪ The Australian pressure-immobilization technique. This technique has proved effective in the management of elapid and sea snake envenomations. Its efficacy in Viperid bites has yet to be fully evaluated clinically. (From Auerbach PS: *Wilderness medicine*, ed 5, Philadelphia, 2007, Mosby Elsevier.)

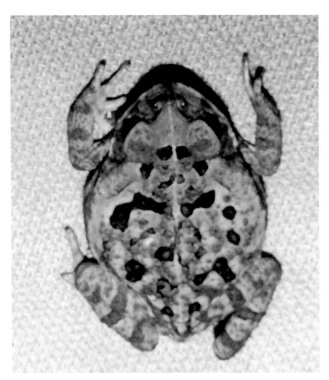

Figure 8-35 ■ *Bufo marinus* (cane or marine toad). (From Peterson ME, Talcott PA: *Small animal toxicology*, ed 2, St Louis, 2006, Saunders Elsevier.)

Poisoning by toads is a significant problem in dogs that try to ingest them. Large toads such as the marine toad (*Bufo marinus;* also known as *cane toads* or *giant neotropical toads*) carry a higher load of venom (Figure 8-35).

Mouthing of the toad by the dog releases toxin into the dog's mouth and contact with mucous membranes, leading to systemic absorption. Poisoned dogs develop excess salivation, anxiety, and vomiting almost immediately, and death can occur within 15 minutes after exposure. Treatment involves decontamination of the oral cavity through irrigation with water and forced emesis if a toad has been swallowed. Endoscopic or surgical removal of the toad may be necessary. If cardiac complications develop in a dog, the use of digoxin-specific Fab fragment should be weighed against its high cost.[10] Bradycardia can be treated with atropine (0.04 mg/kg IM, SC).

MARINE ENVENOMATIONS

Marine envenomations are more of a threat to human health than animal health (Table 8-21), although a case of a horse envenomation by a stingray has been reported.[16] A number of invertebrate and vertebrate organisms are capable of significant envenomations (Color Plate 8-15).

Coelenterates

Jellyfish can cause significant envenomations when encountered in the water or washed up on a beach. Jellyfish belong to two main groupings: Scyphozoa (true jellyfish) and Hydrozoa. Scyphozoa found in U.S. waters include stinging nettles, the chirodropid box jellyfish (*Chironex* spp.; Figure 8-36), and the purple jellyfish (*Pelagia noctiluca*). The class Hydrozoa includes both the Portuguese man-o-war (*Physalia physalis*) and fire coral. The types of jellyfish associated with fatal envenomations in the United States are the box jellyfish and Portuguese man-o-war. In Australia, jellyfish of the Carybdeid family cause a systemic syndrome called *Irukandji syndrome*, with catecholamine release leading to tachycardia, muscle cramps, hypertension, and cerebral edema.[1]

The venom of jellyfish is released by nematocysts—stinging organelles found in cells on the tentacles that are capable of stinging even when a tentacle has become detached (Figure 8-37). The venom is a complex mixture of proteins and polypeptide compounds that have antigenic and toxic effects. One of the toxic effects is disturbance of the sodium-potassium pump of cell membranes.[1] The effects of jellyfish stings range from local pain and rash to tissue necrosis (Color Plate 8-16), cardiac effects, fatal anaphylaxis, and other systemic reactions.

Treatment of jellyfish envenomation involves rinsing the skin with sea water to remove any nematocysts. If a box jellyfish sting is suspected, the skin can be decontaminated first with 5% acetic acid (vinegar) for 5 to 10 minutes to inactivate any undischarged nematocysts before attempting to remove tentacles (Figure 8-38).

For stings from other jellyfish, the skin can be decontaminated by flooding the skin with vinegar, baking soda, or ¼-strength ammonia. After decontamination, any remaining tentacles should be removed by scraping and the area should be treated again with the decontamination solution. Pain can be treated with topical lidocaine and allergic reactions controlled with antihistamines. For persistent pain, a hot shower may inactivate heat-labile venom.[1]

Anthozoa (Sea Anemones)

Sea anemones live in tidal pools and have tentacles that contain nematocysts. An anemone sting presents as an erythematous ring around a pale center. Such lesions usually resolve within 48 hours, although vesicles can form and ulceration can occur.

Larvae (Sea Bather's Eruption)

Larvae of certain jellyfish such as thimble jellyfish, as well as sea anemones, can get under a swimmer's bathing suit or a diver's wet suit. Trapped by the clothing, the nematocysts of the larvae release venom, create stinging and a rash known as *sea bather's eruption* that spares uncovered areas (Color Plate 8-17). Treatment is similar to that for jellyfish stings.

Echinodermata (Sea Urchins)

Sea urchin spines can inject venom if a person inadvertently makes contact with them. The spines can break off in the skin. Sea urchin venom contains heat-labile proteins that can have neurotoxic activity. Clinical manifestations include immediate pain at the site, followed in some cases by systemic effects

Table 8-21 ▪ Marine Envenomations in Human Beings

Organism	Geographic Distribution	Clinical Manifestations	Treatment
Scyphozoa (true jellyfish)	U.S.: stinging nettles, box jellyfish (*Chironex* spp.) purple jellyfish (*Pelagia noctiluca*)	*Local tissue effects*: stinging, redness, swelling, sometimes with necrosis Systemic envenomation with potentially fatal effects (box jellyfish)	Rinse area with sea water *Chironex suspected*: flood with vinegar *Others*: use vinegar, baking soda, or dilute ammonia,[1] then remove tentacles, immerse limb in hot water (45° C) to inactivate toxin; antivenin available for *Chironex* poisoning[13]
	Carybdeid species: Australia	Irukandji syndrome (catecholamine release—tachycardia, muscle cramps)	First-aid as above, supportive care
Hydrozoa (Portuguese man-o-war)	Atlantic, Indopacific ocean	Local tissue effects, stinging, redness, swelling, sometimes with necrosis Systemic envenomation with potentially fatal effects: GI distress, altered mental status, respiratory arrest	Decontaminate skin (vinegar, baking soda, dilute ammonia), remove tentacles,[1] immerse in hot water, pain control, other supportive measures including steroids for skin irritation[13]
Anthozoa (sea anemones)	Worldwide	Local pain, redness, swelling Larval forms (under bathing suits): sea bather's eruption: tingling, burning, pain, itching, redness (spares exposed areas)	Often no treatment required; topical steroids, pain control, remove clothing, shower, skin decontamination with vinegar, topical steroids if necessary for itching
Echinodermata (sea urchins)	Worldwide	Sea urchins associated with spine puncture wounds: pain, swelling at site of puncture Systemic envenomation can occur with multiple wounds	Hot shower, remove spines, antiinflammatory if necessary[1]
Fish	Stingrays: worldwide in oceans, some freshwater species South America: Weever fish Mediterranean and eastern Atlantic: lionfish (aquariums, introduced into the Atlantic), toadfish, scorpion fish (non-U.S.), stone fish (non-U.S.), catfish	Stingray most common source of fish envenomation in U.S.[1] Pain, tissue damage, systemic effects Wound infection can occur	Immerse stung limb in hot water (45° C) for 30 min Antivenin for stone fish sting, tetanus prophylaxis, surgery if necessary for retained fragments of spines, supportive care for systemic envenomation[13]
Sea snakes (Elapidae)	Subtropical and tropical waters of Indian Ocean and Pacific Ocean	Originally painless, then pain, paralysis, respiratory difficulty, myoglobinuria with rhabdomyolysis, and renal failure[13]	Pressure immobilization, antivenin, supportive measures (dialysis if necessary)

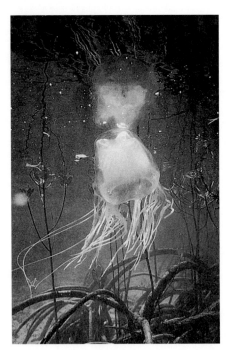

Figure 8-36 ■ Box jellyfish (*Chironex fleckeri*), swimming just beneath the surface of the water. (From Auerbach PS: *Wilderness medicine*, ed 5, Philadelphia, 2007, Mosby Elsevier. Courtesy John Williamson, MD.)

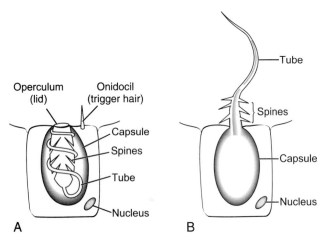

Figure 8-37 ■ Structure of a typical nematocyst from a cnidarian shown before (**A**) and after (**B**) discharge. (From Ford MD, Delaney KA, Ling L et al: *Clinical toxicology*, Philadelphia, 2001, Saunders.)

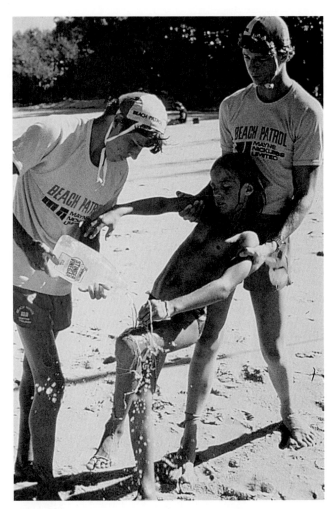

Figure 8-38 ■ Surf lifesavers pour vinegar on the leg of a simulated box jellyfish envenomation. Note how they restrain the victim's arms to prevent him from handling the harmful tentacles. (From Auerbach PS: *Wilderness medicine*, ed 5, Philadelphia, 2007, Mosby Elsevier. Courtesy John Williamson, MD.)

of the envenomation including weakness, muscle spasms, and difficulty breathing. Immersion in hot water may inactivate the venom. Spines should be removed with care because they can break easily. Surgical removal may be necessary if joints or nerves are involved. Tetanus prophylaxis should be given if indicated.

Poisonous Fish

Fish with significant venom include stingrays, lion fish, scorpion fish, stone fish, weever fish, and catfish. All of these fish species possess heat-labile toxins. The stingray has a barbed tail that can puncture skin and inject venom, while the other fish deliver venom injections through their spines. Although most marine fish envenomations occur in waters outside the United States, some of these poisonous fish, including lion fish (Color Plates 8-18 and 8-19) and catfish, are popular aquarium fish, and envenomations have occurred during handling of captive fish.

Clinical manifestations of fish envenomation can include severe local pain, nausea, vomiting and, in severe cases, cardiac arrhythmias. Allergic reactions can occur. Treatment of fish envenomations involves removal of the barb or spine and supportive care. Hot water may inactivate the toxin. An antivenin is available for stone fish envenomations, which tend to produce the most severe reactions.

Sea Snakes

Sea snakes are members of the Elapid family that are found in the Indian and Pacific oceans. They are perhaps the most abundant reptiles on earth, and all 52 species are venomous, with several species capable of severe envenomation. Their venom is highly toxic but the actual bite may be painless. Fishermen may be bitten when encountering sea snakes in nets. Signs and symptoms develop in minutes to hours and include dizziness, nausea, weakness, difficulty speaking or swallowing, pain, altered mental status, coma, and respiratory collapse. Rhabdomyolysis can occur with myoglobinuria and renal failure. Treatment involves pressure administration as for other Elapid bites (see Figure 8-33), supportive measures, administration of sea snake antivenin if available, and dialysis if necessary.[11]

References

1. Singletary EM, Rochman AS, Bodmer JC, et al. Envenomations. *Med Clin North Am.* 2005;89(6):1195–1224.
2. Peterson ME. Snake bite: pit vipers. *Clin Tech Small Anim Pract.* 2006;21(4):174–182.
3. Warrell DA. Treatment of bites by adders and exotic venomous snakes. *BMJ.* 2005;331(7527):1244–1247.
4. Rein JO. Exotic invertebrates—a health problem? [in Norwegian]. *Tidsskr Nor Laegeforen.* 2002;122(30):2896–2901.
5. Fitzgerald KT, Newquist KL. Poisonings in reptiles. *Vet Clin North Am Exot Anim Pract.* 2008;11(2):327–357.
6. Kuo HY, Hsu CW, Chen JH, et al. Life-threatening episode after ingestion of toad eggs: a case report with literature review. *Emerg Med J.* 2007;24(3):215–216.
7. McNally J, Boesen K, Boyer L. Toxicologic information resources for reptile envenomations. *Vet Clin North Am Exot Anim Pract.* 2008;11(2):389–401.
8. Lai MW, Klein-Schwartz W, Rodgers GC, et al. 2005 Annual report of the American Association of Poison Control Centers' national poisoning and exposure database. *Clin Toxicol (Phila).* 2006;44(6–7):803–932.
9. Rangan C. Emergency department evaluation and treatment for children with arthropod envenomations: immunologic and toxicologic considerations. *Clin Ped Emerg Med.* 2007;8(2):104–110.
10. Gupta RC. *Veterinary toxicology: basic and clinical principles.* New York: Academic Press; 2007.
11. Auerbach PS. *Wilderness medicine.* 5th ed. Philadelphia: Mosby Elsevier; 2007.
12. Chippaux J-P. Snake-bites: appraisal of the global situation. *Bull WHO.* 1998;76(5):515–524.
13. Junghanss T, Bodio M. Medically important venomous animals: biology, prevention, first aid, and clinical management. *Clin Infect Dis.* 2006;43(10):1309–1317.
14. Kahn CM, Line S. *The Merck veterinary manual.* 9th ed. Whitehouse Station, NJ: Merck; 2005.
15. Landolt GA. Management of equine poisoning and envenomation. *Vet Clin North Am Equine Pract.* 2007;23(1):31–47.
16. Riggs CM, Carrick JB, O'Hagan BJ, et al. Stingray injury to a horse in coastal waters off eastern Australia. *Vet Rec.* 2003;152(5):144–145.

HARMFUL ALGAL BLOOMS*

Julia Zaias, Lorraine C. Backer, and Lora E. Fleming

(ICD-10: Note: There is no specific ICD-10 code for many of the harmful algae blooms (HAB) illnesses; therefore the following injury codes should be considered as possible HAB illnesses)

E928 Other and Unspecified Environmental and Accidental Causes

E928.6 Environmental Exposure to Harmful Algae and Toxins; Algae Bloom NOS

- Blue-green algae bloom
- Brown tide
- Cyanobacteria bloom
- Florida red tide
- Harmful algae bloom
- *Pfiesteria piscicida*
- Red tide

E860-E869 Accidental Poisoning by Other Solid and Liquid Substances, Gases, and Vapors

E865 Accidental Poisoning from Poisonous Foodstuffs and Poisonous Plants

E865.1 Shellfish

E865.2 Other Fish

988 Toxic Effect of Noxious Substances Eaten as Food

988.0 Fish and Shellfish

E865 Accidental Poisoning from Poisonous Foodstuffs and Poisonous Plants

E865.2 Other Fish

*This work was funded in part by the following sources: the National Center for Environmental Health (NCEH); CDC; Florida Department of Health (FL DOH); Florida Department of Environmental Protection (FL DEP); Florida Red Tide Control and Mitigation; the National Science Foundation (NSF) and the National Institute of Environmental Health Sciences (NIEHS); Oceans and Human Health Center at the University of Miami Rosenstiel School (NSF 0CE0432368, NIEHS 1 P50 ES12736); and the NIEHS Aerosolized Florida Red Tide PO1 (P01 ES 10594).

V70-V82 Persons Without Reported Diagnosis Encountered During Examination and Investigation of Individuals and Populations

V82.5 Chemical Poisoning and Other Contamination, Poisoning from Contaminated Water Supply

Algal blooms are exuberant growths of microalgae such as dinoflagellates, diatoms, and cyanobacteria (blue-green algae; Color Plate 8-20). Harmful algal blooms (HABs) are intense blooms that cause harm to people, animals, or the local ecology, for example, by producing toxins or by inducing hypoxia. HABs occur in all aquatic environments, including freshwater, estuaries, and the oceans. In marine environments, they are also generally called *red tides,* although the causative organism, the color of the water, the particular threats, and subsequent effects of the HABs vary greatly.[1-4]

The primary effects of HABs on human beings and other animals occur through exposure to the toxins produced by the HAB-forming organisms. These toxins are some of the most potent natural substances known, creating untoward effects in nanogram to picogram doses. These toxins can target multiple organ systems, including the nervous system, the liver, the skin, and the respiratory tract. The HAB toxins are most infamous for their acute health effects that range from severe gastroenteritis to respiratory illness, and even death from respiratory paralysis. However, these toxins can also induce chronic illnesses, including long-term neurologic disease and genotoxic damage. Some of the toxins can act as tumor promoters, thus increasing cancer risks.[1-5]

Although it has been known for decades, if not centuries, that exposure to certain HAB toxins causes adverse health effects, studies designed to more fully characterize these acute and chronic effects have only recently begun. Until recently, it has been difficult to measure these potent toxins because even picogram doses can cause adverse health effects. Furthermore, the symptoms of the illnesses associated with exposure to HABs and their toxins are common symptoms associated with other acute diseases, including upper respiratory tract infections, food poisoning, and perhaps even chronic diseases, including chronic fatigue syndrome. Thus unless a physician or veterinarian considers HAB-related poisonings as part of a patient's differential diagnosis, it is likely that the event will be misdiagnosed and thus not identified as HAB related. For example, ciguatera fish poisoning is often diagnosed only as "food poisoning." Despite the difficulties in collecting accurate information about HAB disease occurrence and diagnoses, recent research suggests that there are measurable and increasing societal impacts from HABs manifested as adverse human and animal health events as well as adverse impacts on economic and social resources.[1-4,6]

From the point of view of the health care provider, the diagnosis, treatment, and reporting of HAB-related illnesses can be improved in a number of ways. One of the most important is increased communication across the human, public health, and animal medical care communities. For example, one of the most common first indicators of a toxin-producing bloom in freshwater lakes and ponds is a report of a dog dying shortly after swimming.[7]

Better communication between veterinarians and local public health officials could mean that not only are people protected from toxic blooms subsequent to observing animal morbidity or mortality, but also that local HAB data from monitoring and bloom detection activities can be shared with the veterinary, public health, and human health communities to protect animals and human beings in the community. This would allow veterinarians and physicians to have a high index of suspicion that HAB-related toxins may be the cause of illness in patients with symptoms related to an environmental exposure, such as swimming.[1] For example, in August 1984 in Montana, people who had been swimming in a lake contacted the local health department to report dead cattle in and near the lake and to ask about their own risks of becoming ill.[8] Investigation of the incident found that wind had concentrated a toxin-producing bloom of several cyanobacteria, *Anabena flos-aquae, Microcystis aeruginosa,* and *Aphanizomenon flos-aquae,* against the shore of the lake where the cattle had been drinking. Because people had been swimming in another part of the lake, their exposure was limited and no bloom-associated human illnesses were reported.

Although we are only beginning to understand the dynamics of bloom formation and senescence, we know enough to make some recommendations. For example, lakes and ponds with a low rate of flushing are likely to experience dense blooms during the summer when temperatures increase, particularly right after rains when excess nutrients can enter the water. Thus the medical and veterinary communities can remind patients and owners to limit exposure to water bodies with dense blooms during the summer.[7]

Key Points for Clinicians and Public Health Professionals

Public Health Professionals

- Educate human health and veterinary clinicians about the need to communicate about suspect cases.
- If animal cases of disease related to HABs are reported in the community, consider whether such cases could be sentinels for human risk.
- Coordinate with agricultural agencies monitoring for paralytic shellfish poisoning (PSP), neurotoxic shellfish poisoning (NSP), amnesic shellfish poisoning (ASP), diarrheic shellfish poisoning (DSP), ciguatera fish poisoning, and other HABs associated with contaminated seafood to educate the public about marine areas to avoid.
- Collect implicated seafood and human/animal samples for testing at FDA laboratories.
- Support policies that discourage the application of potential nutrients, such as fertilizers, in areas where runoff can affect the nearby aquatic environment.
- Educate the public about avoiding swimming in ponds or lakes with visible "pond scum."

- Monitor the National Oceanographic and Atmospheric Administration (NOAA) HAB Bulletin; see http://tidesandcurrents.noaa.gov/hab/bulletins.html.

Human Health Clinicians

- Have a high index of suspicion in persons who consume seafood or who are exposed to water bodies.
- Report suspected cases to state or local public health officials.
- Be aware of cases in the community of adverse effects of HABs in human beings and animals.

Veterinary Clinicians

- Discourage pet owners from allowing their animals to swim or drink water containing any pond scum.
- Report suspected cases to state or local public health officials.

PRIMARY PREVENTION

Primary prevention of HAB-related illness in human beings and other animals consists of preventing exposure to the HAB organisms and their toxins. In some cases, this is relatively easy if it is known that HAB organisms and their toxins are in the environment. For example, given the ubiquity of the cyanobacteria in all aquatic environments, it is reasonable to warn people that they, their pets, and other animals may be at risk of exposure to cyanobacteria and their toxins if they swim or drink from areas with obvious pond scums (even though not all pond scums are necessarily toxic). As another example, in areas with frequent HABs, such as coastal New England and the Pacific Northwest (from the dinoflagellate *Alexandrium* spp.) and the Gulf of Mexico (from the dinoflagellate *Karenia brevis*), local governments have instituted shellfish monitoring programs. If the organisms or toxins are detected in the shellfish beds at concentrations above specific limits, the beds are closed to commercial harvest. These closures are the primary prevention of cases of PSP and NSP, respectively. However, even when shellfish beds are closed to commercial harvesting, tourists or isolated ethnic groups may be unaware of these closures and unknowingly harvest toxic seafood.[1-4,9] In addition, HAB organisms can occur in previously unaffected geographic regions; even in areas where blooms are anticipated, local resources for expensive environmental monitoring may be limited or intermittent. Thus monitoring alone cannot protect public health.

Primary prevention is possible for companion animals, but it is particularly difficult for wild animals, even highly protected ones such as marine mammals. Millions of fish die every year in all aquatic environments from exposure to a range of HAB organisms and their toxins. Even more distressing are the acute and chronic illnesses and deaths of aquatic birds and marine mammals through the inadvertent or unavoidable consumption of HAB toxin–contaminated food and/or exposure to contaminated aerosols and water (Box 8-4). Some evidence also indicates that the combination of exposures to the HAB toxins, microbes (including antibiotic-resistant pathogens), and anthropogenic chemicals

---

BOX 8-4   *FLORIDA RED TIDE AND MARINE MAMMALS AS SENTINEL SPECIES*

Shellfish can bioaccumulate brevetoxins during Florida red tides. By contrast, until recently it was assumed that exposure to brevetoxins from Florida red tide instantly killed all fish by paralyzing their gills. Thus it was also assumed that exposure to brevetoxins would not occur through the fin-fish food web, and public health advisories did not recommend against eating fresh fish caught during established Florida red tides. However, between 2002 and 2004 in two separate but large mortality events, 34 Florida manatees (*Trichechus manatus latirostris*) and 107 bottlenose dolphins (*Tursiops truncatus*) died in waters off the Florida coast. In both of these unusual mortality events, extensive water surveys revealed only low concentrations of *Karenia brevis* and brevetoxins. However, analysis of the stomach contents of the dead animals detected high concentrations of brevetoxins in the fish and seagrasses eaten by the dolphins and manatees, respectively. This bioaccumulation was verified in laboratory experiments. Although most of the brevetoxins were found in the fish organs and not in the muscle (the part of the fish usually eaten by people), these findings suggest the need to revise the public health recommendations for eating fresh fish caught in waters affected by established Florida red tides. [10,11]

---

may adversely affect the health of marine mammals. Because people are exposed to a similar array of environmental contaminants, these marine mammals may serve as sentinels for potential human combination exposures and subsequent disease.[4,5]

Another component of primary prevention is identification and prevention of the actual causes of the blooms and of toxin production. There is no single reason why HAB organisms bloom and produce these potent natural toxins. Some organisms, such as the cyanobacteria, seem to bloom when high nutrient concentrations (such as nitrates or phosphates) exist in the aquatic environment; thus there is growing interest in preventing the dispersion of nutrients into waterways. Unfortunately, the environmental factors associated with blooming and toxin production for most HAB organisms are still unknown. However, even when solid evidence linking HAB formation with high nutrient concentrations is lacking, repeatedly affected communities may institute regulations (e.g., Ordinance 2007–062 Sarasota County, FL, Fertilizer and Landscape Management Code) and outreach programs to discourage the application of potential nutrients, such as fertilizers, in areas where runoff can affect the nearby aquatic environment.[12-14]

EARLY DETECTION, SURVEILLANCE, AND EDUCATION

In addition to ongoing and periodic environmental HAB monitoring programs (Figure 8-39), the oceanographic and public health communities continue to develop partnerships directed at the early detection and forecasting of HABs. These efforts were originally aimed at predicting local effects of Florida red tides, HABs that seem to be annual events (Box 8-5). These efforts have been extended to the early detection and forecasting of Florida red tides (*K. brevis*) in the Gulf of Mexico, red tides (*Alexandrium* and *Pseudo-Nitzschia*) in the Pacific Northwest, and now cyanobacteria in Florida; they

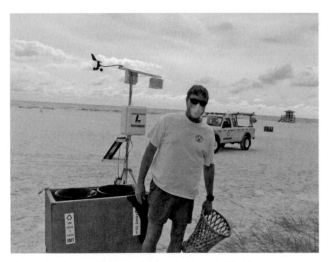

Figure 8-39 ■ Lifeguard during Florida red tide bloom. (Courtesy Florida Red Tide Research Group.)

BOX 8-5   *FLORIDA RED TIDE: HAB DETECTION, SURVEILLANCE, OUTREACH, AND EDUCATION*

Florida red tides are annual blooms of the marine dinoflagellate *Karenia brevis* in the Gulf of Mexico. The organism produces a group of highly potent natural neurotoxins called *brevetoxins*. Brevetoxins cause massive fish kills, neurotoxic shellfish poisoning, and respiratory distress, particularly in people with asthma. The public health challenge is to provide timely preventive information for Florida's dynamic resident and tourist populations about the exposures and health effects of Florida red tide.[15] In a unique collaboration, the Florida Department of Health (FDOH), CDC, NOAA, and public and private partners have established a linked network of public health information resources and exposure and disease surveillance on Florida red tide.

NOAA (coastwatch.noaa.gov/hab/bulletins_ns.htm) and Florida Fish and Wildlife Research Institute (FWRI) (telephone 866-300-9399) produce weekly reports of red tide locations based on remote sensing, oceanographic conditions, and extensive water monitoring for *K. brevis* available by phone and Internet.[16,17] Dead fish reports can be given and received via Florida FWRI Marine Fish Kill Hotline (telephone 800-636-0511). The South Florida Poison Information Center Aquatic Toxins Hotline (telephone 888-232-8635) provides 24-hour/day toll-free health information on exposure and health effects in human beings and other animals of Florida red tide and other HABs in multiple languages; the Hotline also reports cases to the FDOH and to the ongoing CDC Harmful Algal Bloom Incidence Surveillance System (HABISS). In addition, daily reports of respiratory irritation, dead fish, and other beach conditions from Gulf Coast beaches can be obtained from the Beach Conditions Reporting of the Mote Marine Laboratory (www.coolgate.mote.org/beachconditions).

Currently researchers are working to incorporate the respiratory irritation reports from the Aquatic Toxins Hotline and from the Beach Conditions Report into the NOAA HAB Bulletin for use in modeling and to provide an early warning system. The early-warning time frame is important because people in coastal areas may experience the respiratory irritation even before *K. brevis* is measured in the water or dead fish are found on the beaches.[18] In addition, the CDC, FDOH, Mote Marine Laboratory, FWRI, the University of Miami, and other collaborators have ongoing research studies into the causes of the Florida red tide and its potential human health effects (www.isurus.mote.org/niehsredtidestudy/). Finally, the FDOH (http://www.doh.state.fl.us/environment/community/aquatic/index.html), the grassroots organization, START (http://www.start1.com), and their partners have developed beach signage, museum displays, information cards, and a traveling exhibit to advertise this up-to-date information to Florida's tourists and residents. There is even education targeted specifically for health care providers on HAB exposure and health effects available through the Florida Poison Information Center (http://www.med.miami.edu/poisoncontrol/x57.xml).

are published as the NOAA HAB Bulletin (see link above). The NOAA HAB Bulletin uses environmental monitoring and oceanographic data to attempt to predict the location and future direction of HABs. The predictions based on these models are available to beach and resource managers and the public health community. In the future, these bulletins could be used to provide early warnings that threatening local HABs are likely to develop as well as track their progress.

In general, health care providers are not legally required to report HAB-related illnesses to local or state health agencies or to the CDC. However, marine toxin seafood diseases are reportable to state health agencies and the CDC as foodborne outbreaks if more than one person becomes ill. In addition, individual cases of ciguatera are reportable in Florida and Hawaii, cases of NSP are reportable in Florida, and cases of PSP are reportable in Washington, Oregon, California, Maine, and Massachusetts.

ACTIONS TO PREVENT EUTROPHICATION

It appears that worldwide, HABs are occurring more frequently, lasting longer, and occurring over larger geographic areas. This may be a response to the overall increase in nutrients and other anthropogenic inputs into all aquatic environments worldwide, global warming, growth of coastal populations, seafood harvesting, and international commerce. Part of this apparent increase could be ascribed to increased detection efforts. However, evidence suggests that these blooms are occurring in areas where they were previously undocumented; again, human beings may have inadvertently introduced these HAB organisms into new areas through mechanisms such as ship ballast water or the transport of living marine organisms.[4,5,13,14]

The medical, veterinary, and public health communities could address eutrophication (the increase in nutrients in water) by reminding patients about good environmental stewardship. For example, the health threats represented by certain local HABs may be mitigated if community members carefully consider their own behavior, including minimizing the use of lawn and garden fertilizers and taking care not to contaminate local streams and rivers with HAB-inducing nutrients.

CAUSATIVE AGENTS

The main effect of HABs on human beings and other animals seen by the medical community is through exposure to their natural toxins (Tables 8-22, 8-23, and 8-24). These toxins are some of the most potent natural substances known and can affect human beings and other animals in nanogram

Table 8-22 ■ HAB Toxin and Disease Information (Not Including Cyanobacteria)

	Saxitoxin	Brevetoxin	Okadaic Acid	Domoic Acid	Ciguatoxin
Associated diseases in human beings	PSP Certain puffer fish poisonings	NSP Aerosolized respiratory irritation Brevetoxin fish poisoning (?) Skin irritation (?)	DSP Cancer (?)	ASP	Ciguatera fish poisoning
Associated diseases in other animals	Fish deaths	Fish deaths Marine bird deaths Brevetoxicosis and deaths in marine mammals (dolphins, manatees) Dog morbidity and mortality (?)	Fish deaths Cancer (?)	Death and severe encephalopathy in sea lions Death in pelicans	Fish behavior changes (?) Illness and death in domestic animals
Main area with endemic disease	Temperate areas worldwide	Gulf of Mexico, southeast U.S. coast, New Zealand	Europe, Japan	East and west coasts of North America, South America, Northern Europe	Tropical coral reefs (although transported through trade and tourism throughout the world)
Associated transvectors	Bivalve shellfish Specific herbivorous fish and crabs	Bivalve shellfish Marine aerosols Fish species (?) Seaweed (?)	Bivalve shellfish	Bivalve shellfish Some fish species	Large reef fish (e.g., barracuda, grouper, red snapper, and amberjack)
Acute signs or symptoms/ conditions	*Gastrointestinal:* diarrhea, nausea, vomiting *Respiratory:* shortness of breath, progressing to paralysis *Cardiovascular:* arrhythmias, hypertension or hypotension *Neurologic:* paresthesias of mouth and lips, weakness, dysphasia, dysphonia	*Gastrointestinal:* diarrhea, nausea, vomiting *Cardiovascular:* arrhythmias, hypertension, or hypotension *Neurological:* paresthesias of mouth, lips, tongue, and throat; dizziness; reversal of hot and cold sensations *Other:* muscular aches, skin rashes With aerosol exposure, respiratory: shortness of breath particularly in asthmatics	*Gastrointestinal:* nausea, vomiting, diarrhea, abdominal pain *Other:* chills, headache	*Gastrointestinal:* diarrhea, vomiting, abdominal pain *Respiratory:* shortness of breath, progressing to paralysis *Cardiovascular:* arrhythmias, hypertension or hypotension *Neurological:* paresthesias (especially reversal of hot and cold sensation), burning in teeth or extremities, confusion, memory loss, disorientation, seizure, and coma	*1-6 hr postexposure:* *Gastrointestinal:* diarrhea, nausea, vomiting *Respiratory:* shortness of breath, progressing to paralysis *3 hr postexposure:* *Neurological:* paresthesias, reversal of hot/cold, pain, weakness, coma *1-5 days postexposure:* *Cardiovascular:* bradycardia, hypotension, increase in T-wave abnormalities (Note: Pacific ciguatera may present with only neurological symptoms)
Chronic signs or symptoms/ conditions	Unknown	Pneumonia, bronchitis (?)	Unknown Possible carcinogen	Amnesia (?)	Paresthesias, extreme fatigue

Continued

Table 8-22 ■ HAB Toxin and Disease Information (Not Including Cyanobacteria)—cont'd

	Saxitoxin	Brevetoxin	Okadaic Acid	Domoic Acid	Ciguatoxin
Treatment	Supportive care Possibly respiratory support	Supportive care Possibly respiratory support Possibly antihistamines, bronchodilators for respiratory symptoms after aerosol exposure Possibly brevenal, particularly for brevetoxicosis in marine mammals Possibly IV mannitol for NSP	Supportive care	Supportive care, Possibly respiratory support especially for elderly and people with underlying chronic diseases such as renal disease	IV mannitol Supportive care Tricyclic antidepressants for chronic symptoms (?) Food avoidance (alcohol, caffeine, nuts, chocolate) (?) Possibly brevenal (?)
Incubation time	5-30 min	30 min-24 hr	<24 hr	<24 hours	<24 hr
Duration	Days	Days	Days	Weeks to years (?)	Weeks to months to years (?)
Death rate	1%-14%	0%	0%	3%	0.1%- 12%
Toxin-producing organism	Dinoflagellates: *Gymnodinium catenatum, Pyrodinium bahamense* var. *compressum, Alexandrium* spp.	Dinoflagellate: *Karenia brevis* (formerly *Gymnodinium breve*)	Dinoflagellates: *Dinophysis* spp., *Prorocentrum lima*	Diatoms: *Pseudo-Nitzschia* spp.	Epibenthic dinoflagellates: *Gambierdiscus toxicus*, possibly *Ostreopsis* spp, *Coolia* spp, or *Prorocentrum* spp
Molecular mechanism(s)	Na+ channel blocker	Na$^+$ channel activator	Phosphorylase phosphatase inhibitor	Glutamate receptor agonist	Na$^+$, Ca^{++} channel activators

Data from Backer LC, Schurz-Rogers H, Fleming LE et al: Marine phycotoxins in seafood. In Dabrowski W, Sikorski ZE, editors: *Toxins in food*, Boca Raton, FL, 2005, CRC Press.

Table 8-23 ■ Cyanobacteria Responsible for Toxic Freshwater HABs Associated With Human Illness[3,19,23]

Toxin	Toxicologic End Points*	Organisms	Acute Effect	Mechanism of Action	Signs and Symptoms of Intoxication	Therapy
Anatoxin-a	1. 250 µg/kg 2. 2.5 mg/kg/day (mouse, short-term studies) 3. 0.5 mg/kg/day (rat, subchronic studies) 4. 3×10^{-3} mg/kg/day	Anabaena flos-aquae Anabaena spiroides Anabaena circinalis Oscillatoria Aphanizomenon Cylindrospermopsis	Neurotoxicity	Blocks postsynaptic depolarization Mimics acetylcholine	Progression of muscle fasciculations, decreased movement, abdominal breathing, cyanosis, convulsions, death (animals); also opisthotonos (S-shaped neck) (birds)	No known therapy Respiratory support may allow time for detoxification and respiratory recovery
Anatoxin-a	40 µg/kg	Anabaena flos-aquae	Neurotoxicity[2]	Anticholinesterase	Hypersalivation, mucoid nasal discharge, tremors, fasciculations, ataxia, diarrhea, recumbency (pigs); also regurgitation, paresis, opisthotonos, clonic seizures (ducks); lacrimation, hypersalivation, urination, defecation, death from respiratory arrest (mice); also red-pigmented tears (rats)	Has not been thoroughly investigated
Cylindrospermopsin	1. 2100 µg/kg[1] 24 hr LD$_{50}$ 200 µg/kg[2] 5-6 d LDµ 2. 0.15 µg/kg/day (mouse) 3. 0.05 mg/kg/day (short-term studies, mouse liver); 0.3 mg/kg/day (short-term studies, mouse spleen) 4. 3×10^{-5} mg/kg/day	Cylindrospermopsis racborskii	Hepatotoxicity Chromosome breakage, aneuploidy	Inhibition of protein, phosphatases Cumulative toxicity	Huddling, anorexia, slight diarrhea, gasping, respiration (mice) Enlarged liver, malaise, anorexia, vomiting, headache (human beings)	Has not been investigated
Microcystins	1. 45-1000 µg/kg 2. 3 µg/kg (nasal lesions, mouse) 3. 200-500 µg/kg (short-term studies, mouse) 4. 6×10^{-6} mg/kg/day	Microcystis aeruginosa Microcystis viridis Microcystis wesenbergii Anabaena	Hepatotoxicity	Alterations of actin microfilaments, destruction of parenchymal cells, lethal hemorrhage or hepatic insufficiency Inhibition of protein phosphatases, tumor-promoter activity	Weakness, reluctance to move, anorexia, pallor of extremities and mucous membranes (animals) mental derangement (animals) Survivors (animals) may experience photosensitization Elevated alanine amino-transferase (mice, human beings) Elevated gamma-glutamyl transpeptidase (human beings) Embryo lethality, teratogenicity (rats)	Powdered charcoal, cholestyramine, therapeutic support

Continued

Table 8-23 ■ Cyanobacteria Responsible for Toxic Freshwater HABs Associated With Human Illness—cont'd

Toxin	Toxicologic End Points*	Organisms	Acute Effect	Mechanism of Action	Signs and Symptoms of Intoxication	Therapy
Nodularin	1. 30-50 µg/kg	*Nodularia spumigena*	Hepatotoxicity	Inhibition of protein phosphatases, tumor-promoter activity	Skin and eye irritation (dermal contact, human beings)	Therapeutic support
Saxitoxin, neosaxitoxin	1. 10-30 µg/kg	*Aphanizomenon flos-aquae* (New Hampshire, U.S.) *Anabaena circinalis* (Australia)	Neurotoxicity	Sodium channel blocker	Incoordination, recumbency, respiratory failure (animals), death; paresthesia and numbness of lips, mouth within 30 min to 3 hr, extending to face, neck, extremities, motor weakness, incoordination, respiratory and muscular paralysis (human beings)	Activated charcoal, artificial respiration

*1. LD$_{50}$ (i.p. mouse) of pure toxin; 2. NOAEL; 3. LOAEL; 4. Estimated short-term RfD.

Table 8-24	Comparative Effects of Selected Harmful Algal Bloom Toxins in Humans and Other Animals		
Species	**Route of Exposure**	**Clinical Manifestations**	**Laboratory Findings**
Brevetoxins			
Human beings	Ingestion	NSP	With NSP, may have brevetoxin metabolites in urine by ELISA
	Inhalation	Shortness of breath	Decreased FEV$_1$
	Skin	Rash, hives	
Dolphins, manatees	Inhalation, ingestion	Neurological signs including muscle fasciculations, incoordination, and inability to maintain righting reflex (e.g., listing in water)	Congestion, edema, and catarrhal inflammation of nasopharyngeal, tracheal, and bronchial mucosa; pulmonary congestion; nonsuppurative leptomeningitis
			May have brevetoxin metabolites in urine by ELISA
Seabirds		Weakness, reluctance to fly, slumping of head, broad-based stance, clear nasal discharge, excessive lacrimation, diarrhea, dyspnea, tachypnea, tachycardia, decreased blood pressure, hypothermia, dehydration, diminished reflexes, seizures, death	Pulmonary hemorrhage and congestion, hepatic and splenic hemosiderosis, cholangitis, nephritis
Cyanobacterial Toxins			
Human beings	Ingestion	Acute hepatitis, kidney failure, death	Increased liver function tests
	Inhalation	Respiratory irritation	
	Skin	Rash, hives, blistering	
Cattle	Ingestion	*Microcystin and nodularins:* diarrhea, vomiting, piloerection, weakness, pallor, death	Toxins in tissues
			Microcystin and nodularins: hepatic congestion, hepatitis, and hemorrhage; hemorrhagic shock; hypoglycemia, hyperkalemia, bilirubinemia
		Anatoxin, saxitoxin: muscle weakness, paralysis, dyspnea, hypersalivation, death	Anatoxin, saxitoxin: few if any
		Lyngbyatoxin, aphysiatoxin: skin, eye, and respiratory irritation	Lyngbyatoxin, aphysiatoxin: dermatitis
		Clindrospermopsin: acute death	
Ducks, eagles	Ingestion	β-methylamino-L-alanine (BMAA) (?): Avian vacuolar myelinopathy	Vacuolar myelinopathy (?)
			BMAA in tissues (?)
Domoic Acid			
Human beings	Ingestion	*Acute:* vomiting, diarrhea, seizures, lethargy, death	Neuronal necrosis
		Chronic: memory loss (?)	
Sea lions	Ingestion	*Acute:* seizures, lethargy, inappetence, vomiting, muscle twitching, blindness, blepharospasm, abnormal behaviors, abortion, stillbirths, premature births, death	Neuronal necrosis, astrocytosis; abnormal EEG, MRI
			Toxin found in placenta and fetus
		Chronic: seizures/epilepsy (1 yr later)	
Pelicans	Ingestion	Disorientation, ataxia, agitation, difficulty swimming, inability to right themselves, death	Neuronal necrosis, astrocytosis

EEG, Electroencephalogram; *ELISA,* enzyme-linked immunosorbent assay; *FEV$_1$,* forced expiratory volume in the first second; *BMAA,* β-methylamino-L-alanine; *MRI,* magnetic resonance imaging.

to picogram doses (Color Plate 8-21 and Figure 8-40). In general, these are tasteless, odorless, and very stable toxins that are highly resistant to heat, acid, and freezing. Thus they cannot be eliminated from foods with normal preparation and storage methods, and the toxin-contaminated food appears to be normal, reportedly smelling and tasting delicious when consumed.

ROUTES OF EXPOSURE AND METABOLIC FATE

Exposure to HABs can occur through a variety of routes, including skin contact, eating contaminated food, drinking contaminated water, and inhaling aerosolized HAB toxins. Some HAB toxins can bioconcentrate in the aquatic food web, exposing top predators to particularly high doses. For example, the

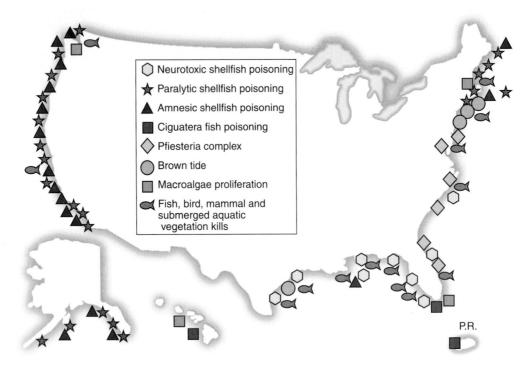

Figure 8-40 ■ Sites and types of harmful algal blooms along U.S. coast. (NOTE: This figure is a summary of verified HABs in marine waters and does not capture HABs verified in the Great Lakes or in inland waters; see Color Plate 8-20). (From Mandell GL, Bennett JE, Dolin R: *Principles and practice of infectious diseases*, ed 6, New York, 2005, Churchill Livingstone.)

ciguatoxins associated with ciguatera fish poisoning bioconcentrate in the food web, making barracuda and other top-reef predators some of the most highly toxic fish.[19] Another example of a HAB toxin that is bioconcentrated is β-methylamino-L-alanine (BMAA), a nonprotein amino acid elaborated by many cyanobacterial species. BMAA is also found in the cycad plant, which is consumed by fruit bats in Guam. Both cycads and fruit bats are eaten by the Chamorro people of Guam, among whom a high number have exhibited degenerative neurologic symptoms. Subsequent studies of these individuals and others support the hypothesis that BMAA may be associated with amyotrophic lateral sclerosis–parkinsonism dementia complex (ALS/PDC). In South Carolina, BMAA elaborated by cyanobacteria is believed to be transferred through water plants eaten by ducks and subsequently to eagles that ate the ducks. Both bird species have developed avian vacuolar myelinopathy (AVM)[20–22] (R. Bidigare, University of Hawaii, personal communication, 2008).

Several HAB toxins are lipophilic and thus pass easily through the blood-brain barrier (including ciguatoxin, brevetoxin, and domoic acid). They are stored in fatty tissues and, during pregnancy, may be mobilized to pass directly into the fetus through the placental barrier. Newborns may be exposed through breast milk.[1,3,19,23]

GROUPS AT RISK

Human beings are exposed to HABs and their toxins through recreational activities (swimming and boating) and occupations (such as lifeguards or fishermen) and through drinking water and possibly irrigation water derived from contami-

nated sources. People who live in coastal areas with aerosolized HABs (such as *K. brevis* and its brevetoxins), particularly those with underlying respiratory diseases, are also at risk. Many of the known HAB toxins are neurotoxins; therefore persons with underlying neurologic disease and infants and young children may be at greater risk from these toxins. Consumers of seafood derived from all aquatic environments are at risk for exposure to HAB toxins. In particular, tourists traveling to areas where HABs are endemic and isolated racial and ethnic groups who are unaware of local HAB-related risks may be particularly at risk for exposure and illness.[1,4]

Domestic animals and pets are at particular risk from exposure to cyanobacterial toxins by dermal contact and by drinking contaminated water from streams, ponds, and lakes.[7] As previously discussed, through consumption of contaminated seagrasses, seafood, and possibly through respiratory contact, marine mammals, marine birds, and fish are particularly vulnerable to coastal HABs that may last for months in large geographic areas (see Box 8-4). Domestic animals are also at risk from marine HABs. For example, dog morbidity and possibly mortality associated with Florida red tide have been reported (J. Landsberg, Florida Fish and Wildlife Commission, personal communication, 2008).

TOXICITY IN HUMAN BEINGS

Skin toxicity, ranging from mild irritation to hives to blistering, has been reported with direct contact with almost all the HAB toxins in contaminated water (Color Plate 8-22). However, this phenomenon has not been well studied and might actually be due to the lipopolysaccharides of some HAB organisms.[1,4]

Many HAB-related illnesses, such as ciguatera fish poisoning and the shellfish-associated diseases (such as PSP, NSP, ASP, and DSP; see Tables 8-22, 8-23, and 8-24), are diagnosed simply as "food poisoning" because victims present with significant GI symptoms within minutes to hours of consuming implicated seafood and usually have no fever. However, because these illnesses have a neurologic component, they may be distinguished from microbial food poisoning or seafood allergy by the concomitant or subsequent onset of neurologic symptoms such as paresthesias and confusion. Other presenting signs and symptoms (also neurologic in origin) can be cardiovascular (including labile hypotension and arrhythmias) and respiratory (including respiratory depression), and may require intensive care unit and respiratory support for several days.[1,4,9,19]

Most HAB toxin–related illnesses present as acute, self-limiting cases of disease. However, there is evidence that ciguatera fish poisoning and possibly ASP produce lingering neurologic symptoms in human beings (i.e., paresthesias and possibly short-term memory loss) that may last from weeks to months and even years.[1,19,24] Although controversial, it is possible that exposure through contaminated food to BMAA may lead to an increased risk for ALS, Parkinson's disease, and even Alzheimer's dementia. However, although the genes needed to produce BMAA have been found in every species of cyanobacteria tested so far, it is not clear that all cyanobacteria produce the toxin. Thus it is not known whether the general population could be exposed via the food web, whether this exposure is limited to specific groups, or whether health effects occur only in sensitive subpopulations.[20,21]

A number of illness outbreaks associated with exposure to cyanobacterial toxins in drinking water have been reported in wild animals, domestic animals, and people. Severe GI illness associated with acute and chronic liver disease and subsequent kidney disease has been reported in people exposed to cyanobacterial toxins in drinking water. In more than one episode in Brazil, dialysis patients received microcystin-contaminated dialysis water. The affected patients experienced severe acute hepatitis and most died. It is important to remember that these dialysis patients received an intraperitoneal dose that was equivalent to the mouse oral median lethal dose (LD$_{50}$).[25]

More recently, upper and lower respiratory tract symptoms (such as cough, shortness of breath, or chest tightness) have been associated with exposure to aerosolized Florida red tide brevetoxins, particularly among those with underlying respiratory disease such as asthma. Some evidence indicates that prolonged exposure to these aerosolized toxins, particularly among coastal residents, is associated with increased emergency department admissions for respiratory illness (including pneumonia, bronchitis, and asthma).[26-28] There have also been anecdotal reports of respiratory illness in persons exposed to aerosols from irrigation systems using pond water with active algae blooms (John Burns, personal communication, 2005).

Several HAB toxins are at least in vitro carcinogens: okadaic acid and microcystin. There is some research to suggest that chronic exposure to microcystin in contaminated drinking water may be associated with an increased risk for hepatocellular carcinoma, whereas okadaic acid may be associated with increased prevalence of tumors in shellfish, which one author speculated might be relevant to an increased risk of tumors in human beings who consume toxin-contaminated seafoods.[1,4,29]

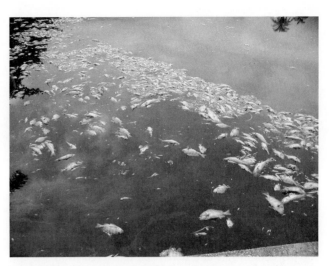

Figure 8-41 ■ Fish kill during Florida red tide bloom. (Courtesy Florida Red Tide Research Group.)

TOXICITY IN ANIMALS

Wildlife

Reports of livestock and wild animals poisoned by toxic cyanobacteria after drinking from small ponds have been in the veterinary literature for years. Affected animals showed neurological signs or died from acute effects.[30] Animals appear to be more frequently and more seriously poisoned by freshwater HABs than are human beings. This may be because thirsty animals are more likely to drink water that people would not use because of foul taste, smell, or presence of surface scum.[31,32] In addition, grooming and licking of their coats also contributes to the toxin load ingested by dogs and other animals.

The most dramatic toxicity in animals from the HAB toxins is the acute death of millions of fish exposed to marine HABs producing saxitoxin or brevetoxins. The first sign of a red tide event along the Florida Gulf coast can be dead fish washing ashore (Figure 8-41). Exposure to these neurotoxins results in loss of equilibrium, erratic swimming behaviors, and rapid respiratory paralysis.[10,33]

Marine seabird deaths (including species such as pelicans, cormorants, mergansers, and scaup) have been reported during HAB events from seabirds inhaling toxic aerosols or eating contaminated fish.[34,35] Typical clinical signs included weakness, reluctance to fly, clear nasal discharge, excessive lacrimation, dyspnea, diminished reflexes, ataxia, seizures, and death. The majority of bird deaths in these events were ascribed to toxicity from the consumption of contaminated fish; many of the affected cormorants were juveniles; as inexperienced foragers, they may have eaten dead or dying fish. This event suggests trophic biotoxin transfer of HAB toxins.[34]

The deaths of numerous marine mammals (e.g., bottlenose dolphins, manatees, sea lions, whales) have been ascribed, at least in part, to intoxication with HAB toxins after both acute and chronic exposure over many years. More recently, with improved toxicologic and necropsy testing, individual and group deaths of many marine mammals have been linked to

HAB toxins, particularly those that accumulate through the food web.[10,11,36,37] It is now clear that toxins such as domoic acid and brevetoxins can enter and be transmitted through the food web (including via seagrasses and fish), be bioconcentrated within the marine mammals over time, and induce subsequent neurological illness and death even when there is not an active bloom (see Box 8-4).[10]

Particularly dramatic episodes of severe neurological illness and death have been reported in California sea lions after they ate fish contaminated with domoic acid. In addition to acute effects of intoxication (e.g., ataxia, seizures, abortion, stillbirths, premature births, death), chronic effects (e.g., seizures that continued to occur more than 1 year after exposure) have been documented in sea lions exposed to domoic acid at relatively low levels over a long period.[38] In addition, both brevetoxins and domoic acid have been shown to cross the placenta in rats and have been recovered from sea lion fetuses and placental tissues.[23,36]

Data from marine mammal strandings during HAB events have also indicated that intoxication may be either a function of current immune status of the animal (i.e., that the animal was immunosuppressed or ill when exposed) or may in fact cause immune suppression. Experimental intratracheal exposure of sheep with purified brevetoxin PbTx-3 demonstrated decreased phagocytic activity by alveolar macrophages in vitro.[39] These findings, in combination with the documentation of lymphoid depletion and uptake of brevetoxin in lymphoid cells from exposed dolphins and manatees in the wild, are suggestive of immune system dysfunction associated with brevetoxin poisoning in marine mammals.[39]

Finally, as noted, it is now believed that consumption of BMAA-contaminated water plants may be the cause of the AVM noted in water fowl and eagles that feed on these waterfowl. However, research on the exposures and acute and chronic health effects of BMAA in human beings and other animals is in its infancy (R. Bidigare, University of Hawaii, personal communication, 2008).[20–22]

Companion Animals

There have been some reports of dogs becoming gravely ill after consuming dead fish they found on a marine beach. In one case, brevetoxins were detected in the dog's urine using ELISA (J. Landsberg, Florida Fish and Wildlife Commission, personal communication, 2008). However, another possible explanation of the dogs' responses is secondary bacterial growth and subsequent bacterial toxin production in the dead fish. Despite the lack of documentation of health effects on pet birds and other animals in areas known for repeated aerosol exposure to toxins (e.g., gulf coast of Florida), pets may be repeatedly exposed to low levels of aerosolized toxin. Clinical veterinarians should be aware of HAB events in their area as this can be a differential diagnosis or compounding factor in pet illnesses.

DIAGNOSIS

The most important aspect of diagnosing HAB-related illness in human beings and other animals is to consider the possibility of HAB toxin exposure and illness in the first place. Many

of these illnesses are misdiagnosed or completely unidentified because of the relatively common presenting signs and symptoms and the specialized toxicologic testing required to make a definitive diagnosis. In addition, the exposure history is crucial, particularly exposure to possibly contaminated aquatic environments and seafood. Reporting suspected HAB-related illnesses to local health authorities may prevent additional cases in other people or animals by alerting local officials to destroy the contaminated seafood or test local water bodies.[1,4]

It is important in all cases of a suspected HAB-related illness to obtain a sample of the contaminated food or water for testing. For example, in the case of suspected HAB food poisoning, a representative from the state or local health agency should obtain a sample of the suspected seafood. The sample should be handled and shipped appropriately for analysis by specialized laboratories such as the FDA. Establishing the link between illness and a contaminated source of exposure is critical not only in terms of the appropriate diagnosis of the etiology in the particular patient, but also in potentially preventing additional cases of illness.[4,19]

In the case of affected animals, stomach contents and tissue samples should also be collected for testing for the HAB toxins. Testing can be done through one of the specialized laboratories at the NOAA or the FDA.[19]

MANAGEMENT OF HAB TOXICITY

No specific antidotes for HAB-related toxins are currently available for general use. In addition, few specific treatments have been identified for HAB-related illnesses. Thus, in general, the treatment of HAB-related illnesses is supportive in both human beings and other animals. Obviously, preventing any additional exposure to the toxins for the patient and for other human beings and animals through the original transvector or environmental pathway is part of the management of and public health response to HAB-related illnesses.[1]

Treatment in Human Beings

In the case of the acute neurological diseases such as PSP, ASP, NSP, and ciguatera fish poisoning, it is important to be aware of the possible need for intensive care and respiratory support, particularly in the first few days of illness.[1,8,19]

Almost no formal research has been conducted regarding the treatment of HAB diseases. Intravenous mannitol (1 g/kg) has been evaluated in two small randomized trials and several case series of ciguatera fish poisoning. This treatment was efficacious in decreasing or even eliminating the symptoms and in preventing the chronic neurological symptoms when used within a few days of exposure. Of note, because brevetoxins and ciguatoxin are structurally very similar, it is possible that intravenous administration of mannitol may also be efficacious for the treatment of acute NSP. Many other medications for ciguatera poisoning have been tried but without appropriate randomized evaluation, such as tricyclic antidepressants and selective serotonin reuptake inhibitors. Anecdotally, avoidance of certain foods (i.e., alcohol, caffeine, nuts, chocolate, and fish) and maintenance of hydration seems to speed recovery from the chronic neurological symptoms.[19]

Based on a sheep model of human asthma, albuterol, diphenhydramine, and corticosteroids have been demonstrated to prevent and mitigate the onset of the bronchoconstriction associated with exposure to aerosolized brevetoxins.[40,41] Recently a natural antagonist to brevetoxin, brevenal, has been demonstrated to prevent the onset of bronchoconstriction caused by inhalation of aerosolized brevetoxins in asthmatic sheep. It is also possible that brevenal may be efficacious in the treatment of ciguatera fish poisoning given the structural similarity between the brevetoxins and ciguatoxin (D. Baden, UNC–Wilmington, personal communication, 2008).[40]

Treatment in Animals

As for human beings, treatment of affected animals involves treating signs and removing the source of exposure. Data from marine mammal deaths during HAB events and from laboratory animal studies indicate that at least brevetoxicosis may be responsible for some immunosuppression[39,42]; thus animals under treatment should be given prophylactic antibiotics for secondary bacterial infections. Restoration of appropriate hydration, fluid support to flush toxins, and medications to treat neurological signs are the most important treatment modalities.

Recently brevenal has been approved as a specific antidote by the FDA for use on a compassionate basis in marine mammals diagnosed with brevetoxicosis. Based on the biologic activity of brevetoxins and brevenal, the drug is likely to be most effective at the very early stages of intoxication (D. Baden, UNC–Wilmington, personal communication, 2008).[40] However, until there is a source of sufficient quantities of brevenal, its use will be limited.

References

1. Fleming LE, Backer L, Rowan A. The epidemiology of human illnesses associated with harmful algal blooms. In: Baden D, Adams D, eds. *Neurotoxicology handbook*. vol. 1. Towata, NJ: Humana Press; 2002.
2. Backer LC, Fleming LE, Rowan AD, et al. Epidemiology and public health of human illnesses associated with harmful marine algae. In: Hallegraeff GM, Anderson DM, Cembella AD, eds. *IOC manual on harmful marine microalgae*. Geneva: UNSECO; 2003.
3. Backer LC, Schurz-Rogers H, Fleming LE, et al. Marine phycotoxins in seafood. In: Dabrowski W, Sikorski ZE, eds. *Toxins in food*. Boca Raton, FL: CRC Press; 2005.
4. Backer LC, Fleming LE. Epidemiologic tools to investigate oceans and public health. In: Walsh PJ, Smith SL, Fleming LE, et al., eds. *Oceans and human health: risks and remedies from the sea*. New York: Academic Press; 2008.
5. Backer LC, McGillicuddy DJ. Harmful algal blooms: at the interface between coastal oceanography and human health. *Oceanography*. 2006;19:94–106.
6. Hoagland P, Anderson DM, Kaoru Y, et al. The economic effects of harmful algal blooms in the United States: estimates, assessment issues, and information needs. *Estuaries*. 2002;25(4b):819–837.
7. Backer LC. Cyanobacterial harmful algal blooms (CyanoHABs): Developing a public health response. *Lake and Reservoir Management*. 2002;18(1):20–31.
8. Spoerke DG, Rumack BH. Blue-green algae poisoning. *J Emerg Med*. 1985;2:353–355.
9. Watkins SM, Reich A, Fleming LE, et al. Neurotoxic shellfish poisoning. *Marine Drugs (special issue on marine toxins)*. 2008;6:431–455.
10. Flewelling LJ, Naar JP, Abbott JP, et al. Red tides and marine mammal mortalities. *Nature*. 2005;435:755–756.
11. Naar JP, Flewelling LJ, Lenzi A, et al. Brevetoxins, like ciguatoxins, are potent ichthyotoxic neurotoxins that accumulate in fish. *Toxicon*. 2007;50:707–723.
12. Viviani R. Eutrophication, marine biotoxins, human health. *Sci Total Environ*. 1992;S1:631.
13. Brand LE, Compton A. Long-term increase in *Karenia brevis* abundance along the southwest Florida coast. *Harmful Algae*. 2006;7:232–252.
14. Vargo GA, Heil CA, Fanninge KA, et al. Nutrient availability in support of *Karenia brevis* on the central west Florida shelf: what keeps *Karenia* blooming? *Cont Shelf Res*. in press.
15. Reich A, Backer LC, Kirkpatrick B, et al. Public health and Florida red tide: from remote sensing to poison information (published abstract). In: *Am Public Health Association Annual Meeting*. Boston, MA, 2006.
16. Stumpf RP, Culver ME, Tester PA, et al. Monitoring *Karenia brevis* blooms in the Gulf of Mexico using satellite ocean color imagery and other data. *Harmful Algae*. 2003;2:147–160.
17. Fisher KM, Allen AL, Keller HM, et al. *Annual report of the Gulf of Mexico Harmful Algal Bloom Operational Forecast System (GOM HAB-OFS). NOAA Technical Report NOS CO-OPS 047*. Silver Spring, MD: NOAA.
18. Kirkpatrick B, Currier R, Nierenberg K, et al. Florida red tide and human health: a pilot beach conditions reporting system to minimize human exposure. *Sci Total Environ*. 2008;402(1):1–8.
19. Friedman MA, Fleming LE, Fernandez M, et al. Ciguatera fish poisoning: treatment, prevention and management. *Marine Drugs* (special issue on marine toxins), in press.
20. Cox PA, Banack SA, Murch SJ. Biomagnification and Chamorro neurodegenerative disease. *PNAS*. 2003;100:13380–13383.
21. Cox PA, Banack SA, Murch SJ, et al. Diverse taxa of cyanobacteria produce Beta-N-methylamino-L-alanine, a neurotoxic amino acid. *PNAS*. 2005;102(14):5074–5078.
22. Rao SD, Banack SA, Cox PA, et al. BMAA selectively injures motor neurons via AMPA/kainate receptor activation. *Exp Neurol*. 2006;201(1):244–252.
23. Benson JM, Gomez AP, Statom GL, et al. Placental transport of brevetoxin-3 in CD1 mice. *Toxicon*. 2006;48:1018–1026.
24. Friedman M, Levin BE. Neurobehavioral effects of harmful algal bloom (HAB) toxins: a critical review. *J Int Neuropsychol Soc*. 2005;11:331–338.
25. Azevedo SMFO, Carmichael WW, Jochimsen EM, et al. Human intoxication by microcystins during renal dialysis treatment in Caruaru—Brazil. *Toxicology*. 2002;181–182:441–446.
26. Fleming LE, Backer LC, Baden DG. Overview of aerosolized Florida red tide toxins: exposures and effects. *Environ Health Perspect*. 2005;113:618–620.
27. Kirkpatrick B, Fleming LE, Backer LC, et al. Environmental exposures to Florida red tides: effects on emergency room respiratory diagnoses admissions. *Harmful Algae*. 2006;5:526–533.
28. Fleming LE, Kirkpatrick B, Backer LC, et al. aerosolized red tide toxins (Brevetoxins) and asthma. *Chest*. 2007;131:187–194.
29. Landsberg J. Neoplasms and biotoxins in bivalves: is there a connection? *J Shellfish Res*. 1996;15(2):203.
30. Briand JF, Jacquet S, Bernard C, et al. Health hazards for terrestrial vertebrates from toxic cyanobacteria in surface water ecosystems. *Vet Res*. 2003;361–377.
31. Senior VE. Algal poisoning in Saskatchewan. *Can J Comp Med*. 1960;24:26–40.
32. Codd GA, Edwards C, Beattie KA, et al. Fatal attraction to cyanobacteria? *Nature*. 1992;359:110–111.
33. Steidinger KA, Landsberg JH, Tomas CR. *Harmful algal blooms in Florida*. Submitted to Florida's Harmful Algal Bloom Task Force by the Harmful Algal Bloom Task Force Technical Advisory Group 1999.
34. Kreuder C, Mazet JAK, Bossart GD, et al. Clinicopathologic features of suspected brevetoxicosis in double-crested cormorants (*Phalacrocorax auritus*) along the Florida Gulf coast. *J Zoo Wildl Med*. 2002;33:8–15.
35. Beltran AS, Palafox-Uribe M, Grajales-Montiel J, et al. Sea bird mortality at Cabo San Lucas, Mexico: evidence that toxic diatom blooms are spreading. *Toxicon*. 1997;35:447–453.
36. Gulland FM, Haulena M, Fauquier D, et al. Domoic acid toxicity in California sea lions (*Zalophus californianus*): clinical signs, treatment and survival. *Vet Rec*. 2002;150:475–480.
37. Lefebvre KA, Powell CL, Busman M, et al. Detection of domoic acid in northern anchovies and California sea lions associated with an unusual mortality event. *Nat Toxins*. 1999;7:85–92.

38. Goldstein T, Mazet JA, Zabka K, et al. Novel symptomatology and changing epidemiology of domoic acid toxicosis in California sea lions (*Zalophus californianus*): an increasing risk to marine mammal health. *Proc R Soc B*. 2008;275:267–276.

39. Zaias J. *Cellular and respiratory effects of aerosolized red tide toxin (brevetoxins)*. PhD dissertation. University of Miami; 2004.

40. Abraham WM, Bourdelais J, Ahmed A, et al. Effects of inhaled brevetoxins in allergic airways: toxin-allergen interactions and pharmacologic intervention. *Environ Health Perspect*. 2005;113:632–637.

41. Abraham WM, Baden DG. Case study: aerosolized Florida red tide toxins and human health effects. *Oceanography*. 2006;19:107–109.

42. Bossart GD, Baden DG, Ewing RY, et al. Brevetoxicosis in manatees (*Trichechus manatus latirostris*) from the 1996 epizootic: gross, histologic, and immunohistochemical features. *Toxicol Pathol*. 1998;26:276–282.

Zoonoses

9

Peter M. Rabinowitz and Lisa A. Conti

OVERVIEW

Key Points for Clinicians and Public Health Professionals

Public Health Professionals

- Establish or refresh lines of communication among the human health and veterinary clinicians within the community (e.g., provide continuing education, update distribution list information).
- Routinely disseminate information about reportable diseases to the human health and veterinary community.
- Consider providing emerging disease exercises that involve the human health and veterinary community.

Human Health Clinicians

- Consider zoonotic diseases in the differential diagnosis of a wide range of medical complaints, and counsel clients about risk.
- Reassure owners about non-zoonoses in terms of human risk.
- Consider inviting veterinary clinicians and veterinary professionals in the community to a joint continuing education meeting regarding zoonoses.

Veterinary Clinicians

- Consider the zoonotic potential of animal infectious diseases and whether an infection in an animal indicates environmental risk shared by humans as well.
- Consider inviting human health clinicians and veterinary professionals in the community to a joint continuing education meeting regarding zoonoses.

INFECTIOUS DISEASES IN HUMANS AND OTHER ANIMALS: FROM "US VERSUS THEM" TO "SHARED RISK"

The history of contact between animals and humans has always involved infectious diseases, and today more than half of the infectious diseases of humans are zoonotic in origin. In fact, the majority of "emerging" infectious diseases in the past three decades are zoonotic. Therefore the control and prevention of these diseases can be accomplished only through improving approaches to reducing disease transmission among humans and other animals.

Despite the great deal of attention that has been focused on emerging infectious zoonotic diseases, including severe acute respiratory syndrome (SARS), West Nile virus, monkeypox, and avian influenza, there has been less discussion and effort targeted at the environmental "drivers" of such diseases. One possible reason is that the traditional approach of the human health community to zoonotic disease has been an "us versus them" approach. The problem is viewed as an infectious animal reservoir that then poses an infectious risk to humans—either through direct contact with infected animals and their excretions, meat, milk, or other tissues, or via a vector transmission bringing the pathogen from the animal population into human hosts. The control of such "us versus them" diseases has traditionally involved measures such as control of the animal reservoir (through culling, quarantine, or vaccination) or vector control (through pesticides and personal protection). For many zoonotic diseases, however, such approaches are limited because the ultimate causes of infection in the animals may not be addressed sufficiently. For example, Nipah virus emerged as a deadly pathogen in Malaysia when pig farms were built close to forest areas frequented by fruit bats (Figure 9-1 and Color Plate 9-1). These fruit bats, natural

105

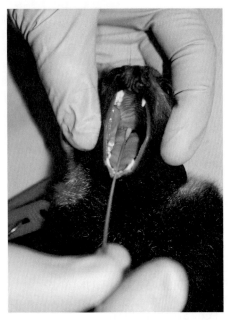

Figure 9-1 ■ Collection of oral swab from anesthetized spectacled flying fox *(Pteropus conspicillatus)* for Hendra virus antigen detection. (From Fowler ME, Miller RE: *Zoo and wild animal medicine: current therapy*, ed 6, St Louis, 2008, Saunders Elsevier. Courtesy Jack Shield.)

hosts for Nipah and other henipaviruses, had sufficient contact with the pig farms to allow the virus pathogen to "spill over" from the wildlife reservoir into the domestic pig population, causing mortality for pigs and humans (and cats) in contact with them.[1]

Therefore, for many infectious diseases that cross between animals and humans, it is advisable for human health professionals to move beyond an "us versus them" view of animals and infections and to instead join veterinarians and public health professionals to examine the environmental forces driving disease emergence that constitute a "shared risk" of infection for both humans and animals.[2] Figure 9-2 outlines these relationships.

This chapter presents this shared risk approach for a number of zoonotic diseases. For each disease, environmental risk factors (drivers) of infectious risk are discussed, as well as practical steps that public health, human health, and animal health professionals can take to prevent, control, diagnose, and treat such infections. A key step with each disease is providing accurate information about risk to clients and other members of the health professions.

NON-ZOONOSES (FOR NOW)

Infection in animals can be a warning signal of infectious disease risk to humans, and sometimes the converse is true. At the same time, many animal diseases currently are not believed to pose a threat to humans, and many human infectious diseases do not appear to infect pets and other animals.

Experience has shown that this situation may change as organisms continue to adapt to new environments and acquire mutations that allow them to cross species barriers. Nonetheless, human health clinicians should (1) be aware of animal diseases that, based on current knowledge, do not appear to cause disease in humans and (2) be able to reassure patients who express such concerns. Similarly, clinicians can correct

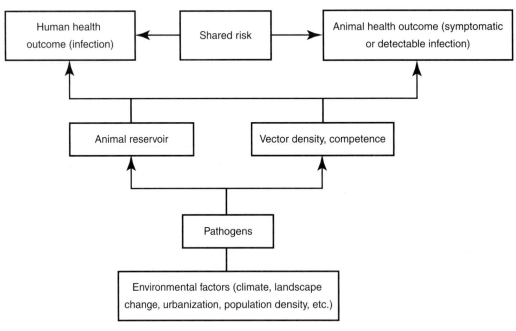

Figure 9-2 ■ Relation between environmental drivers of infectious disease and health outcomes in humans and animals. (From Rabinowitz PM, Odofin L, Dein FJ: From "us vs. them" to "shared risk": can animals help link environmental factors to human health? *Ecohealth* 5(2):224, 2008.)

Table 9-1 ▪ Common Infectious Diseases of Companion Animals Not Currently Believed to Be Zoonotic

Disease	Agent	Species Affected	Signs/Comment
Feline immunodeficiency virus infection (feline AIDS)	Feline immunodeficiency virus: retrovirus in the same genus as HIV, the causative agent of AIDS in humans[3]	Cats	Infected cats are at risk of opportunistic infections. FIV is used as a research model for HIV.
Canine parvovirus infection	Canine parvovirus 2 (CPV-2), DNA virus	Dogs (especially puppies)	Cause of acute debilitating diarrhea and death in untreated young dogs. Related to feline panleukopenia virus causing "feline distemper." In humans, a different strain of parvovirus (parvovirus B19) causes fever and rash (fifth disease) in children and serious infection in pregnancy.
Canine distemper	Canine distemper virus (CDV): Morbillivirus (Paramyxovirus family), related to measles virus	Dogs and other carnivores, including ferrets, raccoons, skunks, foxes, large felines, seals	Febrile disease, often fatal neurological involvement; respiratory signs can occur. Humans may become subclinically infected.[3] "Feline distemper" of domestic cats is a panleukopenia virus, similar to canine parvovirus.
Feline leukemia virus infection	Feline leukemia virus (FeLV)	Cats	Used as natural model for human cancer; zoonotic potential is controversial.

misinformation regarding species-specific human diseases that patients may believe come from animal contact. For example, human pinworm infection is not a zoonotic disease. Table 9-1 lists some of these non-zoonoses. As this list shows, many of these agents, while currently not considered zoonotic to any significant degree, bear some relation to human pathogens.

DISEASES TO WATCH

The sections in this chapter present individual descriptions of zoonotic diseases that human health and veterinary clinicians and public health professionals in the United States may encounter in their clinical work. It has been estimated, however, that there are more than 1600 known zoonotic pathogens, some of which are considered to be "emerging" in terms of expanding their geographical range or pathogenicity to other species. Our knowledge of the zoonotic potential of many infectious pathogens is continually changing as new evidence, some based on improved techniques of molecular diagnosis, appears.

Table 9-2 presents a number of pathogens and diseases for which clinicians and public health professionals should maintain an awareness of possibly increasing zoonotic disease risk. Table 9-3 lists a number of currently recognized zoonotic pathogens and some of the species for which the pathogen has been reported.

References

1. Daszak P, Cunningham AA, Hyatt AD. Anthropogenic environmental change and the emergence of infectious diseases in wildlife. *Acta Trop.* 2001;78(2):103.
2. Rabinowitz PM, Odofin L, Dein FJ. From "us vs. them" to "shared risk": can animals help link environmental factors to human health? *EcoHealth.* 2008;5(2):224.
3. Barr SC, Bowman DD. *5-minute veterinary consult clinical companion canine and feline infectious disease and parasitology.* Ames, IA: Wiley-Blackwell; 2006.
4. Theis JH. Public health aspects of dirofilariasis in the United States. *Vet Parasitol.* 2005;133(2–3):157.
5. Kahn CM, Line S, eds. *The Merck veterinary manual.* 9th ed. Whitehouse Station, NJ: Merck; 2005.
6. Liu W, Chemaly RF, Tuohy MJ, et al. *Pasteurella multocida* urinary tract infection with molecular evidence of zoonotic transmission. *Clin Infect Dis.* 2003;36(4):E58.
7. Dvorak GA, Rovid-Spickler A, Roth JA, eds. *Handbook for zoonotic diseases of companion animals.* Ames, IA: The Center for Food Security & Public Health; Iowa State University; 2006:234.

Table 9-2 ■ Diseases and Agents "to Watch" in Terms of Zoonotic Potential

Disease	Agent	Animal Hosts	Zoonotic Transmission Route	Clinical Manifestations	Comments
Bordetella	*Bordetella bronchiseptica* bacteria	Dogs, rabbits, guinea pigs	Respiratory	Cough, fever; disease seen mostly in immune-compromised humans	A cause of "kennel cough" in dogs
Chagas disease	*Trypanosoma cruzi* protozoa	Rodents rabbits, opossums, dogs, cats, armadillos	Organism in feces of *Triatoma* bug ("kissing" bug or "assassin" bug) can enter wound; blood transfusion	Fever, myocarditis, hepatosplenomegaly	Dogs exhibit clinical signs similar to those in humans Other animals are carriers; dogs infected in southern United States; dogs may be extending the range of this disease
Chikungunya	Chikungunya virus	Humans, rodents, birds, primates	*Aedes* mosquito vector (present in United States)	Fever, rash, arthralgia	Seen in returning travelers, new cases in Europe
Dirofilariasis ("heartworm" in dogs)	*Dirofilaria immitis* roundworm	Dogs, cats, ferrets, raccoons, bears	Mosquito vector	Fever, cough, "coin lesion" in lung due to vasculitis, reported involvement of extrapulmonary sites (CNS, liver)[4]	Parasite not known to complete its life cycle in humans
Erysipeloid (human disease)	*Erysipelothrix rhusiopathiae* bacteria	Pigs, sheep, turkeys, pigeons, marine mammals, fish	Direct contact	Cellulitis	Occupational disease of farmers, butchers, cooks
Feline cowpox	Feline cowpox virus	Cats are principal host; rodents, cows, and humans are accidental hosts	Direct contact	Skin ulcer resembling anthrax	Distribution is Eurasia
Pseudomembranous colitis	*Clostridium difficile* bacteria	Cattle	Ubiquitous organism; may preset with overuse of antibiotics	Diarrhea, abdominal pain	Emerging community-acquired infection Strains in humans recently found to match those in cattle
Glanders	*Burkholderia mallei* bacteria	Horses, mules, donkeys	Direct contact	Four forms of disease: septicemia, pulmonary infection, local infection, chronic infection	Category B bioterrorism agent

Disease	Organism	Reservoir/Host	Transmission	Symptoms	Comments
Helicobacter infection	*Helicobacter:* gram-negative bacteria: *H. pylori* (humans), *H. felis* (cats), *H. canis* (dogs)[3]	Dogs, cats, birds	Ingestion	Peptic ulcer disease, gastritis, gastric neoplasia in humans	
Monkeypox	Monkeypox virus	African rodents (able to infect prairie dogs, rats, mice, squirrels), primates, rabbits	Bites, aerosols, direct contact	Flulike symptoms, rash	Caused outbreak in humans and pet prairie dogs related to importation of Gambian rats and other African rodents intended as exotic pets
Melioidosis (pseudoglanders)	*Pseudomonas pseudomallei* bacteria	Rodents, goats, sheep, horses, swine, primates, dogs, birds, dolphins, tropical fish	Acquired from the environment	Infection of skin, lung, hepatitis	Category B bioterrorism agent, occurs in zoo animals[5]
Pasteurellosis	*Pasteurella multocida* bacteria	Dogs, cats, other animals	Scratch, bite, but also secretions	Wound infection, but UTI recently reported[6]	
Rat-bite fever (Haverhill fever)	*Streptobacillus moniliformis* bacteria	Rodents, including laboratory and wild animals	Bites and scratches, ingestion	Uncommon; risk to laboratory animal workers	
Streptococcosis	*Streptococcus suis* (and other species) bacteria	Pigs	Direct contact, aerosols, fomites	Fever, endocarditis	35 serotypes; type 2 is most frequently isolated from pigs with clinical signs and from humans[7]; occupational disease of pig handlers
Yersiniosis	*Yersinia enterocolitica* bacteria	Pigs	Ingestion, especially of undercooked pork	Diarrhea, abdominal pain	

CNS, Central nervous system; UTI, urinary tract infection.

Table 9-3 ■ Chart of Species and Associated Pathogens

Note: Columns 1–15 (Dogs through Mink) are grouped under the heading **Domestic**.

Disease	Dogs	Cats	Ferret	Reptiles and amphibians	Caged birds	Rabbits	Pocket pets (rodents)	Fish	Horses	Cattle	Goats	Sheep	Swine	Poultry	Mink	Nonhuman primates	Camels, llamas, alpacas	Raccoons	Squirrels	Other wild rodents	Wild birds	Marine mammals	Wild cats	Foxes, coyotes, wild canids	Bats	Skunks	Opossums	Elephants	Beavers	Deer	Other wild herbivores
Arthropods																															
Scabies	×	×	×				×										×														
Other acariasis	×	×	×	×	×	×																									
Bacterial																															
Anthrax	×	×					×			×	×	×	×		×		×		×	×	×		×		×		×			×	×
Bartonellosis	×	×																					×								
Bordetella bronchiseptica	×					×	×																								
Botulism	×							×	×	×		×		×	×						×										
Brucellosis	×									×	×	×	×		×		×			×				×						×	×
Campylobacteriosis	×	×	×	×	×		×		×	×	×	×	×	×							×										
Chlamydophila infection	×	×		×	×		×		×	×	×	×		×							×									×	
Ehrlichiosis and anaplasmosis	×								×	×		×		×		×	×			×	×			×						×	×
Escherichia coli O157 infection	×									×	×	×		×																×	
Erysipeloid								×					×	×								×									
Leptospirosis	×	×				×	×		×	×	×	×	×					×	×	×			×				×			×	
Lyme disease	×	×					×		×	×									×	×							×			×	
Melioidosis									×	×	×	×	×	×		×			×	×											
MRSA	×	×			×	×		×	×	×			×																		
Mycobacteriosis other than TB	×	×	×	×	×			×																							
TB	×	×								×			×			×														×	×

Continued

Disease	1	2	3	4	5	6	7	8	9	10	11	12	13	14	15	16	17
Pasteurellosis	×	×															×
Plague	×	×			×		×	×		×		×	×				
Q Fever	×	×	×		×		×		×		×	×		×		×	
Rat-bite fever	×	×	×		×		×	×		×	×	×		×		×	×
Rocky Mountain spotted fever	×		×					×				×					
Salmonellosis	×	×	×	×	×	×	×	×	×	×	×	×	×	×	×	×	×
Tularemia	×	×	×	×	×	×	×	×		×		×	×	×	×	×	×
Yersiniosis	×	×	×	×	×	×		×		×	×	×					
Fungal																	
Cryptococcosis	×	×			×	×	×	×	×	×	×	×		×		×	
Dermatophytosis	×	×	×	×	×	×	×	×	×	×	×	×		×	×	×	×
Sporotrichosis	×	×			×	×	×	×		×		×		×			
Histoplasmosis								×				×					
Parasitic																	
Baylisascariasis	×	×		×	×	×	×	×	×	×	×	×		×			×
Chagas' disease (trypanosomiasis)	×	×			×	×	×	×	×	×	×	×		×		×	
Cysticercosis (*Taenia* infection)					×			×	×	×	×			×		×	
Cryptosporidiosis	×	×	×	×	×	×	×	×	×	×	×	×	×	×	×	×	×
Dipylidiasis	×	×			×			×	×	×		×					
Dirofilariasis	×	×			×			×	×	×				×			
Echinococcosis	×	×	×	×	×	×	×	×	×	×	×	×		×		×	×
Giardiasis	×	×	×	×	×	×	×	×	×	×	×		×	×			×
Hookworm infestation	×	×	×	×	×	×	×		×			×	×	×	×		
Leishmaniasis	×	×	×	×		×		×		×							
Toxocariasis	×	×	×	×	×	×	×	×	×	×	×	×	×	×	×	×	
Toxoplasmosis	×	×	×	×	×	×	×	×	×	×	×	×	×	×	×	×	×
Trichinellosis	×				×			×	×	×		×					
Prion																	
Transmissible spongiform encephalopathy	×				×		×	×	×	×		×				×	×
Viral																	
Hantavirus infection					×			×								×	
Herpes B																×	

Table 9-3 ■ Chart of Species and Associated Pathogens—cont'd

Disease	Domestic																														
	Dogs	Cats	Ferret	Reptiles and amphibians	Caged birds	Rabbits	Pocket pets (rodents)	Fish	Horses	Cattle	Goats	Sheep	Swine	Poultry	Mink	Nonhuman primates	Camels, llamas, alpacas	Raccoons	Squirrels	Other wild rodents	Wild birds	Marine mammals	Wild cats	Foxes, coyotes, wild canids	Bats	Skunks	Opossums	Elephants	Beavers	Deer	Other wild herbivores
Influenza (human)	X	X	X										X																		
Influenza (avian)	X	X	X		X								X	X	X	X					X	X	X								
Lymphocytic choriomeningitis	X						X									X				X											
Monkeypox						X	X									X				X											
Orf											X	X																			X
Rabies	X	X	X			X			X	X	X	X	X		X	X	X	X					X	X	X	X		X			
Rift Valley fever	X								X	X	X	X				X	X		X	X											
West Nile virus infection	X	X			X				X							X	X		X	X	X				X	X					X

Adapted from Kahn CM, Line S (eds): *The Merck veterinary manual*, ed 9, Whitehouse Station, NJ, 2005, Merck; Dvorak GA, Rovid-Spickler A, Roth JA (eds): *Handbook for zoonotic diseases of companion animals*, The Center for Food Security & Public Health, Ames, IA, 2006, Iowa State University; Forrester DJ: *Parasites and diseases of wild mammals in Florida*, Gainesville, FL, 1992, University Press of Florida.
MRSA, Methicillin-resistant *Staphylococcus aureus*; *TB*, tuberculosis.

ANTHRAX

Peter M. Rabinowitz and Lisa A. Conti

Cutaneous anthrax (ICD-10 A22.0), Pulmonary anthrax (A22.1), Gastrointestinal anthrax (A22.2)

Other names in humans: wool sorter's disease, charbon, malignant carbuncle, Siberian ulcer

Other names in animals: splenic fever, Milzbrand

Anthrax is a fatal disease of herbivores. Most human cases result from direct contact with sick or dead animals or contaminated animal products. The causative agent, *Bacillus anthracis*, is a Centers for Disease Control and Prevention (CDC) Category A bioterrorism agent, and the anthrax-tainted letters mailed in the United States in 2001 were a reminder of its potential for deliberate release. In the United States, anthrax outbreaks in wildlife and livestock occur annually but human cases are rare.[1] Veterinary and human health care professionals need to recognize the clinical signs of disease and report suspected cases to public health authorities.

Key Points for Clinicians and Public Health Professionals

Public Health Professionals

- Characterize the risk in the community, including whether cases have been reported in livestock or wildlife and whether there is a possibility of environmental contamination.
- Work with veterinary authorities to control disease in animals.
- Conduct immediate investigation of human cases to determine whether they are related to zoonotic transmission or deliberate toxin release.
- Ensure that potentially exposed individuals receive postexposure prophylaxis (PEP).
- Counsel people who contact spores to wash hands with soap and water, followed by an organic iodine solution immersion. Clothing should be washed and boiled.
- Recommend that imported animal hides be disinfected before use. The U.S. Department of Agriculture (USDA) Animal and Plant Health Inspection Service (APHIS) regulates importation of all animal hides but does not mandate screening of imported hides for *B. anthracis*. In addition, some hides may be imported illegally.[2]
- Reduce environmental exposure risk through disinfection where possible.
- Provide guidance for environmental sampling and environmental cleanup.[3,4]

Human Health Clinicians

- Consider the diagnosis in all patients with livestock contact or travel to endemic countries.
- Report suspicion of disease immediately to public health authorities.
- Counsel travelers to endemic areas about risk reduction and monitoring for symptoms.
- If providing occupational health services to workers at risk, ensure that they are educated about symptoms of the disease, use adequate protective equipment, and that efforts are taken to reduce potential of infection (such as disinfection of animal hides with formalin).
- Consider vaccine for high-risk groups,[5] including laboratory workers and persons who handle potentially infected animals and animal products in high-incidence areas where safety standards are insufficient to prevent exposure to anthrax spores.[6] Military personnel[7] deployed to areas with high risk for biological warfare may require vaccination.

Veterinary Clinicians

- Do not perform a necropsy on suspected animal cases.
- Annually vaccinate cattle, sheep, horses, goats, and swine in endemic areas using the Sterne strain vaccine.[8] Treat infected and potentially infected animals. During quarantine these animals should not be used as food.
- Report suspected cases to agricultural health authorities who can quarantine premises to prevent spread of disease.
- Veterinarians who work with potentially infected animals in high-incidence areas should consider vaccination.
- Avoid contact with blood and bloody discharges. Keep flies and scavengers from carcasses. Infected carcasses should be burned (preferred) to destroy spores or buried in quick lime. To kill spores use 2% glutaraldehyde or 5% formalin for several hours. Heat sterilization at 121°C for 30 minutes can also be used.
- Notify health department immediately if cases are diagnosed in animals. Such cases could both pose a risk to humans and be a sentinel warning of deliberate release of toxin.

Agent

The bacterium *B. anthracis* is a spore-forming, nonmotile, gram-positive bacillus 3 to 5 microns long. When the vegetative form is exposed to air, it sporulates to form infectious spores. The spores may survive for decades in soil (Figure 9-3).

Geographical Occurrence

National disease control programs have reduced the global incidence of anthrax. It remains common in some Mediterranean countries, localized areas of Canada and the United States, parts of Central and South America, central Asia, parts of sub-Saharan Africa, and western China.[9] An epizootic among cattle in South Dakota in 2000 resulted in 157 cattle deaths and one human case of cutaneous anthrax.[10] Human anthrax resulting from exposure to infected livestock remains rare in the United States but occurs more commonly in less-developed countries. In many regions, the true incidence is not known because many cases in animals and humans probably go unreported.

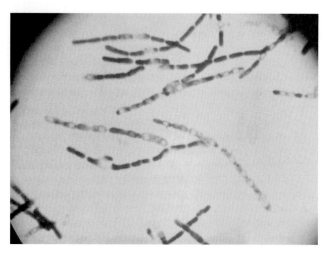

Figure 9-3 ■ Photomicrograph depicting a number of gram-positive, endospore-forming *Bacillus anthracis* bacteria.

Groups at Risk

Anthrax can be an occupational disease of workers who process carcasses and hides of infected animals, including farmers, abattoir workers, butchers, and workers in factories that process hides. Veterinarians who handle sick animals are also at risk, as are laboratory workers who routinely work with *B. anthracis*. Cases of both inhalation and cutaneous anthrax have developed in travelers and drum makers who have bought drums or hides originating from infected animals. In 2007, two cases of cutaneous anthrax in Connecticut were tied to importation of infected goat hides for drum-making (Figure 9-4).[2]

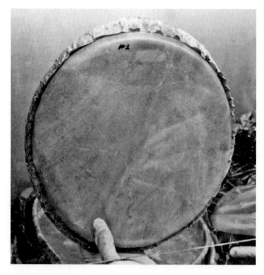

Figure 9-4 ■ *Bacillus anthracis*–contaminated drum head made from goat hide from Guinea; Connecticut, 2007. (From Centers for Disease Control and Prevention: Cutaneous anthrax associated with drum making using goat hides from West Africa—Connecticut, 2007, *MMWR Morbid Mortal Weekly Rep* 57(23):628, 2008.)

In the 2001 intentional use of anthrax in mail, postal workers were an occupational risk group. No animals were affected in these attacks.

Hosts, Reservoir Species, Vectors

The reservoir for anthrax is the environment, where the spores can survive for years in alkaline calcium-rich soil. Anthrax is principally a disease of livestock, including cattle, sheep, goats, and camels. Wild ruminants such as antelope and bison can also be infected and pose a risk to livestock.[11] However, all mammals are susceptible,[12] and horses, pigs, dogs, cats, and humans can be incidentally infected. Because of their higher body temperatures birds are normally resistant, but ostriches are susceptible. In some settings, biting flies may serve as vectors for anthrax transmission.[9]

In the 1979 accidental release of aerosolized anthrax in Sverdslovsk, Russia, cattle and sheep died as far as 50 km downwind from the release site, while human cases of inhalation anthrax occurred only up to 4 km downwind from the release.[13] The fact that animals became sickened over a wider geographical area than did humans may reflect their increased susceptibility and increased exposure risk, making animal cases sentinels for human risk.

Mode of Transmission and Life Cycle

Infected animals release vegetative bacteria into the environment. As the bacteria are exposed to air, they sporulate and the spores can survive for years. Ruminant animals grazing on areas contaminated by spores can ingest the spores and become infected. This can lead to further contamination of the environment and additional animal cases (Figure 9-5). Biting flies appear to play a role in large outbreaks by facilitating animal-animal transmission, sometimes over significant distances (5 to 15 km). Direct animal-animal transmission among herbivores is considered insignificant,[9] but if carnivores eat the flesh of infected animals, they can become infected.

Transmission from animal to human usually involves direct contact with spores because the vegetative form of the microbe is not as infectious. Spores may be present on an infected animal's hide, in meat that has been in contact with air and has developed spores, or as an aerosol from infected animal hide or tissues or from the environment.

Most human infection occurs through direct contact with animals or animal products. Such transmission is more likely when there are breaks in the skin and leads to the cutaneous form of the disease (Figure 9-6).

Airborne transmission from animals to humans can occur when spores are aerosolized during the processing or handling of contaminated animal hair, wool, hides, and bones. Improvements in working conditions have reduced this risk. Airborne transmission can also occur during the deliberate release of the agent.

Humans can also become infected through ingestion of tissue from an infected animal, leading to development of gastrointestinal or oropharyngeal anthrax. Human-to-human transmission is considered rare and has been reported only with cutaneous anthrax.

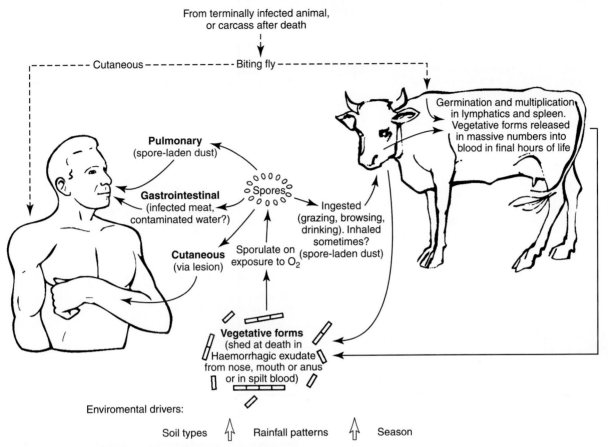

Figure 9-5 ▪ Cycle of anthrax infection. (Modified from *Guidelines for the surveillance and control of anthrax in humans and animals*, ed 4, Geneva, 2008, World Health Organization. Available at http://www.who.int/csr/resources/publications/anthrax/whoemczdi986text.pdf.)

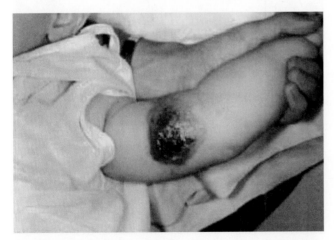

Figure 9-6 ▪ Cutaneous anthrax in a child. (From Roche KJ, Chang MW, Lazarus H: Images in clinical medicine: cutaneous anthrax infection, *N Engl J Med* 345:1611, 2001.)

Environmental Risk Factors

The persistence of spores in the environment depends on a number of factors, including temperature, humidity, soil pH, calcium and other cations in soil, and the abundance of soil bacteria that could break down spores.[14] Outbreaks in wild-life species have been linked to climate factors such as hot, dry weather following spring flooding.[11] Heavy rainfall may increase the population of biting flies that can amplify animal outbreaks and may lead to spores being brought to the soil surface.[9,12]

Anthrax spores can contaminate indoor environments. One of the recent cases in Connecticut tied to imported drum hides was the child of the drum maker, who became infected through contamination of the household environment.[2]

Disease in Humans

There are three main forms of the disease: cutaneous, inhalational, and gastrointestinal. In naturally occurring human disease, more than 95% of cases are the cutaneous form. Inhalational anthrax is the next most common form. Gastrointestinal anthrax has never been reported in the United States. Table 9-4 shows the comparative clinical presentations of anthrax in humans and animals.

Cutaneous Anthrax

Cutaneous anthrax begins 1 to 7 days after inoculation with a small, painless, pruritic papule that is often asymptomatic and does not lead to an infected individual seeking medical

Table 9-4 ▪ Anthrax: Clinical Presentations in Humans and Other Animals

Species	Risk Factors	Incubation Period	Signs and Symptoms	Diagnostic Findings
Humans: *cutaneous* (95% of naturally occurring human cases)	Contact with infected animal or animal products	2-6 days	Painless, pruritic papule followed by vesicles, edema, ulcer, and eschar; bacteremia	Organisms seen on methylene blue stain, culture, or by PCR or ELISA
Inhalational	Aerosol from processing hides, wool, deliberate release	4-6 days	Malaise, fever, cough, followed by acute onset of respiratory distress	Chest radiograph may show widened mediastinum, pleural effusion
Gastrointestinal	Ingestion of infected meat	3-7 days[9]	Fever, abdominal pain, nausea, vomiting, bloody diarrhea, oropharyngeal swelling	Identification of bacteria in blood or other fluid samples
Cattle, sheep goats, other herbivores	Grazing on areas contaminated by spores, biting flies	1-20 days	Fever, depression, staggering, collapse, edema, abortion, sudden death	Demonstration of bacteria by culture, PCR, fluorescent antibody of blood or tissue
Pigs	Contact with contaminated soil	7-14 days	Often a milder form of disease with systemic symptoms and cervical lymphadenopathy Acute septicemia with oropharyngeal swelling and death may occur	Demonstration of bacteria by culture, PCR, fluorescent antibody of lymphoid or other tissue
Dogs, cats, wild carnivores	Ingestion of tissue from infected animal	1-14 days	Resembles disease in pigs	
Horses	Grazing on contaminated pasture	1-20 days	Fever, colic, diarrhea, swelling of neck, belly, genitalia	

ELISA, Enzyme-linked immunosorbent assay; *PCR,* polymerase chain reaction.

care. Over a period of days, vesicles develop with surrounding edema, which then rupture to form an ulcer covered by a black eschar. A significant degree of edema develops around the eschar and can be severe. Most cutaneous lesions are on the hands and arms. If the head and neck are involved, breathing may be compromised by the swelling. Bacteremia can develop, leading to systemic complications. Without antibiotic treatment the mortality rate is approximately 20%.[15] Figure 9-6 shows cutaneous anthrax in a child.

Inhalational Anthrax

Inhalational anthrax often begins with nonspecific malaise, mild fever, and nonproductive cough 1 to 6 days after exposure. After several days, a second phase of the disease begins abruptly with high fever, dyspnea, cyanosis, and stridor. A hemorrhagic lymphadenitis can develop with mediastinal widening (Figure 9-7). Without treatment, respiratory decompensation soon occurs. In up to half of cases, anthrax meningitis may also be present, with meningeal signs and altered consciousness.[15] Mortality rate is high even with antibiotic treatment.

Gastrointestinal Anthrax

Gastrointestinal anthrax is characterized by fever, abdominal pain, and bloody diarrhea that develop 2 to 5 days after ingestion of contaminated meat (to date, it has not been reported in the United States). Oropharyngeal involvement can produce swelling with respiratory compromise. The mortality rate can be 25% to 75%.[16]

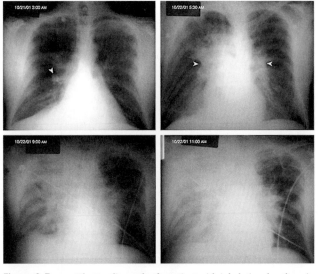

Figure 9-7   ▪   Chest radiograph of a patient with inhalational anthrax in 2001. The *arrows* emphasize the widened mediastinum caused by the characteristic mediastinal adenopathy. (From Borio L, Frank D, Mani V et al: Death due to bioterrorism-related inhalational anthrax: report of 2 patients, *JAMA* 286:2554, 2001.)

Disease in Animals

Cattle and sheep develop an acute form of anthrax that is usually rapidly fatal. Clinical signs include fever, depression, staggering, difficulty breathing, and collapse. Subcutaneous edema may be present. Pregnant animals may abort before dying.

Infected horses can also develop acute disease with fever, colic, diarrhea, weakness, and swelling of the neck, sternum, belly, and genitalia. The disease is also rapidly fatal.

Pigs are considered to be more resistant to the disease compared with ruminants. Although pigs may develop an acute septicemia with sudden death and/or oropharyngitis with throat swelling and suffocation, a chronic form of disease is more common, with mild systemic signs and cervical lymphadenopathy.

Dogs, cats, nonhuman primates, and wild carnivores can develop disease resembling that in pigs (Figure 9-8).[15]

Diagnosis

Diagnosis in Humans

The differential diagnosis of cutaneous anthrax in humans includes boils, cellulitis, spider bite, rickettsial disease, ulceroglandular tularemia, rat-bite fever, leishmaniasis, and human orf. A history of exposure to livestock or livestock products, the presence of extensive edema, and the lack of pus and pain can provide clues to the diagnosis.

Inhalational anthrax can present with nonspecific symptoms and may be confused with other causes of pneumonitis, including community-acquired pneumonia and influenza. In the second, severe stage of illness, possible considerations include aortic dissection, pneumonic plague, and hantavirus pulmonary syndrome. A screening protocol for

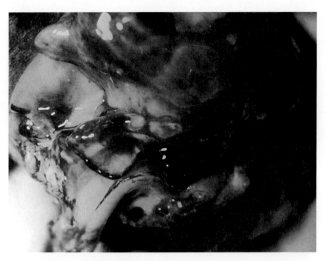

Figure 9-8 ■ Gross pathologic posterior oblique view of inhalation anthrax in a chimpanzee's lungs. (From Centers for Disease Control and Prevention Public Health Image Library, Atlanta, Ga. Courtesy U.S. Army, Arthur E. Kay.)

inhalation anthrax has been proposed by a consensus report (Figure 9-9). This protocol is based on history of exposure and the presence of clinical signs.

Gastrointestinal anthrax, though rare, typically presents as a cluster of cases of acute abdominal pain and diarrhea following ingestion of food from a common source. It can

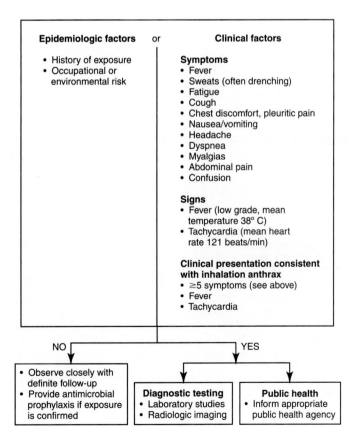

Figure 9-9 ■ Revisions to the Centers for Disease Control and Prevention (CDC) interim inhalation anthrax screening guidelines. (From Stern EJ, Uhde KB, Shadomy SV et al: Conference report on public health and clinical guidelines for anthrax, *Emerg Infect Dis* 14(4):pii: 07-0969, 2008.)

therefore be confused with other causes of food-borne illness.

The differential diagnosis of oropharyngeal anthrax includes streptococcal pharyngitis and Ludwig's angina.[9]

The laboratory diagnosis of anthrax involves identification of the capsulated organism in blood or tissues using methylene blue (M'Fadyean)-stained smears or through bacterial culture of blood or other specimens.[16] Rapid tests that are increasingly available include polymerase chain reaction (PCR), enzyme-linked immunosorbent assay (ELISA), and immunohistochemical staining. Diagnostic testing for suspected inhalation anthrax in humans should include chest radiography and/or chest computed tomographic (CT) scanning to look for mediastinal widening.[1]

Diagnosis in Animals

In cattle, anthrax can be confused with other causes of sudden death, including lightning strikes, poisonings, leptospirosis, anaplasmosis, and clostridial infections. In pigs, other diagnoses to consider include classical or African swine fever and pharyngeal malignant edema. In dogs, other systemic infections or causes of pharyngeal edema should be considered.

Diagnostic testing can be performed on a swab of blood that is allowed to air-dry, resulting in sporulation of the bacteria and death of other bacteria and contaminants. In pigs, lymph tissue should be sent for studies. Bacterial culture, PCR, and fluorescent antibody stains can demonstrate the organism in blood and tissues.[17]

Treatment

Treatment in Humans

Treatment of anthrax in humans involves treatment with antibiotics as soon as the disease is suspected or as PEP.

Table 9-5 shows the recommended initial treatment regimens. Although quinolones or doxycycline are first-line agents, if the infecting strain is found to be susceptible to penicillin, penicillin can be substituted.

Treatment in Animals

Control of anthrax in animals may involve a combination of vaccination, quarantine, PEP of subclinically exposed animals, antibiotic treatment, or euthanization of sick animals and disposal of carcasses by burning. Cattle at risk should receive a full course of antibiotics, followed by vaccination 7 to 10 days later. Vaccination and antibiotics should not be given concurrently. Animals under treatment should be moved to a new pasture that is free from possible contamination.

Carcasses of animals that have died of anthrax should not be necropsied or otherwise opened to prevent sporulation of the bacteria and further cycles of infection.

ADDITIONAL RESOURCES

CDC Advisory Committee on Immunization Practices Recommendations for Use of Anthrax Vaccine

- *Use of Anthrax Vaccine in Response to Terrorism* (2002)
  http://www.cdc.gov/mmwr/preview/mmwrhtml/mm5145a4.htm
- *Use of Anthrax Vaccine in the United States* (2000)
  http://www.cdc.gov/mmwr/preview/mmwrhtml/rr4915a1.htm
- *MMWR Notice to Readers: Occupational Health Guidelines for Remediation Workers at* Bacillus anthracis–contaminated Sites—United States, 2001-2002 (*MMWR* 6;51(35), 786-789, 2002)

Table 9-5 ■ Initial Treatment of Anthrax in Human Beings and Animals		
Species	**Primary Treatment**	**Alternative Treatment**
Humans:		
Cutaneous	Ciprofloxacin 500 mg PO bid *or* levofloxacin 500 mg IV/PO bid × 60 days *Children <50 kg:* ciprofloxacin 20-30 mg/kg/day divided q12h PO (maximum 1 gm/day) × 60 days *or* levofloxacin 8 mg/kg PO q12h × 60 days	Doxycycline 100 mg PO bid × 60 days *Children >8 yr and >45 kg:* doxycycline 100 mg PO bid × 60 days *<8 yr:* doxycycline 2.2 mg/kg PO bid × 60 days[18]
Inhalational and gastrointestinal	*Adult:* Ciprofloxacin 400 mg IV q12h or levofloxacin 500 mg IV q24h *PLUS* clindamycin 900 mg IV q8h *and/or* rifampin 300 mg IV q12h; treatment duration 60 days; switch to PO when able	*Children:* ciprofloxacin 10 mg/kg IV q12h or 15 mg/kg PO q12h *or* doxycycline (>8 yr and >45 kg) 100 mg IV q12h, *PLUS* clindamycin 7.5 mg/kg IV q6h and/or rifampin 20 mg/kg (maximum 600 mg) IV q24h; treatment duration 60 days[19]
Postexposure prophylaxis	Ciprofloxacin 500 mg PO bid *or* levofloxacin 500 mg PO q24h × 60 days *Children:* ciprofloxacin 20-30 mg/kg/day divided q12h × 60 days	Doxycycline 100 mg PO bid × 60 days *Children >8 yr and >45 kg:* doxycycline 100 mg PO bid *<8 yr:* doxycycline 2.2 mg/kg PO bid × 60 days
Cow, sheep, goat, horse	Penicillin	Oxytetracycline
Dog[19]	Oxytetracycline 5 mg/kg IV q24h Potassium penicillin G at 20,000 U/kg IV q8h	Enrofloxacin 5 mg/kg q24h

http://www.cdc.gov/mmwr/preview/mmwrhtml/
mm5135a3.htm
- Bacterial Agents: Anthrax. In *Biosafety in microbiology and biomedical laboratories*, ed 5, pp. 122-124, 2007) http://www.cdc.gov/OD/OHS/biosfty/bmbl5/BMBL_5th_Edition.pdf

Antimicrobial Prophylaxis

- Antimicrobial Prophylaxis to Prevent Anthrax Among Decontamination/Cleanup Workers Responding to an Intentional Distribution of *Bacillus anthracis* (2002): http://emergency.cdc.gov/agent/anthrax/exposure/cleanupprophylaxis.asp
- Responding to Detection of Aerosolized *Bacillus anthracis* by Autonomous Detection Systems in the Workplace (*MMWR* 2004/53(early release);1-11, April 30, 2004) http://www.cdc.gov/mmwr/preview/mmwrhtml/rr53e430-2a1.htm

Personal Protective Equipment

- Protecting Investigators Performing Environmental Sampling for *Bacillus anthracis:* Personal Protective Equipment (Nov. 6, 2001): http://emergency.cdc.gov/agent/anthrax/environment/investigatorppe.asp
- Interim Recommendations for the Selection and Use of Protective Clothing and Respirators Against Biological Agents (Oct. 25, 2001): http://www.bt.cdc.gov/documentsapp/Anthrax/Protective/10242001Protect.asp

References

1. Shadomy, TLSmith SV. Zoonosis update: Anthrax. *J Am Vet Med Assoc.* 2008;233(1):63.
2. Centers for Disease Control and Prevention (CDC). Cutaneous anthrax associated with drum making using goat hides from west Africa—Connecticut, 2007. *MMWR Morb Mortal Wkly Rep.* 2008;57(23):628.
3. Meehan PJ, Rosenstein NE, Gillen M, et al. Responding to detection of aerosolized *Bacillus anthracis* by autonomous detection systems in the workplace. http://www.cdc.gov/mmwr/preview/mmwrhtml/rr53e-30-2a1.htm; Accessed August 11, 2008.
4. National Institute for Occupational Safety and Health. *NIOSH respiratory diseases research program: evidence package for the National Academies' Review 2006–2007: 6.2 Anthrax.* http://www.cdc.gov/niosh/nas/RDRP/ch6.2.htm; Accessed August 11, 2008.
5. Use of anthrax vaccine in the United States: recommendations of the Advisory Committee on Immunization Practices. *MMWR Recomm Rep.* 2000;49(RR15):1.
6. Notice to readers. Use of anthrax vaccine in response to terrorism: supplemental recommendations of the Advisory Committee on Immunization Practices. *MMWR.* 2002;51:1024. Available at http://www.cdc.gov/mmwr/preview/mmwrhtml/mm5145a4.htm.
7. Military Vaccine Agency. *Anthrax vaccine immunization program.* http://www.anthrax.osd.mil; Accessed August 11, 2008.
8. United States Department of Agriculture. Animal and Plant Health Inspection Service: APHIS factsheet: *anthrax—general information and vaccination.* http://www.aphis.usda.gov/publications/animal_health/content/printable_version/fs_ahanthravac.pdf. Accessed August 11, 2008.
9. World Health Organization. Anthrax in humans and animals. http://www.who.int/csr/resources/publications/anthrax/whoemczdi986text.pdf.
10. Centers for Disease Control and Prevention. Human anthrax associated with an epizootic among livestock—North Dakota, 2000. *MMWR Morb Mortal Wkly Rep.* 2001;50(32):677.
11. Nishi JS, Dragon DC, Elkin BT, et al. Emergency response planning for anthrax outbreaks in bison herds of northern Canada. *Ann N Y Acad Sci.* 2002;969:245.
12. Hugh-Jones ME, de Vos V. Anthrax in wildlife. *Rev Sci Tech Off Int Epiz.* 2002;21:359.
13. Meselson M, Guillemin J, Hugh-Jones M, et al. The Sverdlovsk anthrax outbreak of 1979. *Science.* 1994;266(5188):1202.
14. Acha PN, Szyfres B. *Zoonoses and communicable diseases common to man and animals: vol. 1: bacterioses and mycoses.* 3rd ed. Washington, DC: Pan American Health Organization; 2001.
15. Swartz MN. Recognition and management of anthrax—an update. *N Engl J Med.* 2001;345(22):1621.
16. Kahn CM, Line S, eds. *The Merck veterinary manual.* 9th ed. Whitehouse Station, NJ: Merck; 2005.
17. US Food and Drug Administration, Center for Biologics Evaluation and Research. *Anthrax.* http://www.fda.gov/cber/vaccine/anthrax.htm Accessed August 11, 2008.
18. Gilbert DN, Moellering RC, Ellopoulos GM, et al. *Sanford guide to antimicrobial therapy 2009.* 39th ed. Sperryville, VA: Antimicrobial Therapy; 2009.
19. Langston C. *Postexposure management and treatment of anthrax in dogs—executive councils of the American Academy of Veterinary Pharmacology and Therapeutics and the American College of Veterinary Clinical Pharmacology.* http://www.aapsj.org/view.asp?art=aapsj070227. Accessed August 11, 2008.

BARTONELLA INFECTIONS

Peter M. Rabinowitz and Lisa A. Conti

Bartonella infection (ICD-10 A28.1)

Other names in humans: cat-scratch fever, cat-scratch disease, benign lymphoreticulosis, Parinaud's oculoglandular syndrome, bacillary angiomatosis, bacillary parenchymatous peliosis (peliosis hepatis), recurrent rickettsemia

Other names in animals: bartonellosis

Bartonella henselae, the causative agent for cat-scratch disease (CSD), is usually associated with self-limited infection in humans and subclinical disease in cats, but it is capable of serious systemic infection in humans. Other *Bartonella* species may be emerging pathogens for humans and other animals.

Bartonella infection is an occupational risk for veterinary workers (including one reported case of *Bartonella clarridgeiae*) and one of the more common infections associated with cat ownership.

Key Points for Clinicians and Public Health Professionals

Public Health Professionals

- Educate community about avoiding cat scratches and bites (particularly kittens), thorough cleaning of wounds to reduce infection, discouraging cats from licking a person's skin or opens wounds, and flea and tick control.[1]

Human Health Clinicians

- Be alert to diagnosis in persons with unexplained lymphadenopathy or fever of unknown origin.
- Counsel immunocompromised patients to avoid cat scratches, thoroughly clean wounds after a scratch or bite, and to not allow cats to lick a person's skin or open wounds.
- Consider risk of infection in any patient bitten or scratched by a cat or with flea or tick bites.
- Counsel occupationally exposed workers (e.g., zookeepers) and persons owning cats to avoid and seek care for bites and scratches and to be alert to signs and symptoms of infection.
- Report cases to health department if required in state.
- No human vaccine is currently available.

Veterinary Clinicians

- Ensure flea control for cats.
- Counsel cat owners, especially immunocompromised patients, about avoiding cat scratches and bites, thorough cleaning of cat infected wounds, and not allowing cats to lick a person's skin or open wound. Although declawing has not been associated with preventing infection, some recommend trimming cats' nails routinely. Some suggest keeping cats indoors.
- A vaccine has been developed (though not currently marketed).

Agent

B. henselae is a gram-negative bacillus in the family Bartonellaceae. This family shares some features with rickettsial organisms but has been removed from the order Rickettsiales. The genus *Bartonella* includes at least 20 species, five of which (*B. henselae, B. quintana, B. bacilliformis, B. vinsonii* subspecies *arupensis,* and *B. elizabethae*) are recognized human pathogens (Table 9-6).[2] At present, no animal reservoirs of *B. quintana* or *B. bacilliformis* have been

identified. *B. henselae, B. vinsonii,* and *B. elizabethae* are known to infect both human and animal hosts.[3]

Geographical Occurrence

B. henselae is found worldwide.

Groups at Risk

CSD can be an occupational disease of veterinarians and others providing care to cats. Studies of zookeepers have revealed seroprevalence rates for past *Bartonella* infection as high as 65%,[4] while a convenience survey of veterinarians and veterinary workers found *Bartonella* species seroprevalence of only 7%.

Hosts, Reservoir Species, Vectors

Bartonella species have been found in a wide range of subclinically infected mammals, including rodents, rabbits, deer, elk, bighorn sheep, cattle, foxes, dogs, and coyotes.[5] Domestic cats are considered the principal reservoir for *B. henselae.*[6] Seroprevalence studies have shown rates of antibody positivity in cats in the range of 40%.[7] However, infection in cats is considered either subclinical or subtle, even in the setting of chronic bacteremia. *B. henselae* has also been isolated from cat fleas, dog fleas, and a number of other vectors.[8] Dogs may also be infected with *B. henselae.* Recent data show that ticks may play a role in transmission to humans.[9]

B. quintana at present is known to have only a human reservoir and is spread by the human body louse. *B. vinsonii* and *B. elizabethae* have been found in asymptomatic rodent reservoirs, including rural mice (*B. vinsonii*)[10] and urban rats (*B. elizabethae*).[11] Infection to humans may occur through vectors or direct contact.

Mode of Transmission and Life Cycle

Despite the fact that *B. henselae* can occur in vectors, transmission to humans is thought to be mainly mechanical

Table 9-6 ■ Pathogenic *Bartonella* Species

Bartonella Species	Disease(s)	Reservoir(s)	Arthropod Vector(s)
B. bacilliformis	Oroya fever and verruga peruana	Humans	Sandflies
B. clarridgeiae	Cat-scratch disease; canine valvular endocarditis	Domestic cats	?
B. elizabethae	Human endocarditis	Norway rat	?
B. grahamii	Human neuroretinitis	Rodents	Fleas
B. henselae	Human, canine cat-scratch fever, endocarditis, peliosis hepatitis	Domestic cats; dogs (?)	Cat flea
B. quintana	Human trench fever	Humans	Body lice
B. vinsonii subsp. *arupensis*	Human endocarditis	Mice, voles	?
B. vinsonii subsp. *berkhoffii*	Human, canine endocarditis; canine granulomatis lymphadenitis, rhinitis, peliosis hepatitis	Rodents, dogs	Ticks
B. washoensis	Human myocarditis	Ground squirrels	?

From Songer JG, Post KW: *Veterinary microbiology: bacterial and fungal agents of animal disease,* St Louis, 2005, Saunders Elsevier.

through a scratch or bite or licking of an open wound or rubbing the eyes with contaminated hands (Figure 9-10). The role of fleas in transmission is not well understood.

Environmental Risk Factors

Flea infestation is a definite risk factor for both feline and zoonotic infection because cats infested with fleas have higher seroprevalence of *Bartonella* infection.

Disease in Humans

Cat scratch infection produces an inoculation at the point of injury, with inflammation of nearby lymph nodes several weeks later (Color Plate 9-2). The lymph swelling often is self-limited over a period of months in immunocompetent hosts (Figure 9-11). In up to one sixth of cases the lymph nodes suppurate. Other symptoms can include malaise, fatigue, fever, and rash.[3]

Atypical presentations of *B. henselae* infection include Parinaud's oculoglandular syndrome (granulomatous conjunctivitis accompanied by pretragal lymphadenopathy).[3] Even in immunocompetent patients, serious complications of *B. henselae* infection can occur, such as central nervous system (CNS) involvement (including encephalopathy and myelitis)[12]

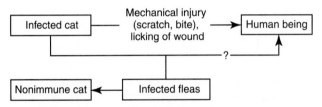

Figure 9-10 ■ Life cycle of *Bartonella henselae* infection.

and hepatic abscesses. In many but not all cases, CSD precedes the development of more serious complications. In the elderly, *B. henselae* endocarditis may be found more frequently (a common cause of culture-negative endocarditis), whereas CSD is less frequent than in younger individuals.[12]

In immunocompromised individuals, complications of infection can include bacillary angiomatosis (Color Plate 9-3). Peliosis hepatis, a condition characterized by fever, chills, hepatosplenomegaly, and gastrointestinal symptoms, can develop in immunocompromised patients. Like *B. henselae*, *B. quintana* causes a number of conditions, including trench fever, endocarditis, bacillary angiomatosis, and peliosis hepatitis.[11]

At present. case reports of bacteremia and endocarditis in humans resulting from infection with *B. vinsonii*[10] and *B. elizabethae* are limited.[13] Antibodies to *B. elizabethae* have been found in urban homeless and drug users,[14] but the clinical significance remains poorly understood.

Disease in Animals

B. henselae causes subclinical infection in cats, including chronic bacteremia. Between 5% and 60% of cats may be seropositive depending on the geographical area. There is a case report of *B. henselae* infection in a Golden Retriever causing pelosis hepatitis (Figure 9-12 and Color Plate 9-4).[15] Table 9-7 provides comparative clinical manifestations in humans and other animals.

Diagnosis

Diagnosis in humans is based on the clinical picture of local lymphadenopathy, especially in the setting of a history of cat contact. *Bartonella* species are difficult to grow in culture; therefore other diagnostic techniques such as PCR and serology are often required (e.g., immunofluorescent antibody [IFA] titer ≥1:64 to *B. henselae*).[19] Cross-reactions can occur among *Bartonella* species and *Chlamydia* and

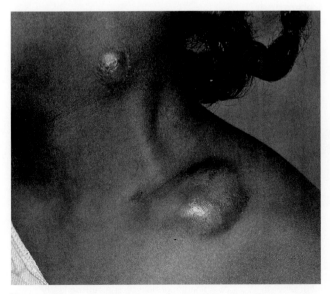

Figure 9-11 ■ Papular lesion and enlarged lymph nodes in a person with cat scratch disease. (From Long SS, Pickering LK, Prober CG (eds): *Principles and practice of pediatric infectious diseases*, ed 3, Philadelphia, 2008, Saunders Elsevier.)

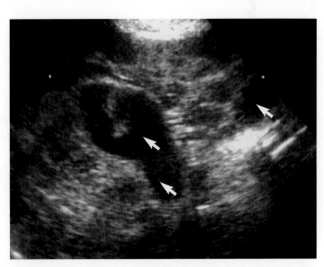

Figure 9-12 ■ Ultrasonographic appearance of the liver of a dog with peliosis hepatis associated with *B. henselae* infection showing hypoechoic areas *(arrows)* representing vascular peliosis. (From Greene CE: *Infectious diseases of the dog and cat*, ed 3, St Louis, 2006, Saunders Elsevier. Courtesy Barbara Kitchell, University of Illinois, Urbana, Ill.)

Table 9-7 ▪ *Bartonella* Infections: Comparative Clinical Presentations in Humans and Other Animals[16]

Species	Risk Factors	Incubation Period	Clinical Manifestations	Laboratory Findings
B. Henselae				
Humans	Cat scratch or bite, immunocompromised individuals at increased risk	3-10 days	Lymphadenopathy, fever, culture-negative endocarditis; rare complications including bacillary angiomatosis, neurological involvement, endocarditis, Parinaud's oculoglandular syndrome	Leukocytosis, elevated sedimentation rate, serology (IFA or ELISA), PCR
Cats		2-16 days (experimental infection)	Subclinical or mild symptoms, uveitis (?)	Blood culture, serology (IFA)
B. Vinsonii Subsp. Berkhoffii				
Humans			Bacteremia and endocarditis reported[17] Isolated in healthy animals	
Dogs and coyotes			Canine granulomatous rhinitis (?), liver disease, endocarditis, fever, death	
B. Vinsonii Subsp. Arupensis				
Humans	Rodent exposure (?)		Bacteremia, endocarditis reported[18]	
Rodents			Subclinical	
B. Elizabethae				
Humans	Rodent exposure[14]		Endocarditis reported[13]	
Rodents			Subclinical	

ELISA, Enzyme-linked immunosorbent assay; *IFA,* immunofluorescent antibody; *PCR,* polymerase chain reaction.

Coxiella. PCR of tissue and fluid obtained from lymph node biopsy can often identify the organism. Disease in animals can be diagnosed by blood culture or serology (IFA or ELISA) and PCR.

Treatment

In humans, some cases of CSD in an immunocompetent host may not require antibiotic treatment.[12] However, any immunocompromised patient, as well as any patient with extralymphatic involvement, should be treated with antibiotics.[20] Table 9-8 outlines treatment guidelines for symptomatic disease in humans. There are no treatment protocols for animals.

References

1. Carr RM, Mohrman L, Arelli V, et al. Update on cause and management of catscratch disease. *Infect Med.* 2008;25:242.
2. Koehler JE, Duncan LM. Case records of the Massachusetts General Hospital. Case 30-2005. A 56-year-old man with fever and axillary lymphadenopathy. *N Engl J Med.* 2005;353(13):1387.

Table 9-8 ▪ *B. Henselae* Treatment in Humans and Other Animals[21]

Species	Primary Treatment	Alternative
Humans		
Cat-scratch disease (immunocompetent)	*Adults:* azithromycin 500 mg × 1, then 250 qd × 4 days *Children* (≤45.5 kg): liquid azithromycin 10 mg/kg ×1, then 5 mg/kg/day × 4 days[12]	Consider no treatment since often self-limited
Bacillary angiomatosis, peliosis hepatitis, immunocompromised patients	Clarithromycin 500 mg bid or clarithromycin ER 1 gm PO q24h *or* azithromycin 250 mg q24h *or* ciprofloxacin 500-750 mg PO bid × 8 wk[12]	Erythromycin 500 mg PO qid *or* doxycycline 100 mg PO bid × 8 weeks, or if severe, combination of doxycycline 100 mg PO/IV bid and rifampin 300 mg PO bid
Cats, Dogs (With Clinical Signs)	Azithromycin 5-10 mg/kg once a day × 7 days and every other day × additional 5 weeks[22]	

3. Mandell GE, Bennett JE, Dolin R. *Principles and practice of infectious diseases.* 6th ed. Philadelphia: Churchill Livingstone Elsevier; 2000.
4. Juncker-Voss M, Prosl H, Lussy H, et al. Screening for antibodies against zoonotic agents among employees of the Zoological Garden of Vienna, Schönbrunn. *Austriac.* 2004;117(9–10):404.
5. Breitschwerdt EB, Kordick DL. Bartonella infection in animals: carriership, reservoir potential, pathogenicity, and zoonotic potential for human infection. *Clin Microbiol Rev.* 2000;13(3):428.
6. Acha PN, Szyfres B. *Zoonoses and communicable diseases common to man and animals: vol. 2: chlamydioses, rickettsioses, and viroses.* 3rd ed. Washington DC: Pan American Health Organization; 2003.
7. Fabbi M, Vicari N, Tranquillo M, et al. Prevalence of Bartonella henselae in stray and domestic cats in different Italian areas: evaluation of the potential risk of transmission of Bartonella to human beings. *Parassitologia.* 2004;46(1–2):127.
8. Maurin M, Birtles R, Raoult D. Current knowledge of Bartonella species. *Eur J Clin Microbiol Infect Dis.* 1997;16(7):487.
9. Breitschwerdt EB, Maggi RG, Duncan AW, et al. Bartonella species in blood of immunocompetent persons with animal and arthropod contact. *Emerg Infect Dis.* 2007;13(6):938.
10. Welch DF, Carroll KC, Hofmeister EK, et al. Isolation of a new subspecies, Bartonella vinsonii subsp. arupensis, from a cattle rancher: identity with isolates found in conjunction with Borrelia burgdorferi and Babesia microti among naturally infected mice. *J Clin Microbiol.* 1999;37(8):2598.
11. Comer JA, Paddock CD, Childs JE. Urban zoonoses caused by Bartonella, Coxiella, Ehrlichia, and Rickettsia species. *Vector Borne Zoonotic Dis.* 2001;1(2):91.
12. Gilbert DN, Moellering RC, Ellopoulos GM, et al. *Sanford guide to antimicrobial therapy 2009.* 39th ed. Sperryville, VA: Antimicrobial Therapy; 2009.
13. Daly JS, Worthington MG, Brenner DJ, et al. Rochalimaea elizabethae sp. nov. isolated from a patient with endocarditis. *J Clin Microbiol.* 1993;31:872.
14. Comer JA, Diaz T, Vlahov D, et al. Evidence of rodent-associated Bartonella and Rickettsia infections among intravenous drug users from Central and East Harlem, New York. *Am J Trop Med Hyg.* 2001;65(6):855.
15. Kitchell BE, Fan TM, Kordick D, et al. Peliosis hepatis in a dog infected with Bartonella henselae. *J Am Vet Med Assoc.* 2000;216(4):519–523 517.
16. Dvorak G, Rovid-Spickler A, Roth JA, et al. *Handbook for zoonotic diseases of companion animals.* Ames, IA: The Center for Food Security and Public Health, Iowa State University; 2008.
17. Roux V, Eykyn SJ, Wyllie S, et al. Bartonella vinsonii subsp. berkhoffii as an agent of afebrile blood culture-negative endocarditis in a human. *J Clin Microbiol.* 2000;38(4):1698.
18. Fenollar F, Sire S, Raoult D. Bartonella vinsonii subsp. arupensis as an agent of blood culture-negative endocarditis in a human. *J Clin Microbiol.* 2005;43(2):945.
19. Heymann DL. *Control of communicable diseases manual.* 19th ed. Washington DC: American Public Health Association; 2008.
20. Boulouis HJ, Chao-chin C, Henn JB, et al. Factors associated with the rapid emergence of zoonotic Bartonella infections. *Vet Res.* 2005;36:383.
21. Rolain JM, Brouqui P, Koehler JE, et al. Recommendations for treatment of human infections caused by Bartonella species. http://www.pubmedcentral.nih.gov/articlerender.fcgi?artid=415619 Accessed September 11, 2008.
22. Breitchwerdt E. Personal communication. August 21, 2008.

BRUCELLOSIS

Peter M. Rabinowitz and Lisa A. Conti

Brucellosis due to Brucella melitensis *(ICD-10 A23),* Brucellosis due to *Brucella abortus (A23.1),* Brucellosis due to *Brucella suis (A23.2),* Brucellosis due to *Brucella canis (A23.3)*

Other names in humans: undulant fever, Mediterranean fever, Malta fever

Other names in animals: Bang's disease (cattle), epizootic abortion, contagious abortion

Brucellosis is an important bacterial disease of ruminants worldwide and an occupational disease for humans working closely with infected animals. Many human cases are related to foodborne exposures to unpasteurized dairy products. Brucellosis prevention demands a "One Health" approach between animal and human health disciplines because the human health risk can be reduced only by controlling the disease in animals.[1] Brucellosis can be passed between domestic cattle and wildlife such as bison, where it can be difficult to control.

Key Points for Clinicians and Public Health Professionals

Public Health Professionals

- Describe the local incidence and prevalence in human, domestic animal, and wildlife populations using cooperative veterinary/human disease surveillance systems.[2]
- In endemic areas, coordinate with local agricultural and wildlife agencies regarding vaccination, testing, and control in domestic livestock and wildlife.

- Educate the public (especially travelers to endemic countries) on risk of infection from unpasteurized dairy products.
- Encourage public health measures to avoid consumption of unpasteurized dairy products.
- Educate hunters of feral swine and other potentially infected wildlife (e.g., elk, bison) about infection control precautions, including gloves and protective clothing while preparing carcasses and burying of all remains to avoid scavenging.
- If disease is present in livestock population, educate farmers and livestock workers regarding personal protection when handling strain 19 vaccine, potentially infected tissue, and adequate ventilation in abattoir environments.
- Sentinel human cases may indicate problems with food safety, infection in local livestock, or inadequate safety controls for workers and require public health follow-up.
- Educate local veterinary and human health clinicians about groups at risk, signs of disease, and to consider the possibility of intentional exposure activity.

Human Health Clinicians

- Screen for exposure risk factors: ingestion of unpasteurized dairy products, contact with potentially infected animals, recent travel to endemic areas, and animal contact during travel.
- Human cases should immediately be reported to local health officials.
- When treating human cases, while rarely transmitted person to person, counsel about safe sex precautions to prevent secondary transmission.
- Ensure that workers in high-risk occupations (including veterinarians and laboratory workers) are using appropriate biosafety procedures.

- Consider brucellosis in workup of fever of unknown origin.
- Offer PEP and management to exposed laboratory workers and veterinary workers with vaccine exposure.
- Counsel patients to avoid consuming unpasteurized dairy products and to use protective clothing (rubber boots, gloves, goggles) if they must come in contact with infected livestock, wild ruminants, or wild dogs.
- Consider a 3- to 6-week prophylactic antibiotic course for a needlestick injury with a veterinary vaccine, laboratory, or bioterrorism exposure.[3]
- No human vaccine is available.

Veterinary Clinicians

- Isolate and screen herd replacements.
- Quarantine infected herds, test and slaughter to eradicate infection, and disinfect facility where infected animals have been housed.
- Report animals with positive screenings to agriculture officials.
- Vaccinate cattle, sheep, and goats against *Brucella*.*
- Ensure proper biosafety procedures are followed in veterinary facility and that staff are aware of symptoms of infection.
- If diagnosing animal case, discuss zoonotic risk with owner; offer direct communication with human health clinician caring for family.
- Disinfect with 1% sodium hypochlorite, 70% ethanol, or iodine solutions. *Brucella* can also be inactivated by several hours of direct sunlight.[3] Replacement swine herds can be placed on ground that has been free of pigs for a minimum of 30 days.

Agent

Brucellosis is caused by *Brucella* species, which are gram-negative coccobacilli. A number of species in the genus have affinities for particular animal hosts. These species have been further subdivided into biologically distinct strains (biovars).[6] At least four species of *Brucella* are found in animals and man; these include *Brucella abortus* (cattle), *B. melitensis* (goats), *B. suis* (swine),* and *B. canis* (dogs). There have been several reported isolations of bacteria from marine mammals, including seals, whales, and dolphins that are currently classified in the genus *Brucella*. However, the human zoonotic potential of these new agents remains to be established.[7]

Geographical Occurrence

Brucellosis is found worldwide, but its prevalence depends largely on the state of control in domestic animals. In the United States, bovine brucellosis control programs have reduced the frequency of infection in both cattle and humans.

Between 1986 and 2007, fewer than 150 human cases were reported annually in the United States.[8,9] As a result, many human health clinicians in the United States have never seen a case. In the United States, the highest incidence rates are in states bordering Mexico, including California and Texas. The most common *Brucella* species for human infections in the United States are *B. abortus* and *B. melitensis*.[10] The occurrence of human brucellosis is higher in other countries where livestock infection is not as well controlled, including Mexico, other Latin American countries, the Mediterranean basin, Eastern Europe, Asia, Africa, and the Middle East. The United Nations' Food and Agriculture Organization has set a goal for worldwide eradication of brucellosis.

Groups at Risk

Worldwide, brucellosis is considered largely an occupational disease of workers exposed to cattle and other large animals through animal husbandry, dairy, and slaughter operations. Such workers include herdsmen, slaughterhouse workers, and veterinarians. Handling of infected aborted fetuses and newborn animals is considered a particularly high-risk activity. Another risk is sharing living spaces with potentially infected animals; high rates of brucellosis infection have been reported among goat-herding families that bring goats into family bedrooms during the winter.[11]

A rare occurrence among veterinarians is the self-inoculation (needlestick, splash or spray to mucous membranes, or broken skin) of vaccine strains of *Brucella* (RB51 or *B. abortus* strain 19, or *B. melitensis* Rev-1) during animal vaccination; this represents one of the rare reported occupational risks of animal vaccination.[12] Outbreaks have occurred in laboratory workers who handled *Brucella* cultures outside biological safety cabinets,[9] and dog handlers are considered to be at risk from *B. canis*. However, analysis of recent cases in the United States indicates that brucellosis is increasingly a foodborne disease associated with ingestion of unpasteurized dairy products from infected animals.[10]

Hosts, Reservoir Species, Vectors

The species and biovars of *Brucella* are adapted to particular animals that serve as definitive hosts. However, as shown in Tables 9-9 and 9-10, cross-species infections can occur, with humans and dogs particularly susceptible to infection by a number of different *Brucella* species.

Table 9-9 ■ Hosts for *Brucella* Species

Species	Animal Hosts
Brucella abortus	Cattle, elk,[13] bison, water buffalo,[14] goats,[4] horses,[15] dogs,[4] coyotes[16]
Brucella melitensis	Goats, sheep, cows, dogs[4]
Brucella suis	Pigs, feral swine and wild boar, horses, cattle,[4] dogs[4]
Brucella ovis	Sheep
Brucella canis	Dogs

*A number of vaccines are available for different animal species. In cattle, vaccination with *B. abortus* strain 19 or RB51 increases resistance to infection.[4] The same vaccines have been used to attempt to control outbreaks in wildlife species, including coyotes, elk, and bison.[5] Goats can be vaccinated with the Rev1 strain of *B. melitensis*. There is no vaccine for Brucellosis in swine. In dogs, brucellosis vaccine has not been found to be effective.[4]

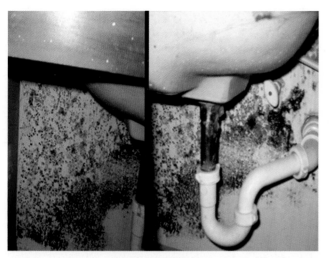

CP 6-1 ■ Mold on drywall under leaky sink. (From Environmental Protection Agency, Washington, DC. Courtesy John Martyny.)

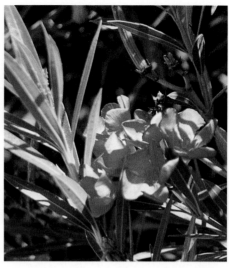

CP 8-2 ■ Oleander *(Nerium oleander)*. (From Plumlee K: *Clinical veterinary toxicology*, St Louis, 2004, Mosby Elsevier. Courtesy K.H. Plumlee.)

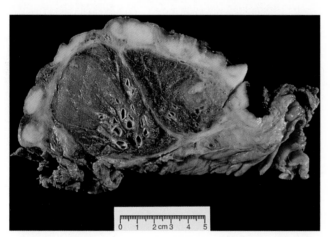

CP 8-1 ■ Malignant mesothelioma. Note the thick, firm, white, pleural tumor that ensheaths this bisected lung. (From Kumar V, Abbas AK, Fausto N et al: *Robbins basic pathology*, ed 8, Philadelphia, 2007, Saunders Elsevier.)

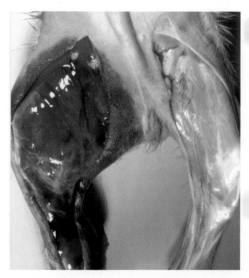

CP 8-3 ■ Hemorrhage, anticoagulant (warfarin-containing) rodenticide toxicosis, skin and subcutis, medial aspect of the right hindleg, dog. There is a large area of extensive hemorrhage in the subcutis. This lesion was attributed to decreased production of coagulation factors II, VII, IX, and X and proteins C and S resulting from a deficiency of vitamin K induced by warfarin. (From McGavin MD, Zachary JF: *Pathologic basis of veterinary disease*, ed 4, St Louis, 2007, Mosby Elsevier. Courtesy D.A. Mosier, College of Veterinary Medicine, Kansas State University.)

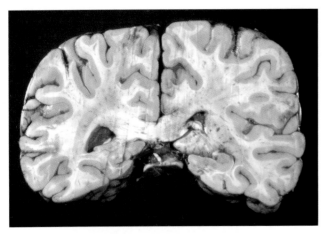

CP 8-4 ▪ Carbon monoxide poisoning, brain, human. The blood in the brain is cherry red from the carboxyhemoglobin formed by the inhalation of carbon monoxide in exhaust gases. (From McGavin MD, Zachary JF: *Pathologic basis of veterinary disease*, ed 4, St Louis, 2007, Mosby Elsevier. Courtesy J.C. Parker, School of Medicine, University of Louisville, Ky.)

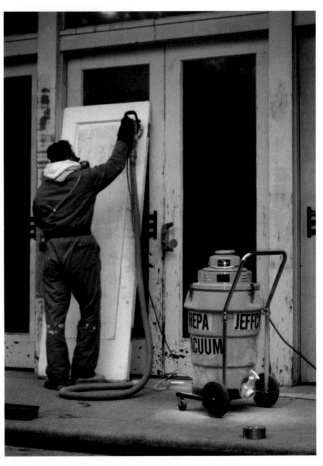

CP 8-6 ▪ Worker using a power sander with a high-efficiency particulate air (HEPA) filter exhaust system that collects paint particulates, demonstrating an exterior renovation method used on residences where lead-based paint was present. This was a low-exposure method. (From Centers for Disease Control and Prevention Public Health Image Library, Atlanta, Ga.)

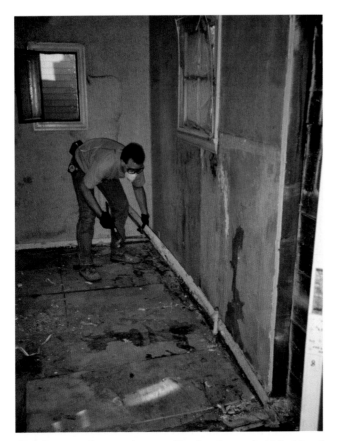

CP 8-5 ▪ Worker removing a wood baseboard covered with lead-based paint, demonstrating renovation methods typically used on residences where lead-based paint was present. (From Centers for Disease Control and Prevention Public Health Image Library, Atlanta, Ga.)

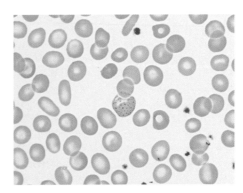

CP 8-7 ▪ Basophilic stippling. Presence of irregular basophilic granules either fine or coarse; commonly seen in increased red blood cell production. Coarse stippling is usually seen in lead poisoning (×1000). (From McPherson RA, Pincus MR: *Henry's clinical diagnosis and management by laboratory methods*, ed 21, Edinburgh, 2006, Saunders Elsevier.)

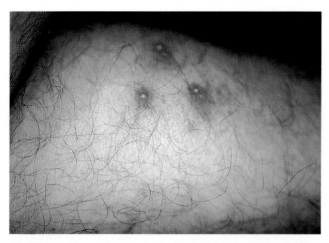

CP 8-8 ■ Fire ant lesions. (From Auerbach PS: *Wilderness medicine*, ed 5, Philadelphia, 2007, Mosby Elsevier.)

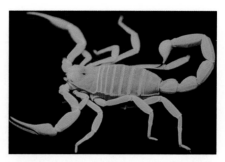

CP 8-11 ■ Scorpions fluoresce in ultraviolet light. (From Auerbach PS: *Wilderness medicine*, ed 5, Philadelphia, 2007, Mosby Elsevier.)

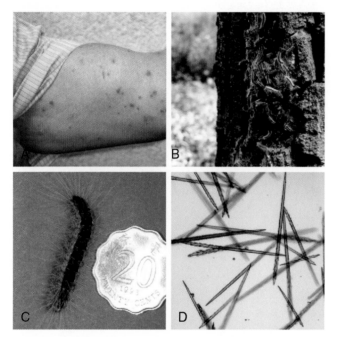

CP 8-9 ■ Lepidopterism. Toxic irritative caterpillar dermatitis. (From Spiegel W, Maier H, Maier M: A non-infectious airborne disease, *Lancet* 363:1438, 2004.)

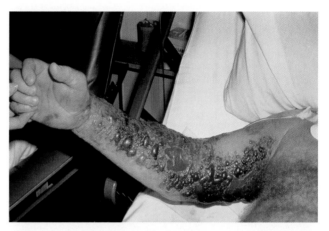

CP 8-12 ■ A case of severe envenomation by a western diamondback rattlesnake *(Crotalus atrox)* 4 days after the bite. Note the soft tissue swelling and hemorrhagic and serum-filled vesicles. (From Townsend CM, Beauchamp RD, Evers BM: *Sabiston textbook of surgery*, ed 18, Philadelphia, 2008, Saunders Elsevier. Courtesy David Hardy.)

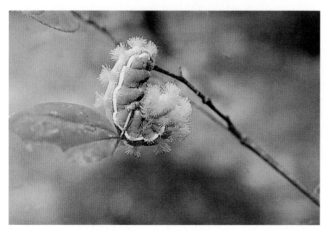

CP 8-10 ■ Caterpillar of the io moth, *Automeris io.* Widespread in the eastern United States, this species can inflict a painful sting. (From Auerbach PS: *Wilderness medicine*, ed 5, Philadelphia, 2007, Mosby Elsevier.)

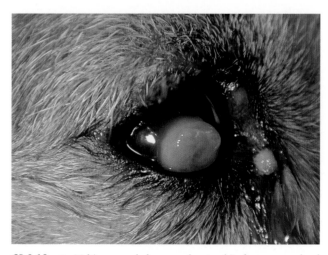

CP 8-13 ■ Melting corneal ulcer secondary to a bite from a copperhead snake to the upper eyelid, which penetrated, but did not perforate, the cornea. (From Dziezyc J, Millichamp NJ: *Color atlas of canine and feline ophthalmology*, St Louis, 2005, Saunders Elsevier.)

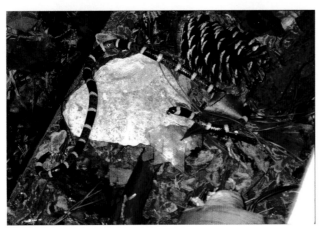

CP 8-14 ■ A Texas coral snake, *Micrurus tener tener*, in Galveston County, Texas. The eastern coral snake, *Micrurus fulvius fulvius*, is similar in appearance and differs primarily in the distribution of black mottling within the red segments. In contrast to the vipers, the fangs of coral snakes and other elapids are short, hollow structures that are permanently fixed in position on the anterior maxillary bones (i.e., proteroglyphous dentition). Because of their small size and short fangs, the North American coral snakes pose little risk to individuals wearing appropriate clothing and footwear. Most human envenomations occur on the hands after a coral snake is erroneously identified as a harmless king snake and intentionally handled. (From Centers for Disease Control and Prevention Public Health Image Library, Atlanta, Ga.)

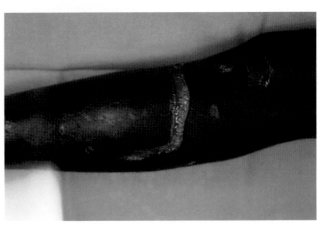

CP 8-16 ■ Skin destruction 3 weeks after an untreated box jellyfish *(Chironex fleckeri)* envenomation. (From Auerbach PS: *Wilderness medicine*, ed 5, Philadelphia, 2007, Mosby Elsevier. Courtesy John Williamson.)

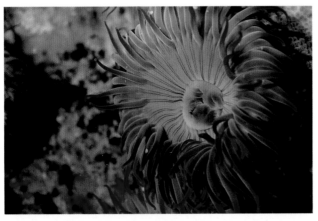

CP 8-15 ■ Many marine invertebrates contain venoms and poisons. Venoms in corals, anemones, and jellyfish are contained within special cellular stinging organelles called *nematocysts*. Nematocysts contain a stinging thread that penetrates the skin and injects venom. Many of these invertebrates are visually attractive, and children are particularly liable to be stung. (From Page C, Hoffman B, Curtis M et al: *Integrated pharmacology*, ed 3, Edinburgh, 2006, Mosby Elsevier. Courtesy Ron Kertesz, permission of the Vancouver Aquarium.)

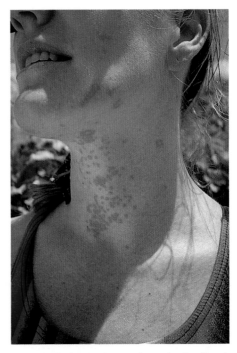

CP 8-17 ■ Seabather's eruption on the neck of a diver in Cozumel, Mexico. (From Auerbach PS: *Wilderness medicine*, ed 5, Philadelphia, 2007, Mosby Elsevier. Courtesy Paul Auerbach.)

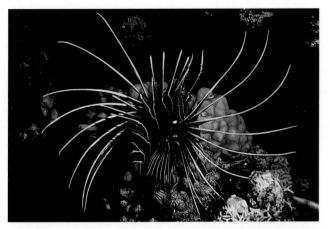

CP 8-18 ▪ Lionfish from the Red Sea. (From Auerbach PS: *Wilderness medicine*, ed 5, Philadelphia, 2007, Mosby Elsevier. Courtesy Paul Auerbach.)

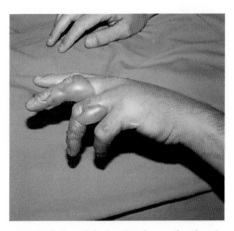

CP 8-19 ▪ Vesiculation of the hand 48 hours after the sting of a lionfish. (From Auerbach PS: *Wilderness medicine*, ed 5, Philadelphia, 2007, Mosby Elsevier. Courtesy Howard McKinney.)

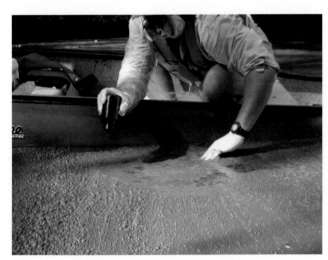

CP 8-20 ▪ Sampling cyanobacteria. (Courtesy Andy Reich, Aquatic Toxins Coordinator, Florida Department of Health.)

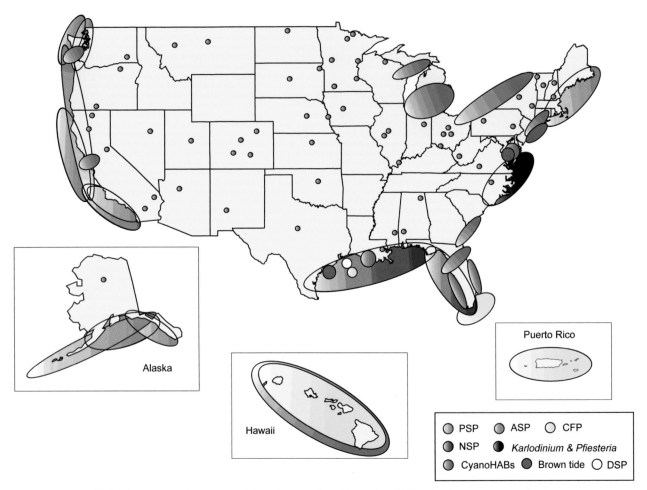

PSP   ASP   CFP

NSP   *Karlodinium & Pfiesteria*

CyanoHABs   Brown tide   DSP

CP 8-21 ■ Approximate areas of the U.S. coast affected by various HAB poisoning syndromes and other effects. Note that cyanoHAB dots portray geographically general representations of outbreaks and may represent events occurring in more than one water body within a state. Note also that not all HABs are depicted in this generalized view of the United States. (From U.S. National Office for Harmful Algal Blooms: Distribution of HABs in the U.S. http://www.whoi.edu/redtide/page.do?pid=14898.)

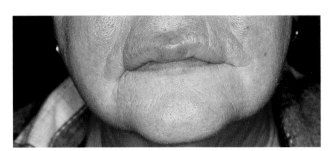

CP 8-22 ■ Blue-green algae. Facial and lip swelling after accidental ingestion of contaminated water. (From Auerbach PS: *Wilderness medicine*, ed 5, Philadelphia, 2007, Mosby Elsevier. Courtesy Edgar Maeyens, Jr.)

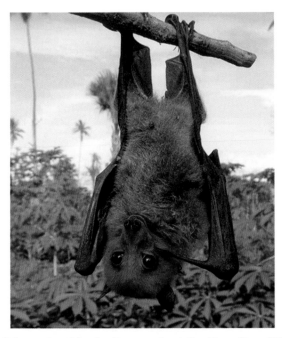

CP 9-1 ■ Gray flying fox *(Pteropus griseus)*, East Timor. Host of Nipah virus. (Courtesy Andrew C. Breed. From Fowler ME, Miller RE: *Zoo and wild animal medicine: current therapy*, ed 6, St Louis, 2008, Saunders Elsevier.)

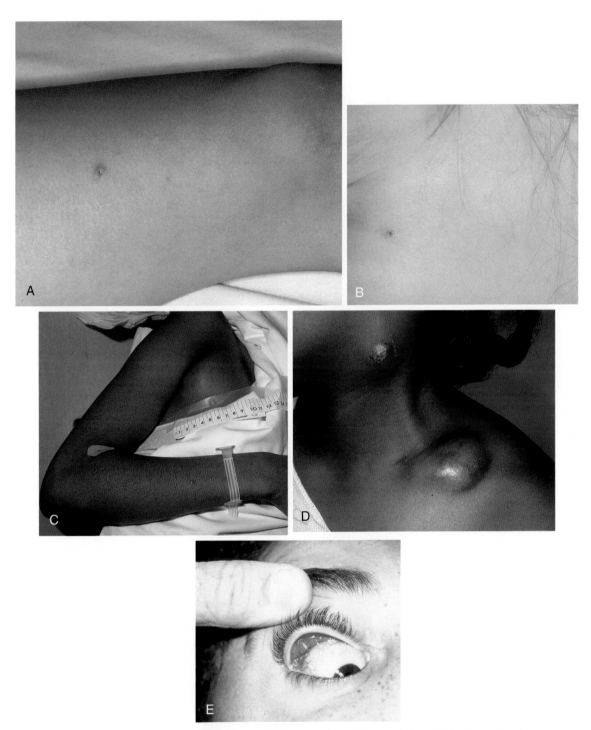

CP 9-2 ■ Typical clinical findings of *Bartonella henselae* infection (cat-scratch disease). Simple papule at the scratch site on the leg (**A**) of a young boy and the face of a young girl (**B**). Papular lesion on the arm and axillary lymphadenopathy in an adolescent (**C**). Papular lesion and fluctuant, enlarged lymph nodes in the supraclavicular and neck areas of an adolescent girl who frequently cuddled her kitten over her chest and shoulder (**D**). Granulomatous conjunctivitis and preauricular lymphadenopathy in a 12-year-old boy (**E**). (From Long SS, Pickering LK, Porber CG: *Principles and practice of pediatric infectious disease*, ed 3, Philadelphia, 2009, Saunders Elsevier.)

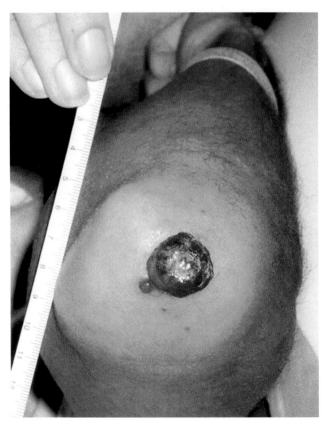

CP 9-3 ■ Cutaneous bacillary angiomatosis lesions on the elbow of a patient with AIDS. (From Mandell GE, Bennett JE, Dolin R: *Principles and practice of infectious diseases*, ed 6, Philadelphia, 2005, Churchill Livingstone Elsevier.)

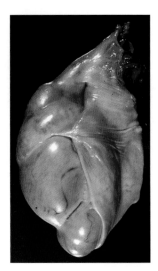

CP 9-5 ■ Epididymitis *(Brucella ovis)*, tunic adhesions, epididymis, ram. Note the dramatic enlargement of the epididymis and the adhesion of the parietal tunica vaginalis to the visceral tunica vaginalis around the affected epididymis. (From McGavin MD: *Pathologic basis of veterinary disease*, ed 4, St Louis, 2007, Mosby Elsevier. Courtesy K. McEntee, Reproductive Pathology Collection, University of Illinois; and J. King, College of Veterinary Medicine, Cornell University.)

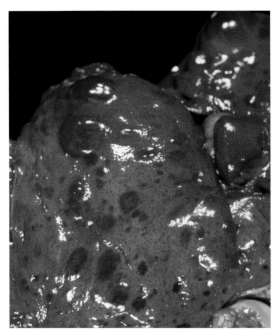

CP 9-4 ■ Liver from a dog with peliosis hepatis associated with *B. henselae* infection. (From Greene CE: *Infectious diseases of the dog and cat*, ed 3, St Louis, 2006, Saunders Elsevier. Courtesy Tim Fan, University of Illinois, Urbana.)

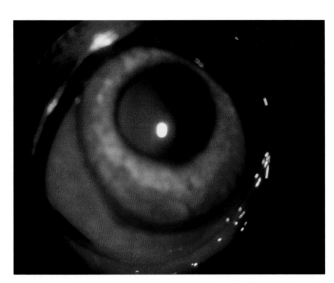

CP 9-6 ■ Anterior uveitis in a 3-year-old female German Shepherd diagnosed with *Brucella canis*. Conjunctival and ciliary injection, corneal edema, and iridal congestion and petechiae are present. (From Maggs DJ, Miller PE, Ofri R (eds): *Slatter's fundamentals of veterinary ophthalmology*, ed 4, St Louis, 2008, Saunders Elsevier.)

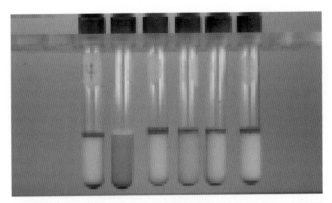

CP 9-7 ■ Milk ring test. Stained *Brucella* remains suspended in the milk in a negative test but rises with the cream in a positive reaction (second tube). (From Tizard IR: *Veterinary immunology: an introduction*, ed 8, St Louis, 2009, Saunders Elsevier. Courtesy John Huff.)

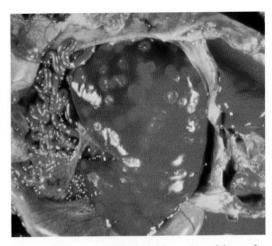

CP 9-9 ■ Ovine abortion resulting from *Campylobacter fetus* spp. *fetus*. (From Songer JG, Post KW: *Veterinary microbiology: bacterial and fungal agents of animal disease*, St Louis, 2005, Saunders Elsevier. Courtesy J. Glenn Songer.)

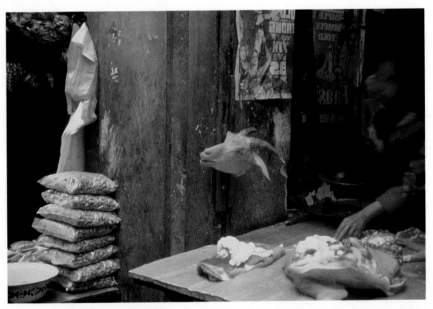

CP 9-8 ■ Foodborne transmission probably accounts for the majority of diarrheal illness in travelers and expatriates. The high rates of shigellosis and campylobacteriosis compared with cholera among travelers in cholera-endemic areas suggest that they may be better able to avoid exposure to contaminated water than to contaminated food. (From Cohen J, Powderly G: *Infectious diseases*, ed 2, Philadelphia, 2004, Mosby Elsevier.)

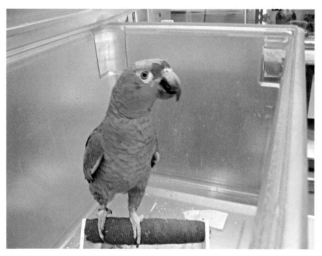

CP 9-10 ■ To many, the Amazon parrot is considered the typical companion psittacine. (From Bewig M: *Manual of exotic pet practice*, St Louis, 2009, Saunders Elsevier.)

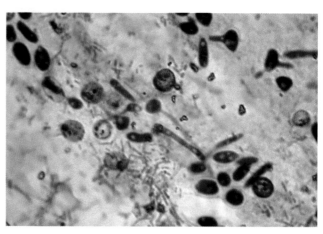

CP 9-12 ■ This micrograph of a direct fecal smear is stained to detect *Cryptosporidium* spp., an intracellular protozoan parasite. Using a modified cold Kinyoun acid-fast staining technique, and under an oil immersion lens, the *Cryptosporidium* oocysts—which are acid-fast—stain red, and the yeast cells, which are not acid-fast, stain green. (From CDC/*Journal of Infectious Diseases*, Vol. 137, no. 5, pp 824-828, May 1983, and Pearl Ma, Director of Microbiology, St. Vincent's Hospital, New York.)

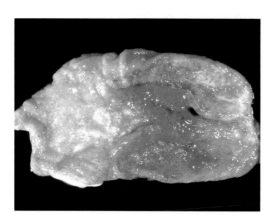

CP 9-11 ■ This snake had severe gastritis develop from a cryptosporidial infection. Infected animals typically vomit their meals 2 to 3 days after ingestion. An animal may commonly keep a meal down, then vomit again on the next feeding, confusing the keeper into thinking that the problem has self-corrected. (From Mader DR: *Reptile medicine and surgery*, ed 2, St Louis, 2006, Saunders Elsevier.)

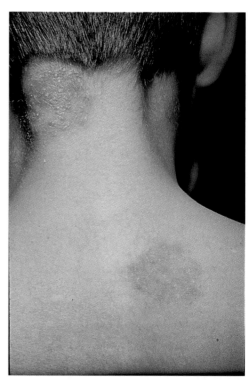

CP 9-13 ■ Tinea corporis due to *T. mentagrophytes.* (From Cohen J, Powderly G: *Infectious diseases*, ed 2, Philadelphia, 2004, Mosby Elsevier.)

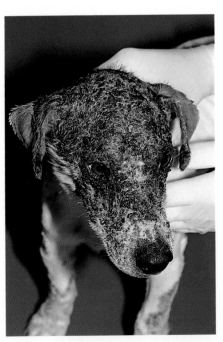

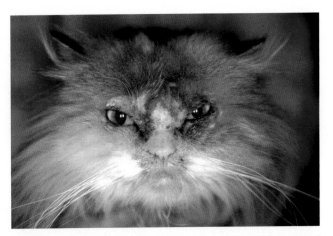

CP 9-15 ■ Dermatophytosis. Crusting alopecic dermatitis typical of dermatophytosis on the face of a cat. (From Medleau L, Hnilica KA: *Small animal dermatology: a color atlas and therapeutic guide*, ed 2, St Louis, 2006, Saunders Elsevier.)

CP 9-14 ■ Dermatophytosis. The severe crusting on the entire head of this Jack Russell Terrier was caused by a *Trichophyton* infection. The furunculosis resulted in severe cellulitis with subsequent scarring. (From Medleau L, Hnilica KA: *Small animal dermatology: a color atlas and therapeutic guide*, ed 2, St Louis, 2006, Saunders Elsevier. Courtesy J. MacDonald.)

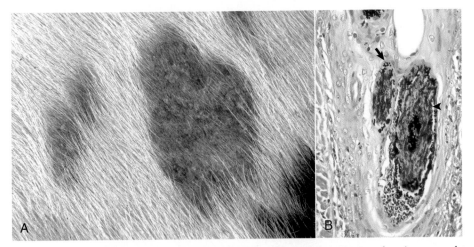

CP 9-16 ■ Dermatophytosis in a cow, luminal folliculitis, skin, haired. **A,** Dermatophytosis, presumed to be *Trichophyton verrucosum*. Note irregularly ovoid, hairless areas with mild surface crusting. **B,** Dermatophyte infection presumed to be *Microsporum canis* involving hair follicle, dog. Note spores *(arrow)* along periphery and hyphae *(arrowhead)* within hair shaft. The hair loss is due to breakage of hair shafts and mural and luminal folliculitis, which interfere with production of new hairs and cause increased loss of old hairs. Gomori's methenamine silver nitrate H&E counterstain. (From McGavin MD, Zachary JF: *Pathologic basis of veterinary disease*, ed 4, St Louis, 2007, Mosby Elsevier. *A,* Courtesy H. Denny Liggitt, University of Washington. *B,* Courtesy Ann M. Hargis, Dermato Diagnostics.)

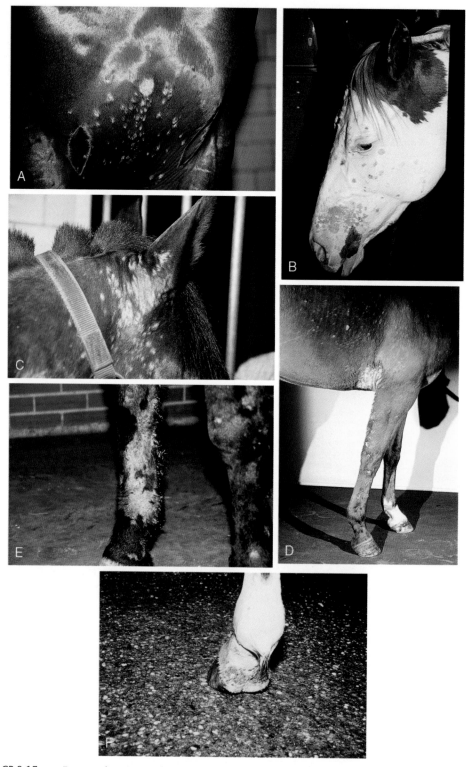

CP 9-17 ■ Dermatophytosis. **A**, Tufted papules and annular areas of crust and alopecia on brisket. **B**, Annular areas of alopecia, scaling, and erythema on the face. **C**, Annular areas of alopecia, scale, and crust near base of ear. **D**, Alopecia and scaling in the girth area. **E**, Alopecia, scaling, and crusting on leg. **F**, Crusting and alopecia on caudal pastern. (From Scott DW, Miller WH: *Equine dermatology*, Philadelphia, 2003, Saunders Elsevier. Courtesy W. McMullen.)

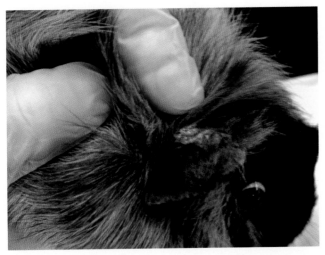

CP 9-18 ■ A guinea pig with a crusted area on the dorsal pinna consistent with dermatophytosis. A *Trichophyton* organism was cultured from the site. (From Mitchell M, Tully TN: *Manual of exotic pet practice*, St Louis, 2008, Saunders Elsevier.)

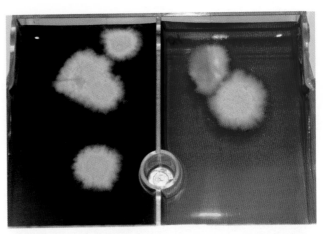

CP 9-19 ■ Dermatophytosis. Close-up of a dermatophyte test medium fungal culture demonstrating the typical white colony growth and red color change. This is suggestive of dermatophytosis, but microscopic identification should be performed to identify *Microsporum canis*. (From Medleau L, Hnilica KA: *Small animal dermatology: a color atlas and therapeutic guide*, ed 2, St Louis, 2006, Saunders Elsevier.)

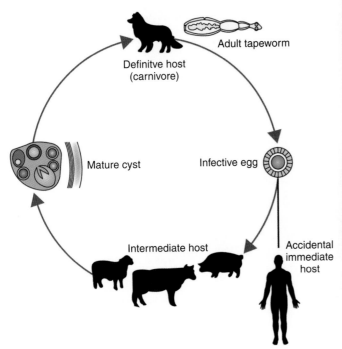

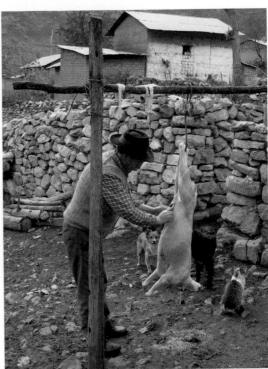

CP 9-20 ■ Slaughtering sheep near dogs. (From Craig PS, McManus DP, Lightowlers MW, et al: Prevention and control of cystic echinococcosis, *Lancet Infect Dis* 7(6):385-94, 2007.)

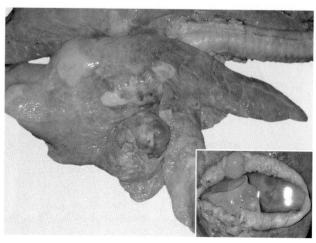

CP 9-21 ■ Hydatidosis (echinococcosis), lung, sheep. A large hydatid cyst is present in the pulmonary parenchyma. *Inset,* Hydatid cyst, cut-open section. The cyst contains fluid and larvae and is often enclosed by a fibrous capsule. (From McGavin MD, Zachary JF: *Pathologic basis of veterinary disease,* ed 4, St Louis, 2007, Mosby Elsevier. Courtesy Manuel Quezada, Universidad de Concepción, Chile.)

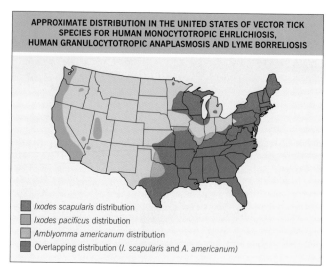

CP 9-22 ■ Approximate distribution in the United States of vector tick species for human monocytotropic ehrlichiosis, human granulocytotropic anaplasmosis, and Lyme borreliosis. (From Chapman AS et al: *MMWR Recomm Rep* 55:1-27, 2006.)

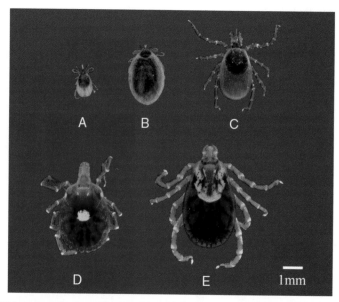

CP 9-23 ■ Tick vectors of agents of human rickettsial diseases. An unengaged nymph *(A),* engorged nymph *(B),* and adult female *(C)* of *Ixodes scapularis* (deer tick), the vector of *Anaplasma phagocytophilum,* the cause of human granulocytic anaplasmosis. An adult female *(D)* of *Amblyomma americanum* (lone star tick), the vector of *Ehrlichia chaffeensis* and *Ehrlichia ewingii,* the causes of human monocytic ehrlichiosis and ewingii ehrlichiosis, respectively. An adult female *(E)* of *Dermacentor variabilis* (American dog tick), the vector of *Rickettsia rickettsii,* the cause of Rocky Mountain spotted fever. (From Siberry GK, Dumler JS: Spotted fever group *Rickettsioses.* In Kliegman RM, Behrman RE, Jenson HB et al (eds): *Nelson textbook of pediatrics,* ed 18, Philadelphia, 2007, Saunders Elsevier.)

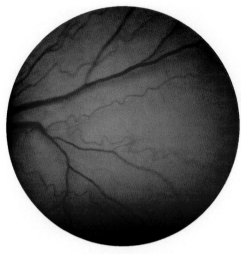

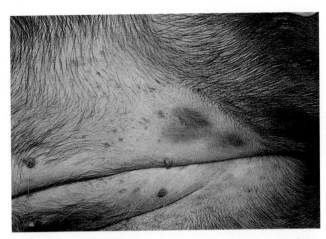

CP 9-26 ■ Canine ehrlichiosis. Petechiae and ecchymotic hemorrhages caused by thrombocytopenia resulting from the infection. (From Medleau L, Hnilica KA: *Small animal dermatology: a color atlas and therapeutic guide*, ed 2, St Louis, 2006, Saunders Elsevier.)

CP 9-24 ■ Flat retinal detachment in a dog with *E. canis* infection. Note the shadowing of retinal vessels. Also note the absence of retinal hemorrhage, which often accompanies the thrombocytopenia that occurs with this disease. (From Dziezyc J, Millichamp NJ: *Color atlas of canine and feline ophthalmology*, St Louis, 2005, Saunders Elsevier.)

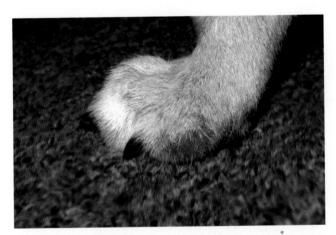

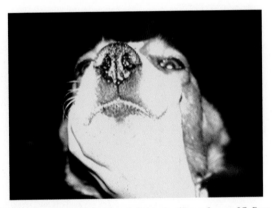

CP 9-27 ■ Epistaxis in canine ehrlichiosis. (From Songer JG, Post KW: *Veterinary microbiology: bacterial and fungal agents of animal disease*, St Louis, 2005, Saunders Elsevier. Courtesy Raymond E. Reed.)

CP 9-25 ■ Canine ehrlichiosis. A focal erythematous, alopecic lesion with superficial erosions in a dog with ehrlichiosis. (From Medleau L, Hnilica KA: *Small animal dermatology: a color atlas and therapeutic guide*, ed 2, St Louis, 2006, Saunders Elsevier.)

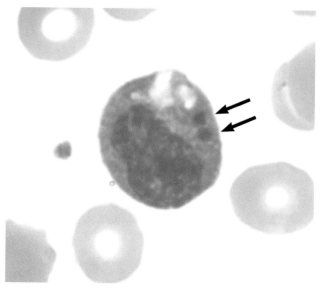

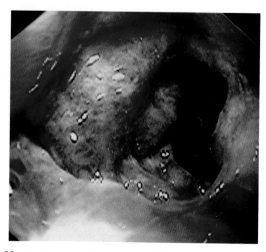

CP 9-29 ■ Colonoscopic appearance of the sigmoid colon in a patient with enterohemorrhagic *Escherichia coli* infection. The mucosa is edematous and violaceous, with diffuse subepithelial hemorrhage. (From Feldman M, et al (eds): *Sleisenger and Fordtran's gastrointestinal and liver disease, vol 1*, ed 8, Philadelphia, 2006, Saunders Elsevier.)

CP 9-28 ■ Peripheral blood smear (buffy coat preparation) showing intracellular inclusions *(arrows)* in mononuclear cells of a patient with ehrlichiosis. (Wright stain, original magnification, ×400.) (From Mandell GL, Bennett JE, Dolin R: *Principles and practice of infectious diseases*, ed 6, Philadelphia, 2005, Churchill Livingstone Elsevier.)

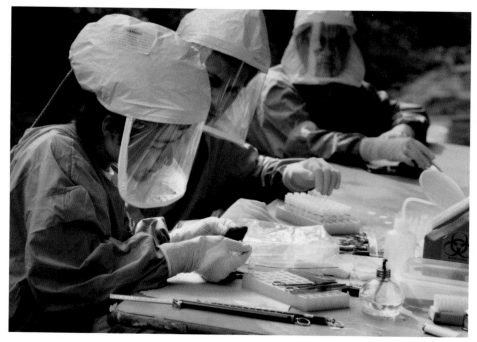

CP 9-30 ■ Field biologists using protective equipment for hantavirus infection while examining wild mice. (From Centers for Disease Control and Prevention, Atlanta, Ga.)

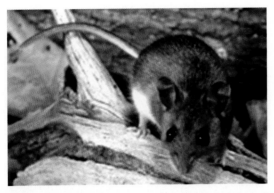

CP 9-31 ■ Deer mouse (*Peromyscus maniculatus*), the principal reservoir species for hantavirus in the United States. (From Centers for Disease Control and Prevention, Atlanta, Ga.)

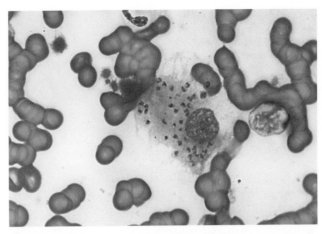

CP 9-34 ■ Leishmaniasis. Microscopic image of the protozoal amastigotes as viewed with a ×100 (oil) objective. (From Medleau L, Hnilica KA: *Small animal dermatology: a color atlas and therapeutic guide*, ed 2, St Louis, 2006, Saunders Elsevier.)

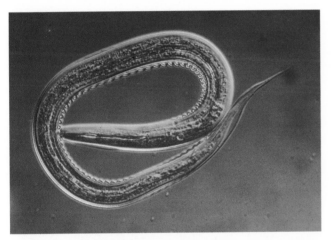

CP 9-32 ■ Third-stage larva of *Ancylostoma caninum*. (From Long SS, Pickering LK, Prober CG (eds): *Principles and practice of pediatric infectious diseases*, ed 2, Philadelphia, 2003, Elsevier. Courtesy E. Gravé.)

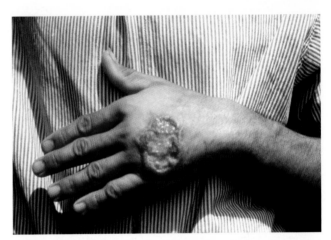

CP 9-35 ■ Skin ulcer due to leishmaniasis on the hand of a Central American adult. (From Centers for Disease Control and Prevention Public Health Image Library, Atlanta, Ga. Courtesy D.S. Martin.)

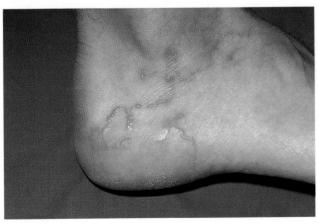

CP 9-33 ■ Cutaneous larva migrans. (From Goldman L, Ausiello DA (eds): *Cecil textbook of medicine,* ed 23, Philadelphia, 2008, Saunders Elsevier.)

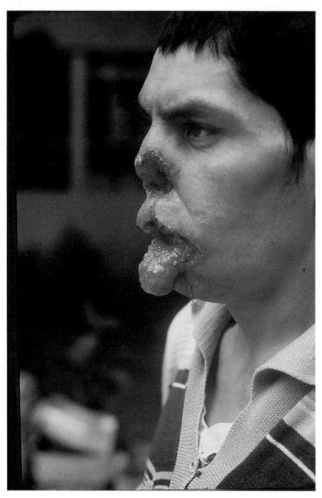

CP 9-36 ■ Mucocutaneous leishmaniasis. (From Cohen J, Powderly WG: *Infectious diseases*, ed 2, Edinburgh, 2003, Elsevier.)

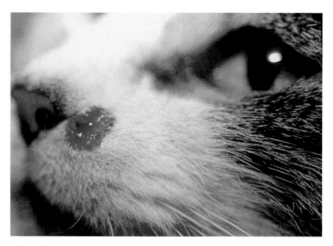

CP 9-38 ■ Cutaneous ulcer in cat with leishmaniasis. (From Greene CE: *Infectious diseases of the dog and cat*, ed 3, St Louis, 2006, Saunders Elsevier. Courtesy Maria Grazia Pennisi, University of Messina, Italy.)

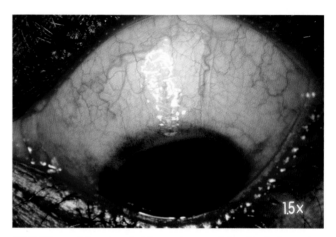

CP 9-39 ■ Subconjunctival hemorrhages and jaundice in leptospirosis. Asymptomatic or atypical infection probably occurs in 90% of cases. In some tropical areas, leptospirosis may account for up to 15% of all patients with undiagnosed pyrexia. Although this form can be mild, the infection may develop into a generalized septic form with confusion within 1 to 2 weeks. This is characterized by fever, myalgia, and often subconjunctival hemorrhages. The patient illustrated was in the second week after the onset of symptoms. The most dangerous form (Weil's disease) may be quite severe and can involve several organs, with jaundice, renal failure, hemorrhagia, vascular collapse, and obtundation. (From Cohen J, Powderly WG: *Infectious diseases*, ed 2, Edinburgh, 2004, Mosby Elsevier.)

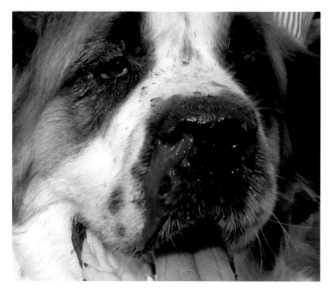

CP 9-37 ■ Epistaxis in a Saint Bernard with leishmaniasis and no dermal lesions. (From Greene CE: *Infectious diseases of the dog and cat*, ed 3, St Louis, 2006, Saunders Elsevier.)

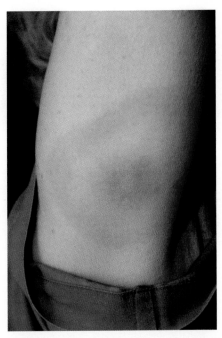

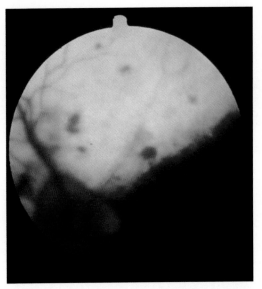

CP 9-42 ■ Preretinal petechiae on the fundus of a 7-year-old blood-hound diagnosed with canine Lyme disease. (From Maggs D, Miller P, Ofri R: *Slatter's fundamentals of veterinary ophthalmology*, ed 4, St Louis, 2008, Saunders Elsevier.)

CP 9-40 ■ Pathognomonic erythematous rash of Lyme disease in the pattern of a bull's-eye, which manifested at the site of a tick bite on this Maryland woman's posterior right upper arm. (From Centers for Disease Control and Prevention Public Health Image Library, Atlanta, Ga. Courtesy James Gathany.)

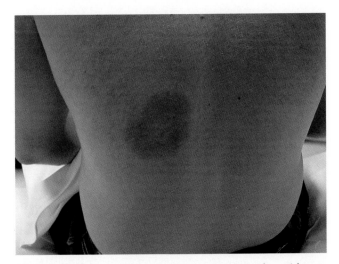

CP 9-41 ■ Rash on patient's back—presumptive southern tick-asso-ciated rash illness, a differential for Lyme disease. (From Auerbach PS: *Wilderness medicine*, ed 5, Philadelphia, 2007, Mosby Elsevier.)

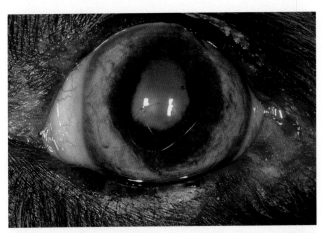

CP 9-43 ■ Posterior synechiae, iris bombé, and cataract associated with a high enzyme-linked immunosorbent assay titer to *Borrelia burgdorferi* in a mixed-breed dog. (The linear opacity on the cornea is a hair.) (From Dziezyc J, Millichamp NJ: *Color atlas of canine and feline ophthalmology*, St Louis, 2005, Saunders Elsevier.)

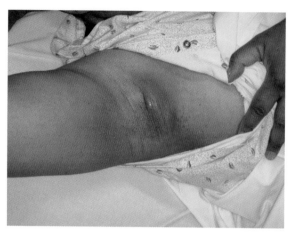

CP 9-44 ■ Necrotizing fascitis. (From Roberts JR, Hedges JR: *Clinical procedures in emergency medicine*, ed 5, Philadelphia, 2010, Saunders Elsevier.)

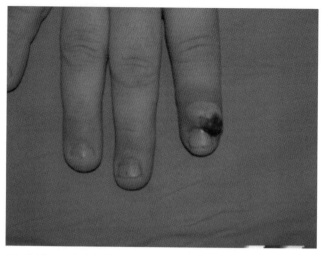

CP 9-47 ■ Orf in finger. (From Centers for Disease Control and Prevention, Atlanta, Ga. Courtesy Sue Meidel, National Center for Zoonotic, Vector-Borne, and Enteric Disease.)

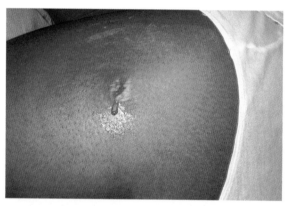

CP 9-45 ■ Methicillin-resistant *Staphylococcus aureus* soft tissue infection. (From Centers for Disease Control and Prevention Public Health Image Library, Atlanta, Ga.)

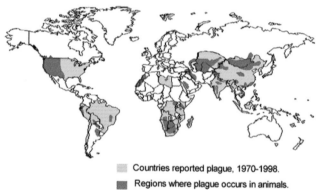

CP 9-48 ■ World distribution of Plague, 1998. (From Centers for Disease Control and Prevention, Division of Vector Borne Infectious Diseases, Atlanta, Ga.)

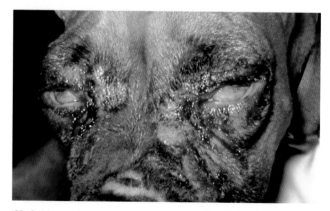

CP 9-46 ■ Severe crusting erosive dermatitis on the face of an adult Boxer. This dog also had a secondary methicillin-resistant *Staphylococcus aureus* infection, possibly obtained from the owner, who worked in the human health care industry. (From Medleau L, Hnilica KA: *Small animal dermatology: a color atlas and therapeutic guide*, ed 2, St Louis, 2006, Saunders Elsevier.)

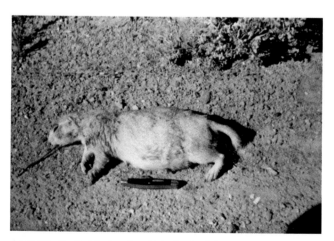

CP 9-49 ■ Prairie dog that died of a *Yersinia pestis* infection. (From Centers for Disease Control and Prevention Public Health Image Library, Atlanta, Ga.)

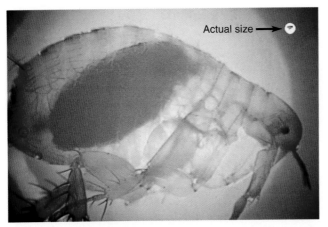

CP 9-50 ■ *Xenopsylla cheopis* (oriental rat flea) engorged with blood. (From Centers for Disease Control and Prevention, Division of Vector Borne Infectious Diseases, Atlanta, Ga.)

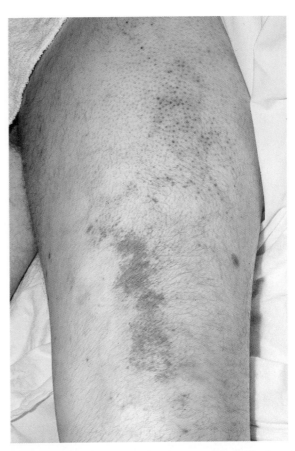

CP 9-52 ■ Septicemic plague with ecchymoses and petechiae from disseminated intravascular coagulation. (From Mandell GL, Bennett JE, Dolin R: *Principles and practice of infectious diseases*, ed 6, Philadelphia, 2005, Churchill Livingstone Elsevier.)

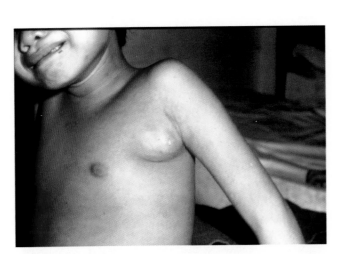

CP 9-51 ■ Axillary bubo in bubonic plague. (From Marx J, Hockberger R, Walls R (eds): *Rosen's emergency medicine: concepts and clinical practice*, ed 6, Philadelphia, 2006, Mosby Elsevier. Courtesy of Frederick M. Burkle, Jr.)

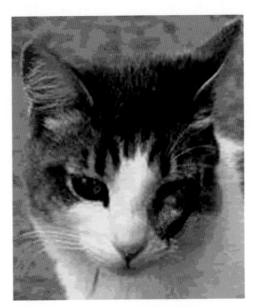

CP 9-53 ■ Cat recovering from bubonic plague. Centers for Disease Control and Prevention: *Emergency preparedness and response: plague: veterinary issues: dogs and ungulates.* http://www.bt.cdc.gov/agent/plague/trainingmodule/7/07.asp.)

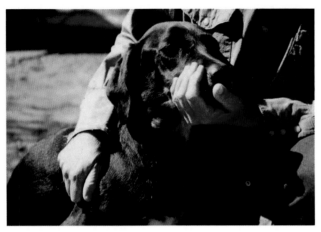

CP 9-54 ■ Dog with submandibular lymphadenopathy. (Courtesy Ted Brown, New Mexico Environment Department.)

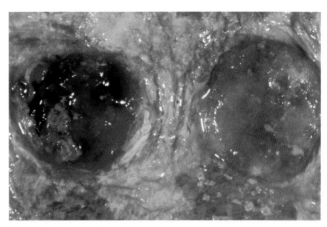

CP 9-56 ■ Intercotyledonary placentitis *(Coxiella burnetii)*, goat. Note the opacity of the intercotyledonary placenta caused by thickening from inflammation and fibrosis. The cotyledons have variable areas of gray discoloration, indicating necrosis and inflammatory exudates. The gross appearance of the lesions of placentitis tends to be similar, regardless of the etiologic agent identified by microbiological examination. (From McGavin MD, Zachary JF: *Pathologic basis of veterinary disease*, ed 4, St Louis, 2007, Mosby Elsevier. Courtesy R.A. Foster, Ontario Veterinary College, University of Guelph.)

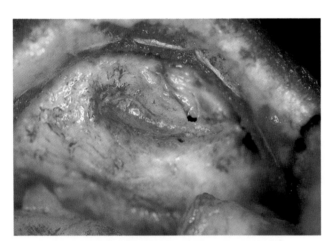

CP 9-55 ■ Q fever endocarditis on bioprosthetic valve leaflet. The ridge in the center of the photograph is the area infiltrated with *C. burnetii.* (From Raoult D, Raza A, Marrie TJ: Q fever endocarditis and other forms of chronic Q fever. In Marrie TJ (ed): *Q fever: the disease*, Boca Raton, FL, 1990, CRC Press.)

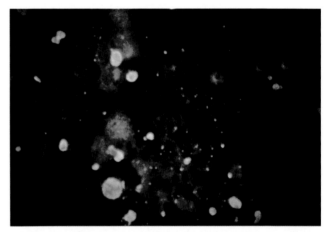

CP 9-57 ■ Immunofluorescent micrograph revealing a positive result for the presence of rabies virus antigens in a specimen. (From Centers for Disease Control and Prevention Public Health Image Library, Atlanta, Ga. Courtesy Dr. Tierkel.)

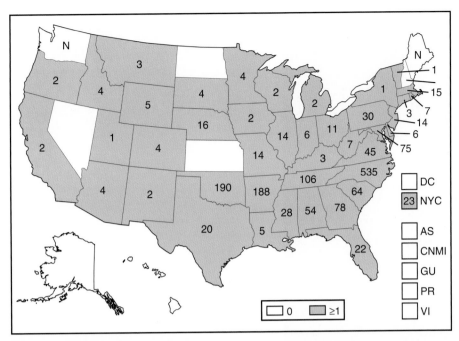

CP 9-58 ■ The number of reported cases of Rocky Mountain spotted fever (RMSF) in the United States and its territories, 2004. Changes in the number of reported cases of RMSF might reflect alterations to surveillance algorithms for this and other tickborne diseases. Biological factors (e.g., changes in tick populations resulting from fluctuating environmental conditions) might also be involved. (From Long SS, Pickering LK, Prober CG: *Principles and practice of pediatric infectious diseases*, ed 3, London, 2009, Churchill Livingstone Elsevier. Data from Centers for Disease Control and Prevention: Summary of Notifiable Disease— United States, 2004, *MMWR Morbid Mortal Wkly Rep* 53:61, 2006.)

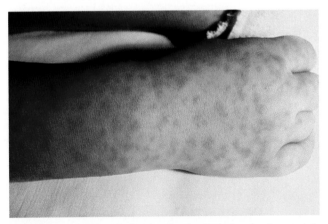

CP 9-59 ■ Child's right hand and wrist displaying the characteristic rash of Rocky Mountain spotted fever. (From Centers for Disease Control and Prevention Public Health Image Library, Atlanta, Ga.)

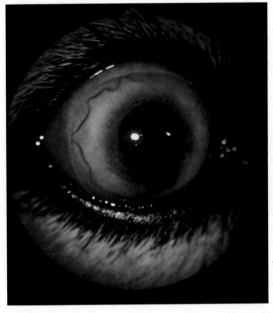

CP 9-60 ■ Anterior uveitis in the left eye of a 9-year-old mixed-breed dog seropositive to *Rickettsia rickettsii*. Iridal congestion, blood, and fibrin in the anterior chamber, and secondary glaucoma (iris bombé) can be seen. (From Maggs D, Miller P, Ofri R: *Slatter's fundamentals of veterinary ophthalmology*, ed 4, St Louis, 2008, Saunders Elsevier.)

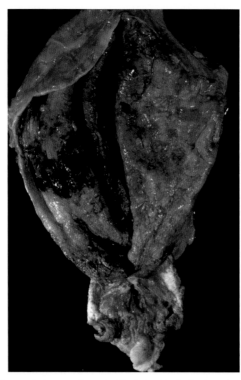

CP 9-61 ▪ Stricture, colon, pig. This lesion in pigs has been attributed to thrombosis of the cranial hemorrhoidal artery from vasculitis and thrombosis caused by salmonella. (From McGavin MD, Zachary JF: *Pathologic basis of veterinary disease*, ed 4, St Louis, 2007, Mosby Elsevier. Courtesy C.S. Patton, College of Veterinary Medicine, University of Tennessee.)

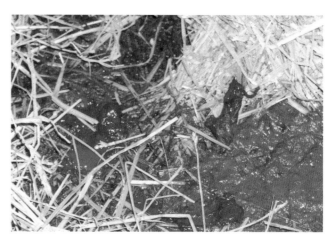

CP 9-63 ▪ Fresh blood clots mixed with feces of a cow that had a type C *Salmonella* spp. enterocolitis. (From Divers TJ, Peek SF: *Rebhun's diseases of dairy cattle*, ed 2, St Louis, 2008, Saunders Elsevier.)

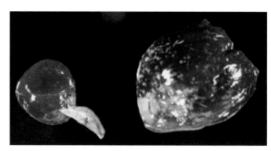

CP 9-64 ▪ Systemic lesions of *Salmonella* infection in a cockatiel. (From Songer JG, Post KW: *Veterinary microbiology: bacterial and fungal agents of animal disease*, St Louis, 2005, Saunders Elsevier. Courtesy Raymond E. Reed.)

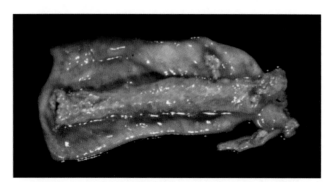

CP 9-62 ▪ Fibrinous cholecystitis, gallbladder, cow. Fibrinous cholecystitis caused by *Salmonella enteritidis* serotype *dublin* has produced a fibrinous cast, which has sloughed into the lumen of the gallbladder. (From McGavin MD, Zachary JF: *Pathologic basis of veterinary disease*, ed 4, St Louis, 2007, Mosby Elsevier. Courtesy D.A. Mosier, College of Veterinary Medicine, Kansas State University.)

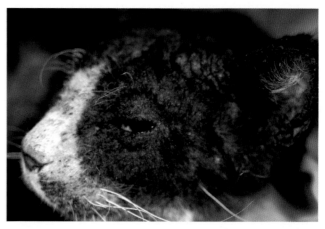

CP 9-65 ▪ Feline scabies. Generalized alopecia and crusting papular dermatitis on the head of an adult cat. (From Medleau L, Hnilica KA: *Small animal dermatology: a color atlas and therapeutic guide*, ed 2, St Louis, 2006, Saunders Elsevier.)

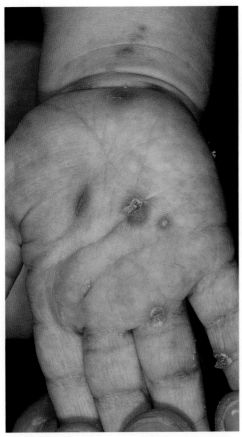

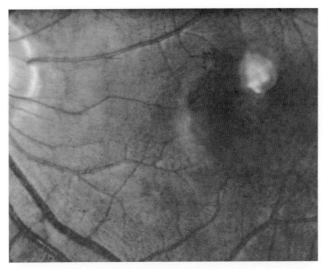

CP 9-68 ■ Larva of *Toxocara* in retina manifesting as granuloma. (From Long SS, Pickering LK, Porber CG: *Principles and practice of pediatric infectious disease*, ed 3, Philadelphia, 2009, Saunders Elsevier.)

CP 9-66 ■ Scabies. Pustules on the palms of an infant. Note the papular lesions on the wrist. (From Habif TP: *Clinical dermatology: a color guide to diagnosis and therapy*, ed 4, St Louis, 2004, Mosby Elsevier.)

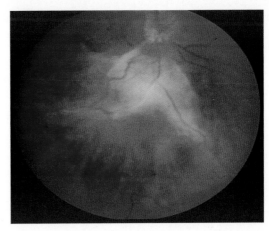

CP 9-69 ■ Chorioretinitis due to toxoplasmosis. (From Cohen J, Powderly WG: *Infectious diseases*, ed 2, Edinburgh, 2004, Mosby Elsevier.)

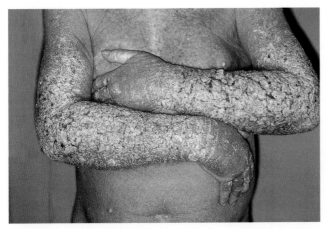

CP 9-67 ■ Marked hyperkeratosis on arms of a patient with crusted ("Norwegian") scabies. (From Mandell GL, Bennett JE, Dolin R: *Principles and practice of infectious diseases*, ed 6, Philadelphia, 2005, Churchill Livingstone Elsevier. Courtesy Kenneth E. Greer, Charlottesville, Va.)

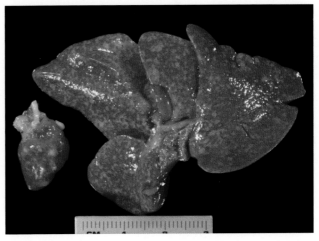

CP 9-70 ■ Pneumonia and necrosis in heart of a kitten congenitally infected with toxoplasmosis. (From Greene CE: *Infectious diseases of the dog and cat*, ed 3, St Louis, 2006, Saunders Elsevier.)

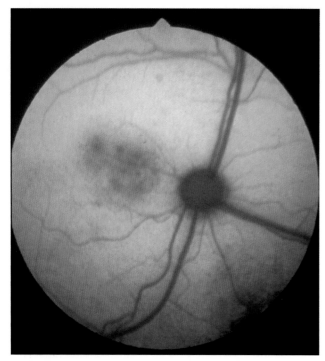

CP 9-71 ■ Punctate chorioretinitis caused by *Toxoplasma gondii* in an experimentally inoculated cat. (From Lappin MR: Polysystemic protozoal infections. In Nelson RW, Couto CG (eds): *Small animal internal medicine*, ed 4, St Louis, 2009, Mosby Elsevier.)

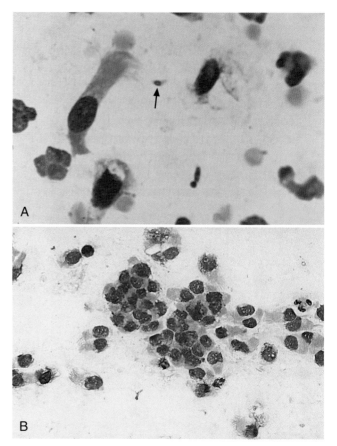

CP 9-72 ■ **A,** Tracheal wash and bronchioalveolar lavage from a dog with toxoplasmosis. A ciliated columnar cell, red blood cells, scattered neutrophils, and an extracellular *Toxoplasma gondii* organism *(arrow)* are shown. (Wright's stain, original magnification ×250.) **B,** Ciliated columnar cells are present both individually and in a cluster. The morphology of the cells in the cluster cannot be discerned. Cilia are evident on the cells that are well spread out. Many of the cells are traumatized, as evidenced by their irregular nuclear outlines. (Wright's stain, original magnification ×160.) (From Cowell RL, Tyler RD, Meinkoth JH, et al: *Diagnostic cytology and hematology of the dog and cat*, ed 3, St Louis, 2008, Mosby Elsevier.)

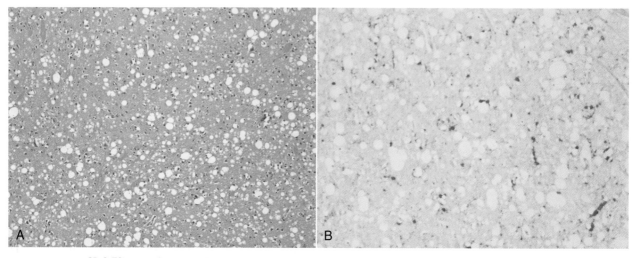

CP 9-73 ■ Feline spongiform encephalopathy. **A,** Area in the thalamus with many small and large vacuoles in the neuropil (H&E stain, ×100). **B,** Area with spongiform change. Punctate and plaquelike deposits *(red)* of the protease resistant PrP (immunocytochemical staining with polyclonal anti-PrP; avidin biotinylated enzyme complex [ABC] technique, ×250). (From Greene CE: *Infectious diseases of the dog and cat*, ed 3, St Louis, 2006, Saunders Elsevier.)

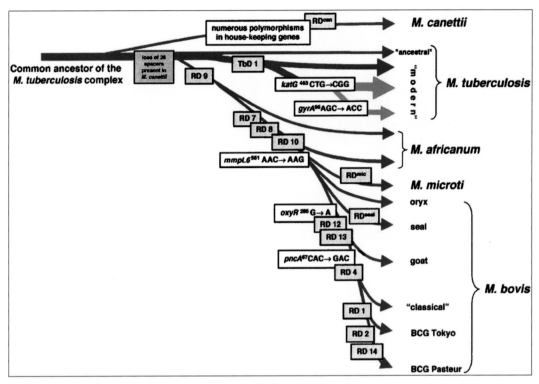

CP 9-74 ■ Scheme of the proposed evolutionary pathway of the tubercle bacilli illustrating successive loss of DNA in certain lineages *(gray boxes)*. (From Brosch R, Gordon SV, Marmiesse M et al: A new evolutionary scenario for the *Mycobacterium tuberculosis* complex, *Proc Natl Acad Sci U S A* 99(6):3684, 2002. Copyright © 2002 The National Academy of Sciences.)

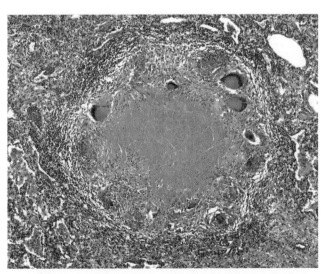

CP 9-75 ■ Typical granuloma resulting from infection with *Mycobacterium tuberculosis* showing central caseous necrosis, activated epithelioid macrophages, many giant cells, and a peripheral accumulation of lymphocytes. (From Kumar V, Abbas AK, Fausto N et al: *Robbins basic pathology*, ed 8, Philadelphia, 2007, Saunders Elsevier.)

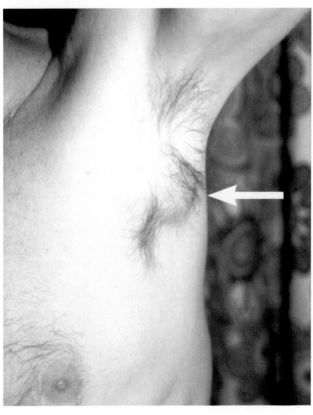

CP 9-76 ■ Axillary lymphadenitis caused by *Mycobacterium tuberculosis* in a patient with AIDS. (From Mandell GL, Bennett JE, Dolin R: *Principles and practice of infectious diseases*, ed 6, New York, 2005, Churchill Livingstone Elsevier.)

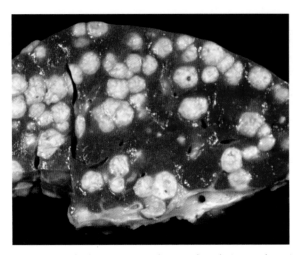

CP 9-77 ■ Multiple caseous granulomas, tuberculosis, *Mycobacterium bovis,* liver, cow. Hepatic tuberculosis is characterized by random, multifocal, pale white to yellow caseous granulomas on the capsular and cut surfaces. (From McGavin MD, Zachary JF: *Pathologic basis of veterinary disease,* ed 4, St Louis, 2007, Mosby Elsevier. Courtesy M. Domingo, Autonomous University of Barcelona, and Noah's Arkive, College of Veterinary Medicine, The University of Georgia.)

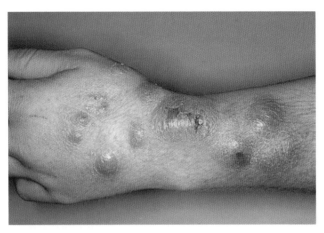

CP 9-78 ■ *Mycobacterium marinum* in a pet store worker. (From Nguyen C: Images in clinical medicine. *Mycobacterium marinum, N Engl J Med* 350(9):e8, 2004.)

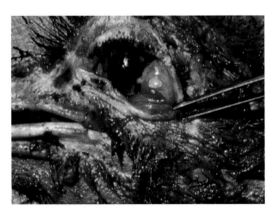

CP 9-79 ■ Conjunctival mycobacteriosis *(Mycobacterium avium)* in an ostrich. (From Songer JG, Post KW: *Veterinary microbiology: bacterial and fungal agents of animal disease,* St Louis, 2005, Saunders Elsevier. Courtesy J. Glenn Songer.)

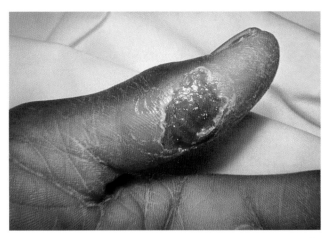

CP 9-80 ■ Thumb with skin ulcer of tularemia. (From Centers for Disease Control and Prevention Public Health Image Library, Atlanta, Ga.)

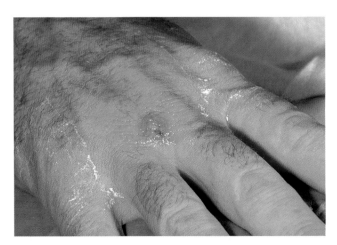

CP 9-81 ■ Ulceroglandular tularemia. (From Reintjes R, Dedushaj I, Gjini A, et al: Tularemia outbreak investigation in Kosovo: case control and environmental studies, *Emerg Infect Dis* 8(1):69, 2002.)

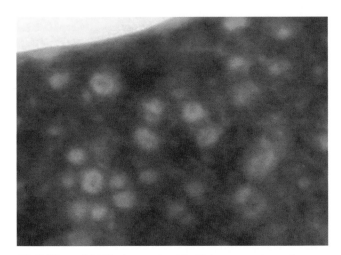

CP 9-82 ■ Multifocal necrosis with fibrinosuppurative and granulomatous inflammation in the spleen of a cat infected with *F. tularensis.* (From Greene CE: *Infectious diseases of the dog and cat,* ed 3, St Louis, 2006, Saunders Elsevier. Courtesy Brad M. DeBey, Department of Veterinary Pathology, Kansas State University, Manhattan.)

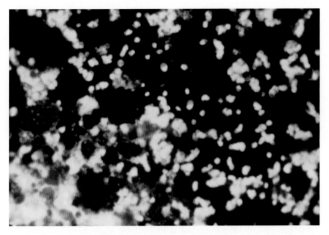

CP 9-83 ▪ Photomicrograph depicting *Francisella tularensis* bacteria as seen with a fluorescent antibody stain. (From Centers for Disease Control and Prevention Public Health Image Library, Atlanta, Ga.)

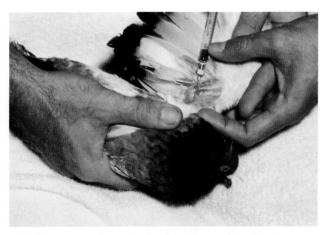

CP 9-85 ▪ Blood being extracted from the wing vein of a pigeon to be tested for the presence of arboviruses. (From Centers for Disease Control and Prevention Public Health Image Library, Atlanta, Ga.)

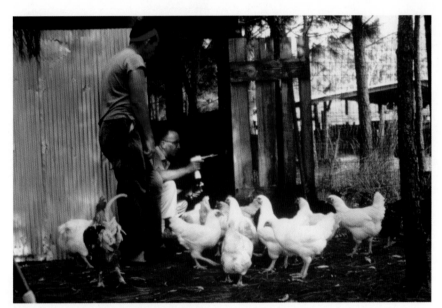

CP 9-84 ▪ Flock of sentinel chickens. (From Scott County Health Department: *Mosquito surveillance program*. http://www.scottcountyiowa.com/health/images/mosquito_surveillance02.jpg.)

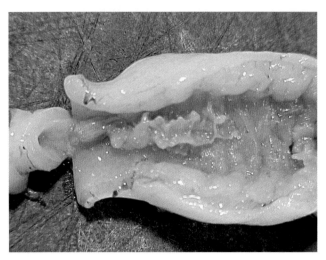

CP 9-86 ■ Fibrinous colitis in an alligator with West Nile virus. This animal was unable to submerge itself. (From Nevarez J: Crocodilians. In Mitchell M, Tully Jr TN (eds): *Manual of exotic pet practice*, St Louis, 2009, Saunders Elsevier.)

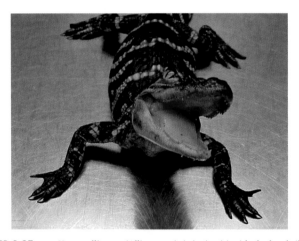

CP 9-87 ■ Young alligator *(Alligator mississippiensis)* with the head tilt typical of those affected with West Nile virus. Notice that it still maintains an aggressive stand with the mouth open. (From Mader DR: *Reptile medicine and surgery*, ed 2, St Louis, 2006, Saunders Elsevier.)

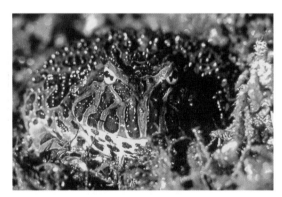

CP 10-1 ■ Many amphibians bite. Some, such as the Argentine horned frog *(Ceratophrys ornata)*, can inflict severe wounds on the human handler. (From Mader DR: *Reptile medicine and surgery*, ed 2, St Louis, 2006, Saunders Elsevier. Courtesy D. Mader.)

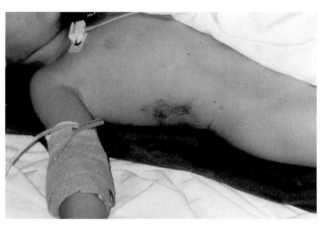

CP 10-2 ■ Toddler victim of moose attack. Hoof mark on chest wall overlies rib fractures and pulmonary contusion. (From Auerbach PS: *Wilderness medicine*, ed 5, Philadelphia, 2007, Mosby Elsevier. Courtesy Luanne Freer.)

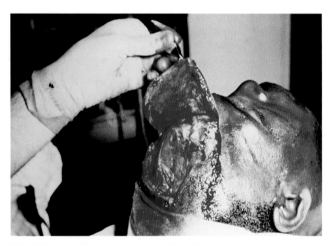

CP 10-3 ■ Lion attack victim. This African victim was rescued by bystanders while his head was in the lion's mouth. His only injury was a degloving scalp laceration. (From Auerbach PS: *Wilderness medicine*, ed 5, Philadelphia, 2007, Mosby Elsevier. Courtesy Harold P. Adolph.)

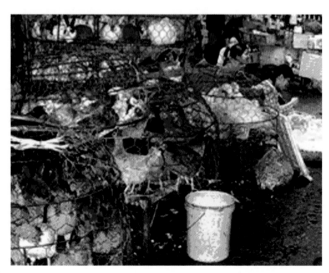

CP 10-4 ■ Live animal market. (From U.S. Agency for International Development: Congress approves $25 million to fight avian flu in Asia, *FrontLines*, July/August 2005.)

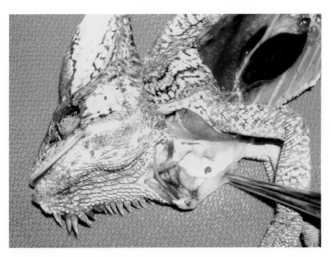

CP 10-5 ■ A nematode in the accessory lung lobe (at tip of forceps) in a chameleon. Small numbers of lung parasites do not usually cause a problem. However, in immunocompromised patients, parasites can lead to inflammation and pneumonia. (From Mader DR: *Reptile medicine and surgery*, ed 2, St Louis, 2006, Saunders Elsevier. Courtesy D. Mader.)

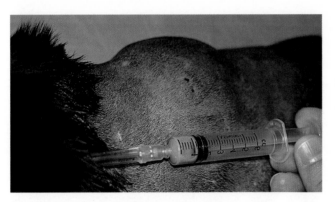

CP 10-6 ■ Subcutaneous abscess. Feline abscess caused by a cat bite. The syringe contains purulent material aspirated from the abscess. (From Medleau L, Hnilica KA: *Small animal dermatology: a color atlas and therapeutic guide*, ed 2, St Louis, 2006, Saunders Elsevier.)

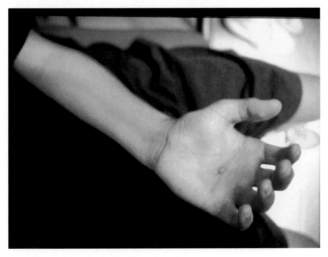

CP 10-7 ■ Infected cat bite. Note the streak of erythema extending proximally along the anterior forearm. (From Zaoutis LB, Chiang VW: *Comprehensive pediatric hospital medicine*, Philadelphia, 2007, Mosby Elsevier.)

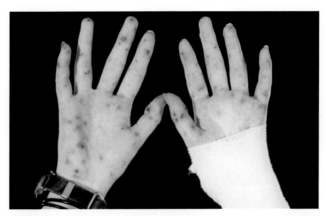

CP 10-8 ■ Maculopapular rash with small, dark-red eruptions on hand of person with rat-bite fever. (From Van Nood E, Peters SH: Rat-bite fever, *Neth J Med* 63:319, 2005.)

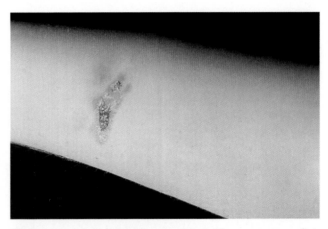

CP 10-9 ■ Localized lesion in sporotrichosis. The most common clinical presentation is a localized cutaneous or subcutaneous lesion, which develops at the site of implantation of the etiologic agent, *Sporothrix schenckii*. (From Cohen J, Powderly WG: *Infectious diseases*, ed 2, London, 2004, Mosby Elsevier.)

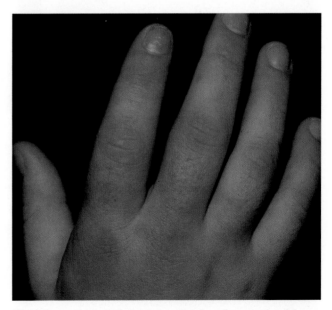

CP 12-1 ■ Erysipeloid. Approximately 3 days after animal or fish contact, a dull red erythema appears at the inoculation site and extends centrifugally. (From Habif TP: *Clinical dermatology: a color guide to diagnosis and therapy*, ed 4, St Louis, 2004, Mosby Elsevier.)

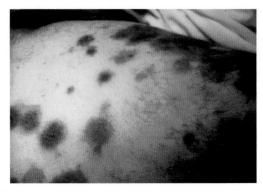

CP 12-2 ■ Torso of a victim with *Vibrio vulnificus* sepsis. (From Auerbach PS: *Wilderness medicine*, ed 5, Philadelphia, 2007, Mosby Elsevier.)

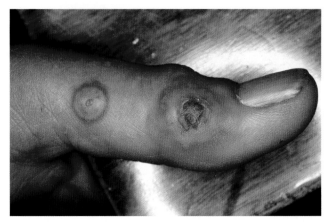

CP 12-3 ■ Seal finger secondary to *Mycoplasma*. (From Auerbach PS: *Wilderness medicine*, ed 5, Philadelphia, 2007, Mosby Elsevier. Courtesy Edgar Maeyens, Jr.)

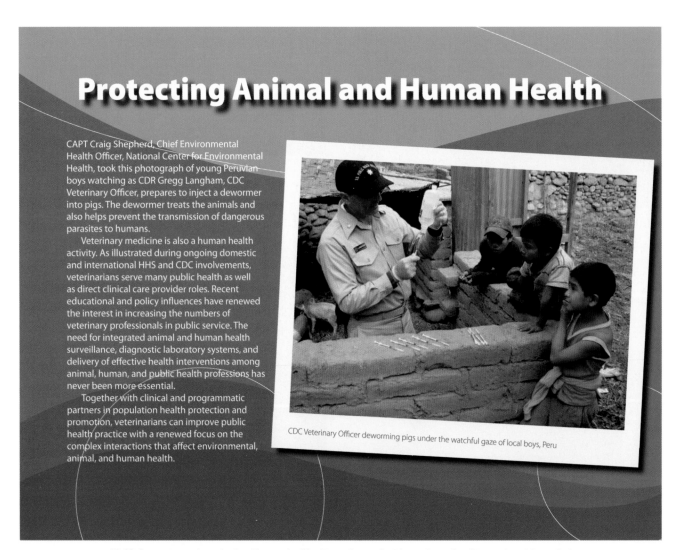

Protecting Animal and Human Health

CAPT Craig Shepherd, Chief Environmental Health Officer, National Center for Environmental Health, took this photograph of young Peruvian boys watching as CDR Gregg Langham, CDC Veterinary Officer, prepares to inject a dewormer into pigs. The dewormer treats the animals and also helps prevent the transmission of dangerous parasites to humans.

Veterinary medicine is also a human health activity. As illustrated during ongoing domestic and international HHS and CDC involvements, veterinarians serve many public health as well as direct clinical care provider roles. Recent educational and policy influences have renewed the interest in increasing the numbers of veterinary professionals in public service. The need for integrated animal and human health surveillance, diagnostic laboratory systems, and delivery of effective health interventions among animal, human, and public health professions has never been more essential.

Together with clinical and programmatic partners in population health protection and promotion, veterinarians can improve public health practice with a renewed focus on the complex interactions that affect environmental, animal, and human health.

CDC Veterinary Officer deworming pigs under the watchful gaze of local boys, Peru

CP 13-1 ■ Protecting animal and human health. (From Centers for Disease Control and Prevention, Atlanta, Ga.)

Table 9-10 ▪ Brucellosis: Comparative Clinical Presentations in Humans and Other Animals

Species	Risk Factors	Incubation Period	Clinical Manifestations	Laboratory Findings
Humans (*B. abortus, B. melitensis, B. suis, B. canis*)	Ingestion of unpasteurized dairy products, occupational exposure to animal tissue, fluids, aerosol	Variable, usually 5-60 days[20]	Fever, joint pain, abdominal pain, weight loss, fatigue, arthritis, endocarditis, epididymitis/orchitis	Elevated IgG; other laboratory values may be normal or leukopenia, thrombocytopenia, abnormal liver function may occur; positive blood culture
Dogs (*B. canis, B. abortus, B. melitensis, B. suis*)	Ingestion of infected tissue Sexual contact Transplacental	Variable, related to stage of gestation, often months	Usually asymptomatic or vague signs, but lethargy, lymphadenopathy, back pain, weakness, glomerulonephritis, discospondylitis may occur[21] *Females:* abortion, infertility *Males:* Epididymitis, testicular atrophy	CBC usually normal, positive serology, positive blood or tissue culture
Sheep, goats (*B. melitensis, B. abortus*) Sheep (*B. ovis*)	Direct contact, sexual transmission	Variable, related to stage of gestation, often months	Abortion Epididymitis	Positive serology
Cattle (*B. abortus*)	Ingestion of contaminated tissue, feed, water	Variable, related to stage of gestation, often months	Abortion, epididymitis, arthritis	Positive serology, *Brucella* ring test
Swine (*B. suis*)	Ingestion of infected tissue, sexual contact	Variable, related to stage of gestation, often months	Abortion, orchitis, spondylitis, sterility[4]	Brucellosis card test

CBC, Complete blood cell count.

Mode of Transmission and Life Cycle

Brucellosis is transmitted by direct contact with infected tissues or secretions and enters the body by breaks in the skin or contact with mucous membranes (Figure 9-13). It can also be acquired by ingestion of contaminated foods. Aerosol transmission can easily occur. It is thought that a small number of inhaled organisms can lead to human infection, as seen in outbreaks

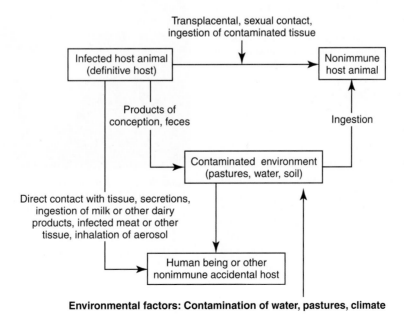

Environmental factors: Contamination of water, pastures, climate

Figure 9-13 ▪ Transmission and life cycle of *Brucellosis.*

of infection among laboratory workers. *Brucella* consequently requires biosafety level 3 containment in laboratories.

Transmission in cattle occurs through ingestion of contaminated pasture forage or water, as well as through licking and other direct contact of infected calves, fetuses, and afterbirths. Transmission in dogs is due to ingestion of or other contact with contaminated tissue, including sexual contact. The risk of transmission of brucellosis from dogs to humans is considered low and related to frequent close contact with blood, birth tissues, or other infected secretions.[17] In humans, person-to-person infection has been reported through breastfeeding, childbirth, bone marrow transplants, sexual contact, and transfusions, but these modes of transmission are considered exceptional.[6]

Environmental Risk Factors

Brucella may survive for months in the environment in water and other media that are not exposed to direct sunlight or heat. Pastures can become contaminated by feces, products of conception, and vaginal discharges of infected animals, leading to spread of infection in herds of grazing animals. *Brucella* organisms have been recovered from cow manure that has remained in a cool environment for longer than 2 months.[4]

Disease in Humans

Five to 60 days after infection, *Brucella* can cause a febrile illness that may be abrupt or gradual. Symptoms are often nonspecific and include fever, headache, night sweats, fatigue, arthralgia, myalgia, joint pain, anorexia, abdominal pain, diarrhea, vomiting, and weight loss. Depression may be a prominent feature. The fever may be "undulant" in patients who remain untreated. Clinical findings may be unremarkable, but in 20% to 30% of patients hepatosplenomegaly and/or lymphadenopathy may develop. Osteoarticular involvement of the spine and large weightbearing joints (Figure 9-14) is common.[18] Rarely, more severe infection can lead to epididymitis, orchitis, uveitis, endocarditis, and meningitis. A review of human cases found *B. melitensis* was more likely than *B. abortus* to cause abdominal pain and tenderness, hepatomegaly, splenomegaly, thrombocytopenia, pancytopenia, and hepatic dysfunction.[10] Laboratory findings are usually mild or absent but may include elevation of liver function test results, thrombocytopenia, and other hematologic abnormalities.

Disease in Animals

In most animals, spontaneous abortion is the most common manifestation of *Brucella* infection. Infection may be chronic and poorly responsive to treatment.

In pregnant cows, *B. abortus* causes placental infection leading to abortion in the second half of gestation. It also causes reduced milk yield, testicular abscesses and epididymitis in bulls, and (rarely) joint involvement with longstanding infection.[4] Infection in goats, sheep, and pigs is similar to that in cattle.

In sheep, *B. ovis* causes epididymitis in rams but abortions and stillbirths in ewes (Color Plate 9-5).[4]

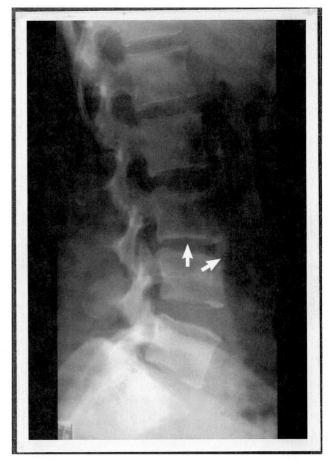

Figure 9-14　■　Radiograph of lumbar spine showing discitis and spondylitis due to brucellosis. Note reduced disk space and the destruction of articular margins at L3-L4 *(arrows)*. (From Cohen J, Powderly WG: *Infectious diseases*, ed 2, St Louis, 2004, Mosby Elsevier.)

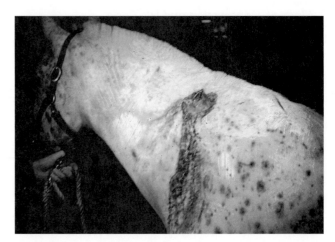

Figure 9-15　■　Fistulous withers in a horse. (From Auer JA: *Equine surgery*, ed 3, Philadelphia, 2006, Saunders Elsevier.)

Horses develop a rare bursitis condition known as *poll evil* or *fistulous withers* that may be caused by *B. abortus* or occasionally *B. suis* (Figure 9-15).[4]

In dogs, the most common recognized sign and symptom are abortion and infertility. Females may have a prolonged vaginal discharge following abortion. Lymphadenitis may be seen. In males, orchitis, epididymitis, and prostatitis may occur. Spondylitis resulting in back pain and weakness, and uveitis are reported complications (Color Plate 9-6).[4]

Cats are apparently resistant to *Brucella* infection.[19]

Diagnosis

The differential diagnosis of brucellosis in humans is extensive and includes other causes of fever, including influenza, mononucleosis, human immunodeficiency virus (HIV), and malaria. A history of contact with animals, laboratory exposure, or consumption of unpasteurized dairy products should make clinicians suspect brucellosis. Diagnosis in humans is based on culturing the organism from blood, bone marrow, or other tissue, and/or serology. Cultures may be slow to grow and require caution in handling. Elevated immunoglobulin G (IgG) antibodies titers by ELISA or other tests including serum agglutination (SAT) are often key to the diagnosis, as active infection titers often exceed 1:160. Infection with *B. canis* may produce antibodies that do not react with standard *Brucella* test antigens; therefore specific *B. canis* serology must be requested if this infection is suspected. PCR techniques have shown promising results but are still in development.[21]

In dogs, cultures of blood and tissue are also used. There are several serological tests. The RSAT test has a high sensitivity but low specificity. The mercaptoethanol test also has low specificity; positive results must be confirmed by other tests such as the agar-gel immunodiffusion (AGID) test.[4]

Possible herd infection in cattle is diagnosed using the *Brucella* milk ring test, which is sensitive but not specific (Color Plate 9-7).[4] Blood samples are collected from slaughtered animals. Further tests are used to confirm positive results.

Postexposure Prophylaxis

Following laboratory or vaccine exposure to *Brucella* species, 100 mg of doxycycline twice daily and rifampin 600 mg/day should be taken for 21 days. Trimethoprin sulfamethoxazole is an alternative for those with a contraindication to doxycycline. Doxycycline alone should be given if the exposure was to *Brucella abortus* strain RB51, which is resistant to rifampin.[9] Baseline serum drawn for *Brucella* serology with repeat serology at 2, 4, 6, and 24 weeks can be used to monitor for evidence of infection. Such monitoring is not recommended for exposures to vaccine RB51, which does not elicit an antibody response on available assays. Exposed pregnant women should consult their obstetric care provider regarding PEP. Exposed persons should be monitored on a regular basis for the development of fever and other clinical signs of infection.[9]

Treatment

Antibiotic therapy for brucellosis infection in humans and other animals is outlined in Table 9-11 below. In humans, relapse and prolonged convalescence may occur after antibiotic treatment. Patients with focal complications including spinal or neurological involvement may require a more prolonged course of treatment.

Table 9-11 ▪ Brucellosis Treatment in Humans and Other Animals

Species	Primary Treatment	Alternative
Humans (adult or child >8 yr[23])	Doxycycline 100 mg bid × 6 wk *PLUS* gentamicin × 7 days *or* doxycycline 100 mg PO bid × 6 wk *PLUS* streptomycin 1 gm IM q24h × 2-3 wk	Doxycycline 100 mg PO bid *PLUS* rifampin 600-900 mg PO q24h × 6 wk *or* trimethoprim-sulfamethoxazole 1 DS tab (160 mg TMP) PO qid × 6 wk *PLUS* gentamicin × 2 wk
Humans (child <8 yr)	Trimethoprim-sulfamethoxazole 5 mg/kg PO q12h × 6 wk *PLUS* gentamicin 2 mg/kg IV/IM q8h × 2 wk[23]	
Postexposure prophylaxis	Doxycycline 100 mg PO bid *PLUS* rifampin 600 mg PO qd × 3 wk (doxycycline alone if exposed to strain *B. abortus* RB51)[9]	Trimethoprim-sulfamethoxazole (160 mg/800 mg) × 3 wk
Dogs	Doxycycline 12-15 mg/kg PO q12h × 4 wk *PLUS* gentamicin 5 mg/kg SC q24h at 0 and 1 wk[21]	

In animals, treatment can be unsuccessful even after prolonged administration of antibiotics. Therefore euthanasia and culling are often used as a means of brucellosis control. Animals may still be infectious to other animals (and humans) despite treatment, and this should be considered before attempting treatment of a pet dog. Neutering of infected dogs is sometimes performed to achieve infection control.

In cattle, antibiotic treatment is considered practical.[4]

References

1. Zinsstag J, Schelling E, Roth F, et al. Human benefits of animal interventions for zoonosis control. *Emerg Infect Dis.* 2007;13(4):527.
2. Food and Agriculture Organization (FAO). *Guidelines for coordinated human and animal brucellosis surveillance.* http://www.fao.org/docrep/006/y4723e/y4723e00.htm; Accessed September 4, 2008.
3. Dvorak G, Rovid-Spickler A, Roth JA, et al. *Handbook for zoonotic diseases of companion animals.* Ames, IA: The Center for food security and public health, Iowa State University College of Veterinary Medicine; 2008.
4. Kahn CM, Line S, eds. *The Merck veterinary manual.* 9th ed. Whitehouse Station, NJ: Merck; 2005.
5. Kreeger TJ, DeLiberto TJ, Olsen SC, et al. Safety of *Brucella abortus* strain RB51 vaccine in non-target ungulates and coyotes. *J Wildl Dis.* 2002;38(3):552.
6. Acha PN, Szyfres B. *Zoonoses and communicable diseases common to man and animals: vol. 1: bacterioses and mycoses.* 3rd ed. Washington, DC: Pan American Health Organization; 2001.
7. Godfroid J, Cloeckaert A, Liautard JP, et al. From the discovery of the Malta fever's agent to the discovery of a marine mammal reservoir, brucellosis has continuously been a re-emerging zoonosis. *Vet Res.* 2005;36(3):313.
8. Chang MH, Glynn MK, Groseclose SL. Endemic, notifiable bioterrorism-related diseases, United States, 1992–1999. *Emerg Infect Dis.* 2003;9:556.
9. Centers for Disease Control and Prevention. Laboratory-acquired brucellosis—Indiana and Minnesota, 2006. *MMWR Morb Mortal Wkly Rep.* 2008;57(2):39.

10. Stephanie B, Troy SB, Rickman LS, et al. Brucellosis in San Diego epidemiology and species-related differences in acute clinical presentations. *Medicine*. 2005;84:174.
11. Acha PN, Szyfres B. *Zoonoses and communicable diseases common to man and animals: vol. 1: bacterioses and mycoses*. 3rd ed. Washington DC: Pan American Health Organization; 2001.
12. Berkelman RL. Human illness associated with use of veterinary vaccines. *Clin Infect Dis*. 2003;37(3):407.
13. Rhyan JC, Aune K, Ewalt DR, et al. Survey of free-ranging elk from Wyoming and Montana for selected pathogens. *J Wildl Dis*. 1997;33:290.
14. Nishi JS, Stephen C, Elkin BT. Implications of agricultural and wildlife policy on management and eradication of bovine tuberculosis and brucellosis in free-ranging wood bison of northern Canada. *Ann N Y Acad Sci*. 2002;969:236.
15. Acosta-Gonzalez RI, Gonzalez-Reyes I, Flores-Gutierrez GH. Prevalence of *Brucella abortus* antibodies in equines of a tropical region of Mexico. *Can J Vet Res*. 2006;70:302.
16. Davis DS, Boeer WJ, Mims JP, et al. *Brucella abortus* in coyotes. I. A serologic and bacteriologic survey in eastern Texas. *J Wildl Dis*. 1979;15(3):367.
17. Centers for Disease Control and Prevention. *Brucellosis*. http://www.cdc.gov/ncidod/dbmd/diseaseinfo/Brucellosis_g.htm#mydog. Accessed July 27, 2008.
18. Mandell GE, Bennett JE, Dolin R. *Principles and practice of infectious diseases*. 6th ed. Philadelphia: Churchill Livingstone; 2000.
19. Colville J, Berryhill D. *Handbook of zoonoses: identification and prevention*. St Louis: Mosby Elsevier; 2007.
20. Heymann DL. *Control of communicable diseases manual*. 19th ed. Washington DC: American Public Health Association; 2008.
21. Barr SC, Bowman DD. *5-Minute veterinary consult clinical companion canine and feline infectious disease and parasitology*. Baltimore: Wiley-Blackwell; 2006.
22. Vrioni G, Pappas G, Priavali E, et al. An eternal microbe: Brucella DNA load persists for years after clinical cure. *Clin Inf Dis*. 2008; 46(12):e131.
23. Gilbert DN, Moellering RC Jr, Eliopoulos GM, et al. *The Sanford guide to antimicrobial therapy, 2009*. 39th ed. Sperryville, VA: Antimicrobial Therapy; 2009.

CAMPYLOBACTERIOSIS

Peter M. Rabinowitz and Lisa A. Conti

Campylobacter *enteritis (ICD-10 A 04.5)*

Other names in humans: Campylobacter *enteritis, vibriosis*

Other names in animals: bovine genital campylobacteriosis, vibriosis, epizootic infertility, epizootic ovine abortion

Campylobacter species (*C. jejuni* and *C. coli*) are now considered the leading cause of bacterial enteritis in humans (*Campylobacter* enteritis).[1] They are also found in a large number of animal species. Collaborative research between human health and veterinary researchers led to the relatively recent discovery of *Campylobacter* species as significant human pathogens. Improving diagnostic methods continue to shed light on the prevalence and clinical importance of *Campylobacter* species, including the high zoonotic potential of these agents.

Campylobacter fetus is associated with less common, but severe, infections in immunocompromised persons. Cattle, sheep, and goats are generally infected by contact with reproductive discharges and feces. *C. fetus* also is a sexually transmitted disease among cattle. Traditional culture methods for other *Campylobacter* may not detect *C. fetus*; therefore its true clinical importance remains poorly understood and probably underestimated.

Key Points for Clinicians and Public Health Professionals

Public Health Professionals

- Educate public (especially travelers to endemic countries) on the risk of infection from untreated drinking water, unpasteurized dairy products, and uncooked poultry, including handwashing and food preparation precautions.

- Educate food handlers to avoid cross-contamination of foods—use separate cutting boards.
- Pursue public health measures to control local consumption of unpasteurized dairy products.
- Prevent infected health care workers from providing direct patient care.
- Educate local human health and veterinary clinicians and public about risk of infection in puppies and kittens. Stress the need for handwashing and other hygiene after contact with pets and poultry. Prevent children from handling sick animals.
- Work with agricultural agencies and local farms to reduce incidence of *Campylobacter* in poultry at all phases of rearing and production.
- Educate local veterinary and human health clinicians about groups at risk and symptoms of disease and importance of handwashing for people with diarrhea.
- Coordinate with agriculture officials and veterinarians to receive information about outbreaks of *C. fetus* in local livestock herds so that agricultural workers can be educated about disease and need for biosafety on farms.

Human Health Clinicians

- Report cases to health department if required in state.
- Interview infected individuals about exposure risk factors, such as recent travel to developing country; ingestion of unpasteurized dairy products or undercooked meat; and contact with poultry or poultry products, dogs and cats (especially kittens and puppies), or other potentially infected animals. Notify public health authorities of ongoing risk to other humans.
- Counsel immunocompromised patients to avoid contact with puppies, kittens, dogs, and cats with diarrhea; poultry; unpasteurized dairy products; or undercooked meat.
- When treating an infected human, ensure enteric infection control precautions are used. Exclude the

symptomatic individual from food handling or care of sick individuals or contact with immunocompromised individuals. Stress proper hand hygiene.

- Ensure that workers in high-risk occupations (including poultry workers and veterinarians) use appropriate biosafety procedures, including handwashing.
- A candidate vaccine has been developed by the Navy Medical Research Institute.[2]

Veterinary Clinicians

- If treating an infected animal, counsel owner regarding zoonotic risk and need for adequate handwashing and disposal of feces. Offer direct communication with human health clinician caring for family.
- Discourage feeding raw diets to pets or allowing pets to hunt.
- Exclude wild birds and rodents and control insects from poultry facilities.
- Ensure disinfection of kennel or other facility where infected animals have been housed. Disinfectants include 1% sodium hypochlorite, 70% ethanol, 2% glutaraldehyde, and iodine-based solutions.[3]
- Ensure proper biosafety procedures are followed in veterinary facility or farm (e.g., sterilization of instruments used on possibly infected animals, proper disposal of potentially infected tissue such as aborted

BOX 9-1   CASE STUDY: CAMPYLOBACTER JEJUNI

Campylobacter jejuni was diagnosed in a child by her physician. The child was exposed to a puppy that was mildly ill a few weeks previously and recovered fine. No specific diagnostic tests were performed on the puppy; it was treated symptomatically and recovered. The physician is concerned about the possibility of the puppy being the source of the *Campylobacter*. The puppy has had all routine dewormers and vaccinations and is in good health now.

Question/concern: The puppy is part of a much larger group of dogs and puppies (~100) that are currently being rehabilitated in foster homes. All were mixed together when they were removed from a common source environment several months ago. There have been no reports of diarrhea in other puppies or human household members among children or parents caring for the puppies over the past several months. Would a fecal culture now reveal *Campylobacter*? Would there be any value in screening other puppies, or should we just have *Campylobacter* on the differential and perform appropriate diagnostics should any other puppies become ill in the future?

Response: There have been several studies demonstrating the link of *Campylobacter* and illness in children. The population attributable risk is in the range of 5% to 7%. *Campylobacter* shedding is more frequent in kittens and puppies versus adult animals. At least in kittens, an average carriage of about 4 to 6 weeks was observed (unknown in dogs). Treatment for animals with diarrhea is appropriate because it likely decreases the days of shedding and the number of organisms shed. Appropriate hand hygiene is critical in households with foster puppies. Treatment for asymptomatic dogs would probably not be appropriate (because of antibiotic resistance issues) even though a fair number of puppies and kittens shed *Campylobacter* when they are asymptomatic. Likely the quantity of organisms is less, and studies seem to support contact with dogs with diarrhea as a source.[23]

placentas and fetuses), and that staff are aware of symptoms of infection.

- Quarantine infected animals. Ensure proper treatment of bulls if indicated.
- No animal vaccine is currently available for enteritis, but *C. fetus* bacterin can prevent abortions in sheep and genital campylobacteriosis in cattle.[4]

Agent

Campylobacter species are spiral, S-shaped, or curved, gram-negative rods (Figures 9-16, 9-17, and 9-18). More than 20 strains have been described, including *C. jejuni, C. coli, C. upsaliensis, C. larii, C. fetus,* and *C. helveticus.*[5] Most cases of *Campylobacter* enteritis in humans are believed to be due to *C. jejuni* or *C. coli.* However, when more sensitive isolation techniques are used, some cases have been found to be

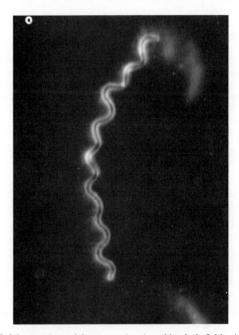

Figure 9-16 ■ *Campylobacter* species viewed by dark-field microscopy. Note the chaining of individual organisms, which are often mistaken for spirochetes. (From Songer JG, Post KW: *Veterinary microbiology: bacterial and fungal agents of animal disease,* St Louis, 2005, Saunders Elsevier. Courtesy J. Glenn Songer.)

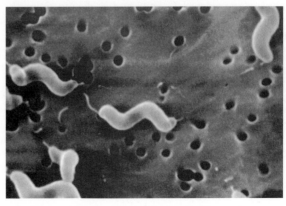

Figure 9-17 ■ Electron micrograph of *Campylobacter.* (From Centers for Disease Control and Prevention, Atlanta, Ga.)

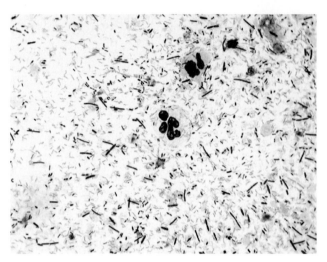

Figure 9-18 ▪ *Campylobacter* species: canine fecal smear (Wright's stain, ×100). Fecal smear shows numerous *Campylobacter* species organisms (lighter-staining smaller bacteria), a mixed population of bacterial rods, and two degenerating neutrophils. The characteristic "gull wing" formations (visible on the surface of the neutrophil) are chains of three to five of these slender, gram-negative, comma-shaped, or curved motile rods. The organisms have the same morphologic characteristics in all species of animals. *Campylobacter* are often overlooked because of their small size. Animals can be carriers, in which case usually only very low numbers are seen. These organisms can be either the primary cause of diarrhea or act as secondary pathogens in conjunction with other enteric bacteria. *Campylobacter* species are difficult to culture. Neutrophils are not seen in normal stool and indicate an active infection. (From Quesenberry K, Carpenter JW: *Ferrets, rabbits and rodents: clinical medicine and surgery*, ed 2, St Louis, 2004, Saunders Elsevier.)

caused by *C. larii* and *C. fetus*. Fluoroquinolone-resistant *Campylobacter* infections are more likely to be severe with bloody diarrhea.

C. fetus is a gram-negative, motile bacteria. Based on current knowledge, it has distinctive epidemiological and clinical features. *C. fetus* has a tendency to invade the vascular endothelium[6] in humans and is an opportunistic pathogen causing mainly systemic infection. In animals, *Campylobacter fetus* subspecies *fetus (intestinalis)* is thought to be primarily an intestinal pathogen (although it has been associated with infertility[4]), whereas *C. fetus venerealis* infects the genital tract. Selective media used to culture other *Campylobacter* species use antibiotics that may inhibit *C. fetus*.[7] *C. fetus* also grows at a lower incubation temperature (25°C vs. 42°C) than other *Campylobacter* species.[8] Normal isolation techniques may not detect *C. fetus*, and as diagnostic methods improve, our understanding of *Campylobacter* infections will continue to evolve.

Geographical Occurrence

C. jejuni, *C. coli*, and *C. fetus* are found worldwide. In the developing world, *C. jejuni* and *C. coli* infections are considered to be mostly diseases of young people. The incidence of *C. fetus* in humans is uncommon but believed to be much higher than recorded.[8]

Groups at Risk

Because poultry flocks have high rates of colonization with *Campylobacter*, persons engaged in poultry raising and processing are at increased risk of infection.[10] Other risk factors

identified have been drinking unpasteurized milk, contact with farm animals, and eating poultry in restaurants.[11] *Campylobacter* is an important cause of travelers' diarrhea in travelers to countries with poor sanitation (Color Plate 9-8). Ownership of cats and dogs (especially puppies and kittens) is considered a risk factor for infection, although the extent of pet-to-human transmission remains unknown.[12]

Most human cases of *C. fetus* to date have occurred in immunocompromised persons, although cases in healthy individuals have been recorded.[13] Risk factors include hepatic cirrhosis, HIV infection, diabetes, and systemic lupus erythematosus.

Hosts, Reservoir Species, Vectors

C. jejuni and *C. coli* occur across a range of species and particular strains appear able to cross species barriers. Surveys of poultry, such as chickens and turkeys, have found colonization rates up to 100%, and contaminated chicken meat is considered a major source of infection for humans.

A survey of dogs and cats in Switzerland found colonization rates of 41% in dogs and 42% in cats.[14] A Taiwan survey reported higher rates in stray dogs versus nonstrays.[15]

C. fetus is widespread in cattle and sheep. It also occurs in reptiles. Unlike *C. jejuni*, it is not commonly recognized in poultry, and therefore poultry may not be a major source of human infection.[16]

Mode of Transmission and Life Cycle

C. jejuni and *C. coli* are transmitted by consumption of contaminated food, such as undercooked poultry or unpasteurized dairy products. It can also be transmitted by fecal-oral contact (Figure 9-19). Waterborne transmission is also possible.

The source of many human *C. fetus* infections is unknown, and the mechanism of transmission from animals to humans remains unclear.[8] In cattle, *C. fetus venerealis* is a sexually transmitted disease. However, cows and ewes may be chronically infected and may have colonization of the gallbladder, leading to fecal elimination. In sheep transmission is fecal-oral, with sexual transmission apparently not playing a role.[8]

Environmental Risk Factors

Environments contaminated by poultry manure, such as occurs in backyard poultry rearing, could propagate *C. jejuni* and *C. coli* infection. Because *Campylobacter* organisms can survive in water, the bacteria circulate in wild bird populations such as waterfowl and shorebirds.[17] Surface water can become contaminated with infected feces of wild and domestic birds; therefore pollution of water bodies is a potential source of infection.

Transmission of *C. fetus* in sheep and cows is thought to involve environmental contamination of grazing areas by infected tissues and feces.[8]

Disease in Humans

Campylobacter enteritis in humans is an acute but usually self-limited diarrheal illness characterized by abdominal cramping, diarrhea, and fever. The incidence is higher among infants and young adults ages 15 to 44 years.

Due to *Campylobacter jejuni* or *Campylobacter coli*

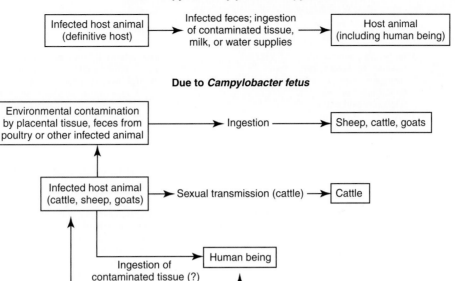

Due to *Campylobacter fetus*

Figure 9-19 ■ Life cycle, campylobacteriosis.

In many cases, blood or mucus is noted in the feces, indicating colorectal inflammation.[18] The abdominal pain may mimic appendicitis. Usually the diarrhea resolves after several days without specific treatment, but other symptoms may persist longer.

Bacteremia and other extraintestinal manifestations are rare, but complications of infection may include erythema nodosum, uveitis, meningitis, and reactive arthritis. Guillain-Barré syndrome occurs in approximately 1 of 1000 cases of *C. jejuni* infection.[19]

C. fetus is an opportunistic pathogen in humans typically presenting as an acute or chronic bacteremia or thrombophlebitis. Complications include myocarditis, endocarditis, meningitis, and abortion (Figure 9-20).

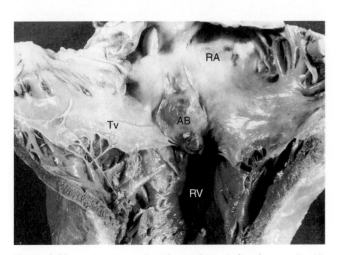

Figure 9-20 ■ Human cardiac abscess from *C. fetus* bacteremia. *AB,* Abcess; *RA,* right atrium; *RV,* right ventricle; *TV,* tricuspid valve. (From Peetermans WE, De Man F, Moerman P et al: Fatal prosthetic valve endocarditis due to *Campylobacter fetus, J Infect Dis* 41(2):180, 2000.)

Disease in Animals

Campylobacter may be present in animals without signs or it may cause diarrhea. Adult animals and poultry older than 1 week are usually subclinical carriers.[3,18,19] The diarrhea is usually most severe in young animals (e.g., in puppies and kittens from birth to 6 months) or in debilitated animals.[4,20] The diarrhea can range from watery to mucus with blood or bile streaking. Affected animals may have reduced appetite and, rarely, vomiting. Tenesmus is common. Diarrhea also occurs after infection in cattle (especially calves), primates, ferrets, and mink.[4] In sheep, *C. jejuni* infection is associated with abortion (Color Plate 9-9).[21]

C. fetus is an important cause of infertility and abortions in cattle and sheep. In cattle, bovine genital campylobacteriosis presents with early fetal death, infertility, and abortion.[4]

Table 9-12 shows comparative clinical presentations of campylobacteriosis in humans and other animals.

Diagnosis

Diagnosis in humans is based on culturing the organism from feces, blood, bone marrow, or other tissue using correct media and incubation procedures. It should be recognized that the selective media may inhibit the growth of certain *Campylobacter* species such as *C. fetus*, leading to false-negative results. Identification of organisms in feces using phase-contrast or dark-field microscopy can be used to make a presumptive diagnosis.[5] PCR techniques have recently been developed and may play a greater role in diagnosis in the future.

In animals, cultures and microscopic examination of feces or reproductive discharges are also used. Agglutination and ELISA tests are used on vaginal mucus of cows suspected to be infected.

Table 9-12 ▪ Campylobacteriosis: Comparative Clinical Presentations in Humans and Other Animals

Species	Risk Factors	Incubation Period	Clinical Manifestations	Laboratory Findings
Humans (*Campylobacter jejuni, C. coli*)	Infants and young adults; travelers to developing countries; ingestion of contaminated meat, unpasteurized dairy products; occupational exposure to animal feces, exposure to sick or colonized pet	2-5 days[18]	Diarrhea, often with mucus or blood, abdominal cramping, fever	Fecal leukocytes, organisms seen on Gram stain, dark-field or phase-contrast microscopy of feces, fecal culture
C. fetus	Immunocompromised, diabetes, cirrhosis infection, SLE, cancer	3-5 days	Gastrointestinal symptoms, bacteremia, endocarditis	Blood culture
Dogs, cats, cattle, sheep, chickens, turkeys, mink, ferrets, pigs, nonhuman primates, others (*C. jejuni, C. coli*)	Ingestion of contaminated food or water Young animals, stressed or debilitated animals at increased risk	3 days[4]	Diarrhea, usually mild, may have mucus or blood; loss of appetite, occasional vomiting, and fever[8] In sheep, abortion near end of pregnancy, stillbirth[16] Mastitis in cattle	CBC may show leukocytosis Fecal leukocytes, organisms seen on Gram stain or phase-contrast microscopy of stool, fecal culture
Sheep (*C. fetus*)	Ingestion of infected material	7-25 days	Abortion near end of pregnancy, stillbirth[8]	Dark-field and phase-contrast microscopy of placenta, fetal abomasums, and uterine discharge[3]
Cattle (*C. fetus*)	Ingestion of infected material, sexual transmission		Subclinical carriage Endometritis, embryonic death, prolonged estrous cycles, abortions	Vaginal mucus agglutination test, ELISA test of vaginal mucus

CBC, Complete blood cell count; *SLE,* systemic lupus erythematosus.

Treatment

Treatment in Humans

Most human enteritis cases are self-limited and resolve with only supportive therapy such as replacement of fluid and electrolytes, lactose-free diet, and avoidance of caffeine. Antibiotic treatment is reserved for more severe cases, including six or more unformed stools per day, and/or temperature of 101.5° F or more, and significant persistent tenesmus, stool blood, and leukocytes. Immunocompromised patients (e.g., individuals who are HIV positive) should be treated with antibiotics to prevent systemic complications[18] Treatment in humans is outlined in Table 9-13. Although in the past ciprofloxacin has been used as a primary therapeutic agent, high rates of resistance to fluoroquinolones have been observed in certain settings.[22]

Treatment in Animals

As in humans, many enteritis cases in dogs and cats are self-limited. When signs are severe (e.g., high fever or dehydration), persist beyond 5 days, or are present in immunocompromised patients, treatment with antibiotics is recommended.

Table 9-13 ▪ Campylobacteriosis Treatment in Humans and Other Animals

Species	Primary Treatment	Alternative
Humans (adults) (*Campylobacter jejuni*)	Azithromycin mg PO q24h × 3 days	Erythromycin stearate 500 mg PO qid × 5 days
(*C. fetus*)	Gentamicin	Ampicillin, chloramphenicol, erythromycin[9]
Dog and cat (*C. jejuni, C. coli*)	Erythromycin 10-20 mg/kg PO q8h × 5 days	Tylosin 11 mg/kg PO q8h × 7 days *or* neomycin 10-20 mg/kg PO q8h × 5 days[13]
Bull (*C. fetus*)	Streptomycin 20 mg/kg SC, 1-2 treatments, streptomycin in oil-based suspension applied to the penis × 3 days	Tylosin 11 mg/kg PO q8h × 7 days *or* neomycin 10-20 mg/kg PO q8h × 5 days

Erythromycin is the drug of choice.[20] Antibiotics may prevent abortions in sheep or prevent the spread of genital campylobacteriosis by treating infected bulls.[3] Good hygiene is critical for prevention. In cattle herds, antibiotic treatment is not considered practical.[4]

References

1. Altekruse SF, Stern NJ, Fields PI, et al. *Campylobacter jejuni*—an emerging foodborne pathogen. *Emerg Infect Dis.* 1999;5(1):28.
2. World Health Organization. http://www.who.int/vaccine_research/diseases/diarrhoeal/en/index2.html. Accessed May 12, 2009.
3. Dvorak G, Rovid-Spickler A, Roth JA, et al. *Handbook for zoonotic diseases of companion animals.* Ames, Iowa: The Center for Food Security and Public Health, Iowa State University College of Veterinary Medicine; 2008.
4. Kahn CM, Line S, eds. *The Merck veterinary manual.* 9th ed. Whitehouse Station, NJ: Merck; 2005.
5. Heymann DL. *Control of communicable diseases manual.* 19th ed. Washington DC: American Public Health Association; 2008.
6. Peetermans WE, De Man F, Moerman P, van de Werf F. Fatal prosthetic valve endocarditis due to *Campylobacter fetus. J Infect.* 2000;41(2):180.
7. Kalka-Moll WM, Van Bergen MA, Plum G, et al. The need to differentiate *Campylobacter fetus* subspecies isolated from humans. *Clin Microbiol Infect.* 2005;11(4):341.
8. Acha PN, Szyfres B. *Zoonoses and communicable diseases common to man and animals: vol. 1: bacterioses and mycoses.* 3rd ed. Washington DC: Pan American Health Organization; 2001.
9. Gilbert DN, Moellering RC, Ellopoulos GM, et al. *Sanford guide to antimicrobial therapy 2009.* 39th ed. Sperryville, VA: Antimicrobial Therapy; 2009.
10. Potter RC, Kaneene JB, Hall WN. Risk factors for sporadic *Campylobacter jejuni* infections in rural Michigan: a prospective case-control study. *Am J Public Health.* 2003;93(12):2118.
11. Friedman CR, Hoekstra RM, Samuel M, et al. Emerging Infections Program FoodNet Working Group. Risk factors for sporadic Campylobacter infection in the United States: a case-control study in FoodNet sites. *Clin Infect Dis.* 2004;38(suppl 3):S285.
12. Damborg P, Olsen KE, Moller Nielsen E, et al. Occurrence of *Campylobacter jejuni* in pets living with human patients infected with *C. jejuni. J Clin Microbiol.* 2004;42(3):1363.
13. Zonios DI, Panayiotakopoulos GD, Kabletsas EO, et al. *Campylobacter fetus* bacteraemia in a healthy individual: clinical and therapeutical implications. *J Infect.* 2005;51(4):329.
14. Wieland B, Regula G, Danuser J, et al. *Campylobacter* spp. in dogs and cats in Switzerland: risk factor analysis and molecular characterization with AFLP. *J Vet Med.* Series B 2005;52(4):183.
15. Tsai HJ, Huang HC, Lin CM, et al. Salmonellae and campylobacters in household and stray dogs in northern Taiwan. *Vet Res Comm.* 2007;31(8):931.
16. Kempf I, Dufour-Gesbert F, Hellard G, et al. Broilers do not play a dominant role in the *Campylobacter fetus* contamination of humans. *J Med Microbiol.* 2006;55(Pt 9):1277.
17. Waldenstrom J, On SL, Ottvall R, et al. Species diversity of campylobacteria in a wild bird community in Sweden. *J App Microbiol.* 2007;102(2):424.
18. Butzler JP. *Campylobacter,* from obscurity to celebrity. *Clin Microbiol Infect.* 2004;10(10):868.
19. Allos BM. Association between *Campylobacter* infection and Guillain-Barré syndrome. *J Infect Dis.* 1997;176(suppl 2):S125.
20. Barr SC, Bowman DD. *5-Minute veterinary consult clinical companion canine and feline infectious disease and parasitology.* Baltimore, MD: Wiley-Blackwell; 2006.
21. Colville J, Berryhill D. *Handbook of zoonoses: identification and prevention.* St Louis: Mosby Elsevier; 2007.
22. Gilbert DN, Moellering RC, Ellopoulos GM, et al. *Sanford guide to antimicrobial therapy 2007.* 37th ed. Sperryville, VA: Antimicrobial Therapy; 2007.
23. NASPHV listserv. Personal communication, August 2008.

CHLAMYDOPHILA PSITTACI AND RELATED INFECTIONS

Peter M. Rabinowitz and Lisa A. Conti

Chlamydophila psittaci *and related infections (ICD-10 A70 Psittacosis; ICD-10 A74 Other diseases caused by chlamydiae)*

Other names in humans: psittacosis, ornithosis, chlamydiosis, parrot fever

Other names in animals: avian chlamydiosis; mammalian chlamydiosis, chlamydial conjunctivitis, feline chlamydial pneumonitis, septic abortion of sheep and goats

Chlamydophila (formerly *Chlamydia*) *psittaci* infection from exposure to birds causes disease in humans ranging from mild flulike signs to severe pneumonia and sepsis. Although fewer than 50 human cases of psittacosis are reported yearly in the United States,[1] it is likely that many cases go undetected. *C. psittaci* commonly infects psittacine (parrot family) birds that are used as pets, but domestic poultry flocks, especially turkeys and ducks, can develop widespread infection with significant flock mortality and occupational risk to poultry workers. Human disease with mammalian chlamydiae (i.e., *C. abortus, C. felis,* and *C. pneumoniae*) is rarely reported. The diagnosis of chlamydiosis can be challenging in humans and other animals.

New molecular evidence is broadening our understanding of the host range and clinical spectrum of *Chlamydophila* infections.[2] Therefore clinicians should maintain a high index of suspicion in the appropriate settings where infection can occur.

Key Points for Clinicians and Public Health Professionals

Public Health Professionals

- Characterize the risk in the community related to pet shops, aviaries, bird ownership, and poultry production.
- Become familiar with the National Association of State Public Health Veterinarians *Compendium of Measures to Control* Chlamydophila psittaci *Infection Among Human Beings (Psittacosis) and Pet Birds (Avian Chlamydiosis).*[3] These measures are summarized in Box 9-2.
- Conduct an investigation of human cases, including surveillance of pet shops and poultry farms, to detect sources of infection and other human cases. If infected birds are found, ensure that they are treated or destroyed and the area is decontaminated with a disinfectant.[4]

BOX 9-2   *MEASURES FOR PSITTACOSIS PREVENTION*

- **Educate persons at risk.** Inform all persons in contact with birds or bird-contaminated materials about the zoonotic nature of the disease.
- **Protect persons at risk.** When cleaning cages or handling infected birds, caretakers should wear protective clothing, which includes gloves, eyewear, a disposable surgical cap, and an appropriately fitted respirator[10] with N-95 or higher rating. Surgical masks might not be effective in preventing transmission of *Chlamydophila psittaci*. When necropsies are performed on potentially infected birds, wet the carcass with detergent and water to prevent aerosolization of infectious particles and work under a biological safety cabinet or equivalent.
- **Maintain accurate records of all bird-related transactions for at least 1 year to aid in identifying sources of infected birds and potentially exposed persons.**
- **Avoid purchasing or selling birds that have signs consistent with avian chlamydiosis** (lethargy, ocular or nasal discharge, diarrhea, ruffled feathers, or low body weight).
- **Isolate newly acquired, ill, or exposed birds.** Isolation should include housing in a separate air space from other birds and non-caretakers.
- **Test birds before they are to be boarded or sold on consignment.**

- **Screen birds with frequent public contact** (e.g., bird encounters, long-term care facilities, schools) routinely for anti-chlamydial antibodies and DNA or bacterial protein.
- **Practice preventive husbandry.** Position cages to prevent the transfer of fecal matter, feathers, food, and other materials from one cage to another. Litter that will not produce dust (e.g., newspapers) should be placed underneath the mesh. Clean all cages, food bowls, and water bowls daily. Soiled bowls should be cleaned with disinfectant. Between occupancies by different birds, cages should be thoroughly scrubbed with soap and water, disinfected, and rinsed in clean running water. Exhaust ventilation should be sufficient to prevent accumulation of aerosols and prevent cross-contamination of rooms.
- **Control the spread of infection.** Isolate birds requiring treatment. Rooms and cages where infected birds were housed should be cleaned immediately and disinfected thoroughly.
- **Use disinfection measures.** *C. psittaci* is susceptible to most disinfectants and detergents as well as heat; however, it is resistant to acid and alkali. Examples of effective disinfectants include 1:1000 dilution of quaternary ammonium compounds (e.g., Roccal-D or Zephiran), 1% Lysol, or freshly prepared 1:32 dilution of household bleach (i.e., 1/2 cup/gallon).

Adapted from *Compendium of measures to control* Chlamydophila psittaci *infection among human beings (psittacosis) and pet birds (avian chlamydiosis),* 2008, National Association of State Public Health Veterinarians.

- Coordinate with agriculture officials to control the disease in bird populations.
- Ensure that poultry workers with occupational risk for *C. psittaci* infection are informed about the disease and its prevention through exposure controls and protective equipment.

Human Health Clinicians

- Consider the diagnosis in all patients with bird contact (avian chlamydiosis) who present with respiratory symptoms or fever, as well as patients with keratoconjunctivitis (or rarely endocarditis and glomerulonephritis) and cat contact (mammalian chlamydiosis).
- Report suspected cases to public health authorities. See CDC case definition: http://www.cdc.gov/ncphi/disss/nndss/casedef/psittacosiscurrent.htm.
- Counsel patients with psittacine birds to take steps to protect their birds from exposure to *C. psittaci* and to seek veterinary care for ill birds, especially if owners are immunocompromized. Other risk reduction measures include avoiding mouth-to-beak contact and appropriate personal protective equipment (PPE) when cleaning cages or handling dead birds (see Box 9-2).
- If caring for workers with occupational exposure to birds (e.g., pet shop workers, poultry workers), ensure that they immediately report symptoms of fever, myalgias, and cough, and that the workplace is adopting preventive practices (see Box 9-2), including respiratory protection for workers who are working with ill or potentially exposed birds.
- Counsel pregnant patients to avoid contact with pregnant or aborting sheep and goats.

Veterinary Clinicians

- Counsel bird owners on the signs of psittacosis, how to protect their birds from exposure, and how to reduce risks to humans, especially if owners are immunocompromised.
- Consider the diagnosis of chlamydiosis in any sick bird with lethargy and nonspecific signs, especially if recently purchased or stressed (e.g., transported).
- Follow local and state reporting regulations; contact local health department or Department of Agriculture.
- Train veterinary personnel in biosafety measures, such as wearing masks and gloves when working with potentially infected birds, and use of strict personal hygiene (e.g., handwashing and cleaning/disinfecting footwear) to prevent spreading the organism to other animals.
- If a case is diagnosed in a cat, immunize cats in the household or cattery using *C. psittaci* vaccine. A live *C. abortus* vaccine may reduce shedding in sheep.

Agent

C. psittaci is an intracellular bacterium closely related to the human pathogen *Chlamydia trachomatis* (causes venereal infection in humans) and other zoonotic Chlamydiae (Table 9-14). A number of different strains (serovars) of *C. psittaci* have been described; the majority are avian pathogens. The strains vary in virulence and zoonotic potential; for example, the turkey strain may be more virulent than serovars that affect pigeons and ducks.[5] Mammalian strains of zoonotic Chlamydiaceae are *Chlamydophila felis*

Table 9-14 ▪ Comparison of Classification of *Chlamydophila* and *Chlamydia*

Hosts	Preferential Tissues	Before 1999	After 1999
Chlamydophila			
Birds	Genital, lung, internal organs	*Chlamydia psittaci*	psittaci
Cattle, sheep	Brain, eye, joints	*Chlamydia pecorum*	pecorum
Humans, koalas, horses	Lung, joints, endothelial	*Chlamydia pneumoniae*	pneumoniae
Sheep, mammals	Intestines, placenta	*Chlamydia psittaci*	abortus
Guinea pigs	Bladder, eye, spleen	*Chlamydia psittaci*	caviae
Cats	Eye, genital, joints, lungs	*Chlamydia psittaci*	felis
Chlamydia			
Humans	Ocular and urogenital, neonatal lung	*Chlamydia trachomatis*	trachomatis
Rodents	Many internal organs	*Chlamydia trachomatis*	muridarum
Swine	Eye, intestines, lung	Novel species	suis

Adapted from Greene CE: *Infectious diseases of the dog and cat*, ed 3, St Louis, 2006, Saunders Elsevier.

(formerly *Chlamydia psittaci*, feline strain, causes conjunctivitis in cats), *C. abortus* (formerly *Chlamydia psittaci*, mammalian abortion strain or serotype 1, causes abortion in ruminants, especially sheep and goats), and *C. pneumoniae* (formerly *Chlamydia pneumoniae*, previously considered a human pathogen, but has been isolated from horses, reptiles, and amphibians).[6]

The CDC considers *C. psittaci* a category B biological warfare agent because of its ability to be produced and disseminated in quantities sufficient to affect large populations.[7]

Geographical Occurrence

Worldwide.

Groups at Risk

Groups at increased risk for *C. psittaci* infection include owners of birds, pet store workers, veterinarians, zookeepers, live poultry and poultry processing workers, and diagnostic laboratorians. Recent studies have found seroprevalence rates as high as 15% in workers at pet bird breeding facilities.[8]

Seroprevalence rates of 15% have been reported in livestock farmers.[9] Pregnant women have developed severe infection with *C. abortus*, including sepsis, stillbirth, and abortion after contact with birth products of sheep and goats, but such cases are considered rare.[10]

Hosts, Reservoir Species, Vectors

C. psittaci occurs in most birds. One serovar is found in a wide range of psittacine birds, including parrots, parakeets, and cockatiels (Color Plate 9-10). Another infects turkeys and ducks and, rarely, chickens. Certain Chlamydiae infect mammals, and a high rate of subclinical carriage has been reported in rodents.[11] Prevalence rates of 5% to 10% in cats have been reported, and exposure to infected cats has been linked to human infection.[12]

Many animals shed the organisms in the absence of clinical signs. Crowding and other stressors appear to increase the rate of fulminant diseases in birds. Wildlife may serve as a reservoir and pose an infectious threat to domestic poultry.[5]

Mode of Transmission and Life Cycle

Chlamydiae exists in two forms, an infectious but metabolically inactive elementary body that is relatively stable in the environment, and the metabolically active but noninfectious reticulate body (Figure 9-21).[5] Infection is initiated by the elementary body attaching to susceptible cell membranes, primarily in the respiratory and later gastrointestinal tracts.[13] Transformation of the elementary body to the reticulate body occurs within several hours, after which the reticulate body creates progeny that differentiate into elementary bodies and are released from infected cells. The bacteria can be shed in the feces, leading to fecal-oral transmission[5]; in addition, nasal, ocular, and uterine discharges can lead to direct inoculation into mucous membranes or aerosol transmission.

Bird species implicated in zoonotic aerosol transmission include psittacine birds, poultry, shorebirds, and raptors.[3] Direct handling of an infected bird or cat followed by self-inoculation of conjunctiva or other mucous membranes is another potential route of animal-human transmission, as is beak-to-mouth contact (kissing a pet bird). Person-to-person transmission has been reported in close contacts of infected persons.[14]

Environmental Risk Factors

Under certain conditions, the bacterial elementary body can persist for prolonged periods in the environment. This can lead to reinfection of poultry flocks or pet birds through both oral and respiratory routes.

Disease in Humans

C. psittaci can cause an acute febrile syndrome with headache, myalgias, cough, and photophobia. Respiratory symptoms may be mild in relation to the chest x-ray findings, which may appear worse than the patient's condi-

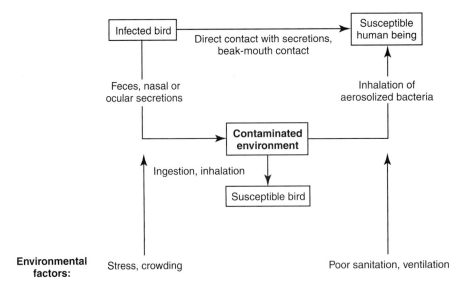

Figure 9-21   ■   Life cycle, *Chlamydophila psittaci* infection.

tion appears (Figure 9-22). Sputum production is often scant. Hepatomegaly and pharyngeal erythema often occur. The pulse may be paradoxically slow in relation to the degree of fever. Skin signs include Horder's spots, a pink, blanching maculopapular rash.[15] Keratoconjunctivitis has been reported in cases of contact with infected cats.[15] Complications of infection include hepatitis, splenomegaly, hemolytic anemia, disseminated intravascular coagulation (DIC), endocarditis, myocarditis, pericarditis, and glomerulonephritis. Neurological complications including hearing loss, cranial nerve palsy, cerebellar symptoms, and confusion can also occur.

In more severe cases, progressive pneumonia and acute respiratory distress syndrome (ARDS) develop with multiorgan failure. Infection in pregnancy can cause severe complications including DIC and fetal death. Past infection does not appear to confer subsequent immunity.[15]

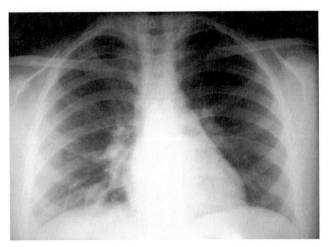

Figure 9-22   ■   Chest radiograph of a 9-year-old girl with a 2-week history of fever, headache, and hacking cough. She was the caretaker of the family's cockatoo. Serum complement fixation antibody titer for *C. psittaci* was 1:256. (From Long SS, Pickering LK, Prober CG (eds): *Principles and practice of pediatric infectious diseases*, ed 3, Philadelphia, 2008, Saunders Elsevier. Courtesy of S.S. Long.)

Many aspects of the disease remain incompletely understood, including an association with ocular adnexal lymphoma, and indolent lymphoma from chronic avian chlamydiosis.[10,16,17] These associations, if true, may lead to preventive therapies for these lymphomas.

Severe complications including sepsis, stillbirth, and miscarriage can develop in pregnant women infected with *C. abortus* from contact with pregnant sheep and goats.[18] The role of other Chlamydiae and *Chlamydia*-like organisms in obstetrical pathology is emerging.[19]

Disease in Animals

Many birds and mammals shed Chlamydiae without any signs. However, *C. psittaci* can cause morbidity and mortality in psittacine birds, with malaise, weight loss, diarrhea, and conjunctivitis. Stress and crowding appear to increase the prevalence of clinical disease.[5] As in humans, previously infected animals may become reinfected.

Cats typically develop conjunctivitis and mild upper respiratory disease. Conjunctivitis may also be seen in other species (Figures 9-23 and 9-24). Kittens 2 to 6 months old are more likely to be infected. *C. abortus* is a major cause of reproductive failure and abortion in sheep and goats. Chlamydial infection has been associated with horses with recurrent airway obstruction.[20] Table 9-15 provides clinical presentations of chlamydiae infections in humans and other animals.

Diagnosis

The differential diagnosis in humans includes other causes of atypical pneumonia, including *Legionella*, *Mycoplasma*, *C. pneumoniae*, *Coxiella*, and influenza. The clinical presentation of an atypical pneumonia in the setting of a history of exposure to birds should lead clinicians to strongly consider the diagnosis of psittacosis.

Confirmation of the diagnosis is usually by serology, using either complement fixation or microimmunofluorescence (MIF). Serology specimens should be obtained acutely and

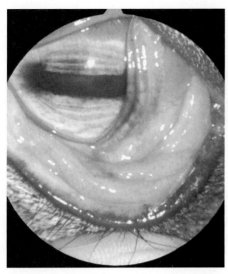

Figure 9-23 ▪ Acute *Chlamydia* species conjunctivitis in a heifer. (From Fubini S: *Farm animal surgery*, Philadelphia, 2004, Saunders Elsevier.)

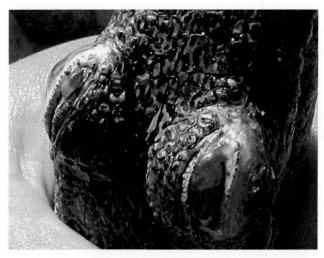

Figure 9-24 ▪ Severe conjunctivitis and periocular edema in a Morelet's crocodile (*Crocodylus moreletii*). (From Bewig M: *Manual of exotic pet practice*, St Louis, 2009, Saunders Elsevier.)

2 to 3 weeks later. Because antibiotics may blunt the antibody response, a third set of serologic tests may be obtained 4 to 6 weeks after the acute sample if the results of the second set are equivocal.

CDC surveillance criteria for a confirmed case of psittacosis are as follows:

- Isolation of *C. psittaci* from respiratory secretions, *or*
- Fourfold or greater increase in antibody against *C. psittaci* by complement fixation or MIF to a reciprocal titer of ≥32 between paired acute- and convalescent-phase serum specimens, *or*

- Presence of immunoglobulin M antibody against *C. psittaci* by MIF to a reciprocal titer of ≥16.[21]

Culture of the organism is difficult and poses a risk to laboratory personnel and therefore should be performed only in qualified laboratories. A PCR test is available through the CDC.

In birds, the diagnosis can be challenging, especially in asymptomatic cases. A combination of culture, antibody testing, and antigen detection is recommended.

For necropsy diagnosis, tissue specimens from the liver and spleen are preferred. In live birds, conjunctival, choanal,

Table 9-15 ▪ Chlamydiae Infections: Comparative Clinical Presentations in Humans and Other Animals

Species	Risk Factors	Incubation Period	Clinical Manifestations	Laboratory Findings
Humans	Contact with sick birds and their environment	5-15 days[15]	Headache, fever, myalgias, cough, photophobia, scant sputum, shortness of breath; rarely endocarditis, hepatitis, neurological complications	Pulmonary infiltrates on x-ray, elevated WBC, erythrocyte sedimentation rate, serology (CF, IFA), PCR, culture
	Contact with cats experiencing keratoconjunctivitis		Conjunctivitis (exposure to *C. felis*)	PCR (may not distinguish species), culture
	Pregnant women working with sheep and goats		Miscarriage (exposure to *C. abortus*)	
Birds	Crowding, other stressors	3 days to weeks Latent infections possible	Often subclinical Lethargy, diarrhea, malaise, conjunctivitis, ruffled feathers, ocular or nasal discharge	Culture and serology (IFA, ELISA) Antigen, PCR
Cats	Crowding	3-10 days[12]	Often subclinical Chronic conjunctivitis, photophobia, pneumonitis, sneezing	Culture, serology, IFA
Sheep, goats	Parturition	Months	May be subclinical Spontaneous abortion	Culture, serology

CF, Complement fixation; *WBC*, white blood cell count.

and cloacal swab specimens or liver biopsy specimens can be used. Fecal specimens can be collected over several days and pooled for increased sensitivity. As with diagnosis of human disease, the culture of *C. psittaci* requires specialized laboratory facilities to minimize risk to laboratory personnel. Conjunctival scrapings of various animals may reveal elementary bodies in epithelial cells (Figure 9-25).

Serological tests available include elementary body agglutination (EBA) for detection of IgM antibodies, and indirect fluorescent antibody test (IFA) to detect IgG antibodies.

Complement fixation (CF) is more sensitive than agglutination methods. Antigen tests include ELISA tests that were originally developed for identification of *Chlamydia trachomatis* in humans and IFAs to detect antigen. PCR is available in a number of diagnostic laboratories to detect C. *psittaci* DNA in samples. Care is necessary in the preparation of samples for PCR testing to prevent environmental contamination.[3]

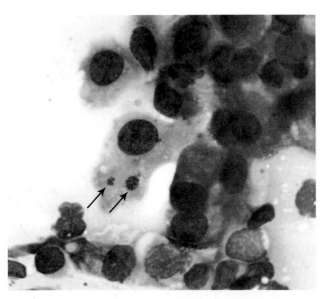

Figure 9-25 ■ Conjunctival scraping from a cat with chlamydial conjunctivitis. Elementary bodies of *Chlamydophila felis* are found in an epithelial cell *(arrows)*. (Wright's stain, original magnification ×1000.) (From Young KM, Taylor J: Laboratory medicine: yesterday, today, tomorrow: eye on the cytoplasm, *Vet Clin Pathol* 35:141, 2006.)

Treatment

Treatment in humans depends on whether the diagnosis is suspected or confirmed. If the diagnosis is not certain, the patient should receive antibiotics to cover the spectrum of organisms causing community-acquired pneumonia, with the regimen adjusted to the severity of disease and existing comorbid conditions such as alcoholism or chronic obstructive lung disease. Once the diagnosis is confirmed, more specific therapy can be given as outlined in Table 9-16. Doxycyline and tetracycline are the mainstay of treatment in humans but are contraindicated in children younger than 8 years and pregnant women, for whom a macrolide antibiotic such as erythromycin may be considered. However, erythromycin may be less efficacious in severe cases and it may not protect the fetus of a pregnant patient.[15]

Treatment in animals also relies on antibiotics of the tetracycline class. Euthanasia may be considered as a control measure during outbreaks. In cats, a vaccine is available that does not prevent disease but may reduce the severity and duration of illness.[12]

References

1. Centers for Disease Control and Prevention. *Disease listing, psittacosis, technical information: CDC bacterial, mycotic diseases.* http://www.cdc.gov/ncidod/dbmd/diseaseinfo/psittacosis_t.htm. Accessed May 30, 2008.
2. Bodetti TJ, Jacobson E, Wan C, et al. Molecular evidence to support the expansion of the hostrange of *Chlamydophila pneumoniae* to include reptiles as well as humans, horses, koalas and amphibians. *Syst Appl Microbiol.* 2002;25(1):146.
3. National Association of State Public Health Veterinarians. Compendium of measures to control *Chlamydophila psittaci* infection among humans (psittacosis) and pet birds (avian chlamydiosis). http://www.nasphv.org/Documents/Psittacosis.pdf. Accessed May 30, 2008.
4. Heymann DL. *Control of communicable diseases manual.* 19th ed. Washington DC: American Public Health Association; 2008.
5. Acha PN, Szyfres B. *Zoonoses and communicable diseases common to man and animals: vol. 2: chlamydioses, rickettsioses, and viroses.* 3rd ed. Washington DC: Pan American Health Organization; 2003.
6. Sykes JE. Feline chlamydiosis. *Clin Tech Small Anim Pract.* 2005;20:129.
7. Biological and chemical terrorism: strategic plan for preparedness and response. Recommendations of the CDC Strategic Planning Workgroup. *Morb Mortal Wkly Rep.* 2000;49:1.
8. Vanrompay D, Harkinezhad T, van de Walle M, et al. *Chlamydophila psittaci* transmission from pet birds to humans. *Emerg Infect Dis.* 2007;13:1108.

Table 9-16 ■ Treatment of *Chlamydophila Psittaci* Infection in Humans and Other Animals		
Species	**Primary Treatment**	**Alternative Treatment**
Humans: adult	Doxycycline 100 mg PO or IV q12h × 10-21 days[22]	Tetracycline 500 mg PO q6h × 10-21 days[22]
<8 yr, pregnancy	Doxycycline, tetracycline contraindicated; consider macrolide (erythromycin), specialist consultation	
Birds	Doxycycline 25-50 mg/kg q24h PO for 30-45 days (dose and time are species dependent)	1% Chlortetracycline in medicated feed; some injectable doxycyclines (consult with avian veterinarian)
Cats	Doxycycline 5 mg/kg PO q12h × 3-4 wk Ophthalmic ointments containing tetracycline q8h	Tetracycline 22 mg/kg PO q8h × 3-4 wk[22] (may affect growing teeth of young kittens)
Sheep, goats	Long-acting oxytetracycline 20 mg/kg, with a second injection 3 weeks later	Tetracycline[21]

9. Fenga C, Cacciola A, Di Nola C, et al. Serologic investigation of the prevalence of *Chlamydophila psittaci* in occupationally-exposed subjects in eastern Sicily. *Ann Agric Environ Med.* 2007;14:93.

10. Walder G, Hotzel H, Brezinka C, et al. An unusual cause of sepsis during pregnancy: recognizing infection with chlamydophila abortus. *Obstet Gynecol.* 2005;106:1215.

11. Cisláková L, Stanko M, Fricová J, et al. Small mammals (Insectivora, Rodentia) as a potential source of chlamydial infection in East Slovakia. *Ann Agric Environ Med.* 2004;11:139.

12. Barr SC, Bowman DD. *5-Minute veterinary consult clinical companion canine and feline infectious disease and parasitology.* Ames, IA: Wiley-Blackwell; 2006.

13. Vanrompay D, Mast J, Ducatelle R, et al. *Chlamydia psittaci* in turkeys: pathogenesis of infections in avian serovars A, B and D. *Vet Microbiol.* 1995;47:245.

14. Hughes C, Maharg P, Rosario P, et al. Possible nosocomial transmission of psittacosis. *Infect Cont Hosp Epidemiol.* 1997;18:165.

15. Baud D, Regan L, Greub G. Emerging role of *Chlamydia* and *Chlamydia*-like organisms in adverse pregnancy outcomes. *Curr Opin Infect Dis.* 2008;21:70.

16. Ferreri AJM, Dolcetti R, Magnino S, et al. *A woman and her canary: a story of chlamydiae and lymphomas.* http://jnci.oxfordjournals.org/cgi/content/extract/99/18/1418. Accessed August 11, 2008.

17. Husain A, Roberts D, Pro B, et al. Meta-analyses of the association between *Chlamydia psittaci* and ocular adnexal lymphoma and the response of ocular adnexal lymphoma to antibiotics. *Cancer.* 2007;110(4):809.

18. Portlock CS, Hamlin P, Noy A, et al. Infectious disease associations in advanced stage, indolent lymphoma (follicular and nonfollicular): developing a lymphoma prevention strategy. *Ann Oncol.* 2008;19:254.

19. Theegarten D, Sachse K, Mentrup B, et al. *Chlamydophila* spp. infection in horses with recurrent airway obstruction: similarities to human chronic obstructive disease. *Respir Res.* 2008;9:14.

20. Centers for Disease Control and Prevention. *Case definitions for infectious conditions under public health surveillance.* http://www.cdc.gov/ncphi/disss/nndss/casedef/psittacosiscurrent.htm. Accessed June 19, 2008.

21. Kahn CM, Line S, eds. *The Merck veterinary manual.* 9th ed.Whitehouse Station, NJ: Merck; 2005.

22. Mandell GL, Bennett JE, Dolin R, eds. *Principles and practice of infectious diseases.* 6th ed. New York: Churchill Livingstone Elsevier; 2005.

CRYPTOSPORIDIOSIS

Peter M. Rabinowitz and Lisa A. Conti

Cryptosporidiosis (ICD-10 A07.2)

Like *Giardia*, *Cryptosporidium* species are a common parasitic cause of infectious diarrhea in humans and are found in many vertebrate species. Many episodes of infection are mild enough that they do not come to medical attention. Yet because of its capability to cause massive human outbreaks through waterborne exposure, it is considered a category B bioterrorism agent. In immunocompromised patients, cryptosporidiosis can cause serious and even fatal disease. A growing body of knowledge supports the importance of cross-species transmission between animals, especially calves, and humans.

Key Points for Clinicians and Public Health Professionals

Public Health Professionals

- Be familiar with CDC guidelines: "Cryptosporidiosis Outbreak and Response Evaluation."[1]
- Analyze and report trends from compulsory reports of human disease.
- In the event of a case report, determine risk factors for infection and conduct additional case finding.
- Public health laboratories should determine the genotype to assist with source tracking.
- Consider zoonotic sources of infection (farm animals/petting zoos, water supplies with animal contact) in addition to human-to-human spread (especially in day care settings).
- Educate the public, veterinarians, and human health clinicians about risk factors for transmission. Highlight the need for strict hygiene measures for, or restrictions on, petting zoos and other animal settings (see the National Association of State Public Health Veterinarians *Compendium of Measures to Prevent Disease Associated with Animals in Public Settings,* 2009; http://www.nasphv.org/Documents/AnimalsInPublicSettings.pdf).

- Disinfect the environment of oocysts using 5% ammonia solution.[2] Recognize the limited efficacy of disinfection procedures and place emphasis on thorough cleaning.
- Provide preventive guidance for day care facilities, recreational water facilities, and boil water notification. Remove reservoirs (recently infected people) from contact with susceptible populations. Exclude children with diarrhea from school or child care centers, water parks, swimming pools, and so on.
- Support policies to keep public areas free of animal feces.
- Consider efficacy of local water treatment procedures with regard to removal of oocysts (i.e., chlorination lacks efficacy; therefore alternative disinfection procedures such as filtration or ozonation may be required).

Human Health Clinicians

- Report cases to public health authorities: http://www.cdc.gov/mmwr/preview/mmwrhtml/00047449.htm.
- Include questions about animal contact for every patient presenting with diarrhea.
- Consider occupational exposure of cattle workers and animal shelter workers.
- Person-to-person transmission is possible; counsel infected persons about hand hygiene and avoiding fecal exposure during sexual activity.

Veterinary Clinicians

- Counsel owners and any others in contact with infected animals about the zoonotic risk, need for hand hygiene after handling pet, feces, pet toys, and other objects that are potentially infected with cysts.

- Decontaminate infected animal's coat with shampoo and kennels or other environments with an 18-hour exposure to 5% ammonia, 10% formol saline, or 3% hydrogen peroxide.[2]
- Counsel persons who work with young ruminants or animal shelters of the increased potential for exposure and provide a clean birthing environment. Neonates should receive colostrum, segregate calves from other calves for the first 2 weeks of life, and maintain hygienic husbandry practices including fly and rodent control.
- Counsel immunosuppressed persons regarding the risks of animal exposures.

Agent

Cryptosporidia are protozoan parasites of the coccidia group in the phylum Apicomplexa (Figure 9-26). At least 30 species of *Cryptosporidium* and multiple genotype variations have been described in a wide number of animal species (Table 9-17). The two species believed to cause most cases of human infections are *C. hominis* (formerly known as *C. parvum* anthroponotic genotype or genotype 1) and *C. parvum*. *C. hominis* is a human pathogen, although infection has

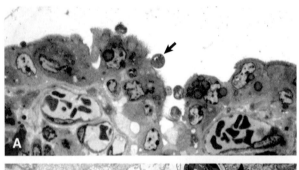
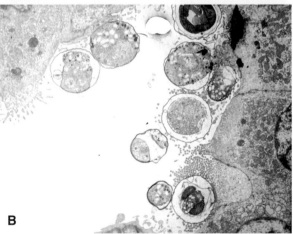

Figure 9-26 ■ Cryptosporidiosis, small intestine. **A,** Cow. Cryptosporidia *(arrow)* are attached to the microvillus border of the enterocyte membrane. Plastic-embedded, toluidine blue–stained section. **B,** Rabbit. The Cryptosporidia form a trilaminated enveloping membrane upon fusion with the enterocyte membrane. Their location is thus intracellular, but extracytoplasmic. Microvilli are effaced. Transmission electron micrograph, uranyl acetate and lead citrate stain. (From McGavin MD: *Pathologic basis of veterinary disease,* ed 4, St Louis, 2006, Mosby Elsevier. *A,* Courtesy Dr. A.R. Doster, University of Nebraska; and Noah's Arkive, College of Veterinary Medicine, The University of Georgia. *B,* Courtesy Dr. H. Gelberg, College of Veterinary Medicine, Oregon State University.)

Table 9-17 ■ *Cryptosporidium* Species Infecting Humans and Other Animals

Host	Major Species	Minor Species
Humans	C. hominis, C. parvum	C. meleagridis, C. felis, C. canis, C. suis, C. baileyi, cervine genotype
Cats	C. felis	
Cattle	C. parvum, C. bovis, C. andersoni deer-like genotype	C. suis
Chickens	C. baileyi	C. meleagridis, C. galli
Deer	C. parvum, deer genotype	
Dogs	C. canis	
Horses	Horse genotype	
Lizards	C. serpentis, C. varanii	Lizard genotype
Mice	C. muris, mouse genotype	
Sheep	Cervine genotypes 1-3, bovine genotype	
Snakes	C. serpentis	C. varanii, snake genotype
Squirrel	C. muris, squirrel genotype	
Swine	C. suis	Pig genotype II
Turkey	C. meleagridis, C. baileyi	

Adapted from Fayer R, Xiao L: *Cryptosporidium and cryptosporidiosis,* Boca Raton, FL, 2007, CRC Press, p 11.

been found in lambs, cattle, and other mammals. *C. parvum* infects humans, cattle, and other ruminants. Other species reported in humans include *C. canis* (dogs), *C. felis* (cats), and *C. meleagridis* (birds).

Cryptosporidia colonize the intestinal and biliary tracts but can also be found in the lungs. The organism reproduces in the intestinal tract to produce oocysts. Oocysts are immediately infectious as shed in feces. The oocysts measure 2.5 to 5 microns in diameter and can survive in moist environments, including water supplies, for several months. They are resistant to chlorination but are inactivated by boiling water or ozonation.

Geographical Occurrence

C. parvum occurs worldwide in animals and humans. Human prevalence is greater in developing countries with poor sanitation practices. Reported rates of infection in human populations range from 20% in developing countries to 1% to 4% in developed countries.[3]

Groups at Risk

Children younger than 2 years, their caregivers, and immunocompromised persons have an increased risk of infection. Other risk groups include animal handlers, travelers, contacts of infected persons, and men who have sex with men.

Hosts, Reservoir Species, Vectors

Humans are the reservoir for *C. hominis*, whereas humans, cattle, and other ruminants (e.g., goats, sheep, deer, elk) appear to be major reservoirs for *C. parvum*.[4] *C. muris* infects mice and cattle gastric glands, and chickens are the reservoir for *C. baileyi*. In many individuals and species, asymptomatic carriage may occur with the ability to transmit the infection to others and the environment. The zoonotic potential of avian Cryptosporidia has not been fully elucidated.

Mode of Transmission and Life Cycle

Each oocyst contains four sporozoites that are the infective phase of the parasite (Figure 9-27). When shed in feces, the oocysts are immediately infective. Upon ingestion by a host,

the sporozoites are released and invade the mucosa of the intestinal tract. Sporozoites mature into trophozoites that multiply asexually first. Then these trophozoites undergo sexual reproduction (meronts) to produce sporozoites, most of which acquire a protective cover to form an oocyst. These oocysts are passed in the feces, where they are immediately infective. Sporozoites that remain in the intestine without developing a cyst wall are able to reinfect the host, perpetuating infection.[5] The infectious dose is about 130 organisms to initiate a *C. parvum* infection in 50% of healthy volunteers.[6] Cattle can shed up to 1 million organisms per gram of feces.

Most transmission appears to occur through ingestion of oocysts. Vehicles of transmission include drinking water, direct fecal-oral contamination, foodborne exposure, or contact with contaminated objects leading to ingestion (Figure 9-28). Infected drinking water and freshwater bathing areas have been the sources of large human outbreaks, such as the

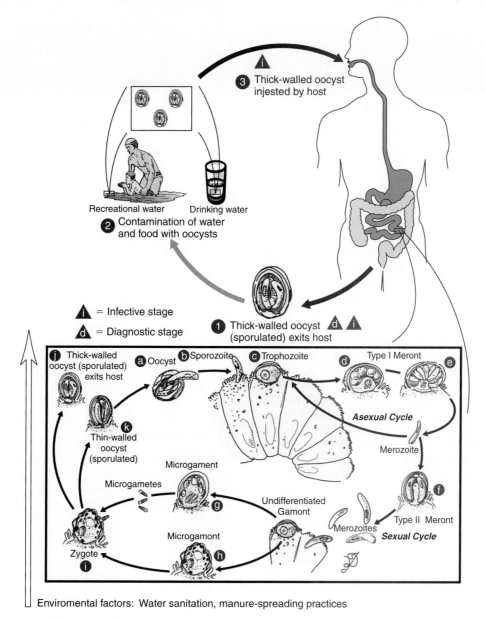

Figure 9-27 ▪ Cryptosporidiosis transmission/life cycle. (Modified from Centers for Disease Control and Prevention Public Health Image Library, Atlanta, Ga.)

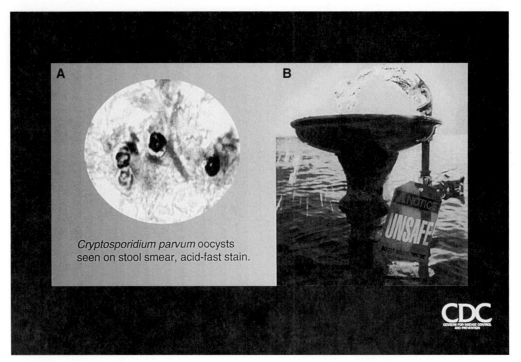

Figure 9-28 ▪ **A,** Photomicrograph of *Cryptosporidium parvum* oocysts in stool smear, acid fast stain. **B,** Water fountain with sign that water is unsafe. (From Centers for Disease Control and Prevention Public Health Image Library, Atlanta, Ga.)

sickening of more than 400,000 people in Milwaukee, Wis., due to improperly treated municipal water supply in 1993.[7] A secondary means of transmission is by inhalation of aerosolized oocysts.

Calves are accepted as a source for human infection. A study in Wisconsin using PCR analysis of human isolates concluded that most sporadic cases of cryptosporidiosis in that state were zoonotic in origin, with cattle and other ruminants the main source.[8] The types of zoonotic transmission that occur appear to differ by geographical area, with less zoonotic transmission occurring in urban areas. The risk of human infection by dogs and cats is believed to be small in industrialized countries. *C. canis, C. felis,* and *C. meleagridis* are responsible for as much as 20% of human infection in some developing countries, but some evidence indicates that although diseases originates in animals, these strains are being transmitted person to person.[4] Data from the Milwaukee outbreak and others suggest two thirds of water-source human outbreaks are not of animal origin. Transmission in animals, as in humans, occurs through ingestion and possibly inhalation of oocysts.

Environmental Risk Factors

Cryptosporidium cysts, like *Giardia,* can contaminate water supplies and other moist environments for months. Environments where manure is spread have been associated with increased risk of human infection.[9]

Disease in Humans

The majority of the North American population has been exposed to the infection at some time. *Cryptosporidium* infection in immunocompetent humans can be asymptomatic.

The major symptom is diarrhea—often explosive, profuse, and watery with mucus—accompanied by abdominal pain and cramping, vomiting, and weight loss.[3] Low-grade fever may occur. The diarrhea is self-limiting in healthy people, lasting 8 to 20 days. In patients infected with HIV and in other immunodeficient patients, symptoms can be more severe and chronic and include massive diarrhea and involvement of the respiratory and biliary tracts.[5]

Disease in Animals

In dogs and cats, the disease is often subclinical. Puppies and kittens are more likely than adults to show intestinal signs of infection. In cats and dogs, most clinical cases are associated with immunosuppression, such as with feline leukemia virus, canine distemper virus, canine parvovirus, and intestinal lymphosarcoma, and can manifest as intestinal, hepatic, pancreatic, or respiratory disease.[10] Calves may exhibit diarrhea, anorexia, and weight loss. Adults are often asymptomatic. Cryptosporidiosis commonly causes vomiting in snakes (Color Plate 9-11). Table 9-18 provides a comparison of clinical manifestations in humans and other animals.

Table 9-18 ■ Cryptosporidiosis: Comparative Clinical Presentations in Humans and Other Animals

Species	Risk Factors	Incubation Period	Clinical Manifestations
Humans	Children and their caretakers Farm animal contact	1-12 days[3]	Asymptomatic *or* acute watery diarrhea, coughing and low-grade fever
Dogs, cats, ruminants, mice, horses (*Cryptosporidium.* spp. can infect reptiles and birds)	Neonates, immunocompromised at increased risk of symptomatic disease	5-10 days	Often asymptomatic in older and immunocompetent animals Small-bowel diarrhea, diarrhea, tenesmus, dehydration, weight loss

Table 9-19 ■ Antibiotic Treatment of Cryptosporidiosis in Humans and Other Animals

Species	Primary Treatment	Alternative Treatment
Humans: immunocompetent	Supportive care Nitazoxanide 500 mg PO bid × 3 days[11]	
Adult with HIV infection	Effective antiretroviral therapy best treatment	
Dogs, cats	Supportive care Paromomycin 125-165 mg/kg PO bid × 5 days (may cause nephropathy in young animals)	Tylosin 11 mg/kg q12h × 28 days
Cattle	Supportive care, hyperimmune bovine colostrum	

Diagnosis

In human beings, cases are diagnosed by IFA visualization of oocysts in feces. An ELISA test is also available. Many laboratories do not routinely test for *Cryptosporidium*, so a special request may be necessary.

Animal diagnosis involves testing for oocysts in feces with sucrose or zinc sulfate solution with visualization after modified acid-fast staining, a procedure typically performed by a veterinary laboratory rather than by the private practitioner (Color Plate 9-12). Routine in-house flotation tests often fail because cysts are small (4 to 5 microns in diameter). To inactivate potential cysts and submit fecal samples to an appropriate laboratory, mix one part 100% formalin with nine parts feces. Oocysts are not shed continuously; therefore repeat samples may be necessary.

Treatment

Acute cryptosporidiosis is treated with supportive care including rehydration. Antibiotics are indicated for symptomatic patients. In patients with HIV infection, adequate antiretroviral therapy is essential to reducing the morbidity of cryptosporidiosis infection (Table 9-19).

In immunocompetent animals the disease is usually self-limiting and may include oral glucose-electrolyte solution. Severe diarrhea warrants parenteral fluids. If there are zoonotic concerns, a trial of antibiotics may be warranted. No antibiotics are registered for treatment of *Cryptosporidium* in animals. Monitor fecal oocyst shedding 14 days after treatment.

References

1. Centers for Disease Control and Prevention. *Cryptosporidiosis outbreak response & evaluation.* http://www.cdc.gov/crypto/pdfs/core_guidelines.pdf.2.
2. Dvorak GA, Rovid-Spickler A, Roth JA, eds. *Handbook for zoonotic diseases of companion animals.* Ames, IA: The Center for Food Security & Public Health, Iowa State University; 2006.
3. Heymann DL. *Control of communicable diseases manual.* 19th ed. Washington DC: American Public Health Association; 2008.
4. Xiao L, Feng Y. Zoonotic cryptosporidiosis. *FEMS Immunol Med Microbiol.* 2008;52(3):309.
5. Acha PN, Szyfres B. *Zoonoses and communicable diseases common to man and animals: vol. 1: bacterioses and mycoses.* 3rd ed. Washington DC: Pan American Health Organization; 2001.
6. Dupont HL, Chappell CL, Sterling CR, et al. The infectivity of *Cryptosporidium parvum* in healthy volunteers. *N Engl J Med.* 1995;332:855.
7. MacKenzie WR, Hoxie NJ, Proctor ME, et al. A massive outbreak in Milwaukee of *Cryptosporidium* infection transmitted through the public water supply. *N Engl J Med.* 1994;331(3):161.
8. Feltus DC, Giddings CW, Schneck BL, et al. Evidence supporting zoonotic transmission of *Cryptosporidium* spp. in Wisconsin. *J Clin Microbiol.* 2006;44(12):4303.
9. Lake IR, Harrison FC, Chalmers RM, et al. Case-control study of environmental and social factors influencing cryptosporidiosis. *Eur J Epidemiol.* 2007;22(11):805.
10. Barr SC, Bowman DD. *5-minute veterinary consult clinical companion canine and feline infectious disease and parasitology.* Ames, IA: Wiley-Blackwell; 2006.
11. Gilbert DN, Moellering RC, Ellopoulos GM, et al. *Sanford guide to antimicrobial therapy 2009.* 39th ed. Sperryville, VA: Antimicrobial Therapy; 2009.

DERMATOPHYTOSIS

Peter M. Rabinowitz and Lisa A. Conti

Dermatophytosis (ICD-10 B35)

Other names in humans: ringworm infection, tinea infection, dermatomycosis, trichophytosis, microphytosis

Other names in animals: ringworm, keratinophilic mycosis

Dermatophytosis is a skin infection caused by members of three genera of fungi: *Epidermophyton, Microsporum,* and *Trichophyton.* Because all domestic animals are susceptible to dermatophytosis and many dermatophytes can pass between species, dermatophytosis is probably one of the most common pet-associated and occupational zoonoses. It has been estimated that approximately 2 million people in the United States are infected each year as a result of contact with animals.[1] The true prevalence is probably greater than recognized; the signs of disease may be mild, so infected individuals may not seek medical care and the condition is often not reported to local health authorities.

Key Points for Clinicians and Public Health Professionals

Public Health Professionals

- Provide descriptive epidemiology about the disease.
- Educate the public on modes of transmission and risk factors for infection.
- Raise awareness of the disease among high-risk groups such as animal workers and in school settings.
- Make recommendations for environmental cleanup of contaminated surfaces and fomites with dilute bleach solution (1:10).

Human Health Clinicians

- When taking a history on a patient with a rash for which dermatophytosis is suspected, inquire about pet and other animal exposures.
- Teach patients to always wash their hands after contact with pets and other animals.[2]
- Encourage infected patients with dogs and cats to seek veterinary evaluation of their pets.
- No human vaccine is available.

Veterinary Clinicians

- Ensure that owners bring affected animals for prompt treatment; be aware that there are inapparent carriers and that use of corticosteroids may prolong infection.
- Counsel clients and veterinary care staff about handwashing and other measures to avoid zoonotic transmission.

- Counsel pet owners and clinic employees to disinfect contaminated equipment, bedding, and the environment with dilute bleach solution (1:10).
- Consider the possibility of rodents spreading the disease to pets and other animals.
- If dermatophytosis is diagnosed in a pet, treat the animal and advise the owner and family members of the zoonotic risk and to seek medical care if symptoms are noticed.
- Isolation may be advisable for an animal that is under treatment due to the zoonotic nature of the disease.
- An attenuated vaccine for cattle is available in Europe, where it has been reported to reduce the incidence of zoonotic disease in animal care workers[3]; it is not currently available in the United States.
- Therapy cats should be tested biannually.[4]

Agent

Fungi that cause dermatophytosis are spore-producing pathogens that may be classified according to mode of transmission as anthropophilic (preferring humans), zoophilic (preferring animals), or geophilic (preferring soil environments). Although zoophilic species often can pass from animals to humans, they tend to not be readily transmissible from human to human. Table 9-20 lists the main species and their type.[5]

Geographical Occurrence

These pathogenic fungi are found worldwide and the incidence is generally higher in hot and humid climates. *Trichophyton tonsurans* is commonly found in urban areas in the eastern United States, Puerto Rico, Mexico, the United Kingdom, and Australia. *T. verrucosum* and *T. mentagrophytes* are common in rural areas[2] as is *Microsporum canis.* *M. audonii* is more common in West Africa.

Groups at Risk

Dermatophytoses from animals are an occupational risk for veterinary health care workers and other animal workers. Pet owners, children, and immunocompromised individuals are at increased risk of infection,[2] as are humans living in close quarters (such as military personnel, athletes, school children, and inner-city residents) who are at risk for human-to-human transmission.

Hosts, Reservoir Species, Vectors

Table 9-20 lists the principal animal reservoir species for the *T. mentagrophytes* zoophilic dermatophytoses. The different species of fungi tend to vary in their host specificity. *M. nanum,* an infection of pigs, tends not to infect other species,[4] whereas *T. mentagrophytes* has a much wider host range, infecting rodents, dogs, cats, rabbits, horses, humans, hedgehogs,[6] and other animals. Mechanical vectors include furniture, animal bedding, hair care articles (scissors, combs, and brushes), clothing, and hats.

Table 9-20 ■ Classification of the Major Dermatophytes

Anthropophilic	Geophilic	Zoophilic	
		Organism	Sources
Trichophyton concentricum	Trichophyton ajelloi	Trichophyton erinacei*	Hedgehogs
T. gourvilii	T. terrestre	T. equinum	Horses
T. mentagrophytes interdigitale*	Microsporum fulvum	T. mentagrophytes*	Rodents
T. megnini	M. gypseum	T. quinckeanum*	Mice
T. rubrum		T. simii	Monkeys
T. schoenleinii		T. verrucosum	Cattle
T. soudanense		Microsporum canis	Cats, dogs
T. tonsurans		M. gallinae	Chickens
T. violaceum		M. nanum	Pigs
T. yaoundei		M. persicolor	Bank voles
Microsporum audouinii			
M. ferrugineum			
Epidermophyton floccosum			

*These organisms are part of the "mentagrophytes" complex and may be classified as a single species.
From Mandell GE, Bennett JE, Dolin R (eds): *Principles and practice of infectious diseases*, ed 6, Philadelphia, 2000, Churchill Livingstone Elsevier.

Mode of Transmission and Life Cycle

Transmission occurs through direct skin-to-skin and skin-to-hair contact with infected animals or humans and indirect contact with the infectious arthrospores in the environment or on fomites (Figure 9-29). An infected human or animal can generate an aerosol of infectious arthrospores.[2] The infectious spores germinate in the keratinized layers of skin, hair, and nails.[7]

The mode of transmission also helps determine the severity of clinical disease. In general, animal-to-human transmission produces some of the most severe clinical syndromes, as shown in Table 9-21.

Environmental Risk Factors

The fungi and infectious spores can survive on surfaces and in desquamated skin for months.[2] Therefore environmental contamination can play an important role in transmission. In general, moist, warm environmental conditions favor the

Table 9-21 ■ Clinical Features of Dermatophytes Based on Mode of Transmission

Mode of Transmission	Clinical Features
Human-to-human	Mild to noninflammatory, chronic
Animal-to-human	Intense inflammation (pustules and vesicles possible), acute
Soil-to-human or animal	Moderate inflammation

From Bolognia JL, Jorizzo JL, Rapini RP (eds): *Dermatology*, ed 2, London, 2003, Mosby Elsevier.)

growth of fungi and persistence of spores on surfaces and articles. Environmental samples such as soil and clothing associated with human and other animal cases have spore positivity rates as high as 100%.[8] Contamination with multiple dermatophyte species has been found on veterinary clinic floors, producing an environmental risk of infection for both animals, clients, and the veterinary staff.[2]

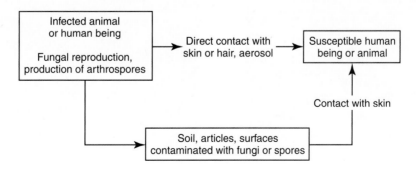

Environmental factors: Climate, temperature, humidity, crowding

Figure 9-29 ■ Transmission of dermatophytosis in animals and humans.

Disease in Humans

The incubation period in humans is 10 to 14 days. Infection in humans usually begins with a small area of erythema that develops into a patch of annular scaling skin with a raised border that then slowly spreads peripherally. Infections are usually accompanied by pruritus, which can lead to excoriation and secondary bacterial infections. As shown in Table 9-21, zoophilic fungi are more likely than anthropophilic or geophilic fungi to produce severe inflammatory changes in humans, often with pustular lesions (kerion).[9] The location of the infection determines the name of the dermatophytosis.

Tinea capitis is an infection of the scalp that occurs most commonly in children. It is caused by only two genera: *Trichophyton* and *Microsporum*. In the United States, *T. tonsurans* is the most common cause and *M. canis* is the second most common.[9] Tinea capitis can produce localized hair loss, pustules, and scarring (Figure 9-30).

Tinea corporis is an infection of the trunk and extremities that does not involve the hair, palms, soles, or groin. Worldwide, it is most commonly caused by *T. rubrum* followed by *T. mentagrophytes*.[9] It can present in a variety of ways dependent in part on the mode of transmission, but classically causes a circular annular lesion with scaling (Color Plate 9-13).

Tinea pedis is an infection of the toes and feet caused *T. rubrum*, *T mentagrophytes*, *Epidermophyton floccosum*, and *T. tonsurans*.[9]

Other dermatophyte infections include tinea barbae, an infection of the beard area; tinea cruris, an infection of the groin and perianal area; and tinea manum, an infection of the hand.

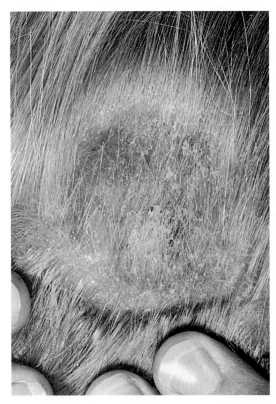

Figure 9-30 ▪ Tinea capitis due to *M. canis* infection. (From Mandell GE, Bennett JE, Dolin R: *Principles and practice of infectious diseases*, ed 6, Philadelphia, 2000, Churchill Livingstone Elsevier.)

In immunocompromised individuals, *T. mentagrophytes* and *M. canis* can cause disseminated skin infection.

Disease in Animals

The incubation period in animals is generally 1 to 2 weeks. The infection in dogs may begin as alopecia (Figure 9-31). Erythema, scaling, and pruritus may develop around the lesions. In some dogs clinical signs do not develop yet the dogs are capable of shedding spores into the environment. In immunocompromised animals, these infections can be severe (Color Plate 9-14).

Up to 90% of infected cats show no clinical signs of disease. Clinical infections are more common in kittens and long-haired breeds of cats. Clinical signs include a poor hair coat or circular skin lesions, usually on the face or paws (Color Plate 9-15).

Infections are more common when cattle are stabled indoors. Lesions often begin as gray-white areas that thicken, scab, and slough, leaving an area of alopecia. Infection is often self-limited over several months (Color Plate 9-16).[3]

Horses tend to become infected at areas of contact with a harness. The disease manifests as areas of localized alopecia with skin thickening (Figure 9-32 and Color Plate 9-17).[3]

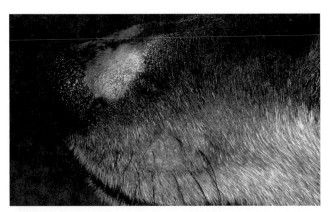

Figure 9-31 ▪ Dermatophytosis. Focal alopecia on the muzzle of a Dachshund. This is a typical location for dogs that frequently dig in soil. (From Medleau L, Hnilica KA: *Small animal dermatology: a color atlas and therapeutic guide*, ed 2, St Louis, 2006, Saunders Elsevier.)

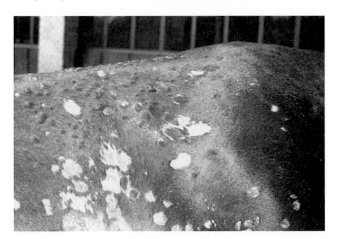

Figure 9-32 ▪ Classic signs of dermatophytosis (ringworm) in a horse. (From Reed SM, Warwick MB, Sellon DC: *Equine internal medicine*, ed 2, St Louis, 2004, Saunders Elsevier.)

Table 9-22 ▪ Dermatophytosis: Comparative Clinical Presentations in Humans and Other Animals

Species	Risk Factors	Incubation Period	Clinical Manifestations	Laboratory Findings
Humans	Children, crowding, contact with animals, immunocompromised	10 days to 2 wk	Erythema, itching, scaling lesion of skin	KOH preparation may show hyphae; Wood's lamp may fluoresce; fungal culture
Dogs or cats	Crowding, young animals, immunodeficiency	1-4 wk	Alopecia or poor hair coat, scales, erythema, asymptomatic	*M. canis* may fluoresce under Wood's lamp, microscopic examination[10] Fungal culture
Cattle	Stabling indoors, calves		Gray-white areas that scab and fall off, leaving alopecia	
Horses	Friction from harnesses		Dry, scaling, thickened areas	
Rodents			Often no clinical signs, white scabby lesions of head and trunk	

KOH, Potassium hydroxide.

Rodents such as mice may show no evidence of disease or may have white scabbing lesions on the head and trunk (Color Plate 9-18).

Table 9-22 shows the comparative clinical presentations in humans and animals.

Diagnosis

In humans the diagnosis can be made clinically based on the typical appearance of lesions and a history of contact with an infected person or animal. The differential diagnosis may include eczema, impetigo, and conditions causing localized alopecia, such as cutaneous lupus. The sensitivity and specificity of the Wood's lamp test is limited because only some dermatophytes will fluoresce; therefore this test should be used only as part of a screening process. Wood's lamp–positive areas can be used to guide scrapings for microscopic examination and/or culture. Samples of skin and hair should be taken from the periphery of lesions where infection is active.

Scrapings or clippings can be placed in 10% to 20% potassium hydroxide solution and examined microscopically. Hyphae can appear as chains (Figure 9-33). Conidae (spores) can also be recognized by microscopy (Figures 9-34 and 9-35).

In addition to microscopy, fungal culture is often worthwhile to confirm the diagnosis and the fungal species (Color Plate 9-19). Similar diagnostic tests are used in other animals.

Treatment

Table 9-23 outlines treatment guidelines in humans and other animals. Many human cases of dermatophytosis are self-limited and do not require treatment. However, treatment

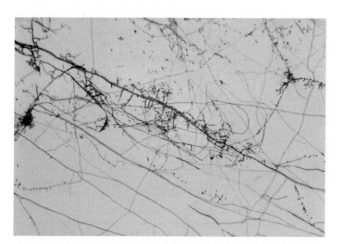

Figure 9-33 ▪ Photomicrograph of the fungus *Trichophyton mentagrophytes*. This dermatophyte is a zoophilic species that commonly inhabits mice, guinea pigs, kangaroos, cats, horses, sheep, and rabbits. Members of the genus *Trichophyton* are common causes of hair, skin, and nail infections in humans. (From Centers for Disease Control and Prevention Public Health Image Library, Atlanta, Ga. Courtesy Dr. Leonor Haley.)

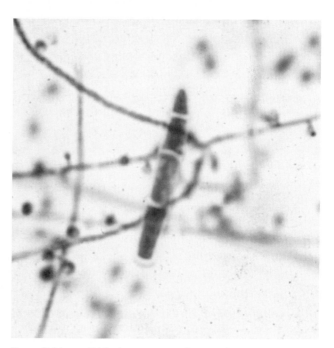

Figure 9-34 ▪ *Trichophyton mentagrophytes* in culture. Spherical microconidia and one thin-walled, multicellular, cigar-shaped macroconidium (lactophenol analine blue, ×2000). (From Greene CE: *Infectious diseases of the dog and cat*, ed 3, St Louis, 2006, Saunders Elsevier. Courtesy Spencer Jang, University of California, Davis.)

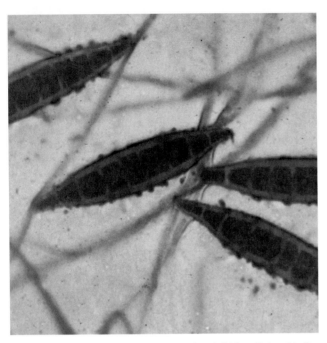

Figure 9-35 ■ *M. canis* in culture. Rough and thick-walled multicellular spindle-shaped macroconidia. Note curved, pointed ends (lactophenol analine blue, ×2000). (From Greene CE: *Infectious diseases of the dog and cat*, ed 3, St Louis, 2006, Saunders Elsevier. Courtesy Richard Walker, University of California, Davis.)

may shorten the duration of infection and reduce the possibility of further transmission.

Companion animals with positive culture findings should be treated because of the zoonotic disease risk.[11] However, eradicating the disease may be a challenge if multiple animals are housed together. Response to therapy is monitored by dermatophyte culture as many animals will remain culture positive while improving clinically.

For mild skin infections, topical medication may be sufficient. More extensive infections may require systemic treatments. In food-producing animals, treatment options may be limited because of food safety concerns.

References

1. Stehr-Green JK, Schantz PM. The impact of zoonotic diseases transmitted by pets on human health and the economy. *Vet Clin N Am Small Anim Pract.* 1987;17:1.
2. Heymann DL. *Control of communicable diseases manual.* 19th ed. Washington DC: American Public Health Association; 2008.
3. Acha PN, Szyfres B. *Zoonoses and communicable diseases common to man and animals: vol. 1: bacterioses and mycoses.* 3rd ed. Washington DC: Pan American Health Organization; 2001.
4. Greene CE. *Infectious diseases of the dog and cat.* 3rd ed. St Louis: Saunders Elsevier; 2006.
5. Mandell GL, Bennett JE, Dolin R, eds. *Principles and practice of infectious diseases.* 6th ed. Philadelphia: Churchill Livingstone Elsevier; 2005.
6. Rosen T. Hazardous hedgehogs. *South Med J.* 2000;93(9):936–938.

Table 9-23 ■ Dermatophytosis Treatment in Humans and Other Animals

Species	Primary Treatment	Alternative
Humans: tinea corporis, tinea cruris, tinea pedis	Topical antifungal, drying powder	Terbinafine 250 mg PO × 4 wk *or* ketoconazole 200 mg PO q24h × 4 wk *or* fluconazole 150 mg PO 1×/wk for 2-4 wk *or* griseofulvin: *Adults:* 500 mg PO q24h × 4-6 wk *Children:* 10-20 mg/kg/day 2-4 wk for T. corporis, 4-8 wk for T. pedis
Humans: tinea capitis	*Adults:* Terbinafine 250 mg PO × 4 wk (*T. tonsurans*) or 4-8 wk (*M. canis*) *Children:* 125 mg or 6-12 mg/kg PO qd[12]	Itraconazole 3-5 mg/kg PO qd × 30 day *or* fluconazole 8 mg/kg (max 150 mg) PO qwk × 8-12 wk griseofulvin: *Adults:* 500 mg PO q24h × 4-6 wk *Children:* 10-20 mg/kg/day until hair regrows[12]
Dogs and cats (NOTE: Spontaneous remission may occur in short-haired cats in a single-cat environment and in dogs; environmental treatment is important; use dilute bleach [1:10]; multi-cat environments can be complicated.)	Topical miconazole or clotrimazole[10] Griseofulvin microsized formulation 25-60 mg/kg PO q12h × 4-6 wk (fed with a fatty meal helps increase absorption) Ultramicrosized formulation 2.5-5.0 mg/kg PO q12-24h Pediatric suspension 10-5 mg/kg PO q12h Lufenuron (Program) 100 mg/kg for 2 doses at 2-week intervals, then treat monthly Clipping and topical therapy: lime sulfur (1:16) or miconazole shampoo	Ketoconazole (not labeled for use in dogs and cats in the United States) 10 mg/kg PO q24h or divided twice per day for 3-4 wk; acid meal (add tomato juice) will enhance absorption Itraconazole 10 mg/kg PO q24h or 5 mg/kg q12h Spot treatment not recommended[11]
Cattle	Washes or sprays of 4% lime sulfur, 0.5% sodium hypochlorite bleach, 0.5% chlorhexidine, 1% povidone-iodine, natamycin, and enilconazole (not available in the United States)	Treat individual lesions with miconazole or clotrimazole lotions
Horses	Topical clotrimazole or miconazole	
Lambs	Sodium hypochlorite washes or enilconazole rinses[11]	

7. Van Rooij P, Detandt M, Nolard N. Trichophyton mentagrophytes of rabbit origin causing family incidence of kerion: an environmental study. *Mycoses.* 2006;49(5):426–430. (Erratum in *Mycoses* 2007;50(2):160.)
8. Cafarchia C, Romito D, Capelli G, et al. Isolation of *Microsporum canis* from the hair coat of pet dogs and cats belonging to owners diagnosed with *M. canis* tinea corporis. *Vet Derm.* 2006;17(5):327–331.
9. Bolognia JL, Jorizzo JL, Rapini RP, eds. *Dermatology.* 2nd ed. London: Mosby Elsevier; 2008.
10. Barr SC, Bowman DD. *5-minute veterinary consult clinical companion canine and feline infectious disease and parasitology.* Ames, IA: Wiley-Blackwell; 2006.
11. Kahn CM, Line S, eds. *The Merck veterinary manual.* 9th ed.Whitehouse Station, NJ: Merck; 2005.
12. Gilbert DN, Moellering RC, Ellopoulos GM, et al. *Sanford guide to antimicrobial therapy 2009.* 39th ed. Sperryville, VA: Antimicrobial Therapy; 2009.

DIPYLIDIASIS

Peter M. Rabinowitz and Lisa A. Conti

Dipylidiasis (ICD-10 B71.1)

Other names in humans: dog tapeworm

Other names in animals: dog tapeworm, dog cestodiasis

The dog tapeworm (*Dipylidium caninum*) is a common parasite of dogs and cats. The cat flea (*Ctenocephalides felis*) and dog flea (*Ctenocephalides canis*, relatively rare in North America)[1] are important intermediate hosts in the life cycle. Human infection is apparently a rare event that occurs when children ingest fleas containing tapeworm eggs.[2] Although infection in both humans and other animals is usually asymptomatic, the white, seedlike, motile proglottids are passed in the stool, causing concern.

Key Points for Clinicians and Public Health Professionals

Public Health Professionals

- Educate the public about the need for routine flea control.
- Ensure policies are in place for proper disposal of animal feces.

Human Health Clinicians

- The veterinarian caring for the family pets should be contacted to ensure that pets receive treatment.
- The appearance of proglottids in the stool of a child may be a sentinel event indicating probable flea infestation in the house as well as infection of a household pet. Human health clinicians should counsel adult patients or parents of pediatric patients to seek veterinary advice and preventive services to ensure that the house and pets of a patient are treated for fleas.
- Children should wash their hands after playing with pets. Children with pica behavior require careful supervision when playing in environments with pets.

Veterinary Clinicians

- Counsel pet owners to practice flea control.
- Deworm all dogs and cats in the household when infection is identified in one animal (typically because of passage of tapeworm segments in stool).
- Counsel owners of pets that have been diagnosed with tapeworms or fleas to watch for signs of infection in children in the household.

Agent

The double-pored dog tapeworm (*D. caninum*) is a Cestode that is the most common tapeworm of dogs and cats.[3] The adult worms may be as long as 70 cm and can live in the small intestine for up to 3 months. The adult worms consist of a head (scolex), neck, and chain of segments known as *proglottids* (Figure 9-36). New segments form at the neck and older segments are pushed back.[4] Each proglottid contains both male and female elements and can become full of eggs (gravid) and break off from the rest of the worm, to be shed in the feces. Fleas play an important role in the life cycle of the worm as intermediate hosts.

Geographical Occurrence

Worldwide.

Groups at Risk

Young children appear to represent most human cases because of their close contact with pets and greater likelihood

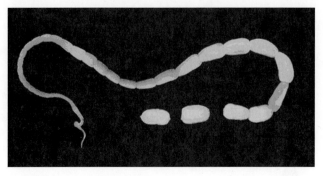

Figure 9-36 ▪ Adult *Dipylidium caninum* with detaching proglottids. (From Centers for Disease Control and Prevention Public Health Image Library, Atlanta, Ga.)

of ingesting fleas directly or in food. A case in a 5-week-old infant has been reported.[5]

Hosts, Reservoir Species, Vectors

Dogs and cats are the principal reservoirs, although wild carnivores have also been found to be infected. Humans are accidental hosts.

Mode of Transmission and Life Cycle

The adult worms live in the intestine of the reservoir host (Figure 9-37). Gravid proglottids are released in the feces (Figure 9-38). In the environment the proglottids break down, releasing the eggs. If the eggs are ingested by a larval cat or dog flea, the eggs hatch and turn into cysticercoids as the flea develops. Dogs and cats may ingest a flea as a defensive behavior. Children may ingest a flea accidentally when playing with or handling a dog or cat or by ingesting food containing a flea (Figure 9-39). Once the flea is ingested, cysticercoids are released into the small intestine, where they develop into adult worms within 20 days.[6]

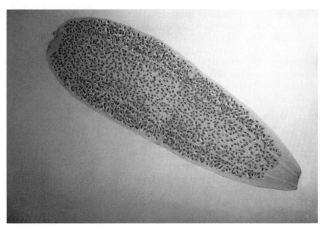

Figure 9-38 ■ Micrograph depicting a proglottid (i.e., a tapeworm segment) from the Cestode *Dipylidium caninum*. Such proglottids, which when mature average 12 mm × 3 mm, are passed with feces and often resemble rice grains when dried. Each proglottid contains egg packets that are held together by an outer embryonic membrane. (From Centers for Disease Control and Prevention Public Health Image Library, Atlanta, Ga.)

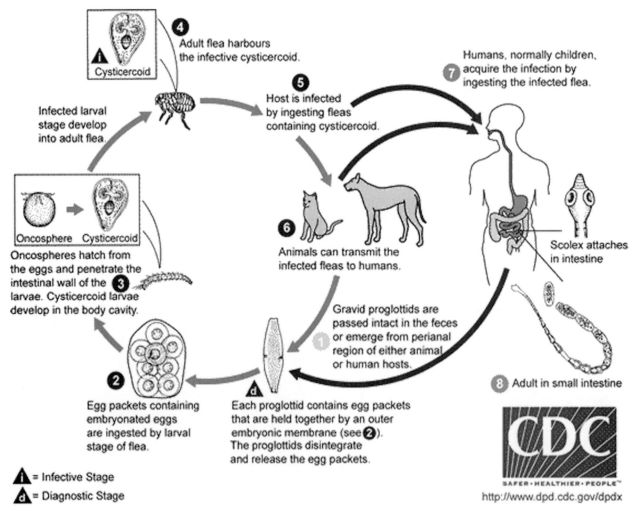

Figure 9-37 ■ Life cycle, dipylidiasis. (From Centers for Disease Control and Prevention Public Health Image Library, Atlanta, Ga.)

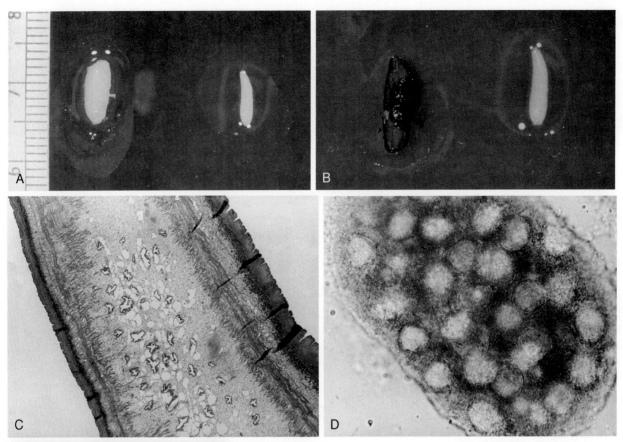

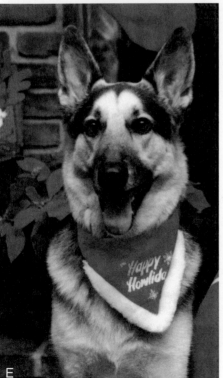

Figure 9-39 ■ A 20-month-old girl was seen in consultation because of "moving rice" in the stool on the diaper. **A,** A grain of rice from the hospital cafeteria is seen on the left, and the patient's "rice" on the right. **B,** A drop of iodine shows the typical carbohydrate blackening of rice on the left. Note the 7-cm vase shape of patient's "rice" on the right. **C,** Histologic section of "rice" shows typical structure of *Dipylidium caninum*. **D,** Typical egg packet of *D. caninum* is seen from patient's stool specimen. **E,** The family dog. (From Long SS, Pickering LK, Prober CG (eds): *Principles and practice of pediatric infectious diseases*, ed 3, Philadelphia, 2008, Churchill Livingstone Elsevier. Courtesy Joel E. Mortensen and Sarah S. Long, St. Christopher's Hospital for Children, Philadelphia, PA.)

Table 9-24 ▪ Dipylidiasis in Humans and Animals

Species	Risk Factors	Incubation Period	Clinical Signs	Diagnostic Findings
Humans	Fleas in house, children at increased risk of ingesting fleas	Adult worms develop in 20 days	Usually asymptomatic, may have abdominal pain	Proglottids in stool
Dogs, cats	Flea contact, ingestion		No symptoms or perianal pruritus	

Environmental Risk Factors

The key environmental risk is flea infestation of a house or other living environment.

Disease in Humans

Based on existing case reports, human infection with dipylidiasis is usually asymptomatic. The proglottids appear in the stool as white, rice-like motile objects and may be shed over a number of months. In one report, dipylidiasis was misdiagnosed as recurrent pinworm (*Enterobius vermicularis*) infection and therefore incorrectly treated.[7] Abdominal discomfort may occur, as well as abdominal distension, appetite disturbances, and insomnia.[6] Accompanying neurological symptoms including vertigo and light-headedness have been described.[8]

Disease in Animals

The infection in dogs and cats is considered to cause few clinical signs. Perianal pruritus may be present. Infected dogs may therefore "scoot," dragging their anus along the ground to relieve the itching. The most significant finding is the sight of proglottids in the feces, emerging from the anus or stuck to perianal hairs. These appear as white, crawling rice-like segments on the fur or in feces or on the perianal area.

Diagnosis

The diagnosis is usually made clinically by identifying the motile proglottids and obtaining a history of contact with fleas or a dog or cat. In animals, visualizing the proglottids of *D. caninum* is diagnostic. Table 9-24 shows the manifestation of disease in humans and other animals.

Treatment

The goal of treatment in humans and other animals is the elimination of the cestodes. Table 9-25 summarizes recommended treatment regimens for dipylidiasis in different species.

Flea control is also important for dogs and cats. This can be accomplished with monthly treatments of selamectin, lufenuron, imadacloprid, fipronil,[10] or spinosad.

Table 9-25 ▪ Treatment of Dog and Cat Tapeworm Infection in Humans and Other Animals

Species	Primary Treatment	Alternative Treatment
Humans	Praziquantel 5-10 mg/kg PO × 1 dose	
Dogs*	Praziquantel 5 mg/kg PO, SC once	Praziquantel*/pyrantel/febantel PO once
	Flea control	Epsiprantel 5.5 mg/kg PO once
		Fenbendazole 50 mg/kg PO q24h × 5 days
Cats*	Praziquantel 5 mg/kg PO, SC once	Praziquantel/pyrantel PO once
	Flea control	Epsiprantel 2.8 mg/kg PO once[10]

*Not for puppies or kittens younger than 3 weeks or weighing less than 2 lb.

References

1. Goddard J. *Physician's guide to arthropods of medical importance.* 5th ed. Boca Raton, FL: CRC Press; 2007.
2. Figueroa HM, Augilar FJ. The first case of dipylidium caninum found and identified in a human being in Guatemala. *Am J Trop Med Hyg.* 1956;5:269-71
3. Kahn CM, Line S, eds. *The Merck veterinary manual.* 9th ed. Whitehouse Station, NJ: Merck; 2005.
4. Colville J, Berryhill D. *Handbook of zoonoses: identification and prevention.* St Louis: Mosby Elsevier; 2007.
5. Minnaganti VR. *Dipylidiasis.* http://www.emedicine.com/med/TOPIC573.htm. Accessed August 13, 2008.
6. Acha PN, Szyfres B. *Zoonoses and communicable diseases common to man and animals: vol 3: chlamydioses, parasitoses.* 3rd ed. Washington DC: Pan American Health Organization; 2003.
7. Samkari A, Kiska DL, Riddell SW, et al. Dipylidium caninum mimicking recurrent Enterobius vermicularis (pinworm) infection. *Clin Pediatr (Phila).* 2008;47:397-9.
8. Cirioni O, Giacometti A, Burzacchini F, et al. Unusual neurological presentation of dipylidiasis in a child. *Eur J Ped.* 1996;155(1):67.
9. Gilbert DN, Moellering RC, Ellopoulos GM, et al. *Sanford guide to antimicrobial therapy 2009.* 39th ed. Sperryville, VA: Antimicrobial Therapy; 2009.
10. Barr SC, Bowman DD. *5-minute veterinary consult clinical companion canine and feline infectious disease and parasitology.* Ames, IA: Wiley-Blackwell; 2006.

ECHINOCOCCOSIS

Peter M. Rabinowitz and Lisa A. Conti

Echinococcosis (ICD10B-67)

Echinococcosis due to Echinococcus granulosus *(ICD-10 B67-67.4), echinococcosis due to* Echinococcus multilocularis *(ICD-10 B67.9)*

Other names in humans: hydatid disease, cystic hydatid disease, alveolar hydatid disease, echinococciasis

Other names in animals: hydatid disease, hydatid cyst, unilocular hydatid disease, cystic echinococcosis, hydatidosis

Echinococcosis is a potentially fatal zoonotic tapeworm infection. Dogs and other canids are the definitive host of *Echinococcus granulosus*; therefore cases in humans are typically related to contact with domestic dogs. The types of human-dog contact and the way that dogs are raised and fed determine the degree of human risk.

Key Points for Clinicians and Public Health Professionals

Public Health Professionals

- Provide descriptive epidemiology regarding the risk in the community.
- Prevent dogs, cats, and foxes from contaminating playgrounds and other public areas with feces.
- Educate the public to thoroughly wash all fruits and vegetables before consuming them.
- Educate pet owners to not allow dogs and cats to roam outside or feed on raw carcasses.
- Ensure that workers with occupational risk for *Echinococcus* infection (e.g., sheep ranchers, wildlife rehabilitators) receive adequate surveillance and reduction of exposure risk through exposure controls and protective equipment.

Human Health Clinicians

- Disease is reportable in some states.
- Counsel dog owners to wash hands after handling pet and to avoid contact with animal feces.
- Counsel all patients to thoroughly wash vegetables and fruits before consumption.
- Ensure that high-risk groups (e.g., veterinarians, laboratory workers, and wildlife rehabilitators) frequently exposed to foxes and wild animals use protective measures (gloves and handwashing).

Veterinary Clinicians

- Counsel clients to avoid feeding raw meat to dogs and cats and to not allow pets to hunt.
- Train veterinary personnel in biosafety measures to reduce risk from infected dogs and wild animals.

- Regularly examine and treat high-risk dogs and cats (e.g., sheep dogs).
- An experimental recombinant vaccine is available for sheep in high-risk areas.

Agent

The causative agent of echinococcosis in humans is the larval (hydatid) phase of Cestodes (tapeworms) in the genus *Echinococcus*, including *E. granulosus, E. multilocularis, E. oligarthrus,* and *E. vogelii* (Figures 9-40 and 9-41).[1] Cystic echinococcosis is causes by *E. granulosus*, whereas *E. multilocularis* causes alveolar echinococcosis.

Geographical Occurrence

E. granulosus is found on every continent except Antarctica. In the United States, human cases are more likely to be found in areas where there is contact between dogs and sheep, such as in the western states. In Alaska, a sylvatic strain of *E. granulosus* is found in caribou and moose; dogs that eat the viscera of these infected animals can then infect humans.[2,3] *E. oligarthus* and *E. vogelii* are found only in Central and South America. Alveolar echinococcosis caused by *E. multilocularis* is restricted to the northern hemisphere.

Groups at Risk

Echinococcosis tends to occur in well-defined groups who have contact with dogs that ingest the raw viscera of infected animals. These include sheepherders who use dogs and persons in Alaska who allow dogs to feed on entrails of wild caribou and moose. Many of the cases diagnosed in the United States are in immigrants from countries where contacts between dogs and sheep and cattle are common.[4] Children may be at greater risk of infection because of close contact with dogs.

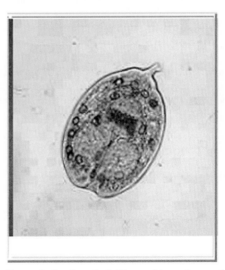

Figure 9-40 ■ Scolex from hydatid cyst. (From Centers for Disease Control and Prevention Public Health Image Library, Atlanta, Ga.)

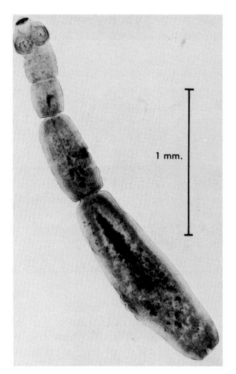

Figure 9-41 ▪ *Echinococcus granulosus* (Taeniidae), entire worm (×44). (From Bowman DD: *Georgis' parasitology for veterinarians,* ed 8, St Louis, 2003, Saunders Elsevier.)

Reported risk factors for *E. multilocularis* infection include owning dogs that kill game or roam outdoors, living in a farmhouse or near a field, growing vegetables, owning outdoor cats, or eating unwashed fruit.[5]

Hosts, Reservoir Species, Vectors

Dogs and wild canids are the definitive hosts for *E. granulosus.* The adult tapeworms reproduce in the dog intestine and shed gravid proglottids or eggs in the feces. These eggs can remain viable in moist conditions with moderate temperatures for months. Intermediate hosts include a wide variety of herbivores as well as mongooses, non-human primates, and humans.

The growing urban populations of red and arctic foxes, the primary definitive host for *E. multilocularis,* increase concern for human risk of infection.[6] The intermediate hosts for *E. multilocularis* are usually rodents, including mice, shrews, lemmings, and voles.[7] In addition to foxes, dogs and cats that hunt such animals can subsequently infect humans.[8]

Mode of Transmission and Life Cycle

The adult tapeworms living in the intestine of a dog or other carnivore release eggs that are shed in the feces (Figure 9-42). Human infection occurs by ingesting these eggs, either through contamination of food or by direct contact with dogs or other definitive hosts. Children are often infected because of more intimate contact with dogs and frequent hand-to-mouth contact. Once ingested, the eggs hatch into larvae (oncospheres) in the small intestine. Migrating through the

intestinal wall, they lodge in the liver, lung, or other tissues. There they form cysts containing protoscolices. *E. granulosus* tends to form large, slowly growing unilocular cysts with a well-defined limiting membrane. By contrast, *E. multilocularis* form multilocular cysts, also known as "alveolar" cysts, without a limiting membrane and grow more aggressively.[4] This results in the potential for *E. multilocularis* to cause more serious complications. When dogs feed on the carcass of an intermediate host containing cysts, the protoscolices develop into adult worms in the dog intestine (Color Plate 9-20).

Environmental Risk Factors

Contamination of the environment by egg-containing feces of infected canids is an important factor in transmission of *Echinococcus.* Feces containing eggs can contaminate grazing areas of sheep and other ruminants, leading to infection of these animals.[8] *Echinococcus* eggs can survive in the environment for weeks to months under optimal conditions.[9]

Dogs that defecate near vegetable gardens or otherwise contaminate sources of food and water can be a source of infection for humans. Factors that increase the abundance of foxes and rodents (potentially infected with *E. multilocularis*) around dwellings can increase the risk of infection to humans and domestic animals; these can include the presence of food sources including pet food and bird seed from bird feeders.

Disease in Humans

Table 9-26 shows the clinical features of *Echinococcus* infection in humans and other animals.

Echinococcosis Caused by E. granulosus (Cystic or Unilocular Hydatid Disease)

The cysts tend to be slow growing, unilocular, and often asymptomatic for many years. The size may reach 15 cm or larger. Many cysts are discovered only during imaging performed for other reasons (Figure 9-43). The severity of disease depends largely on the organ involved and cyst size and number. Most hydatid cysts are found in the liver (50% to 70%) and lungs (20% to 30%) but more rarely can involve spleen, muscles, heart, kidney, and even the brain. Symptoms develop if a cyst becomes large enough to affect organ function or cause pain or if cysts rupture or become superinfected. Liver cysts can cause abdominal pain, whereas lung cysts can cause chest pain, cough, hemoptysis, and embolism.[7] Cyst rupture or leak suddenly, producing anaphylactic reactions, release of protoscolices, eosinophilia, and secondary infectious complications.[8]

Echinococcosis Caused by E. multilocularis

Cysts tend to grow more aggressively than those of *E. granulosus,* almost always involving the liver, but capable of forming metastases in other organs (Figure 9-44). Symptoms can include pain, jaundice, weight loss, and hepatic obstruction, with sometimes fatal complications. The clinical picture can thus resemble hepatic carcinoma. The World Health

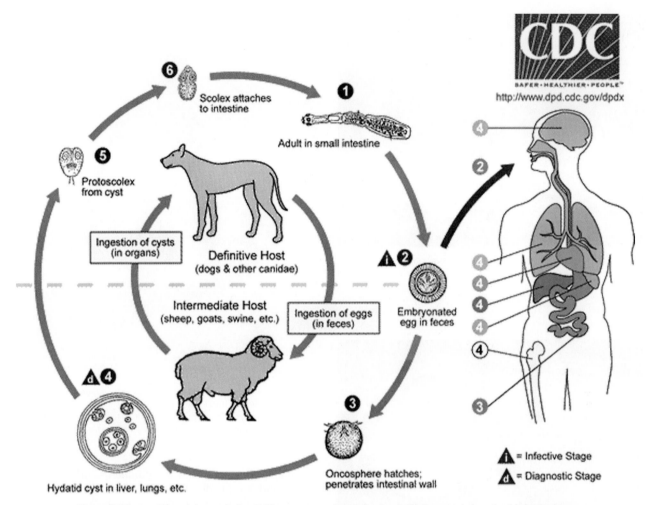

Figure 9-42 ▪ Life cycle/transmission, *Echinococcus granulosus* infection. *1*, Adult worms in bowels of definitive host. *2*, Eggs passed in feces, ingested by humans or intermediate host. *3*, Onchosphere penetrates intestinal wall, carried via blood vessels to lodge in organs. *4*, Hyatid cysts develop in liver, lungs, brain, and heart. *5*, Protoscolices (hydatid sand) ingested by definitive host. *6*, Attached to small intestine and growth to adult worm. (Modified from Centers for Disease Control and Prevention Public Health Image Library, Atlanta, Ga.)

Table 9-26 ▪ Clinical Presentation of Echinococcosis in Humans and Other Animals

Species	Risk Factors	Incubation Period	Clinical Manifestations	Diagnostic Findings
Humans: hydatid cyst disease	Children in rural areas, sheep herders with contact with dogs that feed on carcasses	12 months to years	Often asymptomatic, abdominal pain	Cyst seen on imaging, serology
Echinococcus multilocularis	Proximity to fox populations, ownership of dogs or cats that roam outside and feed on rodents		Pain, jaundice, weight loss, hepatic obstruction	Elevated bilirubin levels Irregular cysts on imaging, may have calcifications
Dogs	Feeding on infected carcasses or rodents	Adult worms produce eggs 27-61 days after infection[1]	Usually asymptomatic, enteritis with high parasite load	Fecal examination for eggs, adult worms, or proglottids
Sheep, goats, pigs, horses	Pastures contaminated with dog feces	Months to years	Usually asymptomatic, bloating may occur	Cysts on necropsy
Wild caribou, moose	Grazing areas contaminated by wolf, dog feces			
Rodents	Areas contaminated by feces of definitive host	Months	Symptomatic, fatal cysts may occur	

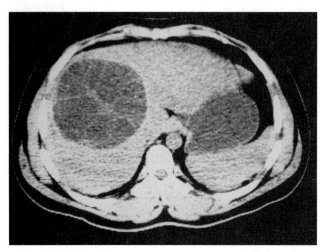

Figure 9-43 ■ CT image of large hydatid cyst in liver caused by *Echinococcus granulosus*. The membranes of multiple internal daughter cysts are visible within the primary cyst structure. (From Kliegman RM, Behrman RE, Jenson HB et al: *Nelson textbook of pediatrics*, ed 18, Philadelphia, 2007, Saunders Elsevier. Courtesy John R. Haaga, University Hospitals, Cleveland, Ohio.)

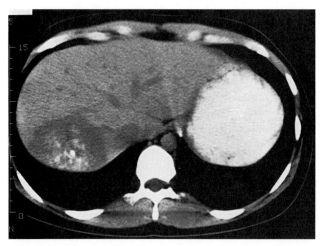

Figure 9-44 ■ CT image of alveolar cyst due *Echinococcus multilocularis* in right lobe of liver. Note irregular densities and areas of calcification. (From Long SS, Pickering LK, Prober CG: *Principles and practice of pediatric infectious disease*, ed 3, Edinburgh, 2008, Churchill Livingstone Elsevier.)

Organization (WHO) has devised a clinical staging system for alveolar echinococcosis based on parasitic mass, nodes, and metastases (PNM) similar to cancer tumor staging.[10]

Polycystic Hydatid Disease Cause by E. vogelii and E. oligarthus

These are comparatively rare infections that usually involve the liver or lungs and are characterized by the development of multiple microcysts.

Disease in Animals

Adult Cestode worms in the intestine of dogs, cats, and other definitive hosts rarely cause serious disease,[11] although large parasite burdens can result in signs of enteritis.

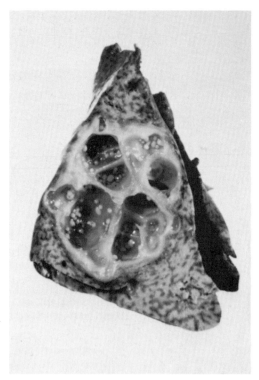

Figure 9-45 ■ A hydatid cyst *(Echinococcus granulosus)* in the liver of a horse (about natural size). This horse displayed no clinical signs of hepatic involvement despite the presence of 20 to 30 cysts like the one illustrated. (From Bowman DD: *Georgis' parasitology for veterinarians*, ed 8, St Louis, 2003, Saunders Elsevier.)

Intermediate hosts for *E. granulosus*, including sheep, goats, and horses, develop cystic disease that is generally subclinical, although jaundice, ascites, bronchopneumonia, decreased growth, and lameness have been reported (Figure 9-45 and Color Plate 9-21).[12] Rodents may develop clinical cystic disease from *E. multilocularis*.[1] Nonhuman primate deaths have been reported from zoologic institutions.

Diagnosis

The initial diagnosis is often made using ultrasound, computed tomography (CT), or magnetic resonance imaging (MRI). The differential diagnosis in human beings includes tumors, abscesses, and tuberculosis. When echinococcosis is suspected, serologic testing is performed using immunoblot or ELISA but is not 100% sensitive. Fine-needle aspiration of cyst contents can help make the diagnosis in equivocal cases by demonstrating protoscolices in the cyst fluid but carries a risk of cyst rupture and leakage.

In definitive host animals, arecoline purgatives can result in finding adult parasites or proglottids. In an experienced laboratory, fecal examination can reveal tapeworm eggs. A stool-based PCR test (copro-PCR) is also available.[13] In intermediate hosts, diagnosis can be made on histologic samples.

Treatment

Treatment of hydatid cyst disease in humans depends on the location of the cyst. While treatment is often surgical, the technique of puncture-aspiration-injection-reaspiration

Table 9-27 ▪ Echinococcus Infection: Treatment in Humans and Other Animals

Disease Agent	Species	Primary	Alternative
E. granulosus	Humans	Puncture-aspiration-injection-reaspiration with albendazole before and after drainage (>60 kg; 400 mg PO bid; <60 kg; 15 mg/kg/day divided bid and for 28 days after[15])	Surgical drainage
E. multilocularis		Wide surgical excision, albendazole as for hydatid disease can be tried but efficacy unclear[15]	
	Dogs*	Praziquantel 5 mg/kg PO, SC once	Epsiprantel 5.5 mg/kg PO once
	Cats*	Praziquantel 5 mg/kg PO, SC once	Epsiprantel 2.8 mg/kg PO once[16]

*Not in animals younger than 4 weeks.

(PAIR) with the adjunctive use of an antihelminthic appears promising as an alternative for the treatment of uncomplicated cysts.[14] Albendazole is given before the procedure; then the cyst is aspirated and injected with hypertonic saline solution or alcohol and is then reaspirated with final irrigation. Albendazole treatment is then continued for 28 days. Such treatment produces cure in more than 90% of cases.[15] The treatment for alveolar echinococcosis is wide surgical excision, although albendazole can be tried in similar doses to that used in *E. granulosus* infection.

In the definitive animal host, tapeworms are treated with antihelminthics. Table 9-27 provides treatment information for humans and other animals.

References

1. Acha PN, Szyfres B. *Zoonoses and communicable diseases common to man and animals: vol 3: chlamydioses, parasitoses.* 3rd ed. Washington DC: Pan American Health Organization; 2003.
2. Moro P, Schantz PM. Cystic echinococcosis in the Americas. *Parasitol Int.* 2006;55(suppl):S181.
3. Schantz PM. Echinococcosis. In: Steele JH, ed. *CRC handbook series in zoonoses, Section C: Parasitic zoonoses. Vol. 1.* Boca Raton, FL: CRC Press; 1982:231–277.
4. Chrieki M. Echinococcosis—an emerging parasite in the immigrant population. *Am Fam Physician.* 2002;66(5):817.
5. Kern P, Ammon A, Kron M, et al. Risk factors for alveolar echinococcosis in humans. *Emerg Infect Dis.* 2004;10(12):2088.
6. Deplazes P, Hegglin D, Gloor S, et al. Wilderness in the city: the urbanization of *Echinococcus multilocularis. Trends in Parasitol.* 2004;20(2):77.
7. Kwan-Gett TS, Kemp C, Kovarik C. *Infectious and tropical diseases: a handbook for primary care.* St Louis: Mosby Elsevier; 2006.
8. Heymann DL. *Control of communicable diseases manual.* 19th ed. Washington DC: American Public Health Association; 2008.
9. Veit P, Bilger B, Schad V, et al. Influence of environmental factors on the infectivity of *Echinococcus multilocularis* eggs. *Parasitology.* 1995;110(Pt 1):79.
10. Kern P, Wen H, Sato N, et al. WHO classification of alveolar echinococcosis: principles and application. *Parasitol Int.* 2006;55(suppl):S283.
11. Kahn CM, Line S, eds. *The Merck veterinary manual.* 9th ed. Whitehouse Station, NJ: Merck; 2005.
12. Dvorak GA, Rovid-Spickler A, Roth JA, eds. *Handbook for zoonotic diseases of companion animals.* The Center for Food Security & Public Health. Ames, IA: Iowa State University; 2006.
13. Craig PS, McManus DP, Lightowlers MW, et al. Prevention and control of cystic echinococcosis. *Lancet Infect Dis.* 2007;7(6):385.
14. Nasseri Moghaddam S, Abrishami A, Malekzadeh R. Percutaneous needle aspiration, injection, and reaspiration with or without benzimidazole coverage for uncomplicated hepatic hydatid cysts. *Cochrane Database Syst Rev.* 2006;(2):CD003623.
15. Gilbert DN, Moellering RC, Ellopoulos GM, et al. *Sanford guide to antimicrobial therapy 2009.* 39th ed. Sperryville, VA: Antimicrobial Therapy; 2009.
16. Barr SC, Bowman DD. *5-minute veterinary consult clinical companion canine and feline infectious disease and parasitology.* Ames, IA: Wiley-Blackwell; 2006.

EHRLICHIOSES AND ANAPLASMOSIS

Peter M. Rabinowitz and Lisa A. Conti

Erlichioses and anaplasmosis (ICD-10 A79.8)

Other names in humans: human monocytic ehrlichiosis (HME), human granulocytic anaplasmosis (HGA), ehrlichiosis ewingii

Other names in animals: canine monocytic ehrlichiosis, canine hemorrhagic fever, tropical canine pancytopenia, canine rickettsiosis, tracker dog disease, canine typhus, tickborne fever, pasture fever, equine anaplasmosis, Potomac horse fever, equine monocytic ehrlichiosis, infectious canine cyclic thrombocytopenia

Ehrlichiosis and anaplasmosis refer to several potentially serious tickborne diseases caused by related members of the family Anaplasmataceae. These diseases are transmitted to people and domestic animals by specific ticks that become infected by feeding on wildlife reservoirs. Recent taxonomic changes have reclassified some of these agents formally broadly called *Ehrlichia* into two genera; *Ehrlichia* and *Anaplasma*. New accepted terminology to describe these diseases in humans includes *ehrlichiosis* to refer to diseases caused by infection with *Ehrlichia chaffeensis* and *Ehrlichia ewingii*, and *anaplasmosis* to describe disease caused by *Anaplasma phagocytophilum*. There are a number of similar diseases in dogs and other animals. Anaplasmataceae provide an excellent example of the need for animal and human health professionals to work together since they were recognized as animal pathogens several decades before being described in human infection.[1] As with several other zoonotic diseases, recent advances in molecular diagnostics are shedding new light on the true prevalence of infection and the degree of overlap between human and animal ehrlichioses. Discoveries using animal models of infection with these agents also may further our understanding of diagnostic and treatment options in humans.

Key Points for Clinicians and Public Health Professionals

Public Health Professionals

- Provide epidemiologic analysis of these reportable diseases and assessment of local ehrlichiosis and anaplasmosis disease risk for the health district.
- Educate the public to:
  - Avoid tick-infested areas, but if this is not possible, wear appropriate clothing (long sleeves, long pants, tuck pants legs into socks, and wear light-colored clothing to visualize ticks). Wash clothes with hot water.[2]
  - Use CDC-recommended tick repellents such as DEET or permethrin (apply to clothes, not skin) where ticks are abundant. Be sure to follow label instructions before using any repellent.
  - Do frequent tick checks to remove even tiny immature-stage ticks.
  - Encourage adults to inspect children at least once daily for ticks. When in heavily infested areas, inspect children every 3 to 4 hours.
  - Use appropriate technique to remove ticks. Wear gloves or grasp tick with tweezers as close to the skin as possible and pull gently, or use a tick-removal spoon. Follow-up by cleaning the area, applying antibiotic topical on tick bite site, and washing hands.[3]
  - Discourage the use of matches, petroleum products, or nail polish as tick removal methods.[3]
  - Implement integrated pest management techniques including landscape management (Box 9-3). Counsel pet owners to discuss tickborne disease prevention strategies with their veterinarian.
- Work with local planning agencies on smart growth to avoid fractionating forested areas (see Chapter 6, Built Environment).

Human Health Clinicians

- Report cases of disease to public health authorities using the appropriate case definition: http://www.cdc.gov/ncphi/disss/nndss/casedef/ehrlichiosis_2008.htm.
- Counsel patients to avoid tick exposure or advise about use of appropriate tick repellents.
- Inquire about occupational risk factors for infection and ensure that workers at risk are educated about

---

BOX 9-3   INTEGRATED PEST MANAGEMENT TO REDUCE TICK POPULATIONS AROUND DWELLINGS

Some actions to consider in an integrated pest management approach include:
- Keep grass mowed.
- Remove leaf litter, brush, and weeds at the edge of the lawn.
- Restrict the use of groundcover, such as pachysandra, in areas frequented by family and pets.
- Remove brush and leaves around stone walls and wood piles.
- Discourage rodent activity. Clean up and seal stone walls and small openings around the home.
- Move firewood piles and bird feeders away from the house.
- Use veterinary-approved tick prevention products on pets; perform daily tick checks on pets and safely remove and dispose of ticks.
- Use plantings that do not attract deer, or exclude deer through various types of fencing.
- Move children's swing sets and sand boxes away from the woodland edge and place them on a wood chip or mulch-type foundation.
- Trim tree branches and shrubs around the lawn edge to let in more sunlight.
- Adopt hardscape and xeriscape (dryer or less water-demanding) landscaping techniques with gravel pathways and mulches. Create a 3-foot or wider wood chip, mulch, or gravel border between lawn and woods or stone walls.
- Consider areas with decking, tile, gravel, and border or container plantings in areas by the house or frequently traveled.
- Widen woodland trails.
- Consider a least-toxic pesticide application to tick-infested areas of high human exposure.

Adapted from Stafford KC: *Tick management handbook: an integrated guide for homeowners, pest control operators, and public health officials for the prevention of tick-associated disease,* revised edition, 2007, The Connecticut Agricultural Experiment Station, The Connecticut General Assembly, Bulletin No. 1010.

---

tickborne disease prevention measures and are taking precautions.
- Ask patients about occurrence of tickborne disease in their pets.
- No ehrlichial vaccine is currently commercially available for humans.

Veterinary Clinicians

- Counsel clients to use protection (e.g., gloves, tick removal devices) when removing ticks from pets.
- Counsel owners about the potential for human infection related to shared environmental exposures, especially upon identification of seropositive pets.
- Treat pets preventively against ectoparasites.
- An equine vaccine against *Neorickettsia risticii* (formerly *Ehrlichia risticii*) is commercially available in the United States.

Agent

A number of related agents cause ehrlichioses and anaplasmosis in humans and other animals. These agents are gram-negative, obligate intracellular coccobacilli bacteria that

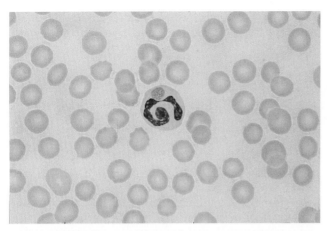

Figure 9-46 ▪ A canine neutrophil containing an *Ehrlichia ewingii* morula. (Wright's stain, original magnification ×250.) (From Cowell RL, Tyler RD, Meinkoth JH et al (eds): *Diagnostic cytology and hematology of the dog and cat*, ed 3, St Louis, 2008, Mosby Elsevier.)

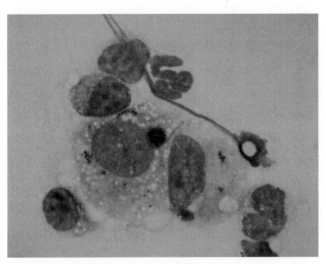

Figure 9-47 ▪ *Ehrlichia* inclusion in the mononuclear cell of a cat. (From Greene CE: *Infectious diseases of the dog and cat*, ed 3, St Louis, 2006, Saunders Elsevier. Courtesy Mike Lappin, Colorado State University, Fort Collins, Colo.)

parasitize leukocytes, erythrocytes, endothelial cells, or platelets (Figures 9-46 and 9-47). The bacteria within the family *Anaplasmataceae* that have been documented to cause disease in humans are *Ehrlichia chaffeensis, Anaplasma phagocytophilum, Ehrlichia ewingii, Ehrlichia canis,* and *Neorickettsia sennetsu.*

E. *chaffeensis* affects monocytic phagocytes, and the disease it causes in humans was formerly termed *human monocytic ehrlichiosis* (HME) but is now most commonly referred to as ehrlichiosis. *E. chaffeensis* is mainly a human pathogen but also causes diseases in dogs. *E. ewingii* is found in neutrophils, especially in immunocompromised patients.[4] It was formerly in the disease category "human ehrlichiosis, unspecified" and now is described as *E. ewingii* ehrlichiosis when it causes disease in humans; it has also been found to cause canine infections. The organism *A. phagocytophilum* (which

now includes the agent formerly called *E. equi*) also infects neutrophils. The disease in humans was formerly termed *human granulocytic ehrlichiosis* (HGE); it is now referred to as *human granulocytic anaplasmosis* (HGA) or, most commonly, simply *anaplasmosis*. Strains of *A. phagocytophilum* also cause disease in dogs, horses, ruminants and, rarely, cats.[5] *A. platys* is a canine pathogen that infects platelets and causes a disease known as *infectious canine cyclic thrombocytopenia*; it is not thought to be a significant human pathogen. Another canine pathogen, *E. canis*, causes ehrlichiosis in dogs; although it is not considered a highly likely zoonotic agent, at least one case of human infection with *E. canis* has been reported.[6] *Neorickettsia sennetsu* causes a febrile syndrome (sennetsu fever) that is rare outside Asia.[7]

Geographical Occurrence

The distribution of both human and domestic animal cases of the various ehrlichioses and anaplasmosis varies largely depending on the distribution of tick vector and reservoir species (Color Plate 9-22). For instance, although human cases of *E. chaffeensis* have been reported in almost every state in the United States, cases are most frequently reported from the southeastern and Midwestern states where whitetailed deer (*Odocoileus virginianus*) and Lone Star ticks (*Amblyomma americanum*) coexist. *E. chaffeensis* is restricted to the United States. *A. phagocytophilum* is found internationally in association with the distribution of *Ixodes* ticks. In the United States, human cases of *A. phagocytophilum* occur particularly in the upper Midwest, Northeast, and West Coast, where the primary vectors *Ixodes scapularis* and *Ixodes pacificus* exist; the distribution of infection is similar to that of Lyme disease. Although dogs seropositive for *E. canis* have been found throughout most of the United States, most canine cases occur in areas with an increased concentration of the brown dog tick (*Rhipicephalus sanguineus*) such as the southeastern states and the Southwest. In the United States, *E. canis* is mainly found in the Gulf Coast states and Eastern Seaboard, Midwest, and California.[8]

Groups at Risk

As in other tickborne diseases, the risk of ehrlichioses and anaplasmosis varies between and within regions and is generally related to the abundance of host ticks that can carry the disease. Individuals living in areas of high tick abundance are at increased risk. Immunocompromised individuals are at risk of infection with severe disease.

Hosts, Reservoir Species, Vectors

Infected animals are not believed to pose a substantial direct zoonotic risk to humans. In general, animal infections serve as a means of sustaining infections in tick vectors, and humans and other animals acquire infection from tick bites. White-tailed deer (*O. virginianus*) are considered a likely major reservoir for *E. chaffeensis* and *E. ewingii*,[4] and dogs may also play a role. The primary reservoir for *A. phagocytophilum* consists of small mammals, including deer mice (*Peromyscus*) and wood rats (*Neotoma*), although deer may also play a role.[9] Vectors of *A. phagocytophilum* are ticks of the genus *Ixodes,* including *I. scapularis, I. ricinus, I. pacificus, I. triangulaceps, I. spinipalpis,* and *I. persulcatus* (Color Plate 9-23).[4] These hard ticks are also the vector for *Borrelia burgdorferi, Babesia microti,* and tickborne encephalitis; therefore coinfection is common. The vector for *E. chaffeensis* and *E. ewingii* is the Lone Star tick (*A. americanum*). In dogs, the brown dog tick (*R. sanguineus*) is the principal vector for *A. platys* and *E. canis.*[10] *Dermacentor variabilis,* the American dog tick, can also be a vector of *E. canis* infection.[11] Accidental hosts for these agents include humans, dogs, cats, and ruminant animals.

Mode of Transmission and Life Cycle

Most ehrlichioses are tickborne infections. The larval, nymphal, and adult forms of the tick vectors are capable of transmitting infections. Figure 9-48 shows the life cycle of

infection for *E. chaffeensis.* Most infections in the United States occur between May and August, coincident with periods of peak tick feeding activity.[9] Direct transmission between humans and other mammals has not been reported.

Environmental Risk Factors

The relation of environmental factors to the risk of anaplasmosis and ehrlichiosis may resemble that for Lyme disease, with landscape modification in the United States related to suburbanization of the human population playing a significant role. These suburban developments encroach into land that was previously forest habitat and result in "fragmentation" of forests (see Chapter 6). This provides habitat for deer and small mammals that can serve as reservoirs for certain *Ehrlichia* and *Anaplasma* and also increases tick abundance and infection rates.

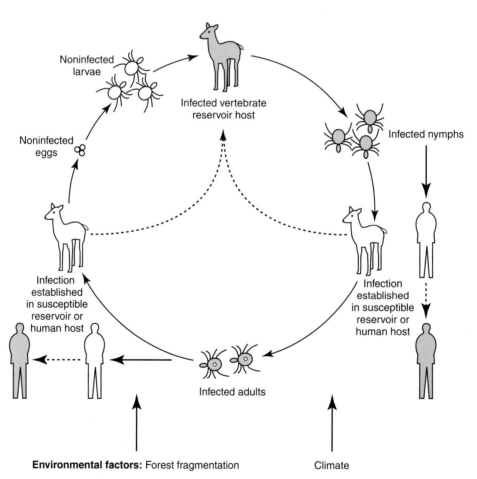

Figure 9-48 ■ Life cycle/transmission, *E. chaffeensis.* Noninfected larvae obtaining blood from a bacteremic vertebrate reservoir host (e.g., white-tailed deer [*shaded*]), become infected, and maintain Ehrlichieae to the nymphal stage. Infected nymphs may transmit *E. chaffeensis* to susceptible reservoir hosts (unshaded) or to humans during acquisition of blood. Infected adult ticks, having acquired Ehrlichieae either by transtadial transmission from infected nymphal stage or during blood meal acquisition as noninfected nymphs on infected deer, may also pass *E. chaffeensis* to humans or other susceptible reservoirs. Transovarial transmission has not been demonstrated, and eggs and unfed larvae are presumably not infected. (From Paddock CD, Childs JE: *Ehrlichia chaffeensis*: a prototypical emerging pathogen, *Clin Microbiol Rev* 16(1):37, 2003.)

Climate change with warmer winters may also be leading to increased tick abundance during the following spring and summer.[12] Wild birds may play a role in dispersing the *Ixodes* tick vectors that can transmit *A. phagocytophilum*.[13]

Disease in Humans

Human ehrlichioses caused by *E. chaffeensis*, *E. ewingii*, or *E. canis* and anaplasmosis (HGA) caused by *A. phagocytophilum* can present as clinical syndromes that share a number of common features, including fever, headache, and myalgias, with laboratory findings of thrombocytopenia, leukopenia, and elevated liver function test results.

Rash is not a common feature of all ehrlichioses and anaplasmosis, although it may occur in up to 30% of children with *E. chaffeensis* infections. When present, it is maculopapular, not petechial.[14] *E. chaffeensis* may cause more severe disease than the other pathogens, and CNS involvement may occur in up to 20% of cases, including meningitis and meningoencephalitis. Septic shock and respiratory distress syndrome can also develop in patients with *E. chaffeensis*. Severe complications and even death are more common among immunocompromised patients. The overall mortality rate of *E. chaffeensis* disease is approximately 3%.[9] Coinfections with other agents sharing the same tick vector are not uncommon; therefore Lyme disease, babesiosis, or tickborne encephalitis may be seen in up to 10% of *E. chaffeensis* cases.[9]

Peripheral neuropathy may develop in patients with *A. phagocytophilum*, but severe complications and fatalities are less common (case fatality rate approximately 0.7%) than with *E. chaffeensis*.

Disease in Animals

Canine ehrlichiosis is a multisystemic disorder that can cause a variety of clinical signs, including fever, anorexia, CNS signs, hemorrhagic conjunctivitis, vasculitis, splenomegaly, and lymphadenopathy (Color Plates 9-24 to 9-27). The course of the infection may be subclinical, acute, or chronic.[15] Although cases of canine ehrlichiosis confirmed via cytology or serology have been attributed to *E. canis*, it is now thought that some cases may have been related to infections with *E. chaffeensis*, *E. ewingii*, or *A. phagocytophilum*.[16] Doberman pinschers and German shepherd dogs are considered by some to be more likely than other breeds to have severe chronic *E. canis* infection.[15] *E. ewingii* causes polyarthritis with fever and hepatosplenomegaly in dogs.[15] Concurrent infection with other *Ehrlichia*, *Anaplasma*, *Babesia*, *Haemobartonella*, or *Hepatozoon* organisms can worsen the clinical course of ehrlichiosis in dogs.

Canine anaplasmosis caused by *A. phagocytophilum* is thought to produce a milder clinical syndrome with fever, lethargy, and thrombocytopenia. *A. platys* causes a moderate to severe cyclic thrombocytopenia in dogs; however, bleeding complications are rare.[15]

Clinical ehrlichiosis has also been described in cats. Although the species of *Ehrlichia* that naturally infects cats has not been fully determined, clinical illness with signs including fever, anorexia, pale mucous membranes, and weight loss has been described.[16] A few cases of feline *A. phagocytophilum* infections, also known as *feline granulocytotropic anaplasmosis*, have been described in cats. Clinical signs associated with these infections include fever, anorexia, and lethargy.

A. phagocytophilum causes tickborne fever (also known as *pasture fever*) in cattle, sheep, and other ruminants, predominantly in Europe (Figure 9-49). The clinical signs are listed in Table 9-28. Equine anaplasmosis (formerly *equine ehrlichiosis*) is also caused by *A. phagocytophilum* (formerly *E. equi*) and consists of a febrile disease resembling human anaplasmosis. Table 9-28 shows the comparative clinical presentations in humans and other animals.

Diagnosis

Diagnosis in Humans

Ehrlichial infections in humans can resemble other tickborne febrile syndromes. A history of a tick bite and thrombocytopenia, leukopenia, and elevated liver function test results favor the diagnosis. Unlike Rocky Mountain spotted fever (RMSF), vasculitis is not present in ehrlichial infections.[14] In HME, rapid laboratory diagnosis is possible when cellular stippling of intracytoplasmic inclusions (morulae) in monocytes are seen, although this is uncommon (see Figure 9-49), while in HGA, morulae in neutrophils and bands can be seen more commonly (in up to 20% to 80% of cases[14]; Color Plate 9-28 and Figure 9-50). A PCR test using ethylenediamine tetraacetic acid (EDTA) or citrate-anticoagulated blood is becoming the standard method of diagnostic confirmation for both conditions.[14] The organisms can also be grown in cell cultures but this may take several weeks. Serologic tests using a fluorescent antibody reaction can be used to compare acute and convalescent titers, and demonstration of a fourfold change in titers is considered the most sensitive method of detecting infection, although the test may cross-react with

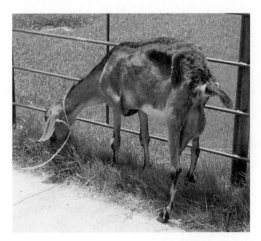

Figure 9-49 ■ Chronic weight loss in a goat as a sequela to anaplasmosis. (From Pugh DG: *Sheep & goat medicine*, St Louis, 2002, Saunders. Courtesy Tom Powe and D.G. Pugh, Auburn University, Auburn, Ala.)

Table 9-28 ▪ Ehrlichioses and Anaplasmosis: Comparative Clinical Presentations in Humans and Other Animals

Species	Agent	Risk Factors	Incubation Period	Clinical Manifestations	Lab Findings
Humans					
Human ehrlichiosis (HME)	Ehrlichia chaffeensis, E. ewingii E. canis[17]	Tick exposures	7-10 days	Fever, myalgias, rash, respiratory distress, CNS and hepatic involvement	Thrombocytopenia, leukopenia, elevated liver function tests, morulae in monocytes (rare)
Human anaplasmosis (HGA)	Anaplasma phagocytophilum		7-14 days[4]	Fever, myalgias, peripheral neuropathies	Thrombocytopenia, leukopenia, morulae seen in neutrophils, bands (20%-80% of cases)[14]; elevated liver function tests[4]
Dogs					
Canine ehrlichiosis	E. canis, E. chaffeensis, E. ewingii	Tick exposures, animals allowed to roam outdoors	1-3 weeks[15]	May be subclinical, acute, or chronic; vasculitis, ataxia, hemorrhagic conjunctivitis, hepatosplenomegaly, lymphadenopathy, polyarthritis	Leukopenia, anemia
Canine anaplasmosis	A. phagocytophilum			Mild illness: fever, lethargy	Thrombocytopenia[15]
Infectious cyclic canine thrombocytopenia	A. platys			Moderate to severe thrombocytopenia, bleeding rare	Thrombocytopenia
Cats	A. phagocytophilum, E. canis	Tick exposures, animals allowed to roam outdoors		Rare; fever, anorexia, lethargy	Thrombocytopenia, leukopenia, anemia
Cattle, Sheep, Goats, Deer					
Tickborne fever (Pasture fever)	A. phagocytophilum	Tick exposures in endemic areas	2-6 days	Fever, lethargy, weight loss, decreased lactation, abortion, lymphadenopathy	Neutropenia, lymphocytopenia, thrombocytopenia[10]
Horses					
Equine anaplasmosis	A. phagocytophilum		10-45 days	Fever, ataxia, depression	Morulae seen in neutrophils

other diseases, including Lyme disease and RMSF.[9] PCR testing may help resolve problems of cross-reactivity between species that can occur with serology testing.

Diagnosis in Animals

In dogs, serology using IFA is commonly used with titers is more reliable 3 weeks after infection. Although IFA is sensitive, the test may not be very specific because of cross-reactivity between *E. ewingii* and *E. canis*, as well as *E. canis* and *A. phagocytophilum*. Standardized serologic tests for feline patients are needed. Depending on the ehrlichial species, cytology may be a useful tool for detecting the presence of morulae in blood or tissue smears. Depending on the type of animal and ehrlichial species, any one or a combination of other testing such as PCR, serology, immunoblotting,

and organism cultivation may be useful in confirming the diagnosis.

Treatment

Antibiotic treatment of ehrlichial infection in humans and other animals is shown in Table 9-29.

Treatment in Humans

Because of the serious nature of *Ehrlichia* and *Anaplasma* infections, early initiation of antibiotic treatment is recommended when the diagnosis is suspected. Doxycycline is considered the first line of treatment (see Table 9-29). In pregnancy, rifampin has been recommended by some authorities.

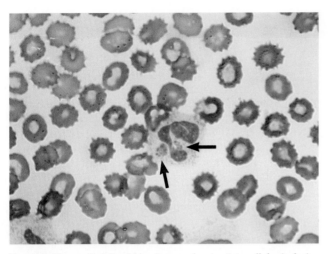

Figure 9-50 ■ Peripheral blood smear showing intracellular inclusion within a neutrophil of a patient with human granulocytic anaplasmosis (*arrows*). (Wright stain, ×1000.) (From Mandell GL, Bennett JE, Dolin R (eds): *Principles and practice of infectious diseases*, ed 6, Philadelphia, 2005, Churchill Livingstone Elsevier.)

Table 9-29 ■ **Antibiotic Treatment of Ehrlichial Infection in Humans and Other Animals**

Species	Primary Treatment	Alternative Treatment
Humans: ehrlichiosis and anaplasmosis	Doxycycline 100 mg PO/IV bid × 7-14 days (not during pregnancy) Children should receive doxycycline per standard guidelines During pregnancy, consider treatment with rifampin[19]	Tetracycline 500 mg PO qid × 7-14 days (not for children or during pregnancy)[19]
Dogs, cats	Doxycycline 5 mg/kg PO q12h *or* 10 mg/kg PO q24h × 28 days (give IV for 5 days if the dog is vomiting)	Imidocarb dipropionate 5 mg/kg IM for 2 doses 14 days apart[15,20] *or* oxytetracycline and tetracycline 22 mg/kg PO q8h × 28 days
Horses	Oxytetracycline 7 mg/kg IV SID × 8 days	

Treatment in Animals

Antibiotics and supportive care are the mainstay of clinical disease in dogs and horses. Antibiotics commonly used in small animals include doxycycline, chloramphenicol, and imidocarb dipropionate. Oxytetracycline can be very effective in reducing the severity of illness in cattle.[18] Adjunctive steroid treatment is sometimes used when thrombocytopenia is life threatening. The prognosis is excellent with

acute disease and prompt treatment. Prognosis is poor for dogs with *E. canis* infection that progresses to hypoplastic marrow; anabolic steroids may be needed to stimulate bone marrow production. In ruminants, administration of oxytetracycline early in the course of the disease may be beneficial. Tick and infection control strategies are considered effective herd health strategies to prevent clinical cases.[18] Previous infection can produce immunity in horses for several years.[10]

References

1. Maeda K, Markowitz N, Hawley RC, et al. Human infection with *Ehrlichia canis*, a leukocytic rickettsia. *N Engl J Med.* 1987; 316(14):853.
2. Centers for Disease Control and Prevention. *Division of Vector Borne Infectious Diseases; Lyme disease.* http://www.cdc.gov/ncidod/dvbid/lyme/Prevention/ld_Prevention_Avoid.htm. Accessed September 28, 2008.
3. Placerville Veterinary Clinic. *Tick removal tools: what should I use to remove ticks?* http://placervillevet.com/ticktools.htm. Accessed December 15, 2008.
4. Heymann DL. *Control of communicable diseases manual.* 19th ed. Washington, DC: American Public Health Association; 2008.
5. Magnarelli LA, Bushmich SL, Ijdo JW, et al. Seroprevalence of antibodies against *Borrelia burgdorferi* and *Anaplasma phagocytophilum* in cats. *Am J Vet Res.* 2005;66(11):1895.
6. Unver A, Perez M, Orellana N, et al. Molecular and antigenic comparison of *Ehrlichia canis* isolates from dogs, ticks, and a human in Venezuela. *J Clin Microbiol.* 2001;39(8):2788.
7. Centers for Disease Control and Prevention. *Tickborne rickettsial diseases, Ehrlichiosis.* http://www.cdc.gov/ticks/diseases/ehrlichiosis. Accessed December 15, 2008.
8. Bockino L, Krimer PM, Latimer KS, et al. *An overview of canine ehrlichiosis, veterinary clinical pathology clerkship program.* http://www.vet.uga.edu/vpp/clerk/Bockino. Accessed October 4, 2008.
9. Dumler JS, Madigan JE, Pusterla N, et al. Ehrlichioses in humans: epidemiology, clinical presentation, diagnosis, and treatment. *Clin Infect Dis.* 2007;45(suppl 1):S45.
10. Kahn CM, Line S, eds. 9th ed. *The Merck veterinary manual.* Whitehouse Station, NJ: Merck; 2005.
11. Waner T. Hematopathological changes in dogs infected with *Ehrlichia canis. Israel J Vet Med.* 2008;63(1). http://www.isrvma.org/article/63_1_3.htm. Accessed December 15, 2008.
12. Bennet L, Halling A, Berglund J. Increased incidence of Lyme borreliosis in southern Sweden following mild winters and during warm, humid summers. *Eur J Clin Microbiol Infect Dis.* 2006;25(7):426.
13. Ogden NH, Lindsay LR, Hanincová K, et al. Role of migratory birds in introduction and range expansion of *Ixodes scapularis* ticks and of *Borrelia burgdorferi* and *Anaplasma phagocytophilum* in Canada. *Appl Environ Microbiol.* 2008;74(6):1780.
14. Mandell GL, Bennett JE, Dolin R, et al. *Principles and practice of infectious diseases.* 6th ed. Philadelphia: Churchill Livingstone Elsevier; 2005.
15. Barr SC, Bowman DD. *5-minute veterinary consult clinical companion canine and feline infectious disease and parasitology.* Ames, IA: Wiley-Blackwell; 2006.
16. Greene CE. *Infectious diseases of the dog and cat.* 3rd ed. St Louis: Saunders Elsevier; 2006.
17. Perez M, Bodor M, Zhang C, et al. Human infection with *Ehrlichia canis* accompanied by clinical signs in Venezuela (Abstract). *Ann N Y Acad Sci.* 2006;1078:110.
18. Howard JL, Smith RA. *Current veterinary therapy: food animal practice.* 4th ed. St Louis: Saunders Elsevier; 1999.
19. Gilbert DN, Moellering RC, Ellopoulos GM, et al. *Sanford guide to antimicrobial therapy 2009.* 39th ed. Sperryville, VA: Antimicrobial Therapy; 2009.
20. Price JE, Dolan TT. A comparison of the efficacy of imidocarb dipropionate and tetracycline hydrochloride in the treatment of canine ehrlichiosis. *Vet Rec.* 1980;107(12):275.

ESCHERICHIA COLI **INFECTION**

Peter M. Rabinowitz and Lisa A. Conti

Escherichia coli *infection (ICD-10 A04.0-A04.4)*

Other names in humans: E. coli *O157:H7, hemorrhagic colitis*

Other names in animals: colibacillosis

The gram-negative bacterium *Escherichia coli* has hundreds of different strains. These strains can be separated into three categories: (1) nonpathogenic, existing as commensal organisms in the normal gut flora; (2) intestinal pathogenic, causing diarrhea in humans, including enterohemorrhagic *E. coli* (EHEC); enterotoxigenic *E. coli* (ETEC); enteroinvasive *E. coli* (EIEC), enteropathogenic, enteroaggregative, and diffuse-adherent[1]; and (3) capable of causing extraintestinal pathologenic *E. coli* (ExPEC). Case reports have linked enteropathogenic *E. coli* causing canine enteritis in a dog to colonization in a child,[2] an outbreak of necrotizing pneumonia in cats to a strain of ExPEC with molecular features resembling human strains,[3] and cases of edema in pigs tied to toxin-producing strains resembling those occurring in humans.[4] Urinary tract infections in humans have been linked with *E. coli* from food sources.[5] It is likely that additional patterns of interspecies transmission of *E. coli* infection will be recognized in the future[6]; however, this chapter emphasizes current knowledge regarding enterohemorrhagic strains, such as O157:H7. Pathogenic *E. coli* strains, particularly those that are antibiotic resistant, from the food supply are a public health and economic concern.

Key Points for Clinicians and Public Health Professionals

Public Health Professionals

- Ensure that health professionals know how to report cases to the local health authorities.
- Exclude infectious patients from child care or patient care facilities and food production facilities.
- Educate the public on modes of transmission and the preventive measures that they can use, including the following:
  o Discourage consumption of undercooked ground meat and unpasteurized dairy products or juices.
  o Encourage washing raw fruits and vegetables before consumption.
- Monitor the chlorination of public water supplies and pools.
- Identify the source of an outbreak and institute control measures to prevent transmission, including transmission by contaminated food, direct animal contact, or person-person transmission.
- Institute environmental cleanup of contaminated areas. The organism can be maintained in the environment for months in feces and soil. Disinfection agents include 1% sodium hypochlorite, 70% ethanol, and iodine-based solutions.[7]
- Ensure that local petting zoos and other areas where the public has contact with animals have policies and procedures in place to reduce the risk of infection. This includes providing access to handwashing stations, proper manure disposal, and separation of animals from food areas.
- Provide descriptive epidemiology of disease in local human and animal populations.
- Coordinate with agriculture officials to ensure that food safety and farm safety measures are in place.

Human Health Clinicians

- Ensure adequate hydration and consider hospitalization to reduce the risk of hemolytic uremic syndrome.[1]
- Report cases immediately to local health authorities.
- Institute enteric precautions for patients.
- Educate patients about personal hygiene and proper handwashing techniques.
- Avoid the use of antibiotics in patients with Shiga toxin–producing *E. coli* infections.

Veterinary Clinicians

- Counsel animal handlers about hygiene, handwashing, and avoiding direct contact with feces.
- Prevent infection in puppies and kittens by cleaning and disinfecting the parturition environment (1:32 dilution of bleach), ensuring adequate colostrum intake, ensuing that the bitch/queen is in good health, and washing hands/changing clothes and shoes before handling neonates.
- Counsel pet owners to avoid feeding raw or undercooked meat to dogs and cats.

Agent

E. coli is a gram-negative bacillus that is a lactose fermenter and a normal inhabitant of the intestinal tract of most mammals (Figure 9-51). The classification into different serogroups is based on the O polysaccharide antigen. Further differentiation into serotypes is based on the H (flagellar) antigen.[8] The most common serotype of EHEC in human infections is O157:H7. This serotype does not ferment sorbitol, so this aids in the identification of the organism. EHEC organisms are capable of producing potent cytotoxins known as *Shiga toxins 1 and 2* (also known as verocytotoxins). Shiga toxin 1 is also produced by *Shigella dysenteriae* (see Chapter 11).

Geographical Occurrence

EHEC strains have been identified in North America and South America, Europe, Japan, and southern Africa. The distribution of these strains in other parts of the world is unknown.[1]

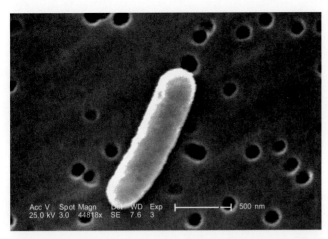

Figure 9-51 ■ At an extremely high magnification (×44,818), this scanning electron micrograph revealed some of the morphologic details displayed by a single gram-negative *Escherichia coli* bacterium. This bacterium was a member of the strain O:169 H41 ETEC (enterotoxigenic *E. coli*). (From Centers for Disease Control and Prevention Public Health Image Library, Atlanta, Ga. Courtesy J.H. Carr.)

Groups at Risk

Although *E. coli* infections can occur in persons of all ages, children younger than 5 years are at increased risk of developing serious complications from EHEC infections, including hemolytic uremic syndrome (HUS). In the elderly, thrombocytopenic purpura may develop.

Hosts, Reservoir Species, Vectors

Cattle are the principal reservoir for EHEC. Other ruminants may also be reservoirs. EHEC strains have been identified in sheep, goats, turkeys, chickens, cats, deer, swine, horses, and dogs.[9,10] Contaminated meat and other food are major vehicles for human infection. Human-to-human transmission is common. When a subclinically infected cat was found to have the same strain of O145:H-EHEC as a child with bloody diarrhea, it was not possible to determine the direction of the transmission, so human-to-animal transmission may be possible as well.[11]

Mode of Transmission and Life Cycle

Transmission occurs through direct contact with feces or through the ingestion of meat, dairy products, produce, or water that is contaminated with feces (Figure 9-52). The infective dose is estimated to be fewer than 10 organisms.[12] Subclinically infected animals may shed organisms in their feces for prolonged periods.

Significant outbreaks have been linked to contaminated beef, vegetables and fruit, and unpasteurized juice and dairy products. Contaminated dust settling into drinks has been suspected in outbreaks associated with fairs and petting zoos. Contaminated swimming pools and drinking water supplies have been associated with waterborne transmission of the bacterium.[13] After the organisms have been ingested, they reproduce in the intestinal tract. The incubation period to clinical illness is between 2 to 10 days.[1] Infected humans may then shed organisms in their feces for several weeks.

Shiga toxin–producing *E. coli* result in cytotoxic effects on intestinal epithelia that cause characteristic bloody diarrhea. Shiga toxins systemically cause renal endothelial damage and possible HUS.

Environmental Risk Factors

E. coli has been shown to persist in contaminated environments for prolonged periods.[14] The organism may persist for longer periods in the soil in cold climates.

Forty-two weeks after an outbreak of human illness at a fair in Ohio, *E. coli* O157:H7 was able to be recovered from the sawdust in the implicated barn.[15] Campers have become infected by camping and contacting mud and soil in pastures where livestock such as sheep have grazed in the past.[12]

Disease in Humans

E. coli O157:H7 and other EHEC strains of *E. coli* cause varying infections that can range from asymptomatic to fatal. Common symptoms include watery diarrhea, often (in more than half of cases[16]) followed by large amounts of blood, abdominal cramping, and colitis (Color Plate 9-29). Fever is either low grade or absent.

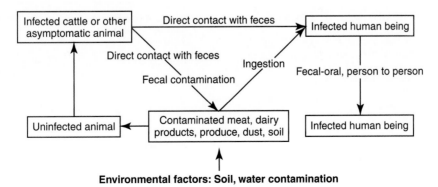

Figure 9-52 ■ Life cycle of *E. coli* O157:H7 infection.

In most cases, the disease can resolve in 5 to 10 days without antibiotics.[17] Severe complications are more common in children and the elderly and include HUS in approximately 10% of cases, acute renal failure, coagulopathies, and anemia.[18] *E. coli* O157:H7 is the major cause of HUS in the United States and the most common cause of acute renal failure in children.

Disease in Animals

Cattle are typically subclinical carriers for *E. coli* O157:H7 (Figure 9-53). Herd prevalence rates in excess of 40% have been reported. Studies of calves have shown EHEC prevalence rates of almost 70%.[19] Sheep (rates in excess of 30%), dogs, deer, swine, and other animals may also subclinically carry EHEC.

ETC, EPEC, uropathogenic *E. coli*, and cytotoxic necrotizing factor *E. coli* have been recovered from dogs, while EPEC, VTEC, and uropathogenic *E. coli* organisms have been recovered from cats. Many of the *E. coli* strains that have been recovered from dogs and cats are hemolytic.

Neonates that have not had adequate amounts of colostrum are more susceptible to enteritis or septicemia caused by β-hemolytic *E. coli*. Sporadic cases of *E. coli* enteritis, cystitis, endometritis, pyelonephritis, prostatitis, or mastitis have also been reported in puppies and kittens, as well as adult dogs and cats. Table 9-30 compares clinical presentations of *E. coli* infection (enterohemorrhagic) in humans and other animals.

Diagnosis

Fecal samples should be cultured on sorbitol/MacConkey's media. All EHEC strains should be sent to a public health laboratory for serotyping to characterize the strain and detect possible outbreaks. There are also commercial assays for Shiga toxins and DNA probe for specific genes.[1] Subtyping of *E. coli* O157:H7 can be done using pulsed gel electrophoresis to further detect outbreaks.

Treatment

Many human cases of EHEC infection are self-limiting and do not require medical intervention. Even in more serious cases, it is believed that antibiotic treatment and antimotility agents may increase the release of toxins and increase the risk of HUS.[16] Supportive measures include fluid and electrolyte replacement and monitoring of hematologic and renal function for the development of HUS. HUS often requires transfusion, dialysis, and intensive care.[20]

In adult animals the disease may be self-limiting; however, animals with clinical signs may need intensive supportive care. Antibiotic therapy protocols should be based on culture results and sensitivity testing. Trimethoprim-sulfa can be used at 30 mg/kg orally every 12 to 24 hours or amoxicillin can be used at 10 to 20 mg/kg orally every 8 to 12 hours. The prognosis for neonates with clinical signs is often poor.

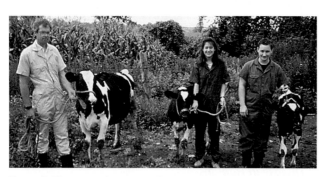

Figure 9-53 ■ Cattle are typically subclinical carriers of *E. coli*. (From Divers TJ, Peek SF (eds): *Rebhun's diseases of dairy cattle*, ed 2, St Louis, 2008, Saunders Elsevier. Courtesy Robert O. Gilbert.)

WEB RESOURCES

- Diagnosis and Management of Foodborne Illnesses: http://www.cdc.gov/mmwr/preview/mmwrhtml/rr5304a1.htm
- *E. coli* Resources for Clinicians: http://www.cdc.gov/ecoli/clinicians.htm

Table 9-30 ■ *E. coli* (Enterohemorrhagic): Comparative Clinical Presentations in Humans and Other Animals

Species	Risk Factors	Incubation Period	Clinical Manifestations	Laboratory Findings
Humans	Children; crowding; contact with feces; consumption of undercooked meat or unpasteurized milk, cider, or juice; ingestion of water from lakes and pools while swimming	2-10 days	Watery diarrhea, bloody diarrhea, abdominal cramping	Positive fecal culture
			HUS, renal failure	Leukocytosis, anemia, thrombocytopenia, abnormal renal function tests
Cattle, poultry, deer, swine	Neonates with inadequate colostrum/immune system		Subclinical carriage; neonates with diarrhea, dehydration, and depression; hypovolemic shock	Positive fecal culture
Dogs, cats	Neonates, inadequate colostrum intake		Subclinical carrier, diarrhea	Positive fecal culture, cytotoxin assays

References

1. Heymann DL. *Control of communicable diseases manual.* 19th ed. Washington DC: American Public Health Association; 2008.
2. Rodrigues J, Thomazini CM, Lopes CA, et al. Concurrent infection in a dog and colonization in a child with a human enteropathogenic *Escherichia coli* clone. *J Clin Microbiol.* 2004;42(3):1388.
3. Sura R, Van Kruiningen HJ, DebRoy C, et al. Extraintestinal pathogenic *Escherichia coli*-induced acute necrotizing pneumonia in cats. *Zoonoses Pub Health.* 2007;54(8):307.
4. Barth S, Tscholshiew A, Menge C, et al. Virulence and fitness gene patterns of Shiga toxin-encoding *Escherichia coli* isolated from pigs with edema disease or diarrhea in Germany. *Berl Munch Tierarztl Wochenschr.* 2007;120(7–8):307.
5. Warren RE, Ensor VM. Imported chicken meat as a potential source of quinolone-resistant *Escherichia coli* producing extended-spectrum β-lactamases in the UK. *J Antimicrob Chemo.* 2008;61(3):504. http://jac.oxfordjournals.org/cgi/content/abstract/61/3/504. Accessed October 2008.
6. Smith JL, Fratamico PM, Gunther NW. Extraintestinal pathogenic *Escherichia coli. Foodborne Pathog Dis.* 2007;4(2):134.
7. Dvorak G, Rovid-Spickler A, Roth JA, et al. *Handbook for zoonotic diseases of companion animals.* Ames, IA: The Center for Food Security and Public Health, Iowa State University College of Veterinary Medicine; 2008.
8. Acha PN, Szyfres B. *Zoonoses and communicable diseases common to man and animals: vol. 1: bacterioses and mycoses.* 3rd ed. Washington DC: Pan American Health Organization; 2001.
9. Colville J, Berryhill D. *Handbook of zoonoses: identification and prevention.* St Louis: Mosby Elsevier; 2007.
10. Doane CA, Pangloli P, Richards HA, et al. Occurrence of *Escherichia coli* O157:H7 in diverse farm environments. *J Food Prot.* 2007;70(1):6.
11. Busch U, Hormansdorfer S, Schranner S, et al. Enterohemorrhagic *Escherichia coli* excretion by child and her cat. *Emerg Infect Dis.* 2007;13(2):348.
12. Strachan NJ, Fenlon DR, Ogden ID. Modelling the vector pathway and infection of humans in an environmental outbreak of *Escherichia coli* O157. *FEMS Microbiol Lett.* 2001;203(1):69.
13. Rangel JM, Sparling PH, Crowe C, et al. Epidemiology of *Escherichia coli* O157:H7 outbreaks, United States, 1982–2002. *Emerg Infect Dis.* 2005;11:603.
14. National Association of State Public Health Veterinarians et al. Compendium of measures to prevent disease associated with animals in public settings, 2007: National Association of State Public Health Veterinarians, Inc. *Morb Mortal Wkly Rep Recomm Rep.* 2007;56(RR-5):1.
15. Varma JK, Greene KD, Reller ME, et al. An outbreak of *Escherichia coli* O157 infection following exposure to a contaminated building. *JAMA.* 2003;290(20):2709.
16. Gilbert DN, Moellering RC, Ellopoulos GM, et al. *Sanford guide to antimicrobial therapy, 2009.* 39th ed. Sperryville, VA: Antimicrobial Therapy; 2009.
17. Centers for Disease Control and Prevention. Disease listing: *Escherichia coli* general information: CDC DFBMD. http://www.cdc.gov/ncidod/dbmd/diseaseinfo/escherichiacoli_g.htm. Accessed February 12, 2008.
18. Kwan-Gett TS, Kemp C, Kovarik C. *Infectious and tropical diseases: a handbook for primary care.* Philadelphia: Mosby Elsevier; 2005.
19. Wieler LH, Sobjinski G, Schlapp T, et al. Longitudinal prevalence study of diarrheagenic *Escherichia coli* in dairy calves. *Berl Munch Tierarztl Wochenschr.* 2007;120(7–8):296.
20. Mandell GL, Bennett JE, Dolin R, eds. *Principles and practice of infectious diseases.* 6th ed. New York: Churchill Livingstone Elsevier; 2005.

GIARDIASIS

Peter M. Rabinowitz and Lisa A. Conti

Giardiasis (ICD-10 A07.1)

Other names in humans: lambliasis, backpacker's disease, beaver fever, traveler's diarrhea

Other names in animals: giardosis, lambliasis, lambliosis

Giardia intestinalis (also known as *Giardia lamblia, Lamblia intestinalis, Giardia duodenalis*)[1] is a common parasitic cause of infectious diarrhea in humans. Human cases are thought to be a result of person-to-person transmission, either directly or through contaminated water supplies. The importance of animals, including dogs and cats, as disease reservoirs and sources of zoonotic transmission of the disease remains incompletely understood and potentially overlooked by human health clinicians and public health authorities. Recent advances in molecular genotyping hold promise for clarifying the risk of *Giardia* infection related to human-animal contact.

Key Points for Clinicians and Public Health Professionals

Public Health Professionals

- Disease is reportable to public health authorities in some states.

- Ensure public water supplies are not contaminated with human or other animal waste and that water treatment includes filtration.
- In the event of a case report, determine risk factors for infection and whether others are at risk.
- Consider zoonotic sources of infection (e.g., pets, farm animals/petting zoos, water supplies with animal contact).
- Educate the public, veterinarians, and human health clinicians about risk factors for transmission, including not drinking untreated surface water.
- Support policies to clean up dog feces and other animal waste in public areas.
- Ensure that day care center staff have proper training to avoid outbreaks.

Human Health Clinicians

- Check with your state health office to determine whether the disease is reportable to public health authorities using the case definition; see http://www.cdc.gov/mmwr/preview/mmwrhtml/ss5607a2.htm.
- Include questions about animal contact in every patient presenting with diarrhea. If pets are in the house, suggest a consultation with the family veterinarian. Human *Giardia* may be able to infect pets.
- Person-to-person transmission is possible. Counsel infected persons about handwashing, avoiding swimming for 2 weeks after symptoms end, and avoiding fecal exposure during sexual activity.

Veterinary Clinicians

- Counsel owners and any others in contact with infected animals about the zoonotic risk, need for handwashing after handling pet, feces, pet toys, and other objects that are potentially infected or contaminated with cysts.
- Decontaminate infected animal's coat with shampoo; also decontaminate kennels or other environments with quaternary ammonium disinfectants that are effective in inactivating *Giardia* cysts.
- Consider vaccinating puppies and kittens at 7 weeks, with booster 3 weeks later, against *Giardia* trophozoites[1] (controversial).
- Decontaminate hard surfaces with 1% sodium hypochlorite, 2% glutaraldehyde, or quaternary ammonium solutions.[1]
- Keep pets indoors to reduce their exposure to the organism.

Agent

Giardia is a genus of flagellated protozoan parasite that lives principally in the upper intestine of vertebrates (Figure 9-54). Recent classification identifies *Giardia intestinalis* as the major species responsible for human infection. *Giardia* species are found in most mammals, and while different strains appear to have adapted to specific host species, molecular tools for typing particular isolates are now allowing an examination of how much zoonotic transmission is taking place. The current classification includes at least seven distinct assemblages (genotypes) of *G. intestinalis*: A and B are found in humans and a number of other animals, and C through G appear to be more host specific.[2,3] *Giardia* organisms exist in two forms, a vegetative trophozoite form capable of causing illness in the host, and a transmissible cyst form that is shed in feces (Figure 9-55). The cysts measure 7 to 10 microns by 8 to 13 microns and can survive up to 2 months in water, where they are resistant to routine chlorination. Upon ingestion by a host, the cysts develop into pathogenic trophozoites that cling to the brush border surface of the intestinal mucosa and reproduce by fission.

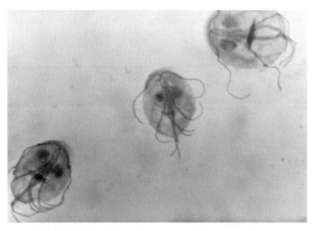

Figure 9-54 ▪ Wet mount of a fresh fecal sample showing motile trophozoites of *Giardia* species. Notice the prominent pair of nuclei containing a single karyosome of condensed chromatin, flagella running longitudinally between the nuclei, and a pair of curved median bodies. The arrangement of the organelles resembles a wide-eyed face. (From Quesenberry K, Carpenter JW: *Ferrets, rabbits and rodents: clinical medicine and surgery*, ed 2, St Louis, 2004, Saunders Elsevier.)

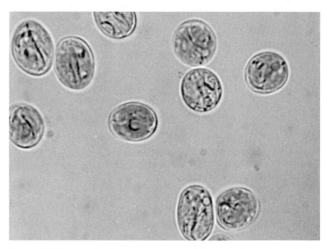

Figure 9-55 ▪ *Giardia* cysts concentrated from the feces of a cat by the zinc sulfate centrifugal flotation technique. Cyst wall, nuclei, axonemes, and median bodies are apparent in several of the cysts (iodine, ×1100). (From Greene CE: *Infectious diseases of the dog and cat*, ed 3, St Louis, 2006, Saunders Elsevier.)

Geographical Occurrence

G. intestinalis occurs worldwide in humans and other animals, with greater human prevalence in regions with poor sanitation practices and crowding. Reported prevalence in human populations ranges from 2% to 4% in developed countries to more than 15% in children from developing countries.

Groups at Risk

Children appear to become infected more frequently than adults. Particular risk groups include children in day care facilities, day care workers, parents of infected children, individuals living in areas without adequate sanitation or who drink from shallow wells, wilderness travelers who drink unfiltered or untreated water, swimmers who swallow water from lakes or ponds, international travelers, and men who have sex with men.[4]

Hosts, Reservoir Species, Vectors

In many host species, *Giardia* infection can produce humoral immunity after 100 days that may result in self-limiting infection.[5] In the United States, the prevalence of *Giardia* in canine kennels has been reported up to 100%.[6] Humans and a wide range of other animals are reservoirs. In many individuals and species, asymptomatic carriage may occur with the ability to transmit the infection to others.

Studies of infection prevalence in animals vary greatly: 20% to 35% in puppies, 10% to 15% in kittens, 5% to 90% in calves, 60% to 80% in lambs, 17% to 32% in foals, and 7% to 44% in young pigs.[7]

Mode of Transmission and Life Cycle

Cysts develop in the intestine and are shed into the environment in feces, where they are immediately infective (Figure 9-56). Transmission occurs when cysts are ingested through drinking water, direct fecal-oral contamination,

Giardiasis
(Giardia intestinalis)

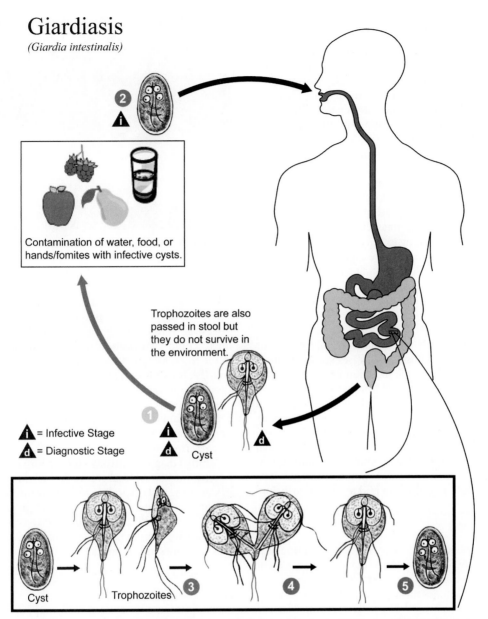

Contamination of water, food, or hands/fomites with infective cysts.

Trophozoites are also passed in stool but they do not survive in the environment.

🔺**i** = Infective Stage

🔺**d** = Diagnostic Stage

Cyst

Cyst   Trophozoites

Figure 9-56 ■ Life cycle, giardiasis. Cysts are resistant forms and are responsible for transmission of giardiasis. Both cysts and trophozoites can be found in the feces (diagnostic stages). *1,* The cysts are hardy and can survive several months in cold water. Infection occurs by the ingestion of cysts in contaminated water, food, or by the fecal-oral route (hands or fomites). *2,* In the small intestine, excystation releases trophozoites (each cyst produces two trophozoites). *3,* Trophozoites multiply by longitudinal binary fission, remaining in the lumen of the proximal small bowel where they can be free or attached to the mucosa by a ventral sucking disk. *4,* Encystation occurs as the parasites transit toward the colon. The cyst is the stage found most commonly in nondiarrheal feces. *5,* Because the cysts are infectious when passed in the feces or shortly afterward, person-to-person transmission is possible. While animals are infected with *Giardia,* their importance as a reservoir is unclear. (From Centers for Disease Control and Prevention: *Giardiasis.* http://www.dpd.cdc.gov/dpdx/HTML/Giardiasis.htm. Accessed September 13, 2008.)

foodborne exposure, or contact with contaminated objects leading to ingestion. Infected drinking water is thought to be the major form of transmission. The infective dose is low, with a median infective dose (ID_{50}) of 10 cysts. Fecal excretion is high—an infected human can secrete 900 million cysts per day.[8]

Once the cysts are ingested, they develop into trophozoites in the small intestine. The trophozoites remain there and, if they cause disease, they do so without invading the mucosa. They have a sucking disk by which they attach to the entero-

cytes and are thus not shed continuously. Reproduction takes place by binary fission and cysts are produced to continue the life cycle.

Circumstantial evidence, such as finding similar genotypes in both children and household dogs, suggests that transmission between pets and people takes place.[9,10] Case control studies have shown increased odds for infection among pet owners and people reporting contact with farm animals.[11] Transmission in animals, as in humans, occurs through ingestion of cysts.

Environmental Risk Factors

Because the *Giardia* cyst can persist for months in the environment, the status of water supplies is a critical environmental factor in sporadic and epidemic outbreaks of giardiasis in both humans and animals. Inadequate filtration of drinking water supplies has been associated with major outbreaks. The degree of contamination of municipal water supplies and shallow wells with animal and human feces is also important. On farms, contamination of water sources could spread infection among animals.

Dogs shedding cysts in feces can contaminate environments such as a lawn or public park for months,[12-14] leading to risks to children who play around soil. Similarly, livestock housing facilities and grazing areas can become contaminated with *Giardia* cysts, leading to infection risk for animals and farmers. Even marine shellfish are capable of being contaminated with *Giardia* cysts, suggesting a foodborne infection risk to humans.[15]

Disease in Humans

Giardia infection in humans is usually asymptomatic or mild enough to escape diagnosis. Most cases are self-limited, yet significant acute and chronic infection can occur. Acute infection can produce bloating, abdominal pain, explosive diarrhea, with pale, frothy, steatorrheic feces often mixed with mucus, but not blood. Symptoms may be continuous or intermittent (with bouts of constipation).

In chronic infections, there can be bloating, abdominal pain, flatulence, steatorrhea, lactose intolerance, and weight loss. In children this can lead to failure to thrive and developmental delays.[16] Rarely, infection can lead to reactive arthritis.

Disease in Animals

In dogs and cats, the disease is often subclinical. Young animals are more likely to show signs of infection and present with frothy diarrhea that may be foul smelling. Calves, lambs, foals, and caged birds (cockatiels, parrots) may also develop diarrhea due to *Giardia*. Table 9-31 provides a comparison of clinical manifestations of giardiasis.

Diagnosis

In humans, the differential diagnosis includes other causes of chronic diarrhea, including bacteria such as *Campylobacter*

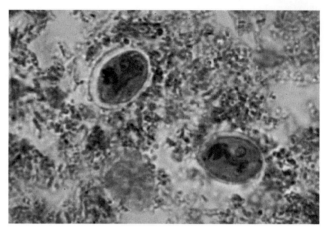

Figure 9-57 ■ *Giardia lamblia* in a reptile. (From Mader DR: *Reptile medicine and surgery*, ed 2, St Louis, 2006, Saunders Elsevier. Photograph courtesy F.L. Frye.)

and *Salmonella*, viral gastroenteritis, and other protozoa including *Cryptosporidium* and *Cyclospora*, and underlying disease such as celiac sprue. Diagnosis is typically by direct microscopic visualization of trophozoites or *Giardia* cysts in the feces. Repeated fecal analysis may be necessary. ELISA and IFA tests for antigen are also commercially available. It should be noted that demonstration of cysts alone in feces does not prove *Giardia* is the cause of a diarrheal episode because many *Giardia* infections are asymptomatic. In questionable cases, a duodenal aspirate, string test, or biopsy may be performed to detect trophozoites.[18]

Animal diagnosis involves testing for *Giardia* trophozoites in direct unstained fecal smears to look for motile trophozoites or using Lugol's iodine to help distinguish the cysts and trophozoites (Figure 9-57).[19] A zinc sulfur concentration test (ZCST) is a fecal flotation method for cysts and is considered a more sensitive test than a newer, fecal ELISA. A direct IFA test may be more sensitive for detecting low numbers of cysts.[20]

Treatment

Acute giardiasis is treated with supportive care including rehydration. Antibiotics are indicated for symptomatic patients. Table 9-32 provides treatment information for giardiasis in humans and other animals.

All drugs for *Giardia* treatment are extralabel in animals. However, a number of drugs are effective. In addition to antibiotic treatment, an animal's coat should be washed

Table 9-31 ■ Giardiasis: Comparative Clinical Presentations in Humans and Other Animals

Species	Risk Factors	Incubation Period	Clinical Manifestations
Humans	Children, day care centers, areas of poor sanitation, international travel, backpackers, pet ownership, farm animal contact	3-25 days[17]	Asymptomatic *or* acute diarrhea with bloating, chronic diarrhea with malabsorption, weight loss
Dogs, cats, calves, rodents, reptiles	Crowding, contaminated environments	5-14 days	Often subclinical
	Young animals at increased risk of clinical disease		Weight loss, intermittent diarrhea; chronic infection can lead to debilitation

Table 9-32 ▪ Antibiotic Treatment of *Giardia* Infection in Humans and Other Animals

Species	Primary Treatment	Alternative Treatment
Humans	Tinidazole 2 gm PO × 1 or nitazoxanide 500 mg PO bid × 3 days	Metronidazole 250 mg PO tid × 5 days If pregnant: paromomycin 500 mg 4×/day × 7 days[21]
Dogs, cats[22]	Fenbendazole 50 mg/kg PO q24h × 3-5 days; a second 5-day course may be necessary	Albendazole 25 mg/kg PO q12h for 2 days; a second 5-day course may be necessary
Cattle	Fenbendazole 5-10 mg/kg PO × 3 days	Albendazole 20 mg/kg 1 PO once daily for 3 days

with an antiseptic shampoo solution to eliminate cysts. Vaccines[19] have been developed for dogs and cats, but their use is controversial.

References

1. Dvorak G, Rovid-Spickler A, Roth JA, et al. *Handbook for zoonotic diseases of companion animals*. Ames, IA: The Center for Food Security and Public Health, Iowa State University College of Veterinary Medicine; 2008.
2. Trout JM, Santín M, Greiner E, et al. Prevalence and genotypes of *Giardia duodenalis* in post-weaned dairy calves. *Vet Parasitol.* 2005;130(3–4):177.
3. Fayer R, Santín M, Trout JM, et al. Prevalence of species and genotypes of *Cryptosporidium* found in 1–2 year old dairy cattle in the eastern United States. *Vet Parasitol.* 2006;135(2):105.
4. Esfandiari A, Swartz J, Teklehaimanot S. Clustering of giardiasis among AIDS patients in Los Angeles County. *Cell Mol Biol.* 1997;43(7):1077.
5. O'Handley RM. Passive immunity and serological immune response in dairy calves associated with natural *Giardia duodenalis* infections. *Vet Parasitol.* 2003;113(2):89.
6. Kirkpatrick CE. Enteric protozoal infections. In: Greene CE, ed. *Infectious diseases of the dog and cat*. Philadelphia: WB Saunders; 1990.
7. Xiao L. Giardia infection in farm animals. *Parasitol Today.* 1994;10(11):436.
8. Acha PN, Szyfres B. *Zoonoses and communicable diseases common to man and animals: vol. III: chlamydioses, parasitoses*. 3rd ed. Washington, DC: Pan American Health Organization; 2003.
9. Volotao AC, Costa-Macedo LM, Haddad FS, et al. Genotyping of *Giardia duodenalis* from human and animal samples from Brazil using beta-giardin gene: a phylogenetic analysis. *Acta Trop.* 2007;102(1):10.
10. Inpankaew T, Traub R, Thompson RC, et al. Canine zoonoses in Bangkok temples. *Southeast Asian J Trop Med Public Health.* 2007;38(2):247.
11. Warburton AR, Jones PH, Bruce J. Zoonotic transmission of giardiasis: a case control study. *Commun Dis Rep CDR Rev.* 1994;4(3):R32.
12. Kahn CM, Line S, eds. *The Merck veterinary manual*. 9th ed. Whitehouse Station, NJ: Merck; 2005.
13. Grimason AM, Smith HV, Parker JF, et al. Occurrence of *Giardia* sp. cysts and *Cryptosporidium* sp. oocysts in faeces from public parks in the west of Scotland. *Epidemiol Infect.* 1993;110(3):641.
14. Graczyk TK, Fayer R, Trout JM, et al. *Giardia* sp. cysts and infectious *Cryptosporidium parvum* oocysts in the feces of migratory Canada geese (*Branta canadensis*). *Appl Environ Microbiol.* 1998;64(7):2736.
15. Robertson LJ. The potential for marine bivalve shellfish to act as transmission vehicles for outbreaks of protozoan infections in humans: a review. *Int J Food Microbiol.* 2007;120(3):201.
16. Kwan-Gett TS, Kemp C, Kovarik C. *Infectious and tropical diseases: a handbook for primary care*. Philadelphia: Mosby Elsevier; 2006.
17. Heymann DL, ed. *Control of communicable diseases manual*. 19th ed. Washington, DC: American Public Health Association; 2008.
18. Mandell GE, Bennett JE, Dolin R. *Principles and practice of infectious diseases*. 6th ed. Philadelphia: Churchill Livingstone Elsevier; 2005.
19. Barr SC, Bowman DD. *The 5-minute veterinary consult clinical companion canine and feline infectious disease and parasitology*. Ames, IA: Blackwell; 2006.
20. Mekaru SR, Marks SL, Felley AJ, et al. Comparison of direct immunofluorescence, immunoassays, and fecal flotation for detection of *Cryptosporidium* spp. and *Giardia* spp. in naturally exposed cats in 4 Northern California animal shelters. *J Vet Intern Med.* 2007;21(5):959.
21. Gilbert DN, Moellering RC, Eliopoulos GM, et al. *Sanford guide to antimicrobial therapy*, 2009 39th ed. Sperryville, VA: Antimicrobial Therapy; 2009.
22. Tilley LP, Francis WK. *Blackwell's five-minute veterinary consult: canine and feline*. 4th ed. Ames, IA: Blackwell; 2008.

HANTAVIRUS INFECTIONS

Peter M. Rabinowitz and Lisa A. Conti

Hantavirus pulmonary syndrome (ICD-10 A), hemorrhagic fever with nephropathy (ICD-10 A)

Other names in humans: hantavirus (cardio-) pulmonary syndrome (HPS); Four-corners' disease; in western Europe, nephropathia epidemica; in parts of eastern Europe and Asia, hemorrhagic fever with renal syndrome (Korean hemorrhagic fever); also many local names

Other names in animals: none

Clinical syndromes of hantavirus infection, including hantavirus pulmonary syndrome (HPS) and hemorrhagic fever with nephropathy, are thought at present to be principally human diseases. However, the presence of domestic animals in, and wildlife around, a household can increase the risk for rodent infestation or contact that can result in hantavirus risk to humans. Limiting contact between humans and rodents (including wild species and laboratory animals) can reduce the risk of infection. However, these interventions are unlikely to prevent sporadic transmission with serious fatal outcomes.

Key Points for Clinicians and Public Health Professionals

Public Health Professionals

- Provide descriptive epidemiology of cases in the health district.
- Educate the public about measures to reduce risk, including the following:
  o Controlling rodents and their fleas near dwellings (flea control should precede rodent control to

CDC "SEAL UP, TRAP UP, CLEAN UP" RECOMMENDATIONS FOR REDUCING RODENT INFESTATION AND RISK OF HPS

- **Seal** rodent entry holes or gaps with steel wool, lath metal, or caulk.
- **Trap** rats and mice using appropriate snap trap.
- **Clean** up rodent food sources and nesting sites.
- Keep woodpiles and compost heaps away from house.
- Take precautions when cleaning rodent-infected areas:
  o Use cross-ventilation when entering a previously unventilated enclosed room or dwelling before cleanup.
  o Use rubber, latex, vinyl, or nitrile gloves.
  o Do not stir up dust by vacuuming, sweeping, or any other means. Instead, thoroughly wet contaminated areas with a bleach solution or household disinfectant. *Hypochlorite (bleach) solution:* Mix 1½ cups of household bleach in 1 gallon of water. Once everything is wet, take up contaminated materials with damp towel and then mop or sponge the area with bleach solution or household disinfectant.
- Spray dead rodents with disinfectant and then double-bag along with all cleaning materials and dispose of bag in an appropriate waste disposal system.
- Remove gloves and thoroughly wash hands with soap and water (or waterless alcohol-based hand rubs when soap is not available and hands are not visibly soiled).

From "Prevent Rodent Infestations" at http://www.cdc.gov/rodents/prevent_rodents/index.htm.

prevent fleas from seeking new hosts): Box 9-4 lists steps for rodent proofing homes
  o Avoiding camping near rodent burrows
  o Avoiding handling wild rodents[1]
- Provide exposure risk reduction guidance to workers with occupational risk (see below).

Human Health Clinicians

- Report disease to public health authorities using the case definition (All About Hantaviruses): http://www.cdc.gov/ncidod/diseases/hanta/hps/noframes/phys/casedefn.htm.
- Ensure that workers in affected areas who are frequently exposed to rodents or who are involved in cleanup of rodent-infested areas are informed of their occupational risk and have a baseline medical screening, including respirator fit testing. They should use protective equipment—including either half-face or supplied air respirators with N100 or P100 filters (Color Plate 9-30)—and gloves while handling rodents or traps containing rodents; they also should disinfect gloves after use.[2,3]
- If fever or respiratory symptoms develop in a worker within 45 days of the last potential exposure, he or she should immediately seek medical attention and inform the health care provider of the potential occupational risk of hantavirus infection. The provider should contact local public health authorities promptly if hantavirus-associated illness is suspected. A blood sample should be submitted to the state health department for hantavirus antibody testing.[4]

Veterinary Clinicians

- Counsel clients about pet-feeding practices that reduce the risk of rodent infestation.
- Dogs and cats are not known to be infected with hantaviruses, but these pets may bring infected rodents into contact with people.
- Train veterinary personnel in biosafety measures to reduce risk from infected rodents.

Agent

Hantaviruses are trisegmented, negative-sense RNA viruses in the Bunyaviridae family. Unlike other bunyaviruses, which are arthropod borne, hantaviruses are rodent borne. A number of species cause human disease, and new hantaviruses and their rodent hosts continue to be described. Like other segmented RNA viruses, hantaviruses appear capable of reassortment when dual infections of target cells occurs, which could lead to the emergence of novel strains.[5]

Geographical Occurrence

In the New World, hantaviruses are found from Canada to Argentina. In North America, Sin Nombre, New York-1, Bayou, and Black Creek Canal hantaviruses have been associated with HPS.[6] In South America, HPS caused by Andes virus may be particularly pathogenic for humans, and rare occurrence of human-human transmission of infection has been linked to this virus in Argentina.[7,8] Old World members of the family, including Seoul virus, Hantaan virus, and Dobrava-Belgrade virus, cause hantavirus hemorrhagic fever with renal syndrome.[9] Another Old World virus, Pumaala virus, causes a somewhat milder disease generally referred to as *nephropathia epidemica.* Pumaala virus is the predominant hantavirus in western and central Europe, whereas Hantaan and Dobrava-Belgrade viruses are found in eastern Europe. Hantaan virus is the major pathogen in Asia and has also been detected in Africa.

Groups at Risk

In the United States, groups at increased risk for hantavirus infection are those with rodent contact, including persons living in endemic areas such as the Southwest, forestry workers, farm workers, construction workers engaged in renovation, wildlife biologists and zoologists, and laboratory animal handlers. Although the risk to such groups is low overall, it may be higher in areas of endemic foci.[2]

Hosts, Reservoir Species, Vectors

Rodents and, in a few instances, insectivores (shrews) are the reservoir host of hantaviruses, and each hantavirus species is associated primarily with a single rodent or insectivore species.[10] Hantavirus infection within individual rodents of a reservoir species is believed to occur horizontally, with males frequently infected at higher prevalence than females.[4] Lifelong persistence of infection with sporadic shedding of virus has been demonstrated for multiple species. HPS is associated with rodents of the subfamily Sigmodontinae.

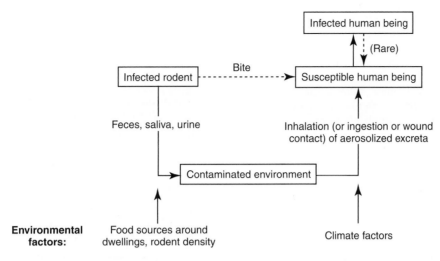

Figure 9-58 ■ Transmission of hantavirus infection.

The principal reservoir for hantavirus in the United States is the deer mouse (*Peromyscus maniculatus*, Color Plate 9-31); other rodents carriers are the cotton rat (*Sigmodon hispidus*), the rice rat (*Oryzomys palustris*), and the white-footed mouse (*Peromyscus leucopus*). Seoul viruses are carried by rats (*Rattus* species).[11] Although most of these reservoir species are usually found in more rural areas, they are capable of infesting buildings in periurban zones near forested areas.[12]

Mode of Transmission and Life Cycle

The spread of virus to humans is believed to occur primarily through inhalation of aerosol of dried feces, saliva, or urine from infected rodents (Figure 9-58). Bites from infected rodents or contact with their feces, saliva, or urine with broken skin, mucous membranes, or through ingestion are other possible transmission pathways.

Person-to-person transmission has been reported only for Andes virus, which has been isolated from human saliva[13]; this transmission required close personal contact in an enclosed space (bus).[8]

Environmental Risk Factors

Contamination of the environment by urine, saliva, and feces of infected rodents is the principal driver of transmission. Under certain conditions, the virus can persist for prolonged periods (several months) in the environment.[14]

Environmental factors that increase the density of rodents around human habitation are critical to human risk. These factors include abundance of food sources (unsecured food in kitchens, seeds from bird feeders, pet/livestock food). A combination of mild winters and increased rainfall related to El Niño cycles has also been associated with increased rodent abundance.[15]

Spatial risk mapping in the American Southwest has identified areas of increased hantaviral transmission related to elevation and precipitation.[16]

Disease in Humans

Hantavirus Pulmonary Syndrome

HPS is a life-threatening disease that begins with a nonspecific prodrome of fever, chills, and myalgia, leading to hypotension and pulmonary edema with accompanying respiratory distress and shock. The incubation period is 1 to 4 weeks.

Radiographs may reveal diffuse alveolar infiltrates (Figure 9-59). Mechanical ventilation is often necessary. Complications may include disseminated intravascular coagulation, myocardial dysfunction, and cardiac arrhythmias. The case fatality rate may reach 40%. In parts of South America, however, milder forms of the disease may occur.[17]

Hantavirus Hemorrhagic Fever with Nephropathy (Hemorrhagic Fever With Renal Syndrome)

This is a disease of variable severity, with a number of different clinical stages.[11]

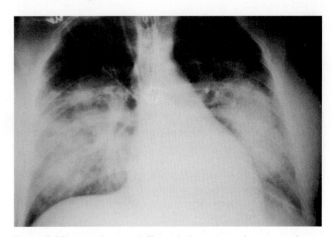

Figure 9-59 ■ Pulmonary infiltrates in hantavirus pulmonary syndrome. (From Centers for Disease Control and Prevention: *Severe hantavirus pulmonary syndrome.* http://www.bt.cdc.gov/agent/plague/trainingmodule/3/12hantavirus.htm. Accessed October 2008.)

1. The *febrile* or *toxic* stage is characterized by the abrupt onset of fever, chills, and headache that may be accompanied by photophobia and other symptoms.
2. The *hypotensive* phase may involve clinical shock and death.
3. The *oliguric* (renal) phase follows the hypotensive phase and includes declining renal function and urine output. Hemorrhagic complications may occur.
4. The *diuretic* phase is characterized by improved urine output and clinical condition.
5. The *convalescent* phase may include long-term abnormalities of renal function, including renal acidosis and renal insufficiency.

Disease in Animals

Rodents appear to have subclinical infection with hantaviruses. Serological studies in the United States have failed to demonstrate significant rates of subclinical infection in dogs or cats.[18]

Diagnosis

The differential diagnosis includes legionella, plague, tularemia, Q fever, leptospirosis, Goodpasture's syndrome (antiglomerular basement antibody disease), and drug-induced noncardiac edema. Typical hematologic findings of hantavirus infection include immature neutrophils (bandemia), atypical lymphocytosis, and thrombocytopenia.[19] An ELISA IgM test is available, and immunohistochemistry can be used for retrospective diagnosis.

Treatment

There is no specific treatment for HPS. Treatment is supportive. Clinicians need to have a high suspicion for the disease because patients require early transfer to an intensive care unit. Mechanical ventilation and support of blood pressure with pressor agents may be necessary. Extracorporeal membrane oxygenation has reportedly provided clinical benefit in some cases.

Hantavirus hemorrhagic fever with nephropathy is also treated with supportive measures, including dialysis if necessary. Ribavirin has been used in some cases.[17]

References

1. Center for Disease Control and Prevention. *Prevent rodents: index: CDC rodent control.* http://www.cdc.gov/rodents/prevent_rodents/index.htm. Accessed May 8, 2008.
2. Fulhorst CF, Milazzo ML, Armstrong LR, et al. Hantavirus and arenavirus antibodies in persons with occupational rodent exposure. *Emerg Infect Dis.* 2007;13(4):532.
3. Mills JN. Regulation of rodent-borne viruses in the natural host: implications for human disease. *Arch Virol.* 2005;45(suppl 19).
4. Mills JN, Corneli A, Young JC, et al. Hantavirus pulmonary syndrome—United States: updated recommendations for risk reduction, Centers for Disease Control and Prevention. *MMWR Recomm Rep.* 2002;51(RR-9):1.
5. Rodriguez LL, Owens JH, Peters CJ, et al. Genetic reassortment among viruses causing hantavirus pulmonary syndrome. *Virology.* 1998;242:99.
6. Monroe MC, Morzunov SP, Johnson AM, et al. Genetic diversity and distribution of *Peromyscus*-borne hantaviruses in North America. *Emerg Infect Dis.* 1999;5:75.
7. Wells RM, Sosa Estani S, Yadon ZE, et al. An unusual hantavirus outbreak in southern Argentina: person-to-person transmission? Hantavirus Pulmonary Syndrome Study Group for Patagonia. *Emerg Infect Dis.* 1997;3(2):171.
8. Martinez VP, Bellomo C, San Juan J, et al. Person-to-person transmission of Andes virus. *Emerg Infect Dis.* 2005;11(12):1848.
9. Acha PN, Szyfres B. *Zoonoses and communicable diseases common to man and animals: vol. II: chlamydioses, rickettsioses, and viroses.* 3rd ed. Washington, DC: Pan American Health Organization; 2003.
10. Arai S, Bennett SN, Sumibcay L, et al. Phylogenetically distinct hantaviruses in the masked shrew (*Sorex cinereus*) and dusky shrew (*Sorex monticulus*) in the United States. *Am J Trop Med Hyg.* 2008;78:348.
11. Heymann DL. *Control of communicable diseases manual.* 18th ed. Washington, DC: American Public Health Association; 2004.
12. Abu Sin M, Stark K, van Treeck U, et al. Risk factors for hantavirus infection in Germany, 2005. *Emerg Infect Dis.* 2007;13(9):1364.
13. Pettersson L, Klingström J, Hardestam J, et al. Hantavirus RNA in saliva from patients with hemorrhagic fever with renal syndrome. *Emerg Infect Dis.* 2008;14(3):406.
14. Clement J, Maes P, Ducoffre G, et al. Hantaviruses: underestimated respiratory viruses? *Clin Infect Dis.* 2008;46(3):477.
15. Miedzinski L. Community-acquired pneumonia: new facets of an old disease—hantavirus pulmonary syndrome. *Resp Care Clin N Am.* 2005;11(1):45.
16. Eisen RJ, Glass GE, Eisen L, et al. A spatial model of shared risk for plague and hantavirus pulmonary syndrome in the southwestern United States. *Am J Trop Med Hyg.* 2007;77(6):999.
17. Kwan-Gett TS, Kemp C, Kovarik C. *Infectious and tropical diseases: a handbook for primary care.* Philadelphia: Mosby Elsevier; 2005.
18. Malecki TM, Jillson GP, Thilsted JP, et al. Serologic survey for hantavirus infection in domestic animals and coyotes from New Mexico and northeastern Arizona. *J Am Vet Med Assoc.* 1998;212(7):970.
19. Center for Disease Control and Prevention (CDC). Hantavirus pulmonary syndrome—five states, 2006. *MMWR Morb Mortal Wkly Rep.* 2006;55(22):627.

HOOKWORM INFECTION

Peter M. Rabinowitz and Lisa A. Conti

Cutaneous larva migrans (ICD-10 B76.9) Disease due to Ancylostoma caninum *or* Ancylostoma braziliense *(B76.0)*

Other names in humans: *ancylostomiasis, creeping eruption, ground itch, dew itch, sandworm, cutaneous larva migrans*

Other names in animals: *ancylostomiasis*

Hookworms of the genus *Ancylostoma* are common parasites that can cause serious infections in dogs and cats and usually milder illness in humans. The classic manifestation of *A. caninum* and *A. braziliense* infection in humans is a dermatitis resulting from the larvae burrowing under the skin, known as *creeping eruption* or *cutaneous larva migrans.* Preventive veterinary care and healthy public policies about pet sanitation can reduce the risk of human disease.

Agent

Hookworms are nematode worms (Color Plate 9-32). Although a number of hookworm species occur in humans and other animals, *A. canium* (dog hookworm) and *A. braziliense* are the species associated with human disease in the United States. *A. braziliense* is considered the most common cause of cutaneous larva migrans.[1] A related species, *A. ceylanicum*, has historically been confused with *A. braziliense*.[2] The adult *A. caninum* worms are 12 to 15 cm in length; the other species are somewhat smaller.

Geographical Occurrence

Because the larvae prefer warm, humid environmental conditions, hookworm infection is more common worldwide in tropical and subtropical regions. *A. caninum* is more widely distributed than *A. braziliense* or *A. ceylanicum*. In the United States, infection with *A. caninum* and *A. braziliense* occurs mostly in the southeast states along the Gulf of Mexico. *A. ceylanicum* is found in tropical regions.

Groups at Risk

Exposure to contaminated soil and sand is a major risk factor; therefore human cases occur among bathers who walk barefoot on contaminated beaches or soils. Other risk groups include gardeners, workers who have to crawl into contaminated crawl spaces under buildings, and travelers to tropical regions.

Hosts, Reservoir Species, Vectors

Dogs are the principal reservoir for *A. caninum. A. braziliense* occurs in cats and dogs. A survey of feral cats in Florida found 33% infected with *A. braziliense. A. braziliense* also is found in wild felids. It is thought that infection in rodents (paratenic hosts) may also play a role in disease transmission.[2]

Mode of Transmission and Life Cycle

Dogs and cats become infected through ingestion of larvae, skin penetration of larvae or from transmission in milk or colostrum of infected bitches (dogs) (Figure 9-60). In puppies and kittens, the larvae migrate through the bloodstream and lymphatics to the lungs, where they are coughed up and swallowed and mature in the small intestine. Approximately 15 to 20 days after infection, the mature worms produce eggs.[3] In older cats and dogs, the life cycle is arrested in the larval stage, but such larvae may become reactivated if adult worms are removed from the intestine or during pregnancy.

After an infected animal sheds eggs into the environment in feces, the eggs complete embryonation, hatch, and larvae begin to develop through a series of stages. The process of developing into infective larvae takes 7 to 10 days in moist, warm soil.[4]

Larvae infect humans through contact with skin, usually of the foot. This produces a characteristic dermatitis (ground itch). The larvae of *A. caninum* and *A. braziliense* burrow under the skin but eventually die. In the process they produce the lesions of cutaneous larva migrans. Larvae of *A. ceylanicum*, however, pass through the lymphatics and bloodstream into the lungs, ascend up the trachea where they are swallowed (similar to infection in dogs and cats), and reach the small intestine, where they attach to the wall and develop to maturity in 3 to 4 weeks.[4]

Environmental Risk Factors

Temperature, humidity, and soil type are important factors determining how well the hookworm eggs hatch and develop into infective larvae. In general, these organisms prefer moist, warm climates and moist, sandy soils. In moist, warm conditions the third-stage (infective) larvae can survive up to 3 weeks.[3] Pet sanitation policies in beaches, parks, and other public places can affect the risk of human infection.

Disease in Humans

Human infection with *A. caninum* or *A. braziliense* causes a linear dermatitis that appears within days to weeks after infection (Color Plate 9-33). The rash is usually accom-

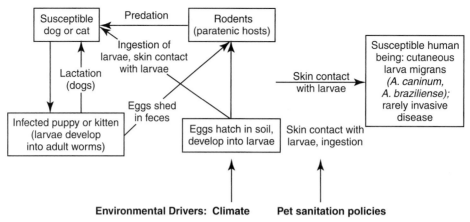

Figure 9-60 ▪ Life cycle of hookworm infection.

panied by intense itching, erythema, and edema. Vesicles may appear. Secondary infection may occur. The infection may last weeks or months. Laboratory findings can include eosinophilia and increased IgE levels.

Rarely, cases of intestinal infection with *A. caninum* have occurred. In such cases, larvae migrate deeper and may reach the intestines causing eosinophilic enteritis. Loeffler's syndrome (eosinophilia, asthma, migratory pulmonary infiltrates, fever, and urticaria) has been described.[5]

Disease in Animals

In young animals, hookworm infection can be an acute disease process with significant blood loss and sudden death. Black, tarry stools may occur. Laboratory tests show anemia that may be accompanied by eosinophilia. The fourth larval stage and adult worms cause a chronic anemia and enteritis. The lung migration phase of the life cycle can rarely cause a dry cough.[6] Because animals may repopulate the bowel with larvae dormant in tissues, infection may continue for months or years. Dogs previously sensitized to *Ancylostoma* may manifest "hookworm dermatitis" at sites of percutaneous larval penetration (Color Plate 9-34). Table 9-33 shows the comparative clinical presentation of hookworm infection in humans and other animals.

Diagnosis

Cutaneous larva migrans in humans is diagnosed clinically by the characteristic linear, slow-moving rash and a history of exposure to potentially contaminated soils. Biopsy may show an eosinophilic infiltrate but usually does not reveal the organism and therefore is not generally indicated to establish the diagnosis.[7] In animals, eggs can be identified in feces by fecal flotation (Figure 9-61).[6]

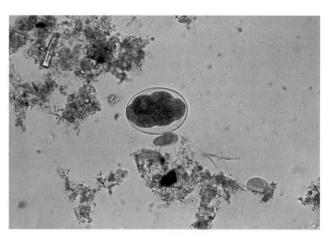

Figure 9-61 ▪ Hookworm ova. (From Centers for Disease Control and Prevention Public Health Image Library, Atlanta, Ga.)

Table 9-33 ▪ Hookworm Infection: Comparative Clinical Presentations in Humans and Other Animals				
Species	**Risk Factors**	**Incubation Period**	**Clinical Manifestations**	**Laboratory Findings**
Humans	Unprotected skin contact with soil, sand	Days to weeks	Linear skin eruption with pruritus, erythema, edema *Rarely*: Loeffler's syndrome, eosinophilic enteritis	Eosinophilia
Dogs	Puppies at increased risk of severe disease	Varies with the number of parasites	Anemia, acute or chronic; weight loss; tarry stools; sudden death	Anemia, iron deficiency Eggs in feces
Cats	More severe signs in kittens		Usually subclinical	Anemia (rare), eggs in feces

Treatment

Treatment in Humans

Many human cases of cutaneous larva migrans are self-limited and do not require medical intervention. However, in symptomatic and persistent infection, anthelmintic therapy is warranted. Topical thiabendazole cream may be effective.[7] Table 9-34 lists choices of oral anthelmintic agents, which are associated with a high cure rate.

Treatment in Animals

Acute illness in dogs and cats is treated with an antihelmintic, as well as supportive care such as blood transfusions. In dogs, adult larvae treatment is sometimes given during the third trimester of pregnancy to reduce transmission to offspring. Pups should be treated at 2 weeks, then every 2 weeks until weaned.

In cats, the queen is given a dewormer before breeding and after littering. Kittens can begin treatment with an adulticide dewormer by 4 weeks of age.[7] Table 9-34 outlines antihelmintic therapy for hookworm infection.

References

1. Georgiev VS. Parasitic infections. Treatment and developmental therapeutics. 1. Necatoriasis. *Curr Pharma Des.* 1999;5(7):545.
2. Acha PN, Szyfres B. *Zoonoses and communicable diseases common to man and animals: vol. 3: Parasitosis.* 3rd ed. Washington, DC: Pan American Health Organization; 2001.
3. Kahn CM, Line S, eds. *The Merck veterinary manual.* 9th ed. Whitehouse Station, NJ: Merck; 2005.
4. Heymann DL. *Control of communicable diseases manual.* 19th ed. Washington, DC: American Public Health Association; 2008.
5. Schaub NA, Perruchoud AP, Buechner SA. Cutaneous larva migrans associated with Loffler's syndrome. *Dermatology.* 2002;205(2):207.
6. Barr SC, Bowman DD. *5-Minute veterinary consult clinical companion canine and feline infectious disease and parasitology.* Ames, IA: Wiley-Blackwell; 2006.
7. Mandell GL, Bennett JE, Dolin R, eds. *Principles and practice of infectious diseases.* 6th ed. New York: Churchill Livingstone Elsevier; 2005.
8. Gilbert DN, Moellering RC, Ellopoulos GM, et al. *Sanford guide to antimicrobial therapy. 2009.* 39th ed. Sperryville, VA: Antimicrobial Therapy; 2009.

Table 9-34 ▪ Treatment of Hookworm Infections in Humans and Other Animals

Species	Primary Treatment	Alternative Treatment
Humans: cutaneous larva migrans	Ivermectin 200 mg PO qd × 1-2 days	Albendazole 200 mg PO bid × 3 days[8]
Dogs		
Adults and larvae	Fenbendazole 50 mg/kg PO × 3 days	Milbemycin oxime 0.5 mg/kg PO once, repeat monthly
Adulticide	Pyrantel pamoate 15 mg/kg PO once, repeat in 14 days	Praziquantel/pyrantel/febantel PO *or* milbemycin oxime 1, repeat in 14 days
		Ivermectin 6 mcg/kg/pyrantel PO once, repeat every month
		Dichlorvos 11 mg/kg PO once, repeat in 14 days
Cats		
Adults and larvae	Milbemycin oxime 2 mg/kg PO q30 days	Praziquantel/pyrantel PO once, repeat in 14 days
Adulticide	Pyrantel pamoate 20-30 mg/kg PO, repeat in 14 days (extralabel)	Dichlorvos 11 mg/kg PO once, repeat in 14 days

INFLUENZA

Carina Blackmore and Peter M. Rabinowitz

Influenza (ICD-9-CM 487.1)

Other names in humans: flu, seasonal flu

Other names in animals: avian flu, bird flu, fowl plague, fowl pest, swine flu, canine flu

Influenza in humans is an acute, usually self-limited febrile respiratory illness caused by influenza virus infections. Bacterial pneumonia is a common complication in persons older than 65 years. Influenza viruses have caused human epidemics and, much less commonly, pandemics (worldwide epidemics) for at least several hundred years,[1] and influenza is still one of the most important causes of morbidity and mortality in the United States.[2] Outbreaks typically occur in the winter months in temperate climates, although they may begin in late autumn and sometimes persist to late spring months. In recent seasons, two and sometimes three different influenza viruses (two type A subtypes, one type B) have co-circulated.

Influenza pandemics can occur when a new influenza virus emerges to which the overall population lacks immunity, typically to a new hemagglutinin subtype (Figure 9-62). The emergence of a pandemic influenza strain has been associated with reassortment of gene segments between human and animal strains. Characteristic traits of pandemics include concurrent, widespread outbreaks of influenza throughout the world, sometimes outside the usual influenza season, with high attack rates in all age groups.[1] Pandemics are usually associated with substantial increases in mortality.

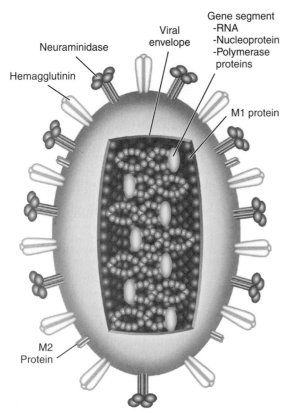

Figure 9-62 ■ Schematic model of an influenza A virus. (From Mandell GL, Bennett JE, Dolin R (eds): *Principles and practice of infectious diseases*, ed 6, Philadelphia, 2005, Churchill Livingstone Elsevier.)

Influenza viruses affect a number of different species, including birds, swine, horses, and dogs, but animal-to-human transmission has been documented only for birds and swine. Humans may transmit human influenza virus to pet ferrets and swine.[3] The epizootic of H5N1 high pathogenicity avian influenza in domestic and wild birds in Asia, Europe, and Africa has focused increased attention on the potential of influenza viruses to cross species barriers and cause human disease, although this is still considered a rare event and the H5N1 epizootic has not, to date, produced a pandemic virus. Dogs and cats have become naturally and experimentally infected with avian influenza viruses but have not as yet been shown to transmit the infection to humans. A swine influenza A H1N1 virus that emerged in Mexico in the spring of 2009 has further underscored the zoonotic nature of this disease. Human cases were identified worldwide within 1 week after the cause of the outbreak had been identified. As of October 25, 2009, the World Health Organization had confirmed more than 440,000 humans infected with the pandemic H1N1 virus and 5700 deaths worldwide (http://www. who.int/csr/don/2009_10_30/en/index.html). Human-to-animal transmission of the virus has also caused outbreaks in swine and turkeys (http://www.fao.org/news/story/en/item/29532/icode/).[4] H1N1 influenza infection has also been documented in ferrets and a cat (http://www.usda. gov/documents/FINAL_RESULTS_2009_PANDEMIC_ H1NI_INFLUENZA_CHT.pdf).

Key Points for Clinicians and Public Health Professionals

Public Health Professionals

- Educate the public and human health care providers about the importance of good cough etiquette (e.g., coughing into your elbow), handwashing practices, and seasonal influenza immunizations for their at-risk patients and for themselves.
- Encourage older individuals to get the pneumococcal (*Streptococcus pneumoniae*) vaccine.
- Educate human health care providers and veterinary clinicians about groups at risk for influenza and its complications, as well as signs and symptoms of the disease in different age groups.
- Educate travelers to countries where avian influenza is circulating about the risk of infection from contact with poultry and environments contaminated with poultry feces and secretions and uncooked poultry, and advise them to seek medical care immediately if signs (e.g., fever, cough) appear.
- Instruct health care workers with influenza-like illness not to provide direct patient care.
- Be aware of pandemic influenza (panflu) planning in your area (http://www.pandemicflu.gov/).

Human Health Clinicians

- Consider testing patients in whom influenza develops early or late in the influenza season, those with unusually severe clinical symptoms, a history of potential exposure to avian or swine influenza, or who are candidates for antiviral treatment.
- Advise symptomatic individuals to avoid caring for sick or immunocompromised individuals.
- Educate ill patients about the importance of covering their cough, keeping their distance from others, and washing their hands.
- Be aware of CDC guidance for detection and testing of avian influenza infections in returning travelers. See Travelers' Health; http://wwwn.cdc.gov/travel/content AvianFluPassengerChecks.aspx.
- Report influenza cases to state or local health department if required in state.
- Recommend influenza vaccinations of high-risk groups. The Advisory Committee on Immunization Practices (ACIP) recommends annual influenza vaccinations for the following groups[5]:
  ○ All persons who want to reduce the risk of becoming ill with influenza or of transmitting influenza to others
  ○ All children aged 6 months to 18 years
  ○ All persons aged 50 years and older
  ○ Women who will be pregnant during the influenza season
  ○ Adults who have chronic pulmonary (including asthma), cardiovascular (except hypertension), renal, hepatic, hematological, or metabolic disorders (including diabetes mellitus)

- Adults who have immunosuppression (including immunosuppression caused by medications or by human immunodeficiency virus
- Adults who have any condition (e.g., cognitive dysfunction, spinal cord injuries, seizure disorders, or other neuromuscular disorders) that can compromise respiratory function or the handling of respiratory secretions or that can increase the risk for aspiration
- Residents of nursing homes and other long-term care facilities
- Health care personnel (Figure 9-63)
- Healthy household contacts and caregivers of children younger than 5 years and adults 50 years and older, with particular emphasis on vaccinating contacts of children younger than 6 months
- Healthy household contacts and caregivers of persons with medical conditions that put them at higher risk for severe complications from influenza

- Two vaccines, a trivalent inactivated influenza vaccine (TIV) and a live, attenuated intranasal vaccine (LAIV) are approved by the Food and Drug Administration (FDA). The TIV is approved for use in people 6 months of age or older. The primary series for children younger than 8 years consists of 2 doses administered 1 month apart. Individuals who only received 1 dose in their first year of vaccination should receive 2 doses in the following year. The TIV is injected into the deltoid muscle of older children and adults. Infants and young children without adequate deltoid muscle mass should be vaccinated in the anterolateral aspect of the thigh. The LAIV is made from a weakened virus and can cause mild illness in some individuals (runny nose, headache, sore throat, or cough). It is approved in healthy people (without underlying health problems predisposing them to complications from influenza) between 2 and 49 years who are not pregnant. Two doses of LAIV administered at least 6 weeks apart are recommended for 2- to 8-year-old children who are receiving an influenza vaccine for the first time. If the child receives only 1 dose in the first year, 2 doses are recommended the following year. The intranasal vaccine comes in a prefilled, single-use sprayer contain-

ing 0.2 mL of the product. Approximately 0.1 mL (i.e., half of the total sprayer contents) is sprayed into one of the nostrils and the second half of the vaccine dose is administered into the other nostril.
- Clinicians should strongly consider seasonal influenza vaccination for poultry and swine workers.[6]
- CDC guidance for detection, testing, and treatment of patients infected with the pandemic H1N1 virus and recommendations for vaccination of people at risk for infection with the novel virus strain can be found at: http://www.cdc.gov/H1N1FLU.

Veterinary Clinicians

- Contact state veterinarian and public health department to report suspected or confirmed cases of animal influenza.
- Wear appropriate PPE when examining animals with suspected influenza infection. This includes gloves and surgical masks—if a highly pathogenic avian influenza, swine influenza, or human influenza strain is suspected, an N-95 respirator should be used.
- Test and isolate sick animals.
- Use appropriate infection control measures in the practice (hospital and clinic) to avoid environmental contamination and nosocomial spread of the virus.[7]
- Educate the animal owner regarding zoonotic risk (where applicable) and need for adequate PPE and handwashing. Offer direct communication with family physician.
- Counsel ferret owners that these pets are susceptible to several human influenza strains.
- Be aware of the USDA's National Highly Pathogenic Avian Influenza (HPAI) Response Plan. Should HPAI be identified in the United States, a team of federal and state officials will be deployed to the area to assess the scope of disease and the resources needed to confine it.
- Veterinarians and veterinary staff should receive annual seasonal influenza vaccinations.
- If an outbreak of HPAI is identified in wild birds, consider diagnosis in domestic birds or bird predators with clinical signs and potential virus exposure.
- Influenza virus vaccines are available for swine, dogs, horses, and domestic birds. Several inactivated whole-virus swine influenza vaccines are currently on the market. The vaccines help reduce the severity of disease in pigs but do not provide complete protection against infection. Many in the swine industry use autogenous vaccines produced against the strain circulating in their herd. Animals are usually vaccinated during the late nursing–early weaning stage to prevent influenza outbreaks in the growth/early finishing animals. Breeding herds are often vaccinated as well.
- All horses in contact with other equines should be vaccinated against equine influenza. Three types of equine influenza virus vaccines are available.[8] Inactivated vaccines and canary pox vector vaccines are administered intramuscularly. The initial series consists of 2 doses of vaccines given 3 to 6 weeks apart followed by boosters every 6 months. Annual influenza vaccine boosters

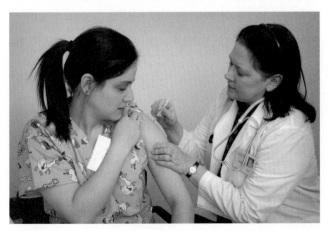

Figure 9-63 ▪ Health care professional receiving an intramuscular vaccination. (From Centers for Disease Control and Prevention Public Health Image Library, Atlanta, Ga.)

may be sufficient for horses at low risk of exposure once they have been primed with 3 doses of vaccine over a 7-month period. The third vaccine type, modified live cold-adapted vaccines, is administered intranasally. One priming dose is recommended followed by boosters every 6 months. The intranasal vaccines are licensed for nonpregnant horses older than 11 months. Inactivated vaccines are licensed for horses older than 6 months, and canary pox virus vaccines are safe for foals 4 months of age or older.

- Vaccination of poultry against avian influenza is not routine because most poultry in developed countries, including the United States, are grown in commercial settings that are free from avian influenza. Vaccines have been used in specific high-risk situations targeting a known hemagglutinin subtype of avian influenza virus, such as in outdoor-reared turkeys in the upper Midwest United States when in contact with avian influenza–infected migratory ducks, or for turkeys in areas of high swine concentration. Avian influenza vaccination requires approval of the state veterinarian, and with H5 and H7 avian influenza, the approval of the USDA. Most licensed vaccines are inactivated whole avian influenza virus in oil-emulsified adjuvant, which requires individual bird handling and subcutaneous or intramuscular injection. One fowl poxvirus recombinant containing an influenza H5 hemagglutinin gene insert is licensed for emergency use. The vaccines protect against clinical disease but HPAI viruses can circulate undetected in a vaccinated flock. Serological tests cannot distinguish between an antibody response to the vaccine and a natural infection.[3]

Agent

Influenza viruses (Family Orthomyxoviridae) are enveloped, segmented, negative-stranded RNA viruses covered with two surface glycoproteins (Figure 9-64).[1] They are divided into three distinct types (A, B, and C) on the basis of their M and nucleocapsid proteins.[9] Influenza A viruses are further divided into subtypes based on the antigenic characteristics of their hemagglutinin (H) and neuraminidase (N) surface glycoproteins. Each virus carries one H and one N glycoprotein type (see Figure 9-63). Sixteen hemagglutinin subtypes (H1 through H16) and 9 neuraminidase (N1 through N9) have been identified from avian hosts.[10] Seasonal human

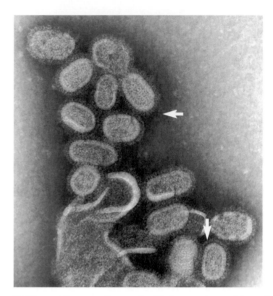

Figure 9-64 ■ Electron micrograph of influenza viruses. (From Centers for Disease Control and Prevention Public Health Image Library, Atlanta, Ga.)

influenza A viruses recognized to date have possessed H1, H2, or H3 and N1 or N2 glycoproteins. Influenza A (H1N1) and A (H3N2) have been circulating worldwide in human populations since 1977. Influenza B, which occurs only in humans and seals, is also responsible for significant human morbidity globally each year.[5] Influenza C is rarely recognized in comparison to A and B viruses but can cause focal human epidemics.

New seasonal influenza viruses evolve from point mutations (antigenic drift) in the surface glycoproteins, particularly the H, which frequently happens during viral replication. Gene segment reassortment among influenza A viruses can also occur. If these reassortments involve human and animal influenza viruses, they may lead to significant antigenic changes (antigenic shifts) that can result in the emergence of a novel virus subtype (Figure 9-65).

Influenza viruses exhibit various degrees of host adaptation with easy transmission between individuals within the same species, and greater difficulty of infection and unsustainable transmission to unrelated host species.[11,12] The basis of this host or species adaptation is unclear, but the presence of the proper constellation of gene segments is critical and may include specific hemagglutinin binding to receptors on host cells,

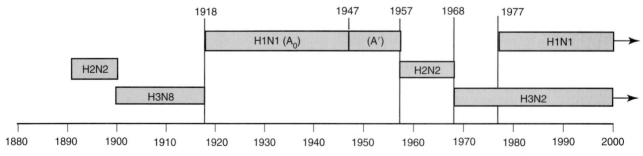

Figure 9-65 ■ Recent pandemics of influenza. The duration of circulation of viruses of various subtypes is shown by the boxes. The nature of influenza epidemics before 1918 is known only by serological means. (From Mandell GL, Bennett JE, Dolin R (eds): *Principles and practice of infectious diseases*, ed 6, Philadelphia, 2005, Churchill Livingstone Elsevier.)

especially respiratory cells, and their differential distribution; cleavability of hemagglutinin protein; presence or absence of glycosylation sites on the hemagglutinin; length of neuraminidase protein and its affinity for the sialic acids; and ability of polymerase complex to function within the host cell.[13]

Strains of avian influenza virus are classified as low pathogenic (LP) or high pathogenic (HP) based on their lethality in chickens.[14] Currently HPAI H5N1 is circulating in Asia, Europe, and Africa. However, other highly pathogenic strains have caused outbreaks in the recent past, including H7N7, H7N3, and H5N2. All HPAI viruses have been H5 and H7, but most H5 and H7 viruses are of low pathogenicity.

Geographical Occurrence

Worldwide.

Groups at Risk

Several population groups are at high risk for complications of seasonal influenza, including people who are 50 years old or older and people with chronic health problems, such as cardiovascular disease, renal and metabolic disorders (including diabetes), and respiratory disorders (including asthma). Other high-risk groups include women who are pregnant during the flu season, children and adolescents who are receiving long-term aspirin therapy, and children younger than 5 years.[15] Severe influenza disease is also often seen in individuals with immunosuppressive disorders such as cancer or HIV/AIDS.[5]

Individuals performing activities involving close contact with animals, such as slaughtering animals and defeathering birds, have been reported to be at increased risk for avian and swine influenza.[16-18]

Hosts, Reservoir Species, Vectors

Avian influenza viruses are maintained in nature by wild birds. The viruses have been isolated from more than 100 bird species in 13 genera; however, the most important avian influenza reservoir hosts belong to the Anseriformes (ducks, geese, and swans) and the Charadriiformes (gulls, terns, and shorebirds) groups.[19] More virus isolations have been reported from Mallards (*Anas platyrhynchos*) than any other bird species. Certain influenza virus strains have adapted to genetically distinct horse, swine, poultry, dog, and human viruses and are self-sustaining in those species.[19-21] Incidental hosts or sporadic infections have been reported in mink, ferrets (Figure 9-66), stone marten, domestic cats, large felids (tigers and leopards), and sea mammals.[19,22]

Swine are susceptible to both human and avian virus strains and are hypothesized to be able to serve as viral mixing vessels where human and avian gene segments may reassort.[1] The 2009 H1N1 swine influenza virus is a novel reassortant of two (parent) swine influenza viruses. It also contains genes of avian and human influenza virus origin incorporated into one of the parent viruses at an earlier time.[23] However, reassortment in swine may not be a requirement for emergence of a pandemic strain if the avian strain can produce infection in a human host.

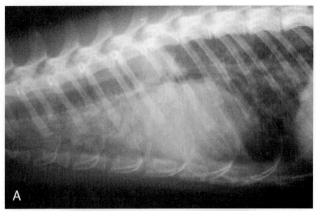
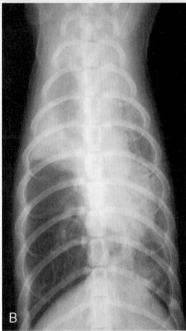

Figure 9-66 ▪ Lateral (**A**) and ventrodorsal (**B**) radiographs of a ferret with bacterial pneumonia as a complication of influenza. (From Quesenberry K, Carpenter JW: *Ferrets, rabbits and rodents: clinical medicine and surgery*, ed 2, St Louis, 2004, Saunders Elsevier.)

Mode of Transmission and Life Cycle

Human influenza is usually spread from person to person in close contact through large-particle respiratory droplet and short-distance small-particle aerosol transmission (coughs, sneezing) (Figure 9-67). Indirect spread via contact with surfaces contaminated with respiratory droplets is also a possible transmission mode, and there is evidence that the virus can persist for 1 to 2 days on some surfaces.[5]

In swine, the virus is found in respiratory secretions and spreads by aerosolization and by direct pig-to-pig contact.[24] Birds can shed high concentrations of influenza virus in feces, and fecal/oral spread is believed to be an important route of virus transmission in wild birds.[19] Infected birds can also shed influenza virus in their saliva and nasal secretions. Poultry can become infected when they have direct contact with infected birds or indirectly through contact with contaminated surfaces (such as equipment or cages) or feed or water. Aerosol transmission may also be possible over short distances.[25]

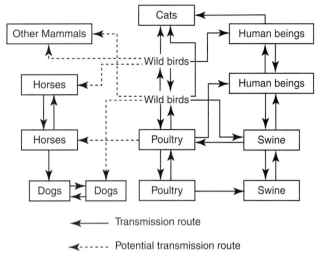

Figure 9-67 ■ Life cycle of influenza.

Touching surfaces contaminated with avian influenza virus in respiratory droplets and handling infected birds or bird manure are hypothesized risk factors for human infection with avian influenza, possibly through contaminated-hand–to–mucous membrane contact or inhalation of contaminated dust particles or aerosols generated during cleaning, slaughtering, defeathering, and other activities.[16,18] Swine influenza transmission appears to occur during close direct or indirect human contact with infected swine.[17]

Environmental Risk Factors

As stated previously, it is believed that contaminated environments such as surfaces, aerosols, and water may play a role in animal-to-animal influenza transmission and may also be important in human-to-human and animal-to-human transmission, although the significance of such environmental spread in each circumstance is not well understood.

Human crowding, such as in nursing homes, is associated with an increased rate of human outbreaks. As in animals, a high density of birds or swine in a production facility or a live animal market, as well as mixing of waterfowl, poultry, and other animal species including swine in a single facility, may facilitate the spread of virus between animals. Farms that have ponds or other water bodies where wild waterfowl can come in contact with domestic animals may also constitute an environmental risk. Whether the seasonal pattern of influenza is related to other environmental variables such as temperature and humidity remains unclear.

Disease in Humans

Influenza virus infections can affect all age groups, although the highest infection rates are seen among infants and children. Upper and lower respiratory tract complications occur across age groups, but hospitalizations and deaths from infection are more common in people older than 65 years.

Uncomplicated influenza typically has a quick onset of fever, myalgia, headache, malaise, sore throat, and nonproductive cough. Rhinitis may also be present. Otitis media, nausea,

and vomiting are other common influenza manifestations among children. Young children may be less likely than other influenza cases to present with fever and cough.[5] The incubation period is short (1 to 4 days) and the morbidity period generally lasts 3 to 7 days. Lassitude and cough may persist for 2 weeks or more.[26] Adults may be infectious the day before through day 5 after disease onset. Young children may shed virus several days before and after symptom onset.[5]

Complications of influenza are common. Patients may develop primary viral pneumonia, viral or secondary bacterial sinusitis and otitis, or pneumonia and experience exacerbations of underlying medical conditions such as pulmonary or cardiac disease. Influenza virus infection also has been uncommonly associated with encephalopathy, transverse myelitis, myositis, myocarditis, pericarditis, and Reye syndrome.[5]

Humans can on rare occasions become infected with avian[27] or swine[19,28] influenza viruses. Symptoms range from a mild conjunctivitis or upper respiratory tract disease to pneumonia, acute respiratory distress, and death. Further human-to-human transmission of these animal influenza viruses has been reported but is uncommon.

Disease in Animals

Avian influenza (AI) viruses are classified into low pathogenicity (LP) and high pathogenicity (HP) based on specific criteria related to their ability to produce high mortality rate in chickens or have a hemagglutinin protein cleavage site sequence compatible with previous HPAI virus.[29] Most AI strains are LP and generally cause no or few clinical signs in poultry. Typical clinical signs associated with LPAI reflect an upper respiratory tract disease or reproductive disease in hens (i.e., drops in egg production with abnormal eggs). However, some H5 and H7 LPAI viruses have mutated into HPAI viruses in the field. Signs of HPAI include high mortality rate; sudden death without premonitory clinical signs; lethargy; severe decrease in egg production; facial edema with swollen eyelids, comb, wattles, and hocks; purple discoloration of the wattles, combs, and legs; upper respiratory tract signs; incoordination; and diarrhea.[30] Turkeys are susceptible to certain strains of H1 and H3 swine influenza viruses.[31,32]

Swine influenza A H1N1 and H3N2 viruses are endemic in swine populations in the United States.[33] Clinical signs of influenza in pigs include fever, coughing, nasal and/or ocular discharge, dyspnea, and depression. Reproductive problems are seen in both males and females. Milk production may also be reduced. The morbidity period is usually 5 to 7 days. Morbidity can reach 100%. Mortality rates are low, usually between 1% and 3%; however, secondary bacterial infections may develop and increase mortality.[25]

Influenza A viruses H3N8 and H7N7 cause equine influenza in horses and other equids. The incubation period is generally 1 to 3 days. Incubation periods as long as 7 days have been reported. Clinical signs include fever; a harsh, dry cough; and serous to mucopurulent nasal discharge. In partially immune or vaccinated animals, one or more of these signs may be absent. Other typical signs include depression, muscle soreness, anorexia, and enlarged submandibular lymph nodes. Young foals lacking maternal antibody protection are susceptible to a fatal viral pneumonia. Horses can also develop a potentially fatal secondary bacterial pneumonia, pleuropneumonia, and myocarditis.[8,34]

Infected horses may shed virus over an extended period starting during the incubation period and ending a week or more after apparent recovery. Peak viral shedding is thought to occur during the first 24 to 48 hours when the animal is febrile.[8] The virus is spread via aerosolized respiratory droplets and fomites with an attack rate that can approach 100% in susceptible populations.

Canine influenza was first recognized in 2004. An equine influenza virus A H3N8 strain has apparently adapted to dogs and causes outbreaks of respiratory disease. Most animals develop a mild cough, purulent nasal discharge, and low-grade fever.[21] Dogs can also develop a more severe disease with high fever and pneumonia. Between 5% and 10% of ill dogs die from the illness.[21,35]

Avian influenza can cause fatal infection in domestic and large cats. Reported signs of HPAI H5N1 in felids include fever, panting, nervousness, and depression.[36] Table 9-35 shows comparative clinical presentations in humans and other animals.

Table 9-35 ■ Influenza: Comparative Clinical Presentations in Humans and Other Animals

Species	Risk Factors	Incubation Period	Clinical Manifestations	Laboratory Findings
Humans	Close contact with infected person, bird, or swine	1-4 days	Fever, myalgia, headache, malaise, sore throat, nonproductive cough and rhinitis, otitis media, nausea and vomiting in children; complications include primary viral pneumonia, secondary bacterial sinusitis, otitis, or pneumonia, exacerbated underlying medical conditions such as pulmonary or cardiac disease	DFA, RT-PCR, EIA, viral cultures, and rapid diagnostic tests such as immunochromatographic assays, paired sera taken 2-4 weeks apart
Birds	Direct contact with secretions or feces from infected birds, contaminated feed, water, equipment, or clothing	1-5 days	LPAI: No or few clinical signs, including inappetence, mild respiratory signs (nasal discharge, coughing, sneezing), and decreased egg production	RRT-PCR and serological screening tests, virus isolation, sequencing, and chicken pathogenicity test needed for confirmation of HPAI; serology by ELISA and AGID are used for monitoring
	Movement of people and birds		HPAI: Sudden death; lethargy; decreased egg production, soft-shelled or misshapen eggs; facial edema with swollen eyelids, comb, wattles, and hocks; purple discoloration of the wattles, combs, and legs; incoordination; and diarrhea	Histopathology findings with HPAI include hemorrhaging and necrosis of multiple organs[19]
Swine	Contact with nasal secretions or aerosol; airborne spread of virus can occur between farms under certain circumstances	<24 hours	Fever; coughing; nasal and/or ocular discharge; dyspnea and depression Reproductive problems such as reduced viability of sperm, first- and second-trimester abortions, delayed return to estrus, and decreased viability of piglets; milk production may also be reduced	Lung or nasal tissues can be evaluated for the presence of live or inactivated virus using immunohistochemistry, DFAs, antigen-capture ELISA, cell culture, or PCR Tests for detecting H1N1 or H3N2 antibodies include the HI, ELISA, immunodiffusion, and IFA
Horses	Aerosolized respiratory secretions; contaminated equipment, brushes, or rugs	1-3 days	Clinical signs include fever; a harsh, dry cough; and serous to mucopurulent nasal discharge; other typical signs include depression, muscle soreness, anorexia, enlarged regional lymph notes, colic, edema of the extremities and scrotum, viral pneumonia in young foals; secondary bacterial pneumonia, pleuritis, and interstitial myocarditis	Viral antigen can be detected from nasopharyngeal swabs, and tracheal and nasal wash samples using virus isolation, RT-PCR, nested RT-PCR, and ELISA Paired acute and convalescent serum samples can be submitted for HI testing
Dogs	Contact with aerosolized respiratory secretions and contaminated objects	2-5 days	Moist or dry cough, purulent nasal discharge, fever, pneumonia	Paired sera taken 2-3 weeks apart, virus detection from nasal swabs by PCR or viral culture[37]
Cats	Predation on diseased birds	2-5 days	Fever, dyspnea, depression, conjunctivitis	Paired sera, pharyngeal swabs[36]

AGID, Agar gel immunodiffusion; *DFA,* direct immunofluorescent antibody; *ELISA,* enzyme-linked immunosorbent assay; *HI,* hemagglutination-inhibition; *IFA,* immunofluorescent antibody; *RT-PCR,* reverse transcriptase polymerase chain reaction; *EIA,* enzyme immunoassay; *RRT-PCR,* real-time reverse transcriptase polymerase chain reaction.

Diagnosis

Diagnosis in Humans

The differential diagnosis for human influenza includes other respiratory pathogens, including *Mycoplasma pneumoniae*, adenovirus, respiratory syncytial virus, rhinovirus, parainfluenza viruses, and *Legionella* species infection.[26] Studies have estimated that 80% to 90% of healthy adults presenting with an acute onset of fever and a cough, the most common presentation of influenza, in areas with confirmed influenza activity have the disease. Young children and older adults are less likely to present with these symptoms. Infants may present with high fevers. A septicemia-like disease, cough, and fever are seen in 64% of children younger than 5 years, and fewer than one in three nonhospitalized patients 60 years or older present with typical influenza signs.[5]

Laboratory confirmation of disease is important. Specimens should be collected the first few days after onset of symptoms or no more than a week after disease onset in young children. The most common diagnostic tests currently used in clinics, doctors' offices, and hospitals are rapid influenza tests using immunochromatography. These tests require no reagent additions or wash steps, usually detect both influenza A and B, and use respiratory tract specimens specified in the manufacturers' instructions.[38] Results are available within 30 minutes. The accuracy of these tests depends on the sensitivity and specificity of the assay, the amount of virus in the sample, and the specimen type used. Infants and young children shed the highest viral titers, and these tests perform best in this patient group. The rapid tests typically have greater than 90% specificity and an average 70% sensitivity for detecting influenza. False-positive results are more common when the prevalence of influenza is low; false-negative results are more likely to occur when disease prevalence is high.

Additional diagnostic tests available in hospital and other clinical laboratories include viral cultures, direct immunofluorescence antibody (DFA) on clinical specimens, reverse transcriptase polymerase chain reaction (RT-PCR), and enzyme immunoassay (EIA). The ideal specimen depends on the test used but may include nasopharyngeal and nasal swabs or aspirates, nasal and bronchial washes, throat swabs, or sputum collected within the first 4 days of illness. Results from antigen tests such as DFA or EIA should be available within a few hours of arrival at the laboratory. Conventional viral cultures can take between 2 and 10 days, whereas rapid centrifugation cultures followed by IFA staining are reported at 1 and 2 days. RT-PCR assays are currently confined to reference laboratories and some large tertiary care hospitals, and where available are performed no more than once a day. Influenza virus infection can be confirmed by serology as well. Paired acute and convalescent sera taken 2 to 4 weeks apart are needed.[5]

Serological and rapid tests for human influenza A may not recognize avian influenza viruses (such as influenza A H5N1).

Diagnosis in Animals

Animal influenza is diagnosed based on clinical signs and laboratory test results. Antigen can be recovered from respiratory secretions in horses, swine, and dogs the first few days after disease onset. Optimal specimens include nasal secretions and lung tissue from swine, nasopharyngeal swabs from horses, nasal swabs from dogs, and oropharyngeal swabs from birds. Serological testing is another valuable diagnostic tool in animals. Acute and convalescent samples taken 2 weeks apart are needed.

In poultry, samples of oropharyngeal and cloacal swabs are preferred for diagnosis. In the United States, matrix gene real-time reverse transcriptase polymerase chain reaction (RRT-PCR) is used to identify influenza A virus and all positives are further tested by H5 and H7 specific RRT-PCR. The hemagglutinin proteolytic cleavage site is sequenced for all H5 or H7 RRT-PCR+ samples to determine LP or HP. The avian influenza virus detection is confirmed by virus isolation in 9- to 11-day embryonating chicken eggs. All influenza A viruses are subtyped by hemagglutination-inhibition (HI) and neuraminidase-inhibition (NI) tests and pathotyped by in vivo chicken pathogenicity testing. Serological monitoring of poultry is done using commercial ELISA and agar gel immunodiffusion (AGID) tests for influenza A, and positives are subtyped by HI and NI tests.

Treatment

Treatment in Humans

Four antiviral medications—amantadine, rimantadine, oseltamivir (Tamiflu), and zanamivir (Relenza)—are approved by FDA for influenza treatment.[39] The first two are not currently recommended because of the widespread presence of antiviral resistance in influenza A (H3N2) viruses and lack of activity against influenza B. The latter two drugs are neuraminidase inhibitors with activity against both influenza A and B viruses. Early treatment reduces illness severity and risk of complications leading to antibiotic use. In hospitalized adults, oseltamivir treatment appears to reduce the likelihood of influenza-related mortality. Antiviral resistance also occurs to the neuraminidase inhibitors, and during the 2007-08 Northern Hemisphere season, community circulation of oseltamivir-resistant H1N1 viruses was noted for the first time.

Treatment should be started as soon as possible after disease onset. Oseltamivir is approved for treatment of people 1 year of age and older. Zanamivir is approved for treatment of people 7 years of age and older. Both drugs can also be used as chemoprophylaxis with a disease prevention efficacy ranging from 70% to 90%. Zanamivir is not recommended for persons with underlying airways disease (e.g., asthma or chronic obstructive pulmonary disease). Table 9-36 outlines treatment guidelines for symptomatic disease in humans.

Treatment in Animals

Treatment of influenza in horses, dogs, and pigs is generally supportive. Antivirals as listed above for humans are not approved for treatment of animal infections, in part due to concern about development of drug resistance.

Table 9-36 ■ Treatment Guidelines for Symptomatic Influenza Disease in Humans

Antiviral Agent		Age Group (yr)					
		1-6	7-9	10-12	13-64	≥65	
Zanamivir*	Treatment, influenza A and B	N/A†	10 mg (2 inhalations) twice daily				
	Chemoprophylaxis, influenza A and B	Ages 1-4 N/A	Ages 5-9 10 mg (2 inhalations) once daily	10 mg (2 inhalations) once daily			
Oseltamivir	Treatment,‡ influenza A and B	Dose varies by child's weight§			75 mg twice daily		
	Chemoprophylaxis, influenza A and B	Dose varies by child's weight‖			75 mg/day		

NOTE: Zanamivir is manufactured by GlaxoSmithKline (Relenza—inhaled powder). Zanamivir is approved for treatment of persons 7 years and older and approved for chemoprophylaxis of persons 5 years and older. Oseltamivir is manufactured by Roche Pharmaceuticals (Tamiflu—tablet). Oseltamivir is approved for treatment or chemoprophylaxis of persons 1 year and older. No antiviral medications are approved for treatment or chemoprophylaxis of influenza among children younger than 1 year. This information is based on data published by the CDC (http://www.cdc.gov/h1n1flu/recommendations.htm).
*Zanamivir is administrated through oral inhalation by using a plastic device included in the medication package. Patients will benefit from instruction and demonstration of the correct use of the device. Zanamivir is not recommended for those persons with underlying airway disease.
†Not applicable.
‡A reduction in the dose of oseltamivir is recommended for persons with creatinine clearance less than 30 mL/min.
§The treatment dosing recommendation for children weighing 15 kg or less is 30 mg twice a day; for children weighing more than 15 kg and up to 23 kg, the dose is 45 mg twice a day; for children weighing >15-23 kg, the dose is 45 mg twice a day; for children weighing >23-40 kg, the dose is 60 mg twice a day; and for children >40 kg, the dose is 75 mg twice a day.
‖The chemoprophylaxis dosing recommendation for children weighing 15 kg or less is 30 mg once a day; for children weighing >15-23 kg, the dose is 45 mg once a day; for children weighing >23-40 kg, the dose is 60 mg once a day; and for children >40 kg, the dose is 75 mg once a day. From http://www.cdc.gov/flu/professionals/antivirals/dosage.htm#table.

References

1. Treanor JT. Influenza Virus. In: Mandell GL, Bennett JE, Dolin R, eds. *Principles and practice of infectious diseases.* 5th ed. Churchill Livingstone; 2000:1823–1849.
2. Centers for Disease Control and Prevention. *Key Facts about Seasonal Influenza (Flu).* http://www.cdc.gov/flu/keyfacts.htm. Accessed May 14, 2009.
3. Thacker E, Janke B. Swine influenza virus: zoonotic potential and vaccination strategies for the control of avian and swine influenza. *J Infect Dis.* 2008;197:S19–S24.
4. Government of Saskatchewan. *Influenza H1N1.* http://www.agriculture.gov.sk.ca/H1N1_Influenza. Accessed May 14, 2009.
5. Fiore AE, Shay DK, Broder K, et al. Prevention and control of seasonal influenza with vaccines: recommendations of the Advisory Committee on Iummunization Practices (ACIP) 2009. *MMWR.* 2009;581-52 Available at http://www.cdc.gov/mmwr/preview/mmwrhtml/rr58e0724a1.htm.
6. Gray GC, Baker WS. The importance of including swine and poultry workers in influenza vaccination programs. *Clin Pharmacol Ther.* 2007;82(6):638–641.
7. Elchos BL, Scheftel JM, et al. Compendium of veterinary standard precautions for zoonotic disease prevention in veterinary personnel. *J Am Vet Med Assoc.* 2008;233(3):415–432.
8. American Association of Equine Practitioners Influenza virus vaccination guidelines. http://www.aaep.org/equine_influenza.htm. Accessed November 1, 2009.
9. Knipe DM, Howley DM, eds. *Fields virology.* 5th ed. Philadelphia: Lippincott Williams & Wilkins; 2007.
10. Capua I, Marangon S. Control of avian influenza in poultry. *Emerg Infect Dis.* 2006;12(9):1319.
11. Gabriel G, Dauber B, Wolff T, et al. The viral polymerase mediates adaptation of an avian influenza virus to a mammalian host. *Proc Natl Acad Sci U S A.* 2005;102(51):18590.
12. Smith GJ, Naipospos TS, Nguyen TD, et al. Evolution and adaptation of H5N1 influenza virus in avian and human hosts in Indonesia and Vietnam. *Virology.* 2006;350(2):258.
13. Mubareka S, Palese P. The biology of a changing virus. In: Rappuoli R, Del Giudice G, eds. *Influenza vaccines of the future.* SpringerLink; 2008:9–30.
14. World Health Organization: *Avian influenza.* http://www.oie.int/eng/normes/mmanual/2008/pdf/2.03.04_AI.pdf. Accessed November 1, 2009.
15. Centers for Disease Control and Prevention. *Influenza vaccine: a summary for clinicians.* http://www.cdc.gov/flu/professionals/vaccination/vax-summary.htm. Accessed November 1, 2009.
16. Dinh PN, Long HT, Tien NTK, et al. Risk factors for human infection with avian influenza A H5N1, Vietnam, 2004. *Emerg Infect Dis.* 2006;12(12):1841.
17. Gray GC, McCarthy T, Capuano AW, et al. Swine workers and swine influenza virus infections. *Emerg Infect Dis.* 2007;13(12):1871.
18. Rabinowitz P, Perdue M, Mumford E. Contact variables for exposure to avian influenza H5N1 virus at the human-animal interface. *Zoonoses Public Health.* March 26, 2009.
19. Stallknecht DE, Nagy E, Hunter B, et al. Avian influenza. In: Thomas NJ, Hunter DB, Atkinson CT, eds. *Infectious diseases of wild birds.* Wiley-Blackwell; 2007:108–130.
20. Song D, Kong B, Lee C, et al. Transmission of avian influenza virus (H3N2) to dogs. *Emerg Infect Dis.* 2008;14(5):741.
21. Payungporn S, Crawford PC, Kouo TS, et al. Influenza A virus (H3N8) in dogs with respiratory disease, Florida. *Emerg Infect Dis.* 2008;14(6):902.
22. U.S. Geological Survey. *Avian influenza.* http://www.nwhc.usgs.gov/disease_information/avian_influenza/index.jsp.
23. Dawood FS, Jain S, et al. Emergence of a novel swine-origin influenza A (H1N1) virus in humans. *N Eng J Med.* 2009;361.
24. Merck Veterinary Manual. *Swine influenza.* http://www.merckvetmanual.com/mvm/index.jsp?cfile=htm/bc/121407.htm. Accessed November 1, 2009.
25. Merck Veterinary Manual. *Avian influenza: introduction.* http://www.merckvetmanual.com/mvm/index.jsp?cfile=htm/bc/206200.htm. Accessed November 1, 2009.
26. Centers for Disease Control and Prevention. *Influenza symptoms and laboratory diagnostic procedures.* http://www.cdc.gov/flu/professionals/diagnosis/labprocedures.htm. Accessed November 1, 2009.
27. Centers for Disease Control and Prevention. *Avian influenza A virus infections of humans.* http://www.cdc.gov/flu/avian/gen-info/avian-flu-humans.htm. Accessed November 1, 2009.
28. Center for Food Safety and Public Health. *Influenza.* http://www.cfsph.iastate.edu/Factsheets/pdfs/influenza.pdf. Accessed November 1, 2009.
29. World Organization for Animal Health. *Avian influenza.* In *Terrestrial Animal Health Code, Article 2.7.12.1, Paris.* Available at: http://www.oie.int/eng/normes/mcode/en_chapitre_2.7.12.htm.
30. Swayne DL, Halvorson DA. Influenza. In: Saif YM, ed. *Diseases of poultry.* 11th ed. Aimes, IA: Iowa State University Press; 2003:135–161.
31. Choi YK, Lee JH, Erickson G, et al. H3N2 influenza virus transmission from swine to turkeys, United States. *Emerg Infect Dis.* 2004;10(12):2156.
32. Wright SM, Kawaoka Y, Sharp GB, et al. Interspecies transmission and reassortment of influenza A viruses in pigs and turkeys in the United States. *Am J Epidemiol.* 1992;136(4):488.
33. Reference deleted in proofs.
34. Merck Veterinary Manual. *Equine influenza.* http://www.merckvetmanual.com/mvm/index.jsp?cfile=htm/bc/121303.htm&word=equine%2cinfluenza. Accessed November 1, 2009.

35. American Veterinary Medical Association. *Influenza updates from the AVMA.* http://www.avma.org/public_health/influenza/canine_bgnd.asp. Accessed November 1, 2009.
36. Marschall J, Hartmann K. Avian influenza A H5N1 infections in cats. *J Feline Med Surg.* 2008;10(4):359–365.
37. Cornell University College of Veterinary Medicine. *Canine influenza virus.* http://www.diaglab.vet.cornell.edu/issues/civ.asp. Accessed November 1, 2009.
38. Centers of Disease Control and Prevention. *Rapid diagnostic testing for influenza.* http://www.cdc.gov/flu/professionals/diagnosis/rapidclin.htm. Accessed November 1, 2009.
39. Centers of Disease Control and Prevention. *Recommended daily dosage of seasonal influenza antiviral medications for treatment and chemoprophylaxis—United States.* http://www.cdc.gov/flu/professionals/antivirals/dosage.htm#table. Accessed November 1, 2009.

LEISHMANIASIS

Peter M. Rabinowitz and Lisa A. Conti

Cutaneous leishmaniasis (ICD-10 B55.1, B55.2)

Other names in humans: Aleppo ulcer, Baghdad or Delhi boil, Oriental sore, Espundia, uta, chiclero ulcer

Visceral leishmaniasis (ICD-10 B55.0)

Other names in humans: kala-azar

Other names in animals: canine visceral leishmaniasis

Leishmaniasis caused by infection with protozoans in the genus *Leishmania* causes millions of infections each year around the world. The infection takes two basic forms: cutaneous and visceral, but disease syndromes may overlap. The severity of human infection ranges from mild skin lesions to severe disfiguring facial involvement or systemic disease with organ failure and death. This zoonotic disease is transmitted by insect vectors, usually of the phlebotomine sand fly family. Leishmaniasis has been transmitted directly from dog to dog in the United States. Worldwide risk of leishmaniasis is increasing in both humans and animals. Factors responsible may include the transboundary movement of humans and animals, global climate change affecting the distribution of vectors, the HIV epidemic,[1] and increasing contact of humans with wilderness areas where the disease is endemic. In addition to being a disease of travelers returning to the United States, there is an expanding focus of human cases of leishmaniasis in Texas, as well as an ongoing outbreak of canine visceral leishmaniasis in foxhounds in the eastern United States. The complex interrelationships of leishmaniasis infection in animals and humans demand ongoing cooperation between animal and human health professionals to detect new cases and better control this challenging disease.

Key Points for Clinicians and Public Health Professionals

Public Health Professionals

- Characterize the risk in the community, including whether the sand fly vector is present and if there is evidence of transmission to humans or domestic animals.
- Educate human health providers that infection could be spread through shared needles.
- Conduct an immediate investigation of a human or veterinary case to determine whether it is related to travel or local transmission.
- In endemic areas, develop a strategy with vector specialists for vector control based on local ecology and transmission patterns. Interventions may include targeted spraying in suspected sand fly habitat, including around doorways of dwellings (if residential transmission suspected), stone walls, animal houses, and garbage dumps.
- In endemic areas where dogs are serving as a reservoir, work with animal control authorities on effective strategies including use of insecticide-impregnated collars. Culling of dog populations has not been proven effective in some areas.[2]
- Ensure that travelers to endemic areas take steps to avoid sand fly bites. Use insect repellent and permethrin-impregnated bed nets and protective clothing.[2]

Human Health Clinicians

- Consider the diagnosis in all patients with a history of recent travel or residence in an endemic area.
- Immediately report disease to public health authorities.
- Counsel travelers to endemic areas about risk reduction in terms of avoiding sand fly bites (see above).

Veterinary Clinicians

- Consider the diagnosis in dogs in the United States, especially foxhounds, who present with constitutional signs.
- Consider the diagnosis in equids with nonhealing cutaneous lesions on the head.
- Counsel clients not to let cats and dogs roam outside and to provide insect repellent for horses in endemic areas.
- Increase index of suspicion of leishmaniasis in animals with a travel history to the Mideast, tropics, or subtropics or with previous blood transfusion.
- Be aware that autochthonous transmission of visceral canine leishmaniasis has occurred in the United States in the absence of insect vectors.[3]
- Vaccine trial work shows promise for use in endemic areas.[4]
- Treat infected dogs using the CDC protocol through the state public health veterinarian. Canine leishmaniasis may be reportable to your state health or agriculture department.

Agent

At least 20 species in the genus *Leishmania* are pathogenic in humans, and are found in a range of mammalian reservoirs and vectors. *Leishmania* are obligate intracellular protozoan parasites, with virulence and types of disease varying between the strains.[5] Visceral leishmaniasis is caused by *L. donovani*, *L. infantum*, and *L. chagasi*. In the United States, *L. mexicana* is the cause of cutaneous leishmaniasis in Texas. In Latin America, *L. braziliensis* causes a more aggressive form of cutaneous leishmaniasis.[6]

Geographical Occurrence

Leishmaniasis occurs in 88 countries, mainly in the tropics and subtropics, with varying patterns of disease and ecological relationships (the disease has not been reported in Australia and Oceania). In the United States, most cases are seen in travelers and their pets returning from endemic regions. There is a small focus of cases of cutaneous leishmaniasis in Texas that appears to be extending northward.[6]

Cutaneous leishmaniasis due to *L. braziliensis* and *L. mexicana* complexes occurs in Latin American countries with the exception of Chile and Uruguay. In the Eastern Hemisphere, cutaneous leishmaniasis is caused by *L. tropica*, *L. major*, and *L. aethiopica*; hotspots include the Indian subcontinent, China, southwestern Asia including Afghanistan and Iran, the Mediterranean region, and sub-Saharan Africa including Sudan.

In the New World, visceral leishmaniasis in humans is due to infection with *L. infantum* and *L. chagasi* and is found across Central and South America. In the Old World, *L. donovani* is the principal cause of visceral leishmaniasis, which occurs in mostly rural areas of India, Bangladesh, China, Nepal, Pakistan, southern regions of the former Soviet Union, the Middle East and Mediterranean, and sub-Saharan and East Africa.[2]

In the United States, *L. infantum* seroprevalence studies of dog kennels have identified positive results in 21 states.

Groups at Risk

Groups at increased risk for leishmaniasis include individuals who encounter the sand fly vector, including forest workers and rural residents. In areas where visceral leishmaniasis is endemic and the sand fly vector is found, dog ownership can be a risk factor for infection.[7]

Hosts, Reservoir Species, Vectors

The vectors and reservoir hosts of leishmaniasis are diverse and vary in part by geographical region and agent. Phlebotomine sand flies are most active dusk through dawn and difficult to see as they are about one third of the size of a mosquito.

In the Americas, New World cutaneous leishmaniasis has zoonotic transmission through bites of a number of sand fly species; mammalian hosts include small rodents and larger mammals. In Texas, the burrowing wood rat (*Neotoma micropus*) is the apparent reservoir for cutaneous leishmaniasis. Zoonotic Old World cutaneous leishmaniasis caused

by *L. major* is spread by bites of the sand fly *Phlebotomus papatasis*.[5] A major reservoir is gerbils (*Meriones unguiculatus*). Hyraxes (*Procavia capensis*) are another mammalian host. Although dogs can be infected, they do not always serve as a competent reservoir for cutaneous leishmaniasis. A human-to-human transmission cycle of cutaneous leishmaniasis in the Old World due to *L. tropica* is spread by *P. sergenti*.

Lutzomyia species sand flies spread visceral leishmaniasis in the New World, whereas *L. donovani* is spread person to person in the Indian subcontinent and Eastern Africa by a number of sand fly species. Dogs and wild canids (foxes and jackals) are the principal animal reservoir for visceral leishmaniasis.[5]

Mode of Transmission and Life Cycle

Transmission is largely vector-borne through bites of the female phlebotomine sand fly injecting the infective, flagellated promastigote forms into the skin of a vertebrate host (Figure 9-68). The parasite then transforms into the non-flagellated amastigote (Color Plate 9-35) and multiplies within macrophages throughout the host's reticuloendothelial system. The vector cycle is complete with sand fly infection from the vertebrate host, where the organisms multiply extracellularly in the sand fly gut over 8 to 20 days to produce infectious promastigotes (see Figure 9-68).[5]

Once infected, a mammalian host appears to retain the ability to be infectious to others even after treatment. The agent may remain dormant in the host animal for years, and then infection can recur when immune status declines, such as in HIV infection, malnutrition, or administration of immunosuppressive drugs for organ transplants or other conditions. Chronically infected individuals, even after receiving treatment, can serve as a reservoir for further infection of sand fly vectors. In addition to vector-borne transmission, person-to-person transmission has been reported through blood transfusions and the sharing of needles between IV drug users.

In an outbreak of canine visceral leishmaniasis among U.S. foxhounds, transmission occurred dog to dog (but not dog to person) through direct contact with blood and secretions and transplacentally from an infected bitch to her pups. There is no evidence of vector transmission to dogs in the United States, and sand flies are not found in many of the regions where dogs are infected.[8] However, in areas where both visceral leishmaniais in dogs and sand flies occur, there is a potential risk of future episodes of vector-borne transmission from dogs to humans.

Environmental Risk Factors

Key environmental factors include the population of reservoir hosts and the population of vectors. Sand fly populations may increase with availability of breeding sites and humid areas around ponds or in tree holes. Factors that increase contact between humans and vectors and reservoirs have been tied to outbreaks, including deforestation and encroachment of human habitation into forested areas. Climate change appears to be playing a role in the extension of the ranges of some vectors and animal reservoirs.

Leishmaniasis
(Leishmania spp.)

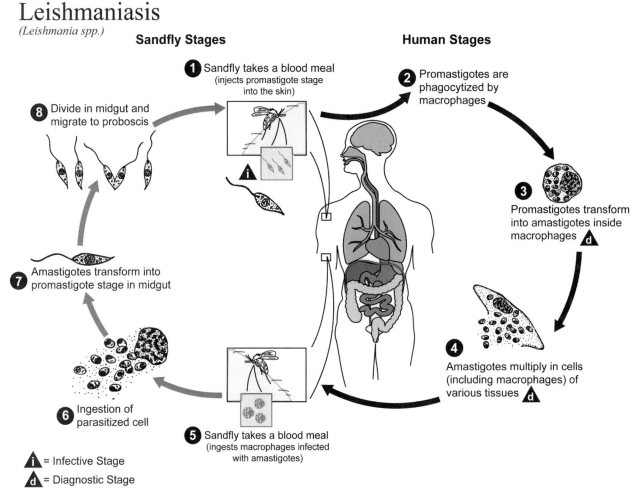

Figure 9-68 ■ Life cycle of *Leishmania* species, the causal agents of leishmaniasis. (From Centers for Disease Control and Prevention Public Health Image Library, Atlanta, Ga. Courtesy Alexander J. da Silva and Melanie Moser.)

Disease in Humans

Table 9-37 provides clinical presentations of leishmaniasis.

Cutaneous Leishmaniasis

Each year cutaneous leishmaniasis occurs in approximately 1.5 million people worldwide. Cutaneous involvement of leishmaniasis infection can take a number of forms, depending on the species involved and the immune status of the host.

Simple *cutaneous* leishmaniasis often begins with a small macule at the site of the fly bite that progresses to a papule. The papule enlarges over time and may ulcerate.[9] In many cases, the lesions resolve spontaneously over a period of months or years (Color Plate 9-36).

Diffuse cutaneous leishmaniasis tends not to ulcerate but instead spreads gradually through the skin, causing chronic nodular lesions especially on the face and extremities. It may be a lifelong infection.

Atypical cutaneous leishmaniasis in Central America caused by *L. infantum* or *L. chagasi* is characterized by cheloid-type lesions without ulceration.[2]

Leishmaniasis recidivans caused by *L. tropica* occurs in Iran and other parts of central Asia. The tuberculoid lesions tend to involve the face, spreading outward and often relapsing. It also tends to be a chronic infection lasting for decades.[9]

Mucocutaneous leishmaniasis due to *L. braziliensis* or related species can develop in individuals years after the lesions of cutaneous leishmaniasis have healed. The symptoms may begin with nasal stuffiness but progress to respiratory and swallowing difficulties as tissue destruction involves the nose, mouth, and laryngopharyngeal regions (Color Plate 9-37).

Visceral Leishmaniasis

Visceral leishmaniasis (kala-azar), occurring in about a half million people each year, is usually due to infection with either *L. donovani* or *L. infantum*. This disease is characterized by systemic signs such as fever and weight loss. Hepatosplenomegaly, pancytopenia, and increased gamma-globulins can occur. Lymphadenopathy and abnormal liver function test results are common. In India, hyperpigmentation is part of the clinical syndrome. Although many cases resolve spontaneously, malnutrition and immunocompromised

Table 9-37 ▪ Leishmaniasis: Clinical Presentations in Humans and Other Animals

Species	Risk Factors	Incubation Period	Clinical Manifestations	Laboratory Findings
Humans				
Simple cutaneous leishmaniasis	Exposure to sand flies, malnutrition, immunosuppression, proximity to reservoir habitat	At least a week, may be many months[2]	Macule progressing to papule with ulceration	Biopsy of lesion may demonstrate intracellular amastigotes; positive leishmanin skin test
Diffuse cutaneous leishmaniasis		At least a week, may be many months[2]	Nodular lesions spreading slowly on face and extremities	
Leishmaniasis recidivans		Develops over months to years	Relapsing lesions on face with central healing	
Mucocutaneous leishmaniasis			Tissue destruction of nose, oropharynx	
Visceral leishmaniasis		Typically 2-6 months, range 10 days to years[2]	Weight loss, fever, hepatosplenomegaly	Anemia, leukopenia, thrombocytopenia, elevated liver function tests, biopsy may show amastigotes
Dogs	Exposure to sand flies, crowding, receipt of blood products from infected donors, parturition (?)	3 months to years	May be subclinical; hyperkeratosis, chapping, weight loss, anorexia, fever, visceral involvement including renal failure	Proteinuria, elevated liver function tests Tissue biopsy and culture
Cats, Horses	Exposure to sand flies	3 months to years	Skin nodules on head	Biopsy may reveal organisms

condition predispose patients to more severe disease and the risk of fatal complications. A post–kala-azar cutaneous leishmaniasis can occur in recovered individuals. These lesions can be a reservoir for continued transmission through sand fly bites.

Disease in Animals

Dogs tend to develop systemic, visceral, and cutaneous involvement (Figures 9-69 and 9-70). Weight loss, anorexia and fever are common. Splenomegaly and lymphadenopathy occur in up to a third of affected dogs. Epistaxis, muscle atrophy, and seizures can also occur (Color Plate 9-38). The skin lesions tend to present as hyperkeratosis and chapping over the head, muzzle, and footpads. These lesions can ulcerate. Renal failure is the most common cause of death and is preceded by nausea and vomiting. Laboratory findings include hyperproteinemia, proteinuria, and elevated liver function test results.[10]

Infection in cats and horses is less common than in dogs and principally involves the skin, typically presenting with nodules on the ears (Color Plate 9-39 and Figure 9-71).[10]

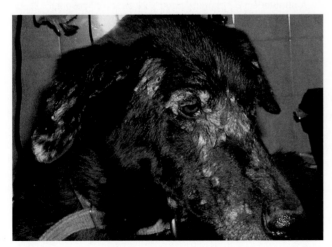

Figure 9-69 ▪ Canine leishmaniasis showing exfoliative dermatitis and scaling on face. (From Greene CE: *Infectious diseases of the dog and cat*, ed 3, St Louis, 2006, Saunders Elsevier.)

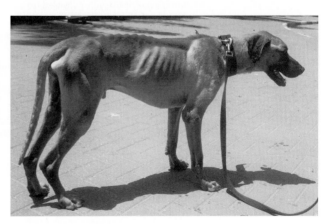

Figure 9-70 ▪ Dog with characteristic features of leishmaniasis. Note cachexia, muscle atrophy, and excessive scaling. (From Greene CE: *Infectious diseases of the dog and cat*, ed 3, St Louis, 2006, Saunders Elsevier.)

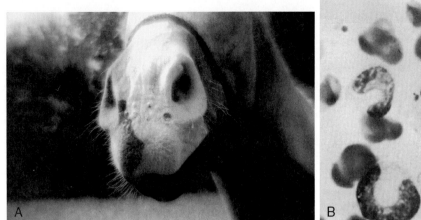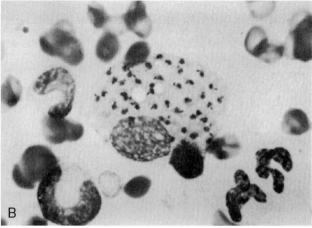

Figure 9-71   ▪   Leishmaniasis. **A,** Nonhealing ulcer on muzzle. **B,** Macrophage containing numerous amastigotes (Leishman-Donovan bodies). (From Scott DW, Miller WH Jr: *Equine dermatology,* St Louis, 2003, Saunders Elsevier. *A,* Courtesy A. Sales; *B,* Courtesy T. French.)

Diagnosis

The differential diagnosis of cutaneous leishmaniasis in humans can be broad and includes sporotrichosis, cutaneous tuberculosis or atypical mycobacterial infection, blastomycosis, sarcoidosis, syphilis, and neoplasia.

The presence of suggestive lesions in the setting of a potential contact such as history of travel to an endemic area should lead one to consider the diagnosis. Definitive diagnosis is often accomplished by a biopsy of the lesion with tissue identification of amastigotes or culture of promastigotes.[9] The leishmanin skin test result is often positive in simple cutaneous leishmaniasis. PCR techniques are in development.[11]

Visceral leishmaniasis in endemic areas can be confused with other causes of fever, chronic weight loss, and splenomegaly such as malaria and schistosomiasis. The diagnosis can be made by isolating amastigotes from macrophages in a bone marrow biopsy or a splenic biopsy. The latter is considered more sensitive but involves a risk of hemorrhage.[9]

In animals, a skin biopsy can reveal the presence of intracellular organisms. Serology with IFA or ELISA is available but cross-reactions with *Trypanosoma cruzi* can occur. Biopsies of skin, spleen, bone marrow, or lymph nodes can be cultured; smears of these samples may reveal the organism.[10] A PCR test is available at some academic institutions.[12]

Table 9-38 ▪ Treatment of Leishmaniasis Infection in Humans and Other Animals

Species	Primary Treatment	Alternative Treatment
Humans (Adult)		
Cutaneous: New World*	Sodium stibogluconate (Pentostam) (available through CDC) *or* meglumine antimoniate 20 mg/kg IV/IM/day in 2 divided doses × 28 days[14]	Amphotericin B 1 mg/kg IV qod × 20 doses *or* liposomal amphotericin 3 mg/kg/day × 6 days (simple cutaneous) *or* 3 weeks (mucocutaneous) *or* miltefosine 2.5 mg/kg PO qd × 28 days[14]
Cutaneous: Old World*	Stibogluconate or meglumine 20 mg/kg/day IV × 10 days[14]	
Visceral*	Liposomal amphotericin 3 mg/kg/day IV once daily days 1-5, then day 14 and 21[14] WHO regimen: 10 mg/kg IV on 2 consecutive days[14]	Stibogluconate or meglumine 20 mg/kg/day IV once daily × 28 days *or* miltefosine 2.5 mg/kg PO qd × 28 days[14]
Dogs	Sodium stibogluconate (Pentostam) 30-50 mg/kg IV/SC q24h × 30 days (available through CDC)	Allopurinol 10 mg/kg PO q8h × 3-24 months (long-term maintenance), works best when combined with amphotericin B 0.25-0.5 mg/kg IV q48h until total cumulative dose of 5-10 mg/kg
Cats	Pinnectomy	Meglumine antimoniate 5 mg/kg SC with 10 mg/kg ketoconazole PO, 4-wk course followed by no therapy for 10 days, repeated three times (used successfully to treat cutaneous lesions in one cat)[15]
Horses	Observation for lesion resolution, pinnectomy	

*Management complex; resistance varies by region; infectious disease consultation recommended.

Treatment

Treatment in humans may involve an often prolonged course of treatment with a variety of agents. The medical management of leishmaniasis is complicated and drug resistance varies by region; therefore infectious disease consultation is advisable. Table 9-38 outlines some currently recommended therapeutic regimens.[14]

In dogs, no drug has been consistently curative. Relapses and the repeated need for treatment are common, although maintenance therapy can reduce parasitemia and reduce the likelihood of transmission.[10]

References

1. World Health Organization. *Leishmaniais and HIV coinfection.* http://www.who.int/leishmaniasis/burden/hiv_coinfection/burden_hiv_coinfection/en/index.html. Accessed August 23, 2008.
2. Heymann DL. *Control of communicable diseases manual.* 19th ed. Washington DC: American Public Health Association; 2008.
3. Schantz PM, Steurer FJ, Duprey ZH, et al. Autochthonous visceral leishmaniasis in dogs in North America. *J Am Vet Med Assoc.* 2005;226(8):1316.
4. Lemesre JM, Holzmuller P, Gonçalves RB, et al. Long-lasting protection against canine visceral leishmaniasis using the LiESAp-MDP vaccine in endemic areas of France: double-blind randomised efficacy field trial. *Vaccine.* 2007;25(21):4223.
5. Desjeux P. Leishmaniasis: current situation and new perspectives. *Comp Immunol Microbiol Infect Dis.* 2004;27(5):305.
6. Wright NA, Davis LE, Aftergut KS, et al. Cutaneous leishmaniasis in Texas: a northern spread of endemic areas. *J Am Acad Dermatol.* 2008;58(4):650.
7. Miró G, Cardoso L, Pennisi MG, et al. Canine leishmaniasis—new concepts and insights on an expanding zoonosis: part two. *Trends Parasitol.* 2008;24(8):371.
8. Duprey ZH, Steurer FJ, Rooney JA, et al. Canine visceral leishmaniasis, United States and Canada, 2000–2003. *Emerg Infect Dis.* 2006;12(3):440.
9. Mandell GE, Bennett JE, Dolin R. *Principles and practice of infectious diseases.* 6th ed. Philadelphia: Churchill Livingstone; 2000.
10. Barr SC, Bowman DD. *The 5-minute veterinary consult clinical companion canine and feline infectious disease and parasitology.* Blackwell; 2006.
11. Weigle KA, Labrada LA, Lozano C, et al. PCR-based diagnosis of acute and chronic cutaneous leishmaniasis caused by *Leishmania (Viannia).* J Clin Microbiol. 2002;40(2):601.
12. North Carolina State College of Veterinary Medicine Veterinary Teaching Hospital. Tick borne diagnostic laboratory. http://www.cvm.ncsu.edu/vth/ticklab.html. Accessed August 23, 2008.
13. Sundar S, Jha TK, Thakur CP, et al. Oral miltefosine for Indian visceral leishmaniasis. *Trans R Soc Trop Med Hyg.* 2006;100(suppl 1):S26.
14. Gilbert DN, Moellering RC, Eliopoulos GM, et al. *Sanford guide to antimicrobial therapy 2009.* 39th ed. Antimicrobial Therapy 2009.
15. Greene CE. *Infectious diseases of the dog and cat.* 3rd ed. St Louis: Saunders Elsevier; 2006.

LEPTOSPIROSIS

Peter M. Rabinowitz and Lisa A. Conti

Leptospirosis ictohemorrhagica (ICD-10 A27.0), Other forms of leptospirosis (A27.8)

Other names in humans: Weil's disease, mud fever, swamp fever, rice field fever, swineherd disease

Other names in animals: redwater of calves, moon blindness (ophthalmia periodica) of horses, Stuttgart disease, canicola disease in dogs

Although leptospirosis is considered a rare disease in the United States, it is one of the most prevalent and important zoonotic diseases worldwide.[1] The epidemiology of this emerging infection appears to be changing due to climate and manmade alterations in the environment. Contamination of water supplies by infected animals is a major source of human exposure, underscoring the importance of waterborne infectious disease risks. The occurrence of leptospirosis in dogs and wildlife living near human habitation and the fact that it is capable of causing both serious disease and outbreaks among groups with high-risk exposure argue for greater awareness of this disease among human and animal health professionals.

Key Points for Clinicians and Public Health Professionals

Public Health Professionals

- Provide descriptive epidemiology of the disease in animal and human populations.
- Educate the public on modes of transmissions (e.g., do not allow animals to drink from contaminated water bodies, maintain good hygiene at kennels and in livestock birthing areas, control rodents).
- Support rodent control efforts in the community.
- Educate local veterinary and human health clinicians in endemic areas about prevention strategies targeted to groups at risk.
- Educate occupational health providers regarding risk groups and how to recognize signs and symptoms of disease.
- Ensure that workers at risk are using appropriate PPE.
- Disinfect with 1% sodium hypochlorite, 70% ethanol, glutaraldehyde, detergents and acid. The organism is killed by pasteurization and moist heat (121° C for 15 minutes).[2]

Human Health Clinicians

- Screen patients for occupational, recreational, housing, and animal (pet and livestock) exposures.
- Treat and report cases to health department if reportable in state.
- Counsel patients on measures to reduce risk of transmission to other humans (direct transmission is rare but possible; e.g., during sexual intercourse and breastfeeding) and from animals (e.g., hygiene regarding urine, reduce rodent exposure).
- Ask patients/family members about any observed illness in pets or other nearby animals; communicate with veterinary professionals animal cases are suspected.
- Counsel immunocompromised patients about risks from animal and environmental contact.

- No human vaccine is available in the United States.
- Exposure prophylaxis: In evaluating an individual who has been exposed to leptospirosis through occupational or environmental contact, consider antibiotics for prophylaxis. A systematic review concluded that prophylactic treatment with doxycycline 200 mg PO weekly for individuals at high risk of exposure (such as individuals training in jungle conditions during the rainy season) was superior to placebo in preventing cases of infection. (evidence-based recommendation: strength B).[3]

Veterinary Clinicians

- Segregate and treat infected animals.
- Vaccinate at-risk dogs and cattle and pigs. Vaccination does not protect against the carrier state. Annual vaccination in closed herds, semiannual vaccination in open herds.[4]
- Counsel owners and veterinary staff about ways to reduce zoonotic risks (precautions with animal urine and other body fluids) and symptoms of disease in humans, advise them to contact medical providers if suspect human cases.
- If veterinary staff experiences occupational exposure to infected animal, consult occupational or infectious disease provider regarding follow-up and possible antibiotic prophylaxis.
- If treating an infected pet, counsel family members regarding zoonotic risk and to contact their health care provider for further advice. Consider directly contacting the medical care provider, especially when immunocompromised patients are in the household or otherwise in contact with an animal case.
- Report animal cases to appropriate animal health authority if indicated in state.

Agent

Leptospirosis is caused by gram-negative spirochete bacteria in the genus *Leptospira*. Based on molecular analysis, there are believed to be at least 13 different species of *Leptospira* and more than 250 serovars.[5] These species and serovars vary widely in pathogenicity. Leptospires can be cultured in polysorbate-albumin media (Figure 9-72).[5]

Geographical Occurrence

Leptospirosis is considered an emerging infectious disease and one of the most common global zoonoses[1]; it is found worldwide except in the polar regions. It is highly prevalent in tropical countries with areas of high rainfall and alkaline soils.[6] The CDC has removed leptospirosis from the list of nationally reportable diseases, and estimates that 1 to 200 cases are identified yearly in the United States (50% of cases occur in Hawaii).[7] However, recent outbreaks and sporadic cases in the United States suggest that leptospirosis remains underdiagnosed and underreported in animals and humans, and that many U.S. health care providers are unfamiliar with the epidemiology and clinical presentation of this disease, which is capable of causing severe morbidity and (rarely) death.

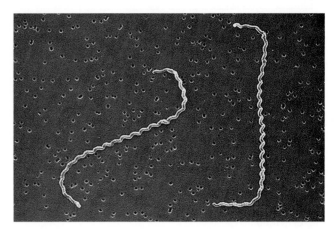

Figure 9-72 ■ Scanning electron micrograph of *Leptospira interrogans* showing helical structure and curved (hooked) ends (original magnification ×60,000). (From Mandell GL, Bennett JE, Dolin R (eds): *Principles and practice of infectious diseases*, ed 6, Philadelphia, 2005, Churchill Livingstone Elsevier. Courtesy of Rob Weyant, Centers for Disease Control and Prevention, Atlanta, Ga.)

Groups at Risk

Leptospirosis is an important occupational disease risk for farmers, dairy and abattoir (slaughterhouse) workers, butchers, hunters, dog handlers, veterinarians, and other veterinary health providers who have direct contact with animals. Workers with exposure to contaminated water, such as military personnel, rice farmers, fishing industry workers, plumbers, and sewer workers, are also at risk.

Recreational exposure to contaminated water leads to infection in campers, sportsmen, freshwater bathers, and travelers returning from highly endemic countries. Urban slum dwellers with rodent exposure are another risk group and infection has been reported in children who handled infected puppies.[5] In the United States, recent reported cases have occurred among cleanup workers at a Hawaiian university campus where a stream had flooded,[8] a returning traveler who had explored caves in Malaysia,[9] an inner-city hospital patient who had recently swum in a creek,[10] and triathletes and community dwellers who had swum in and ingested water from a contaminated lake.[11]

HIV-infected and other immunocompromised patients are at risk of severe disease.[12]

Hosts, Reservoir Species, Vectors

Hosts who exhibit clinical infection with leptospirosis include humans, dogs (where the incidence is reported to be increasing),[13] horses, cattle,[14] sheep, and swine. *Leptospira* species appear to exist subclinically in a large number of wildlife species, including rats and other rodents, raccoons, opossums, reptiles, and frogs. However, in some wildlife species, such as sea lions, periodic epidemics of clinical disease can occur.[15] In the northeastern United States and Canada increasing rates of infection among reservoir hosts, such as skunks, raccoons, and squirrels, that are common in suburban settings has been reported.[16]

Mode of Transmission and Life Cycle

Leptospira enter the body through breaks in the skin or contact with mucous membranes (Figure 9-73). Humans are commonly infected by exposure to water, moist soil, or food contaminated by urine or secretions, or by direct contact with infected animals. Venereal transmission occurs in swine and has been suspected in humans.[17] Eating infected rodents or other animals can result in infection through mucous membrane contact. Direct person-to-person transmission has been reported between soldiers working in close proximity in swampy areas, and in relation to breastfeeding.[6]

Environmental Risk Factors

Outbreaks in humans and animals have been linked to heavy rains resulting in flooding, moist soils, and standing water. Other environmental risk factors include alkaline soils and alkaline freshwater, rodent infestation, and suburban encroachment on wildlife habitat. A case control study of dogs found that seropositive dogs were more likely to live in periurban environments.[18] Inner-city households with cats have been associated with a decreased risk of leptospirosis, possibly through a reduction in rodent exposure.[19]

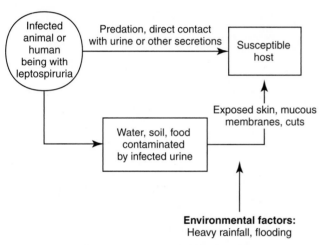

Figure 9-73   ■   Life cycle of leptospirosis.

Disease in Humans

Leptospirosis in humans has protean manifestations, depending in part on the infecting serovar. Infection leads to a systemic vasculitis. The majority of human infections are mild and self-limited; however, in approximately 10% of cases, severe and even fatal illness can develop. The two main severe forms of the disease are Weil's disease (a triad of jaundice, acute renal failure, and bleeding) and severe pulmonary hemorrhagic syndrome (SPHS) (Table 9-39).

After the bacteria enter the body, there is an incubation period of approximately 10 days, followed by the abrupt onset of the leptospiremic phase or febrile phase, which can last 4 to 9 days. In addition to fever, conjunctival suffusion, uveitis, myalgias, and a pretibial rash can be seen. A convalescent (leptospiruric or immune) phase follows. During this period, which often lasts several weeks or longer, secondary transmission may occur through excretion of the leptospires in urine. Aseptic meningitis is a common occurrence during this phase of illness.[5] Figure 9-74 shows the biphasic nature of the illness.

Weil's disease may develop during the immune phase or progress directly from the acute phase of infection. Prominent features include renal failure caused by nephritis, hepatic dysfunction, and thrombocytopenia with hemorrhagic complications.

In some cases, hemorrhagic pneumonitis and severe respiratory distress leading to circulatory collapse can occur without hepatic or renal failure. Mortality is high in severe cases of Weil's disease and SPHS (Color Plate 9-40).

Species	Risk Factors	Incubation Period	Clinical Manifestations	Laboratory Findings
Humans	Exposure to fresh water, flooding, contact with animals	10 days (2-30)[22]	Acute onset of uveitis, conjunctival suffusion, myalgias, fever, renal failure, jaundice	Leukocytosis, liver, renal function test abnormalities
Dogs	Rural/suburban exposure to wildlife, peridomestic rodents, contaminated water	4-12 days[4]	Acute renal failure, fever, depression, lethargy, uveitis	Leukocytosis, renal and liver function test abnormalities, proteinuria, hematuria
Sheep	Rare, exposure to infected animals of other species		Lambs with more severe disease, fever, anorexia	
Horses	Exposure to contaminated urine, water, soil	2-8 months for chronic symptoms	Most asymptomatic[6] Uveitis (moon blindness), abortions	
Cattle			*Calves:* fever anorexia, dyspnea,[4] *Adults:* abortion, stillbirth, hemoglobinuria	
Pigs			Abortions, stillbirth	

Table 9-39 ■ **Leptospirosis: Comparative Clinical Presentations in Humans and Other Animals**

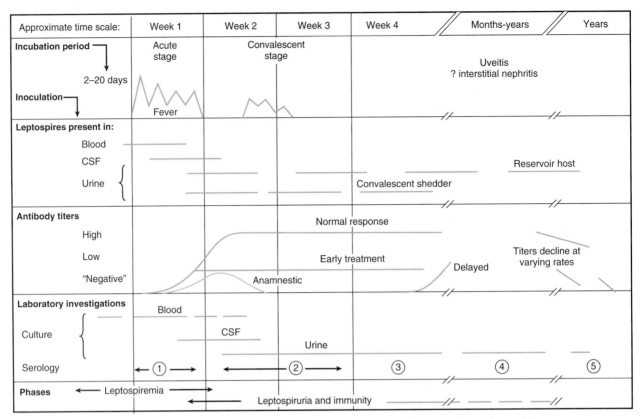

Figure 9-74 ■ Biphasic nature of leptospirosis. The serology numbers refer to specimens taken at different phases of illness to either diagnose acute illness or document chronic or past infection. (From Mandell GL, Bennett JE, Dolin R (eds): *Principles and practice of infectious diseases*, ed 6, Philadelphia, 2005, Churchill Livingstone Elsevier. Adapted from Turner LH: Leptospirosis, *Br Med J* 1:231, and reproduced from Levett PN: Leptospirosis, *Clin Microbiol Rev* 14:296, 2001, with permission of ASM Press.)

Disease in Animals

Although many cases of leptospirosis in dogs are subclinical and chronic, dogs can develop acute disease with fever, anorexia, jaundice, vomiting, and hematuria. Other features of infection can include injected mucous membranes, uveitis, and cough.[20] The most common serious complications in dogs appear to be acute renal failure, vasculitis, and hepatic dysfunction.[21] The disease is much rarer in cats, but similar clinical features to dog leptospirosis may be seen.[20]

Cattle and other livestock including sheep, pigs, and horses can develop either acute or chronic forms of infection. The acute form is more common in young animals and can include fever or respiratory involvement. Adult livestock are more likely to develop the chronic form of the disease and manifest infection as abortion or stillbirth.

The disease is often subclinical in wild animals including rodents. Seals and sea lions may have depression, fever, and abortion.

Diagnosis

The differential diagnosis in humans includes acute causes of fever and jaundice such as hepatitis and malaria. Leptospirosis should be suspected in a patient who presents with exposure risk factors and fever, uveitis/conjunctival suffusion, and abnormal liver and renal function test results. Leptospires can be cultured from blood and cerebrospinal fluid (CSF) during the acute phase of illness and in urine after the first week of illness. Most laboratory diagnosis of human leptospirosis is currently based on serology using the microagglutination test (MAT) or ELISAs. Antibodies develop after about 1 week of illness. The MAT has a high specificity for specific serovars. However, it may lead to underdiagnosis if a person is infected with an unusual serovar not well covered by the standard test. Serial serology titers are required to document seroconversion—a fourfold increase in titer is considered evidence of recent infection.[6] The use of PCR techniques for diagnosing human leptospirosis has been reported.[23]

In animals, the MAT and ELISA are also used; paired sera are preferred. Diagnosis can be affected by a history of immunization, and the results of serology must be interpreted with caution in vaccinated animals. A milk ELISA can be used on a single cow or for bulk tank sampling.

Exposure Prophylaxis

A study of antibiotic prophylaxis for soldiers during jungle military training showed a protective benefit of doxycycline, 200 mg/week, in preventing infection with leptospirosis.[24] Therefore individuals with high-risk exposures for short periods can consider such prophylaxis. However, the efficacy of prophylaxis in other situations, such as after exposure, remains unclear.

Treatment

Antibiotic treatment in people and animals is not always curative but should be started as early in the course of disease

Table 9-40 ▪ Leptospirosis Treatment in Humans and Other Animals

Species	Primary Treatment	Alternative
Humans	Penicillin G 1.5 million units IV q6h *or* ceftriaxone 1 gm q24h × 7 days	Doxycycline 100 mg IV/PO q12h *or* ampicillin 0.5-1 gm IV q6h[27]
Dogs	Doxycycline 5 mg/kg q12h PO/IV × 14 days	Penicillin G 25,000-40,000 units/kg q12h IM/SC/IV × 14 days *or* ampicillin 22 mg/kg PO/IV/SC q6-8h × 14 days *or* amoxicillin 22 mg/kg q8-12h PO × 14 days[20]
Swine	Tetracycline 800 gm/ton of feed × 8-11 days[26]	
Cattle	Tetracycline 40 mg/kg IM qd × 3-5 days, oxytetracycline[4,26]	Amoxicillin 15 mg/kg 1 or 2 (q48h) doses[26]

as possible because of a possible benefit (Table 9-40). Recommended agents include penicillin G, doxycycline, ceftriaxone, and amoxicillin. The serovar may affect the efficacy of the selected antibiotic. Supportive care may be indicated, and hemodialysis is correlated with improved prognosis in severe acute renal failure cases.[25]

References

1. Bharti AR, Nally JE, Ricaldi JN, et al. Peru-United States Leptospirosis Consortium. Leptospirosis: a zoonotic disease of global importance. *Lancet Infect Dis.* 2003;3(12):757.
2. Dvorak G, Rovid-Spickler A, Roth JA, et al. *Handbook for zoonotic diseases of companion animals.* Ames, IA: The Center for Food Security and Public Health, Iowa State University College of Veterinary Medicine; 2008.
3. Guidugli F, Castro AA, Atallah AN. Antibiotics for preventing leptospirosis. *Cochrane Database Syst Rev.* 2000;4.
4. Kahn CM, Line S, eds. *The Merck veterinary manual.* 9th ed. Whitehouse Station, NJ: Merck; 2005.
5. Mandell GL, Bennett JE, Dolin R, eds. *Principles and practice of infectious diseases.* 6th ed. Philadelphia: Churchill Livingstone Elsevier; 2005.
6. Acha PN, Szyfres B. *Zoonoses and communicable diseases common to man and animals: vol. 1: bacterioses and mycoses.* 3rd ed. Washington, DC: Pan American Health Organization; 2001.
7. Centers for Disease Control and Prevention. *Disease listing, leptospirosis, technical information.* http://www.cdc.gov/Ncidod/dbmd/diseaseinfo/leptospirosis_t.htm. Accessed December 5, 2007.
8. Gaynor K, Katz AR, Park SY, et al. Leptospirosis on Oahu: an outbreak associated with flooding of a university campus. *Am J Trop Med Hyg.* 2007;76(5):882.
9. Mortimer RB. Leptospirosis in a caver returned from Sarawak, Malaysia. *Wilderness Environ Med.* 2005;16(3):129.
10. Shaukat A, Pohlel K, Rubin Z, et al. Case of Weil's disease in an inner-city hospital in the USA. *J Gastroenterol Hepatol.* 2004;19(10):1221.
11. Morgan J, Bornstein SL, Karpati AM, et al. Leptospirosis Working Group, Outbreak of leptospirosis among triathlon participants and community residents in Springfield, Illinois, 1998. *Clin Infect Dis.* 2002;34(12):1593.
12. Jones S, Kim T. Fulminant leptospirosis in a patient with human immunodeficiency virus infection: case report and review of the literature. *Clin Infect Dis.* 2001;33(5):e31.
13. Ward MP, Glickman LT, Guptill LE. Prevalence of and risk factors for leptospirosis among dogs in the United States and Canada: 677 cases (1970–1998). *J Am Vet Med Assoc.* 2002;220(1):53.
14. Talpada MD, Garvey N, Sprowls R, et al. Prevalence of leptospiral infection in Texas cattle: implications for transmission to humans. *Vector Borne Zoonotic Dis.* 2003;3(3):141.
15. Lloyd-Smith JO, Greig DJ, Hietala S, et al. Cyclical changes in seroprevalence of leptospirosis in California sea lions: endemic and epidemic disease in one host species. *BMC Infect Dis.* 2007;7:125.
16. Barry M, Wisnewski AV, Matthias MA, et al. Suburban leptospirosis: atypical lymphocytosis and gamma-delta T cell response. *Clin Infect Dis.* 2006;43(10):1304.
17. Harrison NA, Fitzgerald WR. Leptospirosis—can it be a sexually transmitted disease? *Postgrad Med J.* 1988;64(748):163.
18. Ward MP, Guptill LF, Wu CC. Evaluation of environmental risk factors for leptospirosis in dogs: 36 cases (1997–2002). *J Am Vet Med Assoc.* 2004;225(1):72.
19. Childs JE, Schwartz BS, Ksiazek TG, et al. Risk factors associated with antibodies to leptospires in inner-city residents of Baltimore: a protective role for cats. *Am J Public Health.* 1992;82(4):597.
20. Barr SC, Bowman DD. *5-Minute veterinary consult clinical companion canine and feline infectious disease and parasitology.* Ames, IA: Wiley-Blackwell; 2006.
21. Langston CE, Heuter KJ. Leptospirosis: a re-emerging zoonotic disease. *Vet Clin North Am Small Anim Pract.* 2003;33(4):791.
22. Heymann DL. *Control of communicable diseases manual.* 19th ed. Washington, DC: American Public Health Association; 2008.
23. Roczek A, Forster C, Raschel H, et al. Severe course of rat bite-associated Weil's disease in a patient diagnosed with a new *Leptospira*-specific real-time quantitative LUX-PCR. *J Med Microbiol.* 2008; 57(Pt 5):658.
24. Sehgal SC, Sugunan AP, Murhekar MV, et al. Randomized controlled trial of doxycycline prophylaxis against leptospirosis in an endemic area. *Int J Antimicrob Agents.* 2000;13(4):249.
25. Adin CA, Cowgill LD. Treatment and outcome of dogs with leptospirosis: 36 cases. http://www.ncbi.nlm.nih.gov/sites/entrez?cmd=Retrieve&db=PubMed&list_uids=10668536&dopt=AbstractPlus). Accessed February 18, 2008.
26. Giguere S. *Antimicrobial therapy in veterinary medicine.* http://books.google.com/books?id=lxmyfSave4IC&pg=PA388&lpg=PA388&dq=leptospirosis+treatment+veterinary&source=web&ots=ekP7_-1Ete&sig=uzSH8exIoc9dUAJCAkYTHe2t-2I. Accessed February 18, 2008.
27. Gilbert DN, Moellering RC, Ellopoulos GM, et al. *Sanford guide to antimicrobial therapy 2009.* 39th ed. Sperryville, VA: Antimicrobial Therapy; 2009.

LYME DISEASE

Peter M. Rabinowitz and Lisa A. Conti

Lyme Disease (ICD-10 A69.2)

Other names in humans: Lyme borreliosis

Other names in animals: Lyme borreliosis, Lyme arthritis

Lyme disease is caused by a bacterial spirochete, *Borrelia burgdorferi,* and is the most commonly reported arthropod-borne human infection in the United States.[1] Lyme disease presents opportunity for collaboration between human and animal health practitioners. The increased environmental exposure of dogs to ticks, as well as the availability of routine in-house screening tests, has provided critical evidence of the geographical incidence and prevalence of the infection in dogs that serves as a sentinel for human Lyme disease infection risk.[2] Although ticks are considered the principal vector for transmission of *Borrelia* species to humans and animals, there have been occasional published reports of the potential for transmission through blood, milk, placenta, or urine, but none of these alternative transmission routs has been confirmed by unambiguous culture results.[3] In addition to dogs, Lyme disease has been reported in cats, horses, cattle, and goats. Tick avoidance and tick control are important prevention measures for both humans and domestic animals. The risk of Lyme disease to humans and other animals is related to landscape change and human advancement on the habitat of local deer and rodent populations that maintain the vector tick *Ixodes scapularis* (formerly known as *I. dammini*). Therefore development of recommendations that focus on environmental factors associated with Lyme disease could decrease infection risk and benefit both humans and companion animals.

Key Points for Clinicians and Public Health Professionals

Public Health Professionals

- Provide descriptive epidemiologic analysis of this reportable disease and assessment of local Lyme disease risk for the health district.
- Educate the public to:
  o Avoid tick-infested areas, but if not possible, wear appropriate clothing (long sleeves, long pants, tuck pants legs into socks, and light-colored clothing to visualize ticks). Wash clothes with hot water.[4]
  o Use CDC-recommended tick repellents such as DEET, picaridin, or alternatives on clothes or bare skin following label instructions.
  o Do frequent tick checks to remove even tiny immature-stage ticks ("seed" ticks). Inspect children at least once daily for ticks. When in heavily infested areas inspect children every 3 to 4 hours.
  o Use appropriate technique to remove ticks. Wear gloves or grasp tick with tweezers as close to the skin as possible and pull gently (do not use a match, petroleum products, or nail polish). Follow up by cleaning the area, applying antibiotic topical on tick bite site, and washing hands.[5]
  o Implement integrated pest management techniques including landscape management (see Box 9-3). Counsel pet owners to discuss Lyme disease prevention strategies with their veterinarian.
- Work with local agencies to control deer and rodent populations.
- Work with local planning agencies on smart growth to avoid fractionating forested areas.

Human Health Clinicians

- Report Lyme disease cases to public health authorities using the case definition; see http://www.cdc.gov/ncphi/disss/nndss/casedef/lyme_disease_2008.htm.
- Counsel patients to avoid tick exposure and use appropriate tick repellents.
- Inquire about occupational risk factors for infection, and ensure that workers at risk are taking precautions.
- Understand that Lyme disease screening tests may provide false-positive or false-negative results and may require a confirmatory analysis at a reference laboratory such as the CDC.
- Become aware of Lyme disease prevalence through discussions with public health authorities.
- Ask patients about pet ownership generally. For those with pets who live in Lyme endemic areas or who may visit endemic areas, ask if they have discussed Lyme disease risk with their veterinarian.
- Judiciously use antibiotics; antibiotics may not be indicated as a prophylaxis for (nonengorged) tick bite alone.
- No vaccine for Lyme disease is currently commercially available for humans.

Veterinary Clinicians

- Educate clients and hospital team members about how to appropriately remove ticks. Have pet owners remove ticks as soon as possible, ideally before attachment. Conduct daily tick checks on dogs, preferably when coming in from outdoors, with particular attention to the head, ears, and warm fold areas (e.g., between toes, groin). Frequent brushing removes unattached ticks from pets that may be transferred to humans.
- In endemic areas, consider screening dogs with a Lyme C6 antibody test to diagnose subclinical dogs. Among infected dogs, 90% to 95% may be subclinical or have vague clinical signs that go unnoticed by owners.[3,6]
- Educate clients to treat dogs and cats preventatively with topical tick control.
- Consider vaccinating dogs that are at risk and in endemic areas annually against Lyme disease with an OspA Lyme vaccine (controversial).[3,6]

Agent

Lyme disease is caused by a number of species of gram-negative, spirochete bacteria belonging to the genus *Borrelia* (Figure 9-75). *Borrelia* species that cause Lyme disease are grouped under the name *Borrelia burgdorferi sensu lato*. In the United States, the predominant genotype associated with Lyme disease is *Borrelia burgdorferi sensu stricto*. This genotype also causes Lyme disease in Eurasia, as do *B. afzelii*, *B. garinii*, and *B. japonica* (Japan). Among these genotypes, there is considerable genetic diversity.[7] *Borrelia* are slow-growing bacteria (Figure 9-76) that require special culture medium and generally are difficult to culture from blood and tissue biopsies.[8] The organisms are sensitive to heat and ultraviolet light and do not survive long outside the body. Effective disinfectants include 1% sodium hypochlorite and 70% ethanol.[9]

Geographical Occurrence

Initially recognized in the Northeastern United States, specifically in Lyme, Connecticut, in 1975, Lyme disease

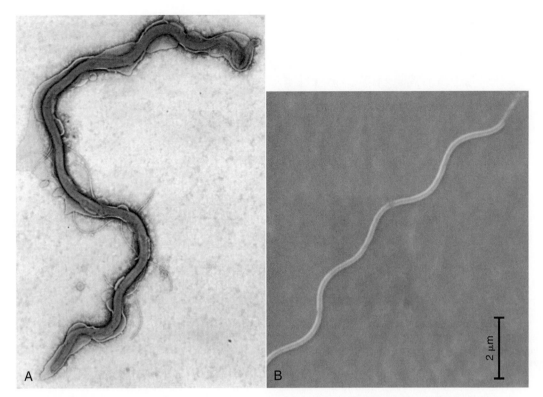

Figure 9-75 ▪ **A**, Transmission electron micrograph of *B. burgdorferi* showing periplasmic flagella that have been released from the confines of the outer membrane secondary to specimen preparation (phosphotungstic acid, ×7100). **B**, Scanning microscopic view of *B. burgdorferi* (×15,000). (From Greene CE: *Infectious diseases of the dog and cat*, ed 3, St Louis, 2006, Saunders Elsevier. Courtesy R. Straubinger, University of Leipzig, Leipzig, Germany.)

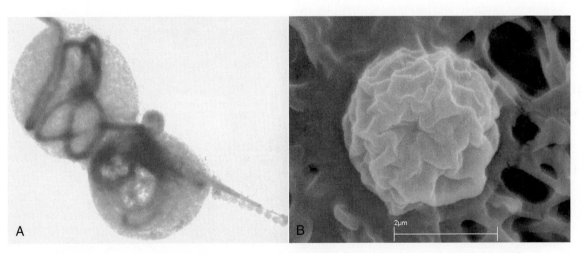

Figure 9-76 ▪ **A**, Transmission electron microscopic (×12,000) and **B**, scanning electron microscopic (×12,000) appearance of cystic form of *B. burgdorferi*, a defense mechanism of organism for survival under adverse conditions such as antimicrobial therapy or host immune defenses. (From Greene CE: *Infectious diseases of the dog and cat*, ed 3, St Louis, 2006, Saunders Elsevier. Courtesy R. Straubinger, University of Leipzig.)

has now been reported in almost every state and in Canada, although the tick vectors have a more restricted distribution. The distribution of Lyme disease in the United States is concentrated, with 12 states accounting for about 95% of reported human cases.[10] Clinical illness from *B. burgdorferi* was first documented in dogs in 1984.[11,12] Geographical foci of higher infection risk are found along the East Coast, Wisconsin, Minnesota, and parts of California and Oregon (Figure 9-77), particularly in peridomestic areas. Areas of endemic Lyme disease activity have been reported in Europe, Russia, China, and Japan.[8]

Reported cases of Lyme Disease – United States, 2007

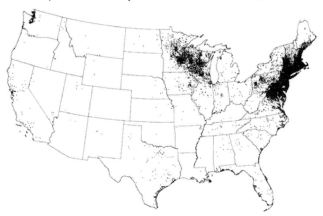

One dot placed randomly within county
of residence for each reported case

Figure 9-77 ■ Distribution of Lyme disease cases in the United States (2007). (From Centers for Disease Control and Prevention: *Lyme disease statistics.* http://www.cdc.gov/ncidod/dvbid/lyme/ld_Incidence.htm.)

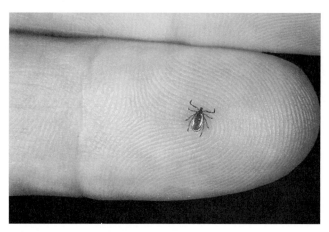

Figure 9-78 ■ The black-legged tick *Ixodes scapularis* (formerly *I. dammini*), one of the vectors for transmitting Lyme disease. This tick is very small and can easily go unnoticed when fixed to the skin in an unengorged state. (From Habif TP: *Clinical dermatology: a color guide to diagnosis and therapy*, ed 4, St Louis, 2004, Mosby Elsevier.)

Groups at Risk

The risk of Lyme disease varies among regions and is generally correlated to the abundance of host ticks that can carry the disease agent. Individuals at most risk for infection are those living in endemic areas of high vector tick density, with a large proportion of the ticks infected, and that are engaged in activities with increased time and exposure to vector ticks.[13] Behavioral factors including frequent outdoor activities such as hunting, camping, and hiking most likely play an important role in disease susceptibility.[14] Higher numbers of cases have been reported in children aged 5 to 14 years and adults aged 35 to 60.[15]

Hosts, Reservoir Species, Vectors

Principal tick vectors include the black-legged (or deer tick) *Ixodes scapularis* (formerly *I. dammini*) in the Northeastern and upper Midwestern United States (Figures 9-78 and 9-79), and *I. pacificus* (western black-legged tick) in the Western United States, as well as *I. ricinus* (Europe) and *I. persulcatus* (Asia).[13] Often, a tick carrying the B. burgdorferi spirochete is also coinfected with other pathogens including *Anaplasma* and *Babesia*. Ixodid ticks attach quickly and feed to repletion without changing hosts.

Wild rodents, including the white-footed mouse (*Peromyscus leucopus*) in the Eastern seaboard (Figure 9-80), and the dusky-footed wood rat (*Neotoma fuscipes*) and kangaroo rats (*Dipodomys californicus*) in the West, serve as disease reservoirs for Lyme disease, remaining persistently infected and capable of infecting naïve ticks. In the West, the life cycle is more complex; the spirochete is maintained in an independent enzootic cycle involving *I. spinipalpis* as the arthropod vector.[13] Lizards may function as reservoirs in some parts of the United States or be a "dilution host," reducing the vector infection prevalence in other areas.[16]

In the United States, the white-tailed deer (*Odocoileus virginianus*) is the preferred host for *I. scapularis* and helps maintain adult tick populations by serving as hosts for the adult ticks. Birds may introduce *I. scapularis* into previously nonendemic areas.[13] Adult male ticks tend to remain on deer, whereas adult females will engorge after mating to drop off and lay about 2000 eggs in the spring.

Humans and domestic animals are accidental hosts for *B. burgdorferi.* Dogs have an increased risk of Lyme disease exposure in endemic areas relative to humans, and this risk can be highly focal with seroprevalence rates as high as 50% to 90% in endemic areas, providing sentinel information for humans.[10] Cats appear to have significant exposure risks as well; a seroprevalence study in Connecticut found more than 45% of cats showed evidence of infection with *B. burgdorferi*, as well as a significant amount of coinfection with *Anaplasma phagocytophilum*; yet most cats did not show clinical signs.[17]

Mode of Transmission and Life Cycle

The life cycle of *B. burgdorferi* is related to the 2-year life cycle of the hard *Ixodes* tick vector. *Ixodes* ticks pass through larval, nymphal, and adult forms (Figure 9-81). To mature from one form to another, they must consume a blood meal. Eggs are laid in the spring and the larvae hatch in the summer. As they feed on the blood of vertebrates, the larvae can become infected with *B. burgdorferi*. After feeding, the larvae become less active and mature into nymphs by the following spring.[18] The majority of human cases occur in the spring and summer as a result of bites by nymphs that are active and seeking a blood meal to allow them to develop into adults.[8] Once they have fed, the nymphs develop into adults. The adult female lays eggs the following spring to continue the cycle. With every feeding, it is possible for a tick to become reinfected with *B. burgdorferi* and also coinfected with other pathogens such as *Babesia* and *Anaplasma*.

When an infected nymphal or adult tick initially bites an animal, it appears that it must remain attached and feed for about 24 hours for upregulation of spirochete outer surface protein C (OSP C) and transmission of organisms to take place. Peak transmission occurs after about 48 hours.[3,19]

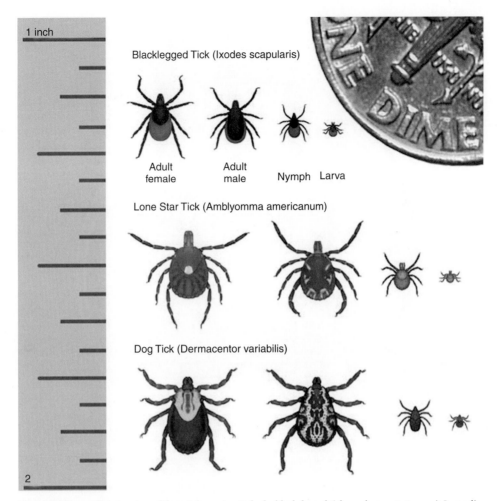

Figure 9-79 ■ Relative sizes of these tick species. Only the black-legged ticks are known to transmit Lyme disease. (From Centers for Disease Control and Prevention: *Lyme disease transmission.* http://www.cdc.gov/ncidod/dvbid/lyme/ld_transmission.htm.)

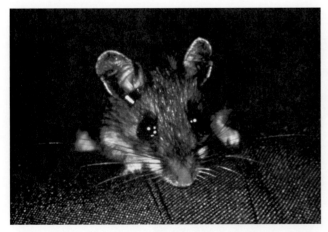

Figure 9-80 ■ White-footed mouse, *Peromyscus leucopus,* a wild rodent reservoir host of ticks, which are known to carry the bacteria *Borrelia burgdorferi,* responsible for Lyme disease. During their larval stage, *Ixodidae,* or "hard ticks," feed on small mammals, particularly the white-footed mouse, which serves as the primary reservoir for *B. burgdorferi.* (From Centers for Disease Control and Prevention Public Health Image Library, Atlanta, Ga.)

Environmental Risk Factors

The relation of environmental factors to the risk of Lyme disease is complex but it appears that landscape modification in the United States related to suburbanization of the human population is playing a significant role. As suburban developments and other human built environments encroach into land that was previously forest habitat, they produce "fragmentation" of forests (Figure 9-82). This breaking up of forested area into patches interspersed with human residential development has caused an increase in deer populations by providing ideal vegetative habitat (including ornamental shrubs for deer to eat) and reduced pressure of being hunted and predators. It also appears to favor increases in populations of peridomestic *Peromyscus,* which are important hosts for *Ixodes* ticks and for *B. burgdorferi.* Such forest fragmentation has been shown to be related to tick abundance and infection rates.[20] However, individual human behavior appears to play an important role in determining human risk, including time spent outdoors and use of protective repellents and clothing.

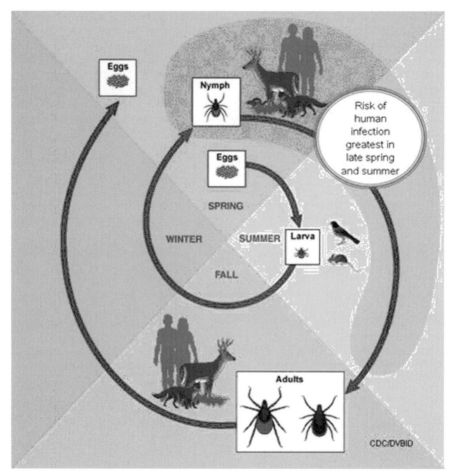

Figure 9-81 ■ Life cycle, Lyme disease. (Modified from Centers for Disease Control and Prevention: *Lyme disease transmission*. http://www.cdc.gov/ncidod/dvbid/lyme/ld_transmission.htm.)

Another environmental factor is climate and climate change. Warmer winters may result in increased tick abundance during the following spring and summer.[21] Because the environment appears to play a role in Lyme disease risk, studies have examined whether environmental modifications can reduce such risk. Area-wide acaricide use reduces tick populations, but many communities are reluctant to use wide-scale pesticides. However, targeting small areas of high human exposure,

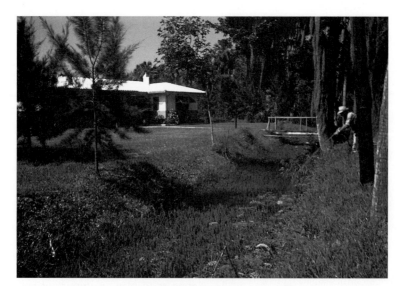

Figure 9-82 ■ Suburban development and other human built environments encroach into land that was previously forest habitat. (From Centers for Disease Control and Prevention: *Learn about Lyme disease*. http://www.cdc.gov/ncidod/dvbid/lyme/index.htm.

such as residential yards, has been highly effective in reducing nymphal tick density.[22] Treating host animals with acaricides, such as the "four poster" method of treating deer with acaricide at feeding stations, has reduced tick populations, but the distribution of bait designed to reduce tick feeding on rodents is less effective. By eliminating the deer population, the maintenance host of ticks, the risk of Lyme disease has been nearly eliminated in an island setting.[23,24] Integrated pest management can be effective to aid in tick control, including landscape modification around dwellings (see "Key Points for Clinicians and Public Health Professionals").

Disease in Humans

In many of the reported cases, the disease begins with early localized infection, consisting of fever and a characteristic skin rash (erythema migrans [EM]) that often starts with a red macule or papule at the site of the tick bite that expands into a circular rash. The rash may develop central clearing, producing a bull's-eye appearance (Color Plate 9-41). The bacterium is sometimes cultured from the leading edge of the rash. Accompanying symptoms may include fatigue, fever, headache, anorexia, arthralgias, myalgias, and lymphadenopathy. Southern tick-associated rash illness (STARI), a differential in the early diagnosis of Lyme disease, manifests with a similar EM rash (Color Plate 9-42), mild clinical signs, and absence of antibodies to *B. burgdorferi*. STARI may be associated with *B. lonestari* rather than *B. burgdorferi* and transmitted by the lone star tick, *A. americanum* (see http://www.cdc.gov/ncidod/dvbid/stari/index.htm).

Days to weeks after the onset of the rash, early disseminated infection may develop, with more severe systemic symptoms. Multiple EM lesions may appear during this phase, as well as borrelial lymphocytomas—blue-red nodules on the earlobes or nipples. Early disseminated infection can involve the nervous system with the development of chronic symptoms including seventh nerve (Bell's) palsy or facial paralysis, meningitis, motor or sensory peripheral neuropathy, and encephalopathy. Cardiac involvement may occur with atrioventricular block. If infection remains untreated, late-stage disease can develop months to years after initial infection, with arthritis of the knees or other weight-bearing joints (Figure 9-83). In late-stage disease, the skin can develop acrodermatitis chronica atrophicans, erythematous plaques and nodules on the extremities. Other complications include encephalopathy and keratitis (Figure 9-84).[25] Previous infection does not confer immunity.

Disease in Animals

Most dogs do not manifest clinical signs after exposure to *B. burgdorferi* or have vague signs that go unnoticed by the owner. Dogs have not been reported to have the bull's-eye rash. Approximately 5% of seropositive dogs develop clinical Lyme disease.[6,26] Clinical signs may not appear for 2 to 6 months after infection and may include lameness, fever, anorexia, myalgia, lethargy, lymphadenopathy, cardiac arrhythmias (rarely), neurological signs, and ocular manifestations (Color Plates 9-43 and 9-44).[3,6] Dogs have also been reported with Lyme arthropathy, a recurrent arthritis with lameness particularly in the tarsal and carpal joints (Figure 9-85). Lyme nephropathy, a chronic protein-losing nephropathy that may

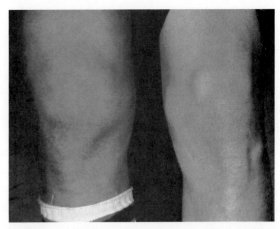

Figure 9-83 ■ Inflammation involving knee joint in Lyme disease. (From Yanoff M, Duker JS: *Ophthalmology*, ed 3, St Louis, 2004, Mosby Elsevier. Adapted with permission of the American Academy of Ophthalmology: *Basic and clinical science course*, San Francisco, American Academy of Ophthalmology, 1998-1999.)

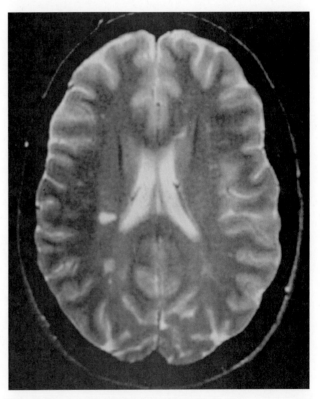

Figure 9-84 ■ T_2-weighted magnetic resonance imaging scan in a patient with Lyme disease reveals areas of increased signal intensity in the cerebral white matter. (From Mandell GL, Bennett JE, Dolin R: *Principles and practice of infectious diseases*, ed 6, New York, 2005, Churchill Livingstone Elsevier.)

be related in part to immune complex deposition, can progress to a fatal acute oliguric or anuric renal failure.[6,26] Some have questioned whether the nephropathy could be related to coinfections with other agents. Coinfection with other tick-borne diseases is common, either transmitted by the same tick vector (*A. phagocytophilum*, *Babesia microti*, or *Bartonella* species) or other tick vectors (*Ehrlichia* species and *Rickettsia rickettsii*).[3,6] Previous infection with *B. burgdorferi* does not appear to confer immunity.

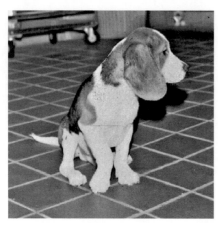

Figure 9-85 ■ Experimentally induced borrelial arthritis in the thoracic limb of beagle dog. Fever and shifting leg lameness develop 60 to 90 days after inoculation. Lameness occurs earliest and is most severe in the limb closest to the inoculation site. (From Greene CE: *Infectious diseases of the dog and cat*, ed 3, St Louis, 2006, Saunders Elsevier. Courtesy R. Straubinger, University of Leipzig.)

Cats appear to be largely asymptomatic but can rarely develop arthritis.[27]

Serosurveys using ELISA antibody screening have reported seroprevalence rates in horses greater than 80% in endemic areas.[28] Although a wide range of clinical conditions have been associated with Lyme infection in horses, clinical infection is considered to be extremely rare and poorly understood.[29] EM lesions have been experimentally caused by infecting rabbits with *B. burgdorferi*. Table 9-41 provides a comparison of Lyme disease clinical presentations in humans and other animals.

Diagnosis

In humans who present with a classic EM rash (described as 5 cm or greater to differentiate it from a hypersensitivity reaction) and a history of a tick bite or tick exposure in a Lyme-endemic area, serological confirmation may not be necessary. However, a search should be performed for possible coinfection with agents such as *Anaplasma* and *Babesia*. When the rash is not present but Lyme disease is suspected and pretest probability is 20% or greater, serological testing using a two-step method is recommended. This consists of a screening ELISA test followed by a confirmatory Western blot if the ELISA is indeterminate or positive. If less than 4 weeks has elapsed since the onset of infection, both IgG and IgM should be tested; if more than 4 weeks have elapsed, only IgG should be tested. The two-step method is considered to have high specificity and a low risk of false-positive diagnosis.[31,32]

In animals, a rapid antibody test has been developed to detect antibodies against the C6 *B. burgdorferi* protein and correlates well with the Western blot immunoassay.[33] This test detects only antibodies against antigen acquired through natural exposures, and therefore will not yield positive results in vaccinated animals.[6] In dogs, testing validates exposure to the *B. burgdorferi* organism but not clinical illness. Supporting evidence for a diagnosis of Lyme disease is based on history of exposure to *B. burgdorferi* through exposure to *Ixodes* ticks in an endemic area, clinical signs, positive C6 peptide and/or Western blot antibody test results, ruling out other differential diagnoses, and response to antibiotics.[6]

Controversy exists in the veterinary literature about whether healthy dogs should be routinely screened for *B. burgdorferi* antibodies.[6] Limitations to serological testing include a long incubation period, presence of subclinical infections, cross-

Table 9-41 ■ Lyme Disease: Comparative Clinical Presentations in Humans and Other Animals

Species	Risk Factors	Incubation Period	Clinical Manifestations	Diagnostic Findings
Humans	Tick exposures	Days to weeks	Early localized form: EM skin lesion, fever *Early disseminated infection:* paralysis of facial muscles, meningitis, numbness in arms or legs *Late-stage infection:* arthritis, cardiac pathology, neuropathy	Positive serology, direct immunofluorescence, rarely isolation from skin biopsy
Dogs	Tick exposures Younger dogs appear to be more susceptible than older dogs, coinfection with other agents	2-5 months in experimentally infected dogs[30]	Often subclinical Arthritis, anorexia, and depression, cardiac disease, nephritis, lymphadenopathy[27]	C6 *Borrelia burgdorferi* ELISA (both qualitative and quantitative) and Western blot antibody test Antibodies generally can be detected 3-5 wk after experimental infection in dogs[6]
Cats	Tick exposures	4-6 weeks	Usually subclinical; fever, arthritis may occur	C6 *B. burgdorferi* ELISA and Western blot antibody test
Horses	Tick exposures	Weeks to months	Fever, lameness, Bell's palsy	Antibodies generally take 4-6 wk to develop in horses; immunoblots may not become positive until 10-12 wk in horses, skin biopsy

ELISA, Enzyme-linked immunosorbent assay; *EM*, erythema migrans.

reactions with other spirochetes, and persistence of antibody titers for months. A positive serological result in the presence or absence of clinical signs should alert the clinician to also search for coinfections commonly associated with *B. burgdorferi* exposure, including *Anaplasma, Babesia, Ehrlichia, Rickettsia, Bartonella, Leptospira, Mycoplasma,* and *Neorickettsia*.[6,10] Clinically normal dogs with positive serological findings should have follow-up by a veterinarian with semiannual or annual health examinations, be monitored for proteinuria, and the owner should be alerted to contact the veterinarian if any clinical signs of Lyme disease develop.

Treatment

Management of *B. burgdorferi* infection in humans and animals involves the use of antibiotics for treatment of disease. Prophylaxis with oral doxycycline may be offered to adults or children if a tick bite is due to an adult or nymphal *I. scapularis* tick that has been attached for at least 24 hours, less than 72 hours has elapsed since removal of the tick, and the use of doxycycline is not contraindicated (doxycycline 200 mg PO for 1 dose; children 8 and older, 4 mg/kg).[1] Following a tick bite, regardless of whether prophylaxis is given, individuals should be monitored for any signs of disease such as development of a fever or an EM rash.

The use of antibiotics for disease treatment depends on the stage of disease. Table 9-42 outlines recommended antibiotics regimens outlined by the Infectious Diseases Society of America (IDSA). The use of macrolides should be reserved for persons who are unable to tolerate tetracyclines, penicillins, or cephalosporins because their efficacy may be lower.

Recommended antibiotic regimens for animals with clinical manifestations of Lyme disease are also shown in Table 9-42. More specific supportive and symptomatic medical treatment should be directed toward the affected organ system. Dogs do not appear to develop natural immunity to infection nor do they develop long-term immunity after vaccination. Therefore after the full course of antibiotic treatment, subsequent exposure to *B. burgdorferi* can result in reinfection.

In the United States there are currently four vaccines for dogs that stimulate antibody production against a single outer surface protein A (OSP A) located on the bacterium when it is attached to the tick's gut.[6] This prevents infection because the vaccinated dog's OSP A antibodies move with the blood to the tick's gut and bind to the bacteria, thus preventing the bacteria from upregulating OSP C and moving to the saliva to infect the dog.[34]

References

1. Wormser GP, Dattwyler RJ, Shapiro ED, et al. The clinical assessment, treatment, and prevention of Lyme disease, human granulocytic anaplasmosis, and babesiosis: clinical practice guidelines by the Infectious Diseases Society of America. *Clin Infect Dis.* 2006;43(9):1089.
2. Duncan AW, Correa MT, Levine JF, et al. The dog as a sentinel for human infection: prevalence of *Borrelia burgdorferi* C6 antibodies in dogs from southeastern and mid-Atlantic states. *Vector Borne Zoonotic Dis.* 2004;4(3):221.
3. Greene CE, Straubinger RK. Borreliosis. In: Green CE, ed. *Infectious diseases of the dog and cat.* 3rd ed. St Louis: Saunders Elsevier; 2006.
4. Centers for Disease Control and Prevention. *Lyme disease prevention and control: protect yourself from tick bites.* http://www.cdc.gov/ncidod/dvbid/lyme/Prevention/ld_Prevention_Avoid.htm. Accessed September 28, 2008.
5. Placerville Veterinary Clinic. *Tick removal tools.* http://placervillevet.com/ticktools.htm. Accessed February 28, 2009.
6. Littmann MP, Goldstein RE, Labato MA, et al. ACVIM small animal consensus statement on Lyme disease in dogs: diagnosis, treatment, and prevention. *J Vet Intern Med.* 2006;20(2):422.
7. Bunikis J, Garpmo U, Tsao J, et al. Sequence typing reveals extensive strain diversity of the Lyme borreliosis agents *Borrelia burgdorferi* in North America and *Borrelia afzelii* in Europe. *Microbiology.* 2004;150(Pt 6):1741.

Table 9-42 ■ Antibiotic Treatment of Lyme Disease in Humans and Other Animals

Species	Primary Treatment	Alternative Treatment
Humans (based on IDSA guidelines[1])		
Oral regimens: Early localized disease, isolated fifth nerve palsy, carditis (if only first-degree block), or arthritis without neurological signs	*Adults:* amoxicillin 500 mg PO tid, doxycycline 100 mg PO bid, *or* cefuroxime axetil 500 mg PO bid *Children:* amoxicillin 50 mg/kg/day (maximum 500 mg/dose) divided q8h, doxycycline if ≥8 yr 4 mg/kg/day divided bid (maximum 100 mg/dose), *or* cefuroxime 30 mg/kg/day (maximum 500 mg/dose) divided bid	*Adults and children:* consider selected macrolide if unable to tolerate penicillins, cephalosporins, or tetracyclines Monitor closely for resolution of clinical manifestations
Parenteral regimens: Lyme meningitis, other acute neurological manifestations, carditis	*Adults:* ceftriaxone 2 gm IV qd *Children:* ceftriaxone 50-75 mg/d IV (maximum 2 gm)	*Adults:* cefotaxime 2 gm, IV 8h *or* penicillin G 18-24 million units/day divided q4h IV *Children:* cefotaxime 150-200 mg/kg/day IV divided tid or qid, maximum 6 gm/day *or* penicillin G 200,000-400,000 units/kg/day, maximum 18-24 million units/day divided into doses q4h
Pregnant women	Same as nonpregnant but avoid doxycycline	
Dogs	Doxycycline 5 mg/kg PO q24h × 28 days[6]	Amoxicillin 20 mg/kg PO q8-12h × 28 days[27]
Horses	Doxycycline 10-20 mg/kg PO q12h[35]	Tetracycline 6.6 mg/kg IV qd[36]

IDSA, Infectious Diseases Society of America.

8. Heymann DL, ed. *Control of communicable diseases manual*. 19th ed.Washington, DC, American Public Health Association; 2008.

9. Center for Food Security and Public Health, Iowa State University. *Lyme disease*. http://www.cfsph.iastate.edu/Factsheets/pdfs/lyme_disease.pdf. Accessed November 2008.

10. Littman MP. Canine borreliosis. *Vet Clin North Am Small Anim Pract*. 2003;33(4):827.

11. Lissman BA, Bosler EM, Camay H, et al. Spirochete associated arthritis (Lyme disease) in a dog. *J Am Vet Med Assoc*. 1984;185(2):219.

12. Kornblatt AN, Urband PH, Steere AC. Arthritis caused by *Borrelia burgdorferi* in dogs. *J Am Vet Med Assoc*. 1985;186(9):960.

13. Fritz CL, Kjemtrup AM. Lyme borreliosis. *J Am Vet Med Assoc*. 2003;223(9):1262.

14. Connally NP, Ginsberg HS, Mather TN. Assessing peridomestic entomological factors as predictors for Lyme disease. *J Vector Ecol*. 2006;31(2):364.

15. Centers for Disease Control and Prevention. Lyme disease—United States, 2003–2005. *MMWR*. 2007;56(23):573.

16. Giery ST, Ostfeld RS. The role of lizards in the ecology of Lyme disease in two endemic zones of the Northeastern United States. *J Parasitol*. 2007;93(3):511.

17. Magnarelli LA, Bushmich SL, IJdo JW, et al. Seroprevalence of antibodies against *Borrelia burgdorferi* and *Anaplasma phagocytophilum* in cats. *Am J Vet Res*. 2005;66(11):1895.

18. Centers for Disease Control and Prevention. Lyme disease transmission. http://www.cdc.gov/ncidod/dvbid/Lyme/ld_transmission.htm. Accessed February 28, 2009.

19. Schwan TG. Temporal regulations of the outer surface proteins of the Lyme-disease spirochaete *Borrelia burgdorferi*. *Biochem Soc Trans*. 2003;31(1):108.

20. Brownstein JS, Skelly DK, Holford TR, et al. Forest fragmentation predicts local scale heterogeneity of Lyme disease risk. *Oecologia*. 2005;146(3):469.

21. Bennet L, Halling A, Berglund J. Increased incidence of Lyme borreliosis in southern Sweden following mild winters and during warm, humid summers. *Euro J Clin Microbiol Infect Dis*. 2006;25(7):426.

22. Curran KL, Fish D, Piesman J. Reduction of nymphal *Ixodes dammini* (Acari: Ixodidae) in a residential suburban landscape by area application of insecticides. *J Med Entomol*. 1993;30(1):107.

23. Rand PW, Lubelczyk C, Holman MS, et al. Abundance of *Ixodes scapularis* (Acari: Ixodidae) after the complete removal of deer from an isolated offshore island, endemic for Lyme disease. *J Med Entomol*. 2004;41(4):779.

24. Piesman J. Strategies for reducing the risk of Lyme borreliosis in North America. *Int J Med Microbiol*. 2006;296(suppl 40):17.

25. Kwan-Gett TS, Kemp C, Kovarik C. *Infectious and tropical diseases: a handbook for primary care*. St Louis: Mosby Elsevier; 2005.

26. Chou J, Wunschmann A, Hodzic E, et al. Detection of *Borrelia burgdorferi* DNA in tissues from dogs with presumptive Lyme borreliosis. *J Am Vet Med Assoc*. 2006;229(8):1260.

27. Barr SC, Bowman DD. *The 5-minute veterinary consult clinical companion: canine and feline infectious diseases and parasitology*. Ames, IA: Blackwell; 2006.

28. Magnarelli L, Fikrig E. Detection of antibodies to *Borrelia burgdorferi* in naturally infected horses in the USA by enzyme-linked immunosorbent assay using whole-cell and recombinant antigens. *Res Vet Sci*. 2005;79(2):99.

29. Butler CM, Houwers DJ, Jongejan F, et al. *Borrelia burgdorferi* infections with special reference to horses. A review. *Vet Q*. 2005;27(4):146.

30. Dvorak G, Rovid-Spickler A, Roth JA, et al. *Handbook for zoonotic diseases of companion animals*. Ames, IA: The Center for Food Security and Public Health, Iowa State University College of Veterinary Medicine; 2008.

31. DePietropaolo DL, Powers JH, Gill JM, et al. Diagnosis of Lyme disease. *Am Fam Physician*. 2005;72(2):297.

32. Centers for Disease Control and Prevention. Notice to readers: caution regarding testing for Lyme disease. *MMWR*. 2005;54(5):25.

33. IDEXX Laboratories. *Lyme Quant C6Test*. http://www.idexx.com/animalhealth/laboratory/c6/. Accessed May 7, 2008.

34. Goldstein RE, Karyn Gavzer K. Lyme disease: what clients need to know. *Clinician's Brief*. 2008;(suppl) April 1.

35. Gilger B. *Equine ophthalmology*. St Louis: Saunders Elsevier; 2005.

36. Sellon DC, Long M. *Equine infectious diseases*. St Louis: Saunders Elsevier; 2007.

LYMPHOCYTIC CHORIOMENINGITIS

Lynda U. Odofin

(ICD-9 049.0 Non-arthropod–borne lymphocytic choriomeningitis (ICD-9 049.0), Unspecified non-arthropod–borne viral diseases of central nervous system (ICD-9 049.9), Viral encephalitis NOS (ICD-10 A87.2)

Other names in humans: none

Other names in animals: none

Lymphocytic choriomeningitis (LCM) is a rodent-borne viral infection that may cause substantial neurological disease,[1,2] especially in immunocompromised individuals. Like other members of the Arenadiviridae family, the causative agent, lymphocytic choriomeningitis virus (LCMV), uses rodents as reservoirs.[3] Although the common house mouse, *Mus musculus,* is the natural host and principal reservoir of LCMV,[4] wild, pet, and laboratory rodents (rats, guinea pigs, hamsters) can be infected also. Infected mice can shed the virus throughout their lives[4]; infected females transmit the virus to their offspring, which may become asymptomatic persistent viral shedders.[5] Human infection is through contact with infected pet rodents or infected wild mice or their droppings. Infected rodents often do not show any signs of illness.[6] LCMV is an emerging neuroteratogen, known to cause diverse congenital defects in children. In addition, because of recent outbreaks in organ transplant patients,[7-9] LCM is a reportable disease in some U.S. states; such states require physicians to report the disease to local health authorities.

Key Points for Clinicians and Public Health Professionals

Public Health Professionals

- Recommend that LCM be reportable in all states.
- Provide descriptive epidemiologic analysis of disease in the community.
- Investigate new cases of disease to determine the source of infection. Search home, place of employment, and immediate surroundings for presence of house mice. Test rodents, including pets found on such premises, for virus.
- Trace the source of infected pets. Work with pet stores to ensure all rodents sold are LCMV free.
- Recommend rodent-proofing homes:
  - Seal rodent entry holes or gaps with steel wool, metal lath, or caulk.
  - Trap rats and mice using appropriate snap trap.
  - Clean rodent food sources and nesting sites.

- Take precautions when cleaning rodent-infected areas:
  - Use cross-ventilation when entering a previously unventilated enclosed room or dwelling before cleanup.
  - Use rubber, latex, vinyl, or nitrile gloves.
  - Do not stir up dust by vacuuming, sweeping, or any other means. Instead, thoroughly wet contaminated areas with a bleach solution or household disinfectant. Hypochlorite (bleach) solution: mix 1½ cups of household bleach in 1 gallon of water. Once everything is wet, take up contaminated materials with damp towel and then mop or sponge the area with bleach solution or household disinfectant.
  - Spray dead rodents with disinfectant and then double-bag along with all cleaning materials and dispose of bag in an appropriate waste disposal system.
  - Remove gloves and thoroughly wash hands with soap and water (or waterless alcohol-based hand rubs when soap is not available and hands are not visibly soiled).
- Counsel people about appropriate rodent pet handling and care:
  - Wash hands with soap and water after handling pet rodents; use waterless alcohol-based hand rubs when soap is not available.
  - Keep rodent cages clean and free of soiled bedding.
  - Clean the cage in a well-ventilated area or outside.
  - Wash hands thoroughly with soap and water after cleaning up pet droppings. Closely supervise young children, especially those younger than 5 years, when cleaning cages, and make sure they wash their hands immediately after handling rodents and rodent caging or bedding.
  - Do not kiss pet rodents or hold them close to the face.
- Recommend that testing for LCMV should be included in the screening protocols for potential organ donors.

- Ensure that potentially exposed immunocompromised persons and pregnant women are given immediate medical attention, and advise such individuals to avoid contact with rodents and rodent droppings and to rodent-proof their homes.
- As part of the history, patients with aseptic meningitis and encephalitis should be asked about contact with rodents or rodent droppings.[10]
- Consider the diagnosis in all patients with rodent contact, such as pet owners, laboratory workers, and people from endemic areas. Work closely with respective state health department to discuss forwarding of samples on patients with disease suggestive of LCM to state laboratories or CDC for testing. (Testing for LCMV infection in asymptomatic persons is not necessary.)
- Consider LCMV infection in organ transplant recipients with unexplained fever, hepatitis, or multisystem organ failure.[10]

- Consider the diagnosis in patients (especially children) presenting with ocular scars regardless of no history of LCM. There have been reports from Europe about such cases.
- Report suspicion of disease immediately to public health authorities. LCM is reportable in some U.S. states.
- Discourage immunocompromised individuals, pregnant women, and families with children younger than 5 years from owning rodent pets. Also educate these individuals and parents about the consequences of owning pet rodents.[11] Consider routine testing of exposed pregnant women for the virus.
- If caring for occupational groups at risk, ensure that they are educated about symptoms of the disease, potential routes of transmission, use of adequate protective equipment, and that efforts are taken to reduce the risk of infection.
- Educate patients on reduction of environmental exposure risk through the elimination of wild rodents. Seal up rodent entry holes or gaps with steel wool, metal lath, or caulk.
- Trap rats and mice by using an appropriate snap trap. Clean up rodent food sources and nesting sites and take precautions when cleaning rodent-infected areas.[11]
- Promote proper handwashing after pet handling, and educate patients on providing a clean environment for pet rodents, such as supplying fresh bedding, food, and water on a regular basis. Clean cages outdoors or in well-ventilated areas.[11]
- Provide an information sheet on LCM prevention and control for at risk patients; a CDC information sheet is available at http://www.cdc.gov/ncidod/dvrd/spb/mnpages/dispages/lcmv.htm.

- Advise clients to consult their physicians if an infected rodent is seen or if they are considering acquiring a rodent as a pet.
- Although the length of LCMV infection in pets varies, it has been shown that hamsters (subfamily Cricetinae) can transmit the virus for at least 8 months. Thus it is advisable to euthanize infected rodents.
- Although LCMV is not reported in animals, it is advisable to report increased incidence of cases to the local health authorities. Disease in animals may serve as an early warning of environmental exposure risk and possible human outbreaks.
- Screening pet rodents is not recommended as serological testing on rodents can be inaccurate and results misleading; however, hygienic practices (handwashing, cage sanitation) should be followed.[12]

Agent

LCMV is an enveloped single-stranded RNA virus belonging to the family Arenaviridae. The virus is serologically related to Lassa, Machupo, Junin, Guaranito, and Sabia viruses[5] and has been referred to as the prototypic member of the family. Along with Lassa and Lassa-related viruses,

LCMV forms the Old World group of the Arenaviridae.[13] Because of its unique properties, the LCMV model has been used to make important contributions to the fields of virology and immunology[14] and further understanding of viral-immune interactions. For instance, a specific glycoprotein (GP1), which is expressed on the envelope of LCMV,[15] mediates attachment of the virus, thereby initiating infection; thus mutations in this protein have the potential to alter viral targeting and influence the course of disease.[14] The immune system plays a major role in the outcome of human LCMV infection, ranging from no disease in healthy individuals to severe neurological disease in immunocompromised individuals.

Geographical Occurrence

LCMV is found worldwide and is endemic in wild mice. The virus has the greatest geographical range potential of any arenavirus and may occur on all land masses where the genus *Mus* has been introduced, including all continents except Antarctica.[7,16] The CDC estimates 5% of the U.S. wild mouse population is infected with LCMV, although epidemiological studies have documented a prevalence ranging from 3% to 21% in various U.S. locations.[11] An overall prevalence rate of 9% (43/468) was determined in wild mice captured in various sites, including residential and park locations in Baltimore, Maryland.[13]

In general, human infection, with the exception of those associated with hamsters,[13] tends to reflect the distribution of house mice.[17-19] Several serological studies conducted in urban areas have shown that the prevalence of LCMV infection among humans ranges from 2% to 5%.[11] In Baltimore, LCMV antibodies were found in 4.7% of 1149 inner-city residents tested,[6,20] and 49% of these reported house mice within their residence.[21]

The true incidence of LCM is unknown because many cases go unreported owing to the self-limiting effect in healthy individuals and lack of recognition by physicians.

Groups at Risk

In general, people who are in contact with rodents are at risk from LCMV infection; these include laboratory workers who routinely work with LCMV and laboratory mice and other rodents, farmers who are in frequent contact with wild mice, homeowners with mouse infestations, veterinarians who handle sick hamsters and other rodents, pet-store keepers, and pet rodent owners. Immunocompromised individuals, children younger than 5 years, and fetuses are particularly vulnerable to LCMV, which usually lead to severe infection in these subpopulations.

Recently LCMV infection has been associated with organ transplants.[8,9] Transmissions of virus between donors and recipients have been documented in the United States and other parts of the world. In one of these cases, the donor had recently acquired a pet hamster.[22]

Hosts, Reservoir Species, Vectors

LCMV has a highly restrictive host range; the house mouse (*M. musculus*) is the natural host and reservoir. Once infected, house mice often become lifelong shedders of the virus. Infection has also been reported in other rodents such as wood mice (*Apodemus sylvaticus*) and yellow-necked field mice (*A. flavicollis*).[23] Pet hamsters and guinea pigs are not known to be natural reservoirs for LCM, but pet rodents can become infected if they have contact with wild house mice in a breeding facility, pet store, or home. The golden hamster (*Mesocricetus auratus*) has become an important linkage host for LCMV transmission in humans and has been the source of recent outbreaks in the United States and abroad.[24-27]

Mode of Transmission and Life Cycle

Infected house mice play a major role in maintaining the life cycle of LCMV, thereby ensuring its persistence in nature (Figure 9-86). Wild mice are usually infected in utero, thereby

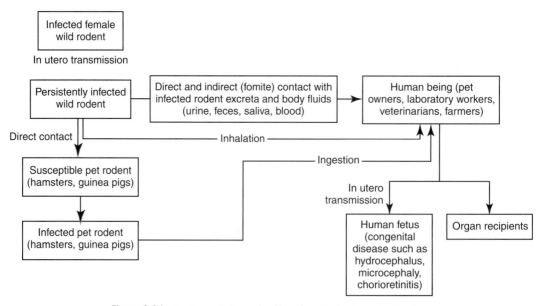

Figure 9-86　■　Transmission cycle of lymphocytic choriomeningitis virus.

becoming chronically or persistently infected. The virus is usually excreted in urine, saliva, and feces of infected mice; transmission to humans occurs through the oral and respiratory contact with virus-contaminated excreta, food, or dust or through the contamination of skin lesions and cuts. Fomites such as bedding materials and other articles contaminated by infected rodents can put nearby humans at infection risk.

Human-to-human transmission occurs vertically between infected mother and fetus and horizontally from organ transplant between infected donors and recipients. Many of the women who gave birth to children with congenital LCM had a known exposure to wild mice or sick hamsters during pregnancy.[28]

Environmental Risk Factors

Most of the human LCMV infection is usually associated with contact with infected rodents (wild and pet rodents); thus the virus persistence in the environment is dependent on the infection rate of mice and frequency of contact between infected rodents and humans. For instance, during the fall there appear to be more mice in residential areas and even commercial areas such as restaurants because the mice look for warmer places to spend the winter. This enables more contact with nearby pet rodents (hamsters, guinea pigs) and even humans.

Disease in Humans

The immune response plays a major role in determining the manifestation and progression of clinical symptoms following LCMV infection. Thus infection in healthy people usually goes unnoticed and the virus is readily cleared. The onset of symptoms in ill individuals occur 8 to 15 days after exposure and is characterized by a biphasic febrile illness. The initial phase, which may last as long as a week, typically begins with any or all of the following flulike symptoms: fever, malaise, lack of appetite, muscle aches, retroorbital headache, nausea, and vomiting. Other symptoms that appear less frequently include sore throat; cough; arthritis; pain in the chest, testicles, and parotid gland; and rarely a rash. Most people recover after this phase. However, some may proceed to the second phase of the disease consisting of symptoms of meningitis or characteristics of encephalitis. The course of the disease is usually short, rarely fatal (about 1% mortality rate), and the prognosis is usually good, although convalescence with fatigue and vasomotor instability may be prolonged. An association between LCMV infection and myocarditis has been suggested.

Immunosuppressed patients such as organ recipients may develop fatal hemorrhagic fever; of 11 organ recipients described in three LCM clusters, 10 died of multisystem organ failure, with LCMV-associated hepatitis the prominent feature.[10]

Congenital LCMV infection first was recognized in Europe half a century ago.[24,29-31] The first U.S. cases were reported in 1993[30,31] and were characterized by severe brain and retinal injury.[15,32-35] Infection of the fetus during the early stages of pregnancy may lead to developmental deficits that are permanent; congenital LCM can be manifested in a variety of neurological signs such as microcephaly, chorioretinitis, hydrocephalus, seizures, and hypertonia (Figure 9-87). These signs are usually evident within 48 hours of birth. Diverse clinical signs have been recorded among 20 children diagnosed with congenital LCMV infection.[36] LCMV was diagnosed in these children at birth with follow-up of 11 years. Clinical signs covered a wide spectrum of neurological disease, but chorioretinitis was the only common presenting sign. In addition, the study suggested that the variability of the disease was related to the gestational timing of infection.

The most common laboratory abnormalities are leukopenia and thrombocytopenia in the first phase of disease with a mild elevation in liver enzymes in the serum. After the onset of neurological disease, an increase in protein levels and the number of white blood cells or a decrease in the glucose levels in the CSF is usually observed. No chronic state has been reported in humans, who usually clear the virus after the acute phase of the disease.

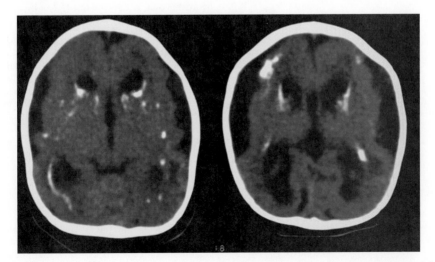

Figure 9-87 ▪ Computed tomography at 5 months of an infant with profound developmental delay and chorioretinitis due to intrauterine lymphocytic choriomeningitis virus infection. The scan shows microencephaly, lissencephaly, and calcifications that are periventricular, intracerebral, and over the convexities of the brain. (From Long SS, Pickering LK, Prober CG: *Principles and practice of pediatric infectious diseases*, ed 3, Philadelphia, 2008, Saunders Elsevier. Courtesy G.L. Rodgers and S.S. Long, St. Christopher's Hospital for Children, Philadelphia, Pa.)

Disease in Animals

Wild mice infected with LCMV in utero or at an early age develop a persistent subclinical infection and likely shed the virus for life. In naturally infected colonies of wild mice, the proportion of mice with persistent infection increases over time and at 4 years almost all the animals will be shedding virus.[37] Although most rodents with LCMV infection are subclinical, there have been reports of illness in infected hamsters characterized by a wasting disease that may run a long course (ranging from several weeks to months). Early signs include loss of activity, loss of appetite, and rough coat. Later the animal may show signs of weight loss, hunched posture, inflammation of the eye lids (blepharitis), clonic convulsions, and eventually death. The effects of LCMV have been studied in laboratory mice and mimic the disease in humans. Mice exposed to the virus at an older age are more likely to develop clinical disease. Gross lesions include necrosis of the liver and lymphoid tissue. LCMV infection has been documented in other animals such as dogs and monkeys; however, this is rare and has been consistently associated with contact to infected rodents.

Diagnosis

In humans, the early stage of disease could be confused with the flu, and at latter stages it must be differentiated from other aseptic meningitides and viral encephalitides, such as those caused by enteroviruses, the arthropod-borne togaviruses, or herpes simplex virus. Drug-induced meningitis is also a differential. In the case of congenital LCM, valid differential diagnoses include TORCH infections (toxoplasmosis, rubella, cytomegalovirus, herpes, and syphilis), parvovirus, and enterovirus. Confirmatory diagnosis usually is by virus isolation in blood or CSF, by PCR, or identification of anti-LCMV IgM and IgG by ELISA or complement fixation. Detection of rising antibody titers in paired sera by IFA, and LCMV antigens by immunohistochemistry in liver biopsy or at autopsy also are considered diagnostic.

In rodents, confirmatory diagnosis is by viral isolation via inoculation in guinea pigs or LCM-free mice, complement fixation, and fluorescent antibody (Table 9-43).

Treatment

Early diagnosis is the key to successful treatment of LCM. Treatment is mainly supportive and involves use of antiinflammatory drugs. As for other cases of aseptic meningitis, suggested treatment regimens include intravenous fluids and analgesics.[38]

Treatment in animals is normally not advocated because they could develop a chronic state and continue to shed the virus, thereby posing a risk for other animals and humans. In general, by the time clinical signs are seen the prognosis is poor.

Table 9-43 ■ Lymphocytic Choriomeningitis: Clinical Presentations in Humans and Other Animals				
Species	**Risk Factors**	**Incubation Period**	**Clinical Manifestations**	**Diagnostic Findings**
Humans	Rodent exposure, immunocompromised	8-13 days; 15-21 days until meningeal symptoms appear[5]	*Adults:* flulike symptoms, myalgia, retroorbital headache, orchitis, parotiditis, arthritis, myocarditis, muscle ache, acute hydrocephalus, occasional rash[5] In rare cases, muscle weakness, paralysis, body sensation changes *Newborns/infants (0-<2 yr):* hydrocephalus, chorioretinitis, seizures, irritability, microcephaly, blistered skin, hypertonia, hypotonia, light perception, blindness, spastic quadriparesis, quadriplegia, hearing loss, cognitive deficits *Children (2-11 yr):* same as in infants, and ataxia, spastic diplegia	*Early stages of disease:* isolation of virus from blood or CSF by PCR or intracerebral inoculation of LCM-free mice (3-5 weeks old) or by cell culture[5] Demonstration of anti-LCMV IgM and IgG in serum or CSF by ELISA or complement fixation; Also demonstration of rising titers by IFA in paired sera Liver biopsy and multiple autopsy specimen stained positive for LCMV antigens by immunohistochemistry
Organ recipients	Infected organ donor	2-4 wk after transplant	Lethargy, anorexia, fever, shock, hepatitis, multisystem organ failure	
Rodents (hamsters, guinea pigs, mice)	Exposure to infected animals	Varies (several weeks to months)	Weight loss, ocular and nasal discharge, hunched posture, inflammation of the eyelids, clonic convulsions	Virus isolation by inoculation of LCM-free mice or guinea pigs, complement fixation, and fluorescent antibody on serum; immunofluorescence test on liver tissue

CSF, Cerebrospinal fluid; *LCM*, lymphocytic choriomeningitis; *LCMV*, lymphocytic choriomeningitis virus.

References

1. Jahrling PB, Peters CJ. Lymphocytic choriomeningitis virus. A neglected pathogen of man. *Arch Pathol Lab Med.* 1992;116(5):486.
2. Peters CJ. Lymphocytic choriomeningitis virus—an old enemy up to new tricks. *N Engl J Med.* 2006;354(21):2208.
3. Rowe WP, Murphy FA, Bergold GH, et al. Arenaviruses: proposed name for a newly defined virus group. *J Virol.* 1970;5(5):651.
4. Buchmeier M, Zajac A. Lymphocytic chiromeningitis virus. In: Ahmed R, Chen I, eds. *Persistent viral infections.* New York: Wiley; 1999.
5. Heymann DL, ed. *Control of communicable diseases manual.* 19th ed. Washington, DC: American Public Health Association; 2008.
6. College of Veterinary Medicine. *University of Minnesota: lymphocytic choriomeningitis virus (LCMV).* www.cvm.umn.edu Accessed August 20, 2008.
7. Enria D, Mills JN, Flick R, et al. Arenavirus infections. In: Guerrant RL, Walker DH, Weller PF, eds. *Tropical infectious diseases: principles, pathogens, and practice.* 2nd ed. Philadelphia: Churchill Livingstone Elsevier; 2006.
8. Fischer SA, Graham MB, Kuehnert MJ, et al. Transmission of lymphocytic choriomeningitis virus by organ transplantation. *N Engl J Med.* 2006;354(21):2235.
9. Palacios G, Druce J, Du L, et al. A new arenavirus in a cluster of fatal transplant-associated diseases. *N Engl J Med.* 2008;358(10):991.
10. Centers for Disease Control and Prevention. Lymphocytic choriomeningitis virus transmitted through solid organ transplantation—Massachusetts, 2008. *MMWR.* 2008;57(29):799.
11. Centers for Disease Control and Prevention. *Lymphocytic choriomeningitis.* http://www.cdc.gov/ncidod/dvrd/spb/mnpages/dispages/lcmv/qa.htm. Accessed on August 27, 2008.
12. Centers for Disease Control and Prevention. Interim guidance for minimizing risk for human lymphocytic choriomeningitis virus infection associated with rodents. *MMWR.* 2005;54(30):747.
13. Childs JE, Glass GE, Korch GW, et al. Lymphocytic choriomeningitis virus infection and house mouse *(Mus musculus)* distribution in urban Baltimore. *Am J Trop Med Hyg.* 1992;47(1):27.
14. Kang SS, McGavern DB. Lymphocytic choriomeningitis infection of the central nervous system. *Front Biosci.* 2008;13:4529.
15. Wright KE, Spiro RC, Burns JW, et al. Post-translational processing of the glycoproteins of lymphocytic choriomeningitis virus. *Virology.* 1990;177(1):175.
16. Sage RD. Wild mice. In: Foster HL, Small JD, Fox J, eds. *The mouse in biomedical research, vol I: history, genetics, and wild mice.* New York: Academic Press; 1981.
17. Armstrong C, Sweet L. Lymphocytic choriomeningitis. Report of two cases, with recovery of the virus from gray mice *(Mus musculus)* trapped in the two infected households. *Public Health Rep.* 1939;54:673.
18. Blumenthal W, Ackermann R, Scheid W. Distribution of the lymphocytic choriomeningitis virus in an endemic area [in German]. *Dtsch Med Wochenschr.* 1968;93(19):944.
19. Smithard EHR, Macrae AD. Lymphocytic choriomeningitis; associated human and mouse infections. *Br Med J.* 1951;1(4718):1298.
20. Childs JE, Glass GE, Ksiazek TG, et al. Human-rodent contact and infection with lymphocytic choriomeningitis and Seoul viruses in an inner-city population. *Am J Trop Med Hyg.* 1991;44(2):117.
21. Childs JE, Glass GE, LeDuc JW. Rodent sightings and contacts in an inner-city population of Baltimore, Maryland, USA. *Bull Soc Vector Ecol.* 1991;16(2):245.
22. Amman BR, Pavlin BI, Albariño CG, et al. Pet rodents and fatal lymphocytic choriomeningitis in transplant patients. *Emerg Infect Dis.* 2007;13(5):719.
23. Lehmann-Grube F. *Lymphocytic choriomeningitis virus, Virology monographs. 10.* Wein and New York: Springer-Verlag; 1971.
24. Ackermann R, Stille W, Blumenthal W, et al. Syrian hamsters as vectors of lymphocytic choriomeningitis [in German]. *Dtsch Med Wochenschr.* 1972;97(45):1725.
25. Biggar RJ, Woodall JP, Walter PD, et al. Lymphocytic choriomeningitis outbreak associated with pet hamsters. Fifty-seven cases from New York State. *JAMA.* 1975;232(5):494.
26. Deibel R, Woodall JP, Decher WJ, et al. Lymphocytic choriomeningitis virus in man. Serologic evidence of association with pet hamsters. *JAMA.* 1975;232(5):501.
27. Hirsch MS, Moellering Jr RC, Pope HG, et al. Lymphocytic-choriomeningitis-virus infection traced to a pet hamster. *N Engl J Med.* 1974;291(12):610.
28. Wright R, Johnson D, Neumann M, et al. Congenital lymphocytic choriomeningitis virus syndrome: a disease that mimics congenital toxoplasmosis or cytomegalovirus infection. *Pediatrics.* 1997;100(1):e9.
29. Komrower GM, Williams BL, Stones PB. Lymphocytic choriomeningitis in the newborn. Probable transplacental infection. *Lancet.* 1955;268(6866):697.
30. Barton LL, Budd SC, Morfitt WS, et al. Congenital lymphocytic choriomeningitis virus infection in twins. *Pediatr Infect Dis J.* 1993;12(11):942.
31. Larsen PD, Chartrand SA, Tomashek KM, et al. Hydrocephalus complicating lymphocytic choriomeningitis virus infection. *Pediatr Infect Dis J.* 1993;12(6):528.
32. Barton LL, Mets MB, Beauchamp CL. Lymphocytic choriomeningitis virus: emerging fetal teratogen. *Am J Obstet Gynecol.* 2002;187(6):1715.
33. Barton LL, Peters CJ, Ksiazek TG. Lymphocytic choriomeningitis virus: an unrecognized teratogenic pathogen. *Emerg Infect Dis.* 1995;1(4):152.
34. Enders G, Varho-Gobel M, Lohler J, et al. Congenital lymphocytic choriomeningitis virus infection: an underdiagnosed disease. *Pediatr Infect Dis J.* 1999;18(7):652.
35. Mets MB, Barton LL, Khan AS, et al. Lymphocytic choriomeningitis virus: an underdiagnosed cause of congenital chorioretinitis. *Am J Ophthalmol.* 2000;130(2):209.
36. Bonthius DJ, Perlman S. Congenital viral infections of the brain: lessons learned from lymphocytic choriomeningitis virus in the neonatal rat. *PLoS Pathog.* 2007;3(11):e149.
37. Acha PN, Szyfres B. *Zoonoses and communicable diseases common to man and animals, vol. II: chlamydioses, rickettsioses and viroses.* 3rd ed. Washington, DC: Pan American Health Organization; 2003.
38. Gilbert DN, Moellering RC, Eliopoulos GM, et al. *Sanford guide to antimicrobial therapy 2009.* 39th ed. Sperryville, VA: Antimicrobial Therapy; 2009.

METHICILLIN-RESISTANT *STAPHYLOCOCCUS AUREUS* INFECTION

Peter M. Rabinowitz and Lisa A. Conti

Staphylococcal infection, unspecified (ICD -10 A49.0)

Other names in humans: MRSA

Other names in animals: MRSA

In recent years, methicillin-resistant *Staphylococcus aureus* (MRSA), long considered a nosocomial infection of hospitalized patients, has emerged as a significant pathogen in the community setting. Although *S. aureus* most commonly causes skin and soft tissue infections, invasive strains of MRSA have been associated with necrotizing pneumonia, sepsis, and necrotizing fasciitis, even in previously healthy persons.[1] This community-acquired MRSA (CA-MRSA) has also been found in companion animals[2-13] and livestock,[14-17] and there is evidence of transmission between animals and humans.[4,8,12,15,18-26] Concern has been expressed in the media about the emergence of a new "superbug" in people and animals. The picture is complex and evolving, reinforcing the need for close cooperation and communication between human and veterinary health professionals.

Key Points for Public Health Professionals and Clinicians

Public Health Professionals

- Provide descriptive epidemiology of infection in human and animal populations.
- Educate the public on prevention strategies, such as not sharing towels, clothes, or razors; frequent handwashing (the Healthcare Infection Control Practices Advisory Committee has specific guidance), bandaging wounds, and disinfecting surfaces[27] (disinfectants include 1% sodium hypochlorite, glutaraldehyde, and iodone/alcohol combinations[28]); and the occurrence of carrier states.[29]
- Educate local veterinary and human health clinicians in risk areas and during high-risk periods about groups at risk and symptoms of disease.
- Educate health providers regarding risk groups and how to recognize clusters of patients.
- Ensure that workers at risk are using appropriate handwashing and PPE, as well as isolation of suspected cases.
- Encourage community members to be immunized against seasonal influenza as MRSA pneumonia can occur when healthy persons get influenza.
- Encourage and facilitate communication among physicians, veterinarians, and public health personnel.
- Ensure that positive aspects of animal contact are not ignored when assessing risk of zoonotic MRSA transmission.[30]

Human Health Clinicians

- Be alert to the possibility of MRSA when diagnosing and treating soft tissue infections.
- Treat and report cases to health department if reportable in state.
- Ensure that adequate hand hygiene practices are used with all patients and isolation procedures are used for suspected MRSA cases.[31]
- Counsel patients in whom MRSA has been colonized regarding measures to reduce risk of transmission to other humans and animals (bandage wounds, avoid direct contact).
- Query patients about animal contact. Ask patients/family members about any observed illness in pets.
- Consider the role of household pets and other animal contacts in situations where MRSA transmission appears to be ongoing in a household.[30] Recommend testing of pets only in situations where the entire household is being tested. All animal testing should be directed by the attending veterinarian, with results reported to the physician with pet owner consent.

Veterinary Clinicians

- Ensure that the clinical laboratory processing bacterial cultures is able to identify S. aureus and MRSA in clinical specimens.

- Isolate and screen all suspected cases. Isolate confirmed cases.
- Consider the role of household pets and other animal contacts in situations where MRSA transmission appears to be ongoing in a household. Recommend testing of pets in situations where the entire household is being tested. Animal results should be reported to the physician with pet owner consent.
- Ensure that adequate hand hygiene procedures and a high standard of environmental cleaning and disinfection are in place for staff in veterinary hospitals, and isolation procedures are used for suspected MRSA cases.
- Consider screening of veterinary personnel[32] during extreme circumstances (i.e., when there is epidemiological evidence of personnel-borne transmission and transmission persists after improvement in infection control practices are made). NOTE: The prevalence of MRSA colonization is higher in general among veterinary personnel than the general population[4,20,23,33] and veterinary staff can be exposed at any time. A negative screening result does not ensure that the person's test result will be negative the following day. A positive result also does not mean the person is involved in transmission, and there is no indication to restrict the duties of a veterinary worker in whom MRSA has been colonized.

Agent

The S. aureus bacterium is a gram-positive coccus that is coagulase positive and exists as a commensal organism in humans and many animal species, typically carried in the nasopharynx. The resistance of S. aureus to β-lactam antibiotics (penicillins and cephalosporins) including methicillin is due to the production of a penicillin-binding protein (PBP2a) encoded by the mecA gene, which is carried on a transposable genetic element called the staphylococcal cassette chromosome mec (SCCmec). There are at least five different SCCmec types (I-V) and several subtypes.[34] The PBP2a protein is expressed in the cell wall and has a low affinity for β-lactam antibiotic binding. Some MRSA also have membrane-bound protein pumps to remove antibiotics. Although strains of S. aureus that are resistant to methicillin have been identified for many years, some recent clones circulating in humans since 2000 include genes coding for Panton-Valentine leukocidin (PVL), a membrane toxin that appears to be related to virulence (Figure 9-88).[29] The bacteria are stable in the environment for 17 hours in sunlight, 46 hours on glass, less than 7 days on floors, 42 days in carcasses and organs, and 60 days in meat products.[35]

Geographical Occurrence

S. aureus is a major human pathogen that is found worldwide. It appears to have a predominantly human reservoir and can be isolated from the nares of about 30% of healthy adults.[36] MRSA has emerged in developing countries, where it remains common.[37] In some parts of the United States, the majority of community isolates of S. aureus from ill patients are now MRSA.[38]

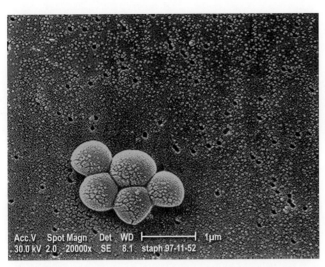

Figure 9-88 ■ Magnified (×20,000), this scanning electron micrograph depicts a grouping of MRSA bacteria. (From Centers for Disease Control and Prevention Public Health Image Library, Atlanta, Ga. Photo Courtesy Janice Carr.)

Groups at Risk

The major risk factor for MRSA infection continues to be contact with the health care system, such as a recent hospitalization, nursing home stay, or surgery.[39] Studies of hospital personnel have found MRSA in nasal carriages in 6% of persons sampled.[1] For cases that arise in the community, reported risk factors include age younger than 2 years, low socioeconomic status, participation in contact sports, injection drug use, men who have sex with men, military personnel, inmates of correctional facilities, veterinarians, pet owners, and pig farmers.[40]

Hosts, Reservoir Species, Vectors

Although humans are considered the primary host for *S. aureus* infection, *S. aureus* is clearly a commensal of many other species. In addition to skin and soft tissue infection, pneumonia, and other pathologic conditions, asymptomatic nasal carriage rates of 30% or greater have been reported. Previous surveys have indicated that human nasal carriage rates of MRSA are much lower than for *S. aureus* in general, but this may be changing.[41]

In animals, *S. aureus* is not as common a pathogen as other *Staphylococcus* species such as *S. pseudintermedius* (previously referred to as *S. intermedius*).[7] However, recent studies have found significant carriage rates of MRSA in dogs and cats from almost all body sites tested (wounds, abscesses, and chronic pyodermas). Other animals that carry MRSA include horses, pigs, elephants, rabbits, cattle, and birds.[4,12,14-15,17,21,42,43] Strain-typed MRSA infections found in dogs and cats are typically indistinguishable from predominant human strains.[3,6,8,44,45] To date, studies have shown transmission of MRSA from people to animals and animals to people, but it is not clear whether animals are a significant reservoir for people. However, evidence suggests that several new MRSA strains may have entered human populations from pigs and cattle.[4] A study in a small animal hospital found 9% of the dogs were MRSA carriers, whereas almost 18% of the staff was infected.[5] Among *S. aureus* isolates from sick animals in veterinary teaching hospitals, 14% were MRSA.[46] Among healthy dogs and cats in the general population, MRSA prevalence has been reported at 1% to 3%, although there was a high rate of infection with methicillin-resistant coagulase-negative *Staphylococcus* (MRCoNS).[14] The epidemiology in pigs may be different. A relatively high prevalence of nasal carriage of MRSA has been reported[47] in agreement with previous studies showing transmission between pigs and farmers.[14]

MRSA infections associated with pigs and calves have emerged as a significant concern in Europe. Studies have identified pig or calf contact as significant risk factors for both colonization or infection with a specific MRSA strain, called ST398, which has been found in pigs in Europe, Asia, and North America.[15-17,42] Astoundingly high rates of colonization have been identified in pig and cattle farmers.[15,16,25] There is concern that this strain is now causing infections beyond direct human contacts and that farm animals may be an important reservoir of this strain for human infections.[25,48,49]

Mode of Transmission

The risk of transmission between humans and other animals may vary by species and type of MRSA (Figure 9-89). One study found evidence of MRSA transmission between dogs and veterinary workers.[50] Equine-human zoonotic transmission has been fairly clearly established.[12]

The mode of transmission in the community is thought to be primarily by hands that become contaminated by contact with colonized or infected body sites of other individuals or fomites contaminated with body fluids containing MRSA. Other factors contributing to transmission include skin-to-skin contact, crowded conditions, and poor hygiene.[51] Risk factors for acquisition of MRSA are likely to include certain antimicrobial use in veterinary medicine.

Environmental Risk Factors

MRSA can persist on environmental surfaces and has been cultured from surfaces in veterinary hospitals.[4] Despite finding MRSA on various environmental surfaces, evidence of surfaces as a source of infection is weak; direct contact with humans or animals is a much more likely route of transmission.

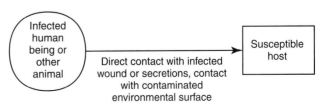

Figure 9-89 ■ Life cycle, MRSA infection.

Disease in Humans

S. aureus typically causes skin and soft tissue infection, including furunculosis, folliculitis, and cellulitis. The more invasive strains of MRSA have been associated with necrotizing pneumonia and necrotizing fasciitis (Color Plate 9-45). Sepsis can occur with any strain. Often the first sign of infection is a small pustule or area of redness. This can rapidly progress to a localized abscess or a more generalized infection (Color Plate 9-46).

Disease in Animals

Infection in animals, while often subclinical, can be associated with a wide range of opportunistic infections, ranging from skin and soft tissue infections to pneumonia and sepsis (Color Plate 9-47). *S. aureus* causes mastitis in cows, and milk is a recognized source of *S. aureus* infection (but not MRSA). Surveys of dairy products have detected MRSA in milk and cheese.[52] Table 9-44 provides comparative clinical presentations in humans and other animals.

Diagnosis

In humans and animals, the cornerstone of diagnosis is culture with appropriate sensitivities. Genotyping can provide information about strain type but does not provide any guidance regarding clinical management. For rapid diagnosis in human patients, a Gram stain showing gram-positive cocci in clusters is suggestive of *S. aureus* infection. This does not apply in animals where other *Staphylococcus* organisms are common.

Some veterinary laboratories may not perform the studies necessary to identify a case of staphylococcal infection as *S. aureus* or MRSA because traditionally *S. pseudintermedius* has been a more important pathogen.

Treatment

Table 9-45 outlines treatment guidelines in humans and other animals. Since clindamycin resistance occurs in some cases, a test for inducible resistance "double D" (double disk diffusion)

Table 9-45 ■ MRSA Treatment in Humans and Other Animals

Species	Primary Treatment	Alternative
Humans (health care–associated)	Vancomycin	Teicoplanin, daptomycin, linezolid, dalbavancin, TMP-SMX (test susceptibility first)
Human (community acquired): abscess, immunocompetent, afebrile (outpatient care)	TMP-SMX double strength	Doxycycline *or* minocycline *or* clindamycin
Abscess with fever (outpatient care)	TMP-SMX double strength ± rifampin	Clindamycin *or* doxycycline
Pneumonia	Vancomycin IV	Linezolid IV
Bacteremia, endocarditis, septic	Vancomycin IV	Daptomycin IV[53]
Dogs	Chloramphenicol 33 mg/kg tid	
Cats	Chloramphenicol 50 mg/kg bid	
Horses	Based on susceptibility testing	
Cattle	Based on susceptibility testing	

D-test, Double-disk diffusion; *quino/dalfo*, quinupristin/dalfopristin; *TMP-SMX*, trimethoprim-sulfamethoxazole.

or D-test should be performed before using this agent.[53] Antimicrobial therapy should be based on antibiogram as well as patient (e.g., age, renal function) and infection factors (e.g., location, organic debris, drug penetration). In most cases, MRSA isolates are susceptible to a variety of antimicrobials, and commonly used antimicrobials such as chloramphenicol may be used. Trimethoprim-sulfamethoxazole is often useful;

Table 9-44 ■ Methicillin-Resistant *Staphylococcus Aureus:* Comparative Clinical Presentations in Humans and Other Animals

Species	Risk Factors for all Species	Clinical Manifestations	Laboratory Findings
Humans	Contact with a colonized or infected person or animal; nosocomial contact; poor hygiene	Soft tissue infection, pneumonia	Gram stain showing gram-positive cocci in clusters, culture and sensitivity, PFGE, spa typing, latex agglutination for PBP2a
Dogs		Soft tissue infection	
Cats		Soft tissue infection	
Horses		Soft tissue infection, joint infections, pleuropneumonia	
Cattle		Mastitis	
Pigs		Subclinical carriage, rare skin infections	

PBP2a, Penicillin-binding protein 2a; *PFGE*, pulsed-field gel electrophoresis.

however, adverse effects (keratoconjunctivitis sicca, arthropathy) must be considered. Aminoglycosides are often effective but must be administered parenterally. Some isolates may appear susceptible to fluoroquinolones in vitro, but this class of drugs should not be used because in vivo response is typically poor and resistance develops quickly.

There is currently controversy about the use of drugs in a veterinary setting that are important in human medicine (i.e., vancomycin, linezolid). Although veterinarians have the ability to use such drugs in an extra-label fashion, ethical issues about the use of these critically important human drugs should be considered, and if used, they should only be used in extreme circumstances when no other options exist and the infection cannot be treated topically or in some other manner.

References

1. Hawkes M, Barton M, Conly J, et al. Community-associated MRSA: superbug at our doorstep. *Can Med Assoc J.* 2007;176(1):54.
2. Boost M, O'donoghue M, Siu K. Characterisation of methicillin-resistant *Staphylococcus aureus* isolates from dogs and their owners. *Clin Microbiol Infect.* 2007;13:731.
3. Leonard FC, Abbott Y, Rossney A, et al. Methicillin-resistant *Staphylococcus aureus* isolated from a veterinary surgeon and five dogs in one practice. *Vet Rec.* 2006;158:155.
4. Loeffler A, Boag A, Sung J, et al. Prevalence of methicillin-resistant *Staphylococcus aureus* among staff and pets in a small animal referral hospital in the UK. *J Antimicrob Chemother.* 2005;56:692.
5. Middleton J, Fales W, Luby C, et al. Surveillance of *Staphylococcus aureus* in veterinary teaching hospitals. *J Clin Microbiol.* 2005;43:2916.
6. O'Mahony R, Abbott Y, Leonard F, et al. Methicillin-resistant *Staphylococcus aureus* (MRSA) isolated from animals and veterinary personnel in Ireland. *Vet Microbiol.* 2005;109:285.
7. Rankin S, Roberts S, O'Shea K, et al. Panton Valentine leukocidin (PVL) toxin positive MRSA strains isolated from companion animals. *Vet Microbiol.* 2005;108:145.
8. Weese J, Dick H, Willey B, et al. Suspected transmission of methicillin-resistant *Staphylococcus aureus* between domestic pets and humans in veterinary clinics and in the household. *Vet Microbiol.* 2006;115:148.
9. Weese JS, Faires M, Rousseau J, et al. Cluster of methicillin-resistant *Staphylococcus aureus* colonization in a small animal intensive care unit. *J Am Vet Med Assoc.* 2007;231:1361.
10. Baptiste K, Williams K, Willams N, et al. Methicillin-resistant staphylococci in companion animals. *Emerg Infect Dis.* 2005;11:1942.
11. Seguin JC, Walker RD, Caron JP, et al. Methicillin-resistant *Staphylococcus aureus* outbreak in a veterinary teaching hospital: potential human-to-animal transmission. *J Clin Microbiol.* 1999;37:1459.
12. Weese J, Archambault M, Willey B, et al. Methicillin-resistant *Staphylococcus aureus* in horses and horse personnel, 2000–2002. *Emerg Infect Dis.* 2005;11:430.
13. Weese J, Rousseau J, Traub-Dargatz J, et al. Community-associated methicillin-resistant *Staphylococcus aureus* in horses and humans who work with horses. *J Am Vet Med Assoc.* 2005;226:580.
14. de Neeling A, van den Broek M, Spalburg E, et al. High prevalence of methicillin resistant *Staphylococcus aureus* in pigs. *Vet Microbiol.* 2007;122:366.
15. Huijsdens X, van Dijke B, Spalburg E, et al. Community-acquired MRSA and pig-farming. *Ann Clin Microbiol Antimicrob.* 2006;5:26.
16. Khanna T, Friendship R, Dewey C, et al. Methicillin resistant *Staphylococcus aureus* colonization in pigs and pig farmers. *Vet Microbiol.* 2008;128(3):298.
17. van Duijkeren E, Ikawaty R, Broekhuizen-Stins MJ, et al. Transmission of methicillin-resistant *Staphylococcus aureus* strains between different kinds of pig farms. *Vet Microbiol.* 2008;126(4):383.
18. Weese J, Caldwell F, Willey B, et al. An outbreak of methicillin-resistant *Staphylococcus aureus* skin infections resulting from horse to human transmission in a veterinary hospital. *Vet Microbiol.* 2006;114:160.
19. Wulf MW, Sørum M, van Nes A, et al. Prevalence of methicillin-resistant *Staphylococcus aureus* among veterinarians: an international study. *Clin Microbiol Infect.* 2007;14(1):29.
20. Hanselman B, Kruth S, Rousseau J, et al. Methicillin-resistant *Staphylococcus aureus* colonization in veterinary personnel. *Emerg Infect Dis.* 2006;12:1933.
21. Juhász-Kaszanyitzky E, Jánosi S, Somogyi P, et al. MRSA transmission between cows and humans. *Emerg Infect Dis.* 2007;13:630.
22. Manian FA. Asymptomatic nasal carriage of mupirocin-resistant, methicillin-resistant *Staphylococcus aureus* (MRSA) in a pet dog associated with MRSA infection in household contacts. *Clin Infect Dis.* 2003;36:e26.
23. Moodley A, Nightingale EC, Stegger M, et al. High risk for nasal carriage of methicillin-resistant *Staphylococcus aureus* among Danish veterinary practitioners. *Scand J Work Environ Health.* 2008;34:151.
24. van Duijkeren E, Wolfhagen MJ, Heck ME, et al. Transmission of a Panton-Valentine leukocidin-positive, methicillin-resistant *Staphylococcus aureus* strain between humans and a dog. *J Clin Microbiol.* 2005;43:6209.
25. van Rijen MM, Van Keulen PH, Kluytmans JA, et al. Increase in a Dutch hospital of methicillin-resistant *Staphylococcus aureus* related to animal farming. *Clin Infect Dis.* 2008;46:261.
26. Wulf M, van Nes A, Eikelenboom-Boskamp A, et al. Methicillin-resistant *Staphylococcus aureus* in veterinary doctors and students, the Netherlands. *Emerg Infect Dis.* 2006;12:1939.
27. Centers for Disease Control and Prevention. *Environmental management of Staph and MRSA in community settings.* http://www.cdc.gov/ncidod/dhqp/ar_mrsa_Enviro_Manage.html. Accessed September 9, 2008.
28. Dvorak G, Rovid-Spickler A, Roth JA, et al. *Handbook for zoonotic diseases of companion animals.* Ames, IA: The Center for food security and public health, Iowa State University College of Veterinary Medicine; 2008.
29. Centers for Disease Control and Prevention. *Healthcare-associated methicillin resistant Staphylococcus aureus.* http://www.cdc.gov/ncidod/dhqp/ar_mrsa_prevention.html. Accessed September 9, 2008.
30. Barton M, Hawkes M, Moore D, et al. Guidelines for the prevention and management of community-associated methicillin-resistant *Staphylococcus aureus*: a perspective for Canadian health care practitioners. *Can J Infect Dis Med Microbiol.* 2006;17(suppl C):4C–24C.
31. Centers for Disease Control and Prevention. *Management of multidrug-resistant organisms in healthcare settings.* http://www.cdc.gov/ncidod/dhqp/pdf/ar/MDROGuideline2006.pdf. Accessed September 9, 2008.
32. Leonard FC, Markey BK. Methicillin-resistant *Staphylococcus aureus* in animals: a review. *Vet J.* 2008;175(1):27.
33. Deurenberg RH, Vink C, Kalenic S, et al. The molecular evolution of methicillin-resistant *Staphylococcus aureus.* *Clin Microbiol Infect.* 2007;13(3):222.
34. Chambers HF. Community-associated MRSA—resistance and virulence converge. *N Engl J Med.* 2005;352(14):1485.
35. Kluytmans J, van Belkum A, Verbrugh H. Nasal carriage of *Staphylococcus aureus*: epidemiology, underlying mechanisms, and associated risks. *Clin Microbiol Rev.* 1997;10:505.
36. Hart CA, Kariuki S. *Antimicrobial resistance in developing countries.* http://www.bmj.com/cgi/content/extract/317/7159/647. Accessed September 9, 2008.
37. Chambers HF. *The changing epidemiology of Staphylococcus aureus.* http://www.cdc.gov/ncidod/eid/vol7no2/chambers.htm. Accessed September 9, 2008.
38. Klevens RM, Morrison MA, Nadle J, et al. Active bacterial core surveillance (ABCs) MRSA investigators. Invasive methicillin-resistant *Staphylococcus aureus* infections in the United States. *JAMA.* 2007;298(15):1763.
39. Kenner Cesur S, Cokca F. Nasal carriage of methicillin-resistant *Staphylococcus aureus* among hospital staff and outpatients. *Infect Cont Hosp Epidemiol.* 2004;25(2):169.
40. Kuehnert MJ, Kruszon-Moran D, Hill HA, et al. Prevalence of *Staphylococcus aureus* nasal colonization in the United States, 2001–2002. *J Infect Dis.* 2006;193(2):172.
41. Morris DO, Rook KA, Shofer FS, et al. Screening of *Staphylococcus aureus, Staphylococcus intermedius,* and *Staphylococcus schleiferi* isolates obtained from small companion animals for antimicrobial resistance: a retrospective review of 749 isolates (2003–04). *Vet Dermatol.* 2006;17(5):332.
42. van Duijkeren E, Jansen MD, Flemming SC, et al. Methicillin-resistant *Staphylococcus aureus* in pigs with exudative epidermitis. *Emerg Infect Dis.* 2007;13:1408.
43. Walther B, Wieler LH, Friedrich AW, et al. Methicillin-resistant *Staphylococcus aureus* (MRSA) isolated from small and exotic animals at a university hospital during routine microbiological examinations. *Vet Microbiol.* 2008;127(1):171.

44. Strommenger B, Kehrenberg C, Kettlitz C, et al. Molecular characterization of methicillin-resistant *Staphylococcus aureus* strains from pet animals and their relationship to human isolates. *J Antimicrob Chemother.* 2006;57:461.
45. van Loo I, Huijsdens X, Tiemersma E, et al. Emergence of methicillin-resistant *Staphylococcus aureus* of animal origin in humans. *Emerg Infect Dis.* 2007;13(12):1834.
46. Vengust M, Anderson ME, Rousseau J, et al. Methicillin-resistant staphylococcal colonization in clinically normal dogs and horses in the community. *Lett Appl Microbiol.* 2006;43(6):602.
47. Voss A, Loeffen F, Bakker J, et al. Methicillin-resistant *Staphylococcus aureus* in pig farming. *Emerg Infect Dis.* 2005;11(12):1965.
48. Wulf M, Voss A. MRSA in livestock animals—an epidemic waiting to happen? *Clin Microbiol Infect.* 2008;14(6):519.
49. Baptiste KE, Strommenger B, Kehrenberg C, et al. Molecular characterization of methicillin-resistant *Staphylococcus aureus* strains from pet animals and their relationship to human isolates. *J Antimicrob Chemother.* 2006;57(3):461.
50. Williams K, Willams NJ, Wattret A, et al. Methicillin-resistant staphylococci in companion animals. *Emerg Infect Dis.* 2005;11(12):1942.
51. Centers for Disease Control and Prevention. *Community-associated MRSA information for clinicians.* http://www.cdc.gov/ncidod/dhqp/ar_mrsa_ca_clinicians.html#8. Accessed September 9, 2008.
52. Normanno G, Corrente M, La Salandra G, et al. Methicillin-resistant *Staphylococcus aureus* (MRSA) in foods of animal origin product in Italy. *Int J Food Microbiol.* 2007;117(2):219.
53. Gilbert DN, Moellering RC, Ellopoulos GM, et al. *Sanford guide to antimicrobial therapy 2009.* 39th ed. Antimicrobial Therapy; 2009.

ORF

Natasha Rabinowitz, Matthew S. Alkaitis, Lisa Conti, and Peter Rabinowitz

Other orthopox infections (ICD-10 B08.0)

Other names in humans: ecthyma contagiosum, contagious ecthyma virus, contagious pustular dermatitis virus, contagious pustular stomatitis, giant orf

Other names in animals: cutaneous ecthyma, scabby mouth disease, sore mouth disease, ovine pustular dermatitis

Infection with orf virus is primarily a disease of sheep and goats that can significantly affect husbandry operations. Transmission of the disease to humans was first recognized in the 1930s[1-3] and remains an occupational risk to those who handle these animals, particularly immunocompromised individuals. It is also a hazard in public settings such as petting zoos and county fairs. Recent outbreaks in the United States have underscored the importance of differentiating orf virus infection from life-threatening or other rare diseases in humans and from other economically significant diseases in animals such as foot and mouth disease (FMD).

Key Points for Clinicians and Public Health Professionals

Public Health Professionals

- Provide descriptive epidemiology for the community.
- Educate local veterinary and human health clinicians in risk areas and during high-risk periods about groups at risk and the signs and symptoms of disease.
- Educate the public, especially parents, on ways to prevent general transmission of infection on farms and petting zoos.
- Encourage handwashing after handling animals.
- Provide animal owners and exhibitors with the *Compendium of Measures to Prevent Disease Associated with Animals in Public Settings.*[4]
- Work with local agricultural authorities to exclude potentially infected animals from fairs, exhibitions, and other locations where cross-infection could occur.

- Encourage barrier protection such as the use of nonporous gloves when handling infected or recently vaccinated animals in addition to handwashing.
- Encourage animal owners and exhibitors to carefully monitor their animals and promptly quarantine those that present lesions or were recently vaccinated.[5]

Human Health Clinicians

- Consider the diagnosis in humans compared with other life-threatening conditions such as cutaneous anthrax.
- Counsel at-risk workers regarding the importance of protecting open wounds, using nonporous gloves, and handwashing when caring for infected or recently vaccinated sheep and goats[5-7] and to use caution when handling the animal vaccine.
- Counsel immunocompromised individuals or those with chronic skin disorders to avoid contact with potentially infected animals.
- No human vaccine is available.

Veterinary Clinicians

- Consider orf in the differential diagnosis of vesicular lesions, including foot and mouth disease.
- Counsel farmers to remove thistle and harsh brush from grazing areas, which can reduce skin trauma to the mouth and muzzle area necessary for transmission of the virus.[6]
- Counsel animal owners to refrain from bringing infected or recently vaccinated animals to public events or shows.
- Advise PPE and sharps injury prevention for veterinary staff and farm workers during vaccination and care of infected animals.
- Ensure that veterinarians and veterinary staff can recognize signs of occupational infection and seek care.
- Report disease to veterinary/agriculture and public health authorities as well as occupational health care providers caring for at-risk workers.
- Live, nonattenuated orf virus vaccines are commercially available.[5] Preparations can also be made from scabs of

previously infected animals. Both types are potentially infectious to humans who handle the vaccine, experience a sharps injury during vaccine administration, or have contact with the vaccine site or recently vaccinated animals.[5] Orf virus vaccines are intended to produce controlled infection in flocks and will ultimately seed the environment with virus-containing scabs.[6] Thus vaccination should be used only in previously infected flocks.[8,9] The immunity conferred by current vaccines is not lifelong and failures have been reported.[5] The 2001 USDA National Animal Health Monitoring System (NAHMS) sheep survey reported that 5% of sheep operations vaccinated replacement or breeding ewes and 14% vaccinated nursing lambs.[10] In counseling animal owners who are considering vaccinating their livestock, veterinary clinicians should:

- o Encourage the vaccination of lambs at ≈1 month of age and a second vaccination at 2 to 3 months for at-risk lambs.[11]
- o Provide proper precaution to prevent outbreaks and transmission to humans associated with vaccine use.
- o Discourage the use of vaccines in flocks that have not previously been infected.

Agent

Orf is caused by *Parapoxvirus ovis*, also known as *orf virus* (Figure 9-90). It is a highly epitheliotropic poxvirus of the family Poxviridae with a double-stranded DNA genome of approximately 140 kb.[12] It can be visualized by electron microscopy of negatively stained samples and appears as a cylinder of roughly 260×160 nm with a crisscross pattern characteristic of poxviruses.[7,13] Several other related parapox viruses cause zoonotic infections. Paravaccinia virus (also known as pseudo-cowpox) infect the teats of cattle and cause nodular lesions on the hands of dairy workers (milker's nodule).[12] Other zoonotic parapox virus infections include bovine papular stomatitis and seal pox.[14]

Geographical Occurrence

Orf virus is found worldwide with a higher prevalence in countries with extensive sheep and goat populations.[6-8] According to the 2001 national USDA NAHMS survey, 40% of U.S. sheep operations reported cases of orf infection within the past 3 years.[10] Human cases in recent years have been reported in Illinois, Tennessee, Missouri, New York, and California.[5,6] The incidence of human cases reflects the prevalence of infection in sheep and goat populations. However, cases in humans are probably underreported because those at risk are often familiar with the disease, recognize that it is self-limiting, and choose not to seek medical attention.[1,2,16,17] The fact that many laboratories lack the diagnostic capability for orf virus testing may further contribute to underreporting of the disease.[6]

Groups at Risk

Orf virus is an occupational risk to those who handle sheep and goats, including farmers, shepherds, veterinarians, butchers, and abattoir workers.[2,16] Wildlife researchers with contact with wild sheep and goat species are also at risk. These groups are especially at risk during the primary lambing season (spring and summer) because young animals are more susceptible to infection.[1,5,12] Those handling orf vaccines or recently vaccinated flocks are at greater risk of developing an infection.[1,5,6] Children may be at greater risk in both occupational (e.g., family farm) or recreational (e.g., petting zoo[4]) settings because common childhood behaviors such as nuzzling animals can lead to significant skin contact or bites.[5] Furthermore, children may be less likely to wash their hands or use gloves than adults.[5] Orf has been reported in conjunction with religious holidays during which families customarily slaughter a sheep or cow.[12,16,17] Contact with wildlife such as deer can also result in transmission to humans.[18] Patients with chronic skin disorders such as eczema are at increased risk for contracting orf infection.[5] Immunocompromised individuals are at risk for more severe disease.[6]

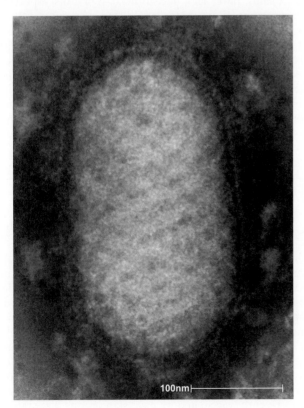

Figure 9-90 ■ Negative-stained transmission electron micrograph image depicted the ultrastructural details of an orf virus, a member of the genus *Parapoxvirus*. (From Centers for Disease Control and Prevention Public Health Image Library, Atlanta, Ga. Photo courtesy A. Likos.)

Hosts, Reservoir Species, Vectors

Small ruminants including sheep and goats are the predominant species affected, although infection has been reported in gazelles, musk oxen, alpacas, camels, deer, reindeer, and dogs.[7,19,20] Wild bighorn sheep (*Ovis canadensis*) and other wild sheep and goats can be infected. Certain breeds such as Boer goats are particularly susceptible to infection.[8,19] Humans are accidental hosts.

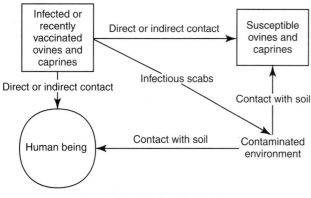

Figure 9-91 ■ Life cycle of orf virus.

Mode of Transmission and Life Cycle

Orf virus is transmitted via direct contact with broken skin or mucous membranes (Figure 9-91). Skin trauma is considered a predisposing factor in both animals[9,19,21] and humans.[5,6,9] Modes of transmission between animals include contact with infected animals or fomites such as bedding, feed, stalls fences, and trailers.[7,8] Because young animals are particularly susceptible due to their developing immune systems, outbreaks often occur during the principal lambing season.[1,5] Suckling can lead to lesions on the mother's teats and cause her to withhold feeding, leading to the spread of the disease to non-mother adults or to humans via tube- or bottle-feeding practices.[5]

Transmission from animals to humans can be facilitated by either minor (thistle pricks, torn cuticle) or severe (animal bite) skin trauma.[5,6] Other human activities that can lead to infection include shearing, petting, and handling infected equipment.[8] Orf virus can persist in wool and hides for over a month after the resolution of lesions, putting butchers, abattoir workers, and shearers at risk.[7,22] Orf virus vaccine is a live, nonattenuated preparation that has been known to cause outbreaks among sheep and human handlers.[6,7] Human-to-human transmission of orf infection has yet to be reported.

Environmental Risk Factors

Infected animals can shed virus-containing scabs that persist in animal housing and other inanimate objects such as harnesses, and pastures.[7,8,12] This environmental contamination can lead to indirect infection of other animals and humans. Although the virus is susceptible to ultraviolet rays, it is resistant to desiccation, temperature drops, and other environmental stressors and can survive in the soil and on surfaces for months.[7,13,22]

Disease in Humans

Initial signs of infection appear at the site of skin penetration after a 2- to 3-day incubation period. Lesions can reach 3 cm in diameter and typically occur on the hands or forearms, although infection of the face has also been reported.[2]

Symptoms of infection progress through several stages, each lasting approximately a week.[2]

The maculopapular stage begins with isolated or multiple erythematous macules and papules appearing at the site of contact that may be pruritic. The target stage features the development of vesiculonodules characterized by a white ring enclosing a red center (Color Plate 9-48). This is followed by an acute stage with an erythematous nodule with weeping, bleeding, and eventual crusting.

In immunocompetent patients, the infection is usually self-limited with full healing without scarring over a 6-week period.[5,6,13,16] Bacterial superinfection of the lesions may occur.[7,13] Other reported complications include pain, fever, malaise, erythema multiforme, blindness from ocular involvement, lymphangitis, and autoimmune pemphigus with bullous eruptions.[1,13,17,22-24] Immunocompromised patients are at greater risk for these complications, in addition to progressive or recurring "giant" lesions.[5,6,8,13] Infection with orf confers immunity, but reinfection has been reported, although it is typically less severe.[1]

Disease in Animals

Although animals of any age are susceptible, the disease is seen primary in animals younger than 1 year because adult animals are typically immune as a result of previous contact.[5] Outbreaks among livestock tend to occur in spring and summer.

Lesions occur primarily on the muzzle, nostrils, ears, lips, eyelids, lower legs, buccal mucosa, or teats, especially when nursing.[2] Boer goats may develop suppurative arthritis, chronic fibrinous pneumonia, and premature thymic involution.[19] No loss of appetite or difficulty in nursing was reported in lambs infected with buccal cavity lesions.[21] Recovery occurs within a month. Some animals may require feeding assistance. Animals can be infected more than once during their lifetime, but infections occur far apart and young animals present with the most severe cases.[8] Table 9-46 shows comparative clinical presentations in humans and other animals.

Diagnosis

Diagnosis in Humans

The diagnosis of orf in humans can be made clinically based on a history of exposure to sheep or goats and the presence of characteristic skin lesions. The differential diagnosis includes a number of potentially life-threatening infections, including cutaneous anthrax,[5] tularemia, and erysipeloid.[5,6] Other similar conditions include milker's nodule, cowpox, pyogenic granuloma, and skin cancer.[3,17] Clues to the clinical diagnosis include a history of exposure to sheep, goats, deer, and alpacas in petting zoos, farms, or other settings such as fairs, especially if animals were recently vaccinated or have skin lesions. Laboratory diagnostic techniques include PCR, electron microscopic histopathological analysis, and viral isolation, but these tests are not widely available.

Table 9-46 ▪ Orf Virus: Comparative Clinical Presentations in Humans and Other Animals

Species	Risk Factors	Incubation Period	Clinical Manifestations	Laboratory Findings
Humans	Direct contact with infected animals; contact with soil and objects contaminated by animals, vaccine exposure	3-7 days	Maculopapular eruption progressing to weeping nodule	PCR, EM, viral isolation
Sheep, goats, alpaca, camels, deer	Contact with infected or recently vaccinated animals or contaminated environments	2-3 days	Papules, vesicles, pustules on the lips, mouth, nostrils, eyelids, ears, extremities	PCR, EM, viral isolation

EM, Electron microscopy; *PCR*, polymerase chain reaction.

Diagnosis in Animals

Lesions in animals can resemble foot and mouth disease because both diseases can present as erythematous, ulcerated papules.[6,9,21] The main clinical sign differentiating orf from foot and mouth disease is the proliferative nature of the lesions.[21] As with humans, the diagnosis can be confirmed with PCR or viral isolation.

Treatment

Orf infections in immunocompetent persons typically resolve spontaneously over 3 to 6 weeks.[2] Some treatments, including 40% topical idoxuridine,[2,5] imiquimod,[12] or cidofovir cream, accelerate the resolution of lesions.[24] Cleaning and antiseptically dressing the lesion can reduce the risk of secondary infection.[2] Surgical treatment may be used in severe cases but can occasionally result in the formation of satellite lesions.[2] The course of treatment usually depends on the location of the lesion.[13]

In animals, repellent should be applied to avoid development of myiasis caused by larvae from the fly *Cochliomyia hominivorax*.[7] Cases of bacterial superinfection can be treated with antibiotics.

References

1. Buchan J. Characteristics of orf in a farming community in mid-Wales. *BMJ.* 1996;313:203.
2. Key SJ, Catania J, Mustafa SF, et al. Unusual presentation of human giant orf (ecthyma contagiosum). *J Craniofac Surg.* 2007;18:1076.
3. Georgiades G, Katsarou A, Dimitroglou K. Human orf (ecthyma contagiosum). *J Hand Surg [Br].* 2005;30:409.
4. National Association of State Public Health Veterinarians. Compendium of measures to prevent disease associated with animals in public settings. *MMWR.* 2007;56(RR-5):1.
5. Lederman ER, Austin C, Trevino I, et al. Orf virus infection in children: clinical characteristics, transmission, diagnostic methods, and future therapeutics. *Pediatr Infect Dis J.* 2007;26:740.
6. Centers for Disease Control and Prevention. Orf virus infection in humans—New York, Illinois, California, and Tennessee, 2004–2005. *MMWR.* 2006;55:65.
7. Acha PN, Szyfres B. *Zoonoses and communicable diseases common to man and animals, vol. II: chlamydioses, rickettsioses and viroses.* 3rd ed. Washington, DC: Pan American Health Organization; 2003.
8. Centers for Disease Control and Prevention. *Frequently asked questions about sore mouth (orf virus).* http://www.cdc.gov/ncidod/dvrd/orf_virus. Accessed September 27, 2008.
9. Büttner M, Rziha HJ. Parapoxviruses: from the lesion to the viral genome. *J Vet Med B Infect Dis Vet Public Health.* 2002;49:7.
10. United States Department of Agriculture, Animal and Plant Health Inspection Service, Veterinary Services, National Animal Monitoring System. *Sheep 2001, part II: reference of sheep health in the United States, 2001.* Fort Collins: USDA; 2003.
11. Kahn CM, Line S, eds. *The Merck veterinary manual.* 9th ed. Whitehouse Station, NJ: Merck; 2005.
12. Haig DM, McInnes CJ. Immunity and counter-immunity during infection with the parapoxvirus orf virus. *Virus Res.* 2002;88:3.
13. Erbağci Z, Erbağci I, Almila Tuncel A. Rapid improvement of human orf (ecthyma contagiosum) with topical imiquimod cream: report of four complicated cases. *J Dermatolog Treat.* 2005;16:353.
14. Becher P, Konig M, Muller G, et al. Characterization of sealpox, a separate member of the parapoxviruses. *Arch Virol.* 2002;147:113.
15. Mandell GL, Bennett JE, Dolin R. *Principles and practice of infectious diseases.* 6th ed. New York: Churchill Livingstone Elsevier; 2005.
16. Gurel MS, Ozardali I, Bitiren M, et al. Giant orf on the nose. *Eur J Dermatol.* 2002;12:183.
17. Al-Salam S, Nowotny N, Sohail MR, et al. Ecthyma contagiosum (orf)—report of a human case from the United Arab Emirates and review of the literature. *J Cutan Pathol.* 2008;35:603.
18. Kuhl JT, Huerter CJ, Hashish H. A case of human orf contracted from a deer. *Cutis.* 2003;71:288.
19. de la Concha-Bermejillo A, Guo J, Zhang Z, et al. Severe persistent orf in young goats. *J Vet Diagn Invest.* 2003;15(423).
20. Vikøren T, Lillehaug A, Akerstedt J, et al. A severe outbreak of contagious ecthyma (orf) in a free-ranging musk ox (*Ovibos moschatus*) population in Norway. *Vet Microbiol.* 2008;127:10.
21. McElroy MC, Bassett HF. The development of oral lesions in lambs naturally infected with orf virus. *Vet J.* 2007;174:663.
22. Heymann DL, ed. *Control of communicable diseases manual.* 19th ed. Washington, DC: American Public Health Association; 2008.
23. White KP, Zedek DC, White WL, et al. Orf-induced immunobullous disease: a distinct autoimmune blistering disorder. *J Am Acad Dermatol.* 2008;58:49.
24. Geerinck K, Lukito G, Snoeck R, et al. A case of human orf in an immunocompromised patient treated successfully with cidofovir cream. *J Med Virol.* 2001;64:543.

PLAGUE

Peter M. Rabinowitz and Lisa A. Conti

Plague (ICD-10 A20)

Other names in humans: bubonic plague, pneumonic plague, septicemic plague, black death

Other names in animals: feline plague, rodent plague, sylvatic plague

Yersinia pestis, the agent of plague in humans and other animals, has caused some of the largest epidemics in history. Plague continues to be an important and potentially fatal zoonotic disease, with 1 to 40 reported cases each year in the United States associated with rodent and flea contact and occasionally contact with sick cats.[1] Worldwide, several thousand cases are reported yearly to the World Health Organization. *Y. pestis* is a category A potential biological warfare agent. Despite its fearsome reputation and sensitivity to prompt antibiotic treatment, delays in diagnosis of plague in both humans and animals are frequent, often with tragic consequences. There is a continuing need for heightened awareness of the disease, especially in enzootic areas.

Key Points for Clinicians and Public Health Professionals

Public Health Professionals

- Provide descriptive epidemiology of the disease in the health district. Use of GIS risk mapping has been helpful in determining areas of high risk for endemic plague.[2]
- Educate the public about measures to reduce risk, including the following:
  - Control rodents and their fleas near dwellings (flea control should precede rodent control to prevent fleas from seeking new hosts); Box 9-5 lists steps for rodent-proofing homes.
  - Avoid camping near rodent burrows.
  - Avoid handling wild rodents (plague in the United States is strongly associated with ground-dwelling sciurid rodents, such as various species of prairie dogs and their fleas).
  - Use flea control on cats and dogs.
  - Prevent pets from hunting.[1]
- Conduct an immediate investigation of human, cat, or dog cases; consider the possibility of deliberate use (biological warfare).
- Ensure flea control in an outbreak situation before initiating rodent control measures.
- Ensure that persons with exposure to cases of pneumonic plague or other high-risk exposures (including exposures to cats with plague) are receiving antibiotic prophylaxis (see below) and are maintained under surveillance for 7 days.

BOX 9-5   *STEPS FOR RODENT-PROOFING HOMES*

- *Seal* rodent entry holes or gaps with steel wool, lath metal, or caulk.
- *Trap* rats and mice using appropriate snap trap.
- *Clean up* rodent food sources and nesting sites.
- Keep wood piles and compost heaps away from the house.
- Take precautions when cleaning rodent-infected areas:
  - Use cross-ventilation when entering a previously unventilated enclosed room or dwelling before to cleanup.
  - Use rubber, latex, vinyl, or nitrile gloves.
  - Do not stir up dust by vacuuming, sweeping, or any other means. Instead, thoroughly wet contaminated areas with a bleach solution or household disinfectant. *Hypochlorite (bleach) solution:* mix 1½ cups of household bleach in 1 gallon of water. Once everything is wet, take up contaminated materials with damp towel and then mop or sponge the area with bleach solution or household disinfectant.
  - Spray dead rodents with disinfectant and then double-bag along with all cleaning materials and dispose of bag in an appropriate waste disposal system.
  - Remove gloves and thoroughly wash hands with soap and water (or waterless alcohol-based hand rubs when soap is not available and hands are not visibly soiled).

- Ensure that workers with occupational risk for *Y. pestis* infection receive adequate surveillance and reduction of exposure risk through exposure controls and protective equipment.
- A plague vaccine is being developed.

Human Health Clinicians

- Consider the diagnosis in all patients with recent travel or residence in an enzootic area, with occupational exposure (such as veterinarians or wildlife workers), history of handling rodents, rabbits, or flea bites, as well as the possibility of deliberate use.
- Report disease immediately to public health authorities using the CDC case definition (see http://www.cdc.gov/ncphi/disss/nndss/casedef/plague_current.htm). CDC, Fort Collins, is a WHO Collaborating Center for Reference and Research on Plague Control, and reports all human plague cases in the United States to the WHO.
- Ensure patients are hospitalized with drainage and secretion precautions (bubonic plague) and maintain droplet precautions until 48 hours of appropriate antibiotic treatment has been completed with clinical improvement (including defervescence).
- Counsel patients in endemic areas with rodent exposure or with cats or dogs in risk reduction measures, including regular use of flea control (see above).

Veterinary Clinicians

- Consider the diagnosis in any sick cat from an enzootic area with fever, lymphadenopathy, and abscesses on the head and neck or progressive respiratory signs accompanied by other systemic signs. The submandibular lymph node is the most common site of lymphadenopathy due to the inoculation of the oral mucosa from ingestion of plague-infected rodents.

- Train veterinary personnel in biosafety measures such as masks and gloves when working with potentially infected animals. N-95 respirators are recommended.[3]
- Treat animals at the veterinary hospital for 48 to 72 hours and observe clinical improvement (including defervescence) before allowing animal to be treated at home. This will ensure that owners will not be exposed to infectious saliva and other secretions when handling or treating their pet.
- Isolate and control fleas on suspected cases while treating with antibiotics.
- Follow local and state reporting regulations; contact local health department immediately regarding suspected animal cases.
- Recommend keeping cats indoors.
- Counsel clients not to let cats and dogs roam outside or otherwise come in contact with wildlife in endemic areas, and to treat monthly to control and prevent flea infestations.
- Store animal food in rodent-proof containers.
- A plague vaccine for use in endangered black-footed ferrets has been developed and used.[4]

Agent

Y. pestis is a gram-negative, bipolar staining, nonmotile bacillus that is a member of the family of Enterobacteraciae.[5] The CDC classifies *Y. pestis* to be a category A biological warfare agent due to its ability to be produced and disseminated in quantities sufficient to affect large populations and its high case fatality rate among untreated persons. It is believed that deliberate use of the agent would be in an aerosol form.[6]

Geographical Occurrence

Plague occurs in localized areas on most continents, with most cases being reported in less-industrialized countries (Color Plate 9-49). Some cases in developing countries are related to rats and their fleas in urban areas (urban plague). In the United States, most cases occur in rural areas west of the Mississippi, where the disease exists in wild (ground-dwelling) rodent reservoirs (sylvatic plague)—New Mexico, Idaho, Colorado, Nevada, Oregon, Texas, Arizona, California, Utah, Washington, and Wyoming. Mapping of rodent habitat in the Southwestern United States has successfully identified areas of increased human risk related to conifer forests and amount of precipitation. Much of the area of increased plague risk in the Southwest overlaps with risk areas for hantaviral infection, another rodent-borne disease.[7]

Groups at Risk

Groups at increased risk for *Y. pestis* infection include hunters, veterinarians, mammalogists, campers, hikers, Native Americans, owners of cats allowed to roam free, and rural residents in enzootic areas. A significant number of cat-associated human cases have occurred among veterinarians and veterinary assistants.[3,8] Most U.S. cases occur between May and October, when temperatures favor transmission from the fleas and potential human and rodent interactions are higher.[5]

Hosts, Reservoir Species, Vectors

Worldwide, an important reservoir for *Y. pestis* is domestic rats (*R. rattus* and *R. norvegicus*), especially in urban settings. In the United States, however, wild rodents are the principal reservoir species, including ground squirrels, rock squirrels, and prairie dogs.[9] In many of these species, susceptible individuals develop the disease and significant die-offs among colonies of some species of prairie dogs are well documented (Color Plate 9-50).[10] Black-footed ferrets, an endangered species, can become infected from preying on prairie dogs.[4] Risk of exposure to fleas infected by *Y. pestis* is elevated in areas adjacent to rodent colonies experiencing widespread mortality, and these die-offs provide a warning of infection risk to humans and domestic animals.

Fleas are the principal vector of plague. Urban plague has been linked to exposure to the oriental rat flea *Xenopsylla cheopis* (Color Plate 9-51), which commonly infests *Rattus* species. Fleas, once infected, may remain infectious for a year or longer.[11] Both male and female fleas can transmit the infection. Wild rodent fleas vary by species in their ability to be effective vectors. Cat fleas (*Ctenocephalides felis*) are considered poor vectors for plague.[3,11] The human flea (*Pulex irritans*) may spread the infection between humans in situations of crowding and poor sanitation.[11]

Mode of Transmission and Life Cycle

Plague is spread through flea bites, direct contact with an infected animal, and by inhalation of infectious aerosols (Figure 9-92).[12,13] Fleas that have ingested a blood meal from an infected host can then infect another animal through a bite.

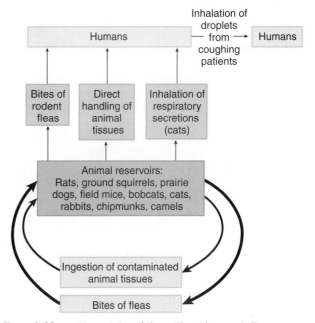

Figure 9-92 ■ Transmission of plague. The *wide arrows* indicate common modes of transmission, the *medium arrows* indicate occasional modes of transmission, and the *thin arrow* indicates a rare kind of transmission. (From Mandell GL (ed): *Mandell, Douglas, and Bennett's principles and practice of infectious diseases*, ed 7, Philadelphia, 2010, Churchill Livingstone Elsevier.)

The usual source of human infection is a bite from an infected flea or direct handling of an infected animal carcass. Dogs and cats may bring fleas into a home where they can bite humans. Infected cats with pneumonic plague are a source of respiratory spread to humans. Person-to-person transmission through infectious aerosols occurs when there is respiratory involvement but has not been documented in the United States since 1924.

Environmental Risk Factors

The bacterium does not appear to survive long outside a mammal host. It can be destroyed by sunlight and drying.[14] Environmental factors influencing the risk of plague include those driving increases in rodent populations. Human habitation encroachment into wildlife habitat is an environmental driver of infection risk, because it leads to contact between wild rodent reservoirs of the infection and their fleas and peridomestic rodents. Dogs and cats may contribute to this wildlife-human contact by bringing fleas into dwellings.

Disease in Humans

There are several forms of human plague infection:
- *Bubonic plague* usually results from a flea bite or direct contact with an infected animal. There can be a local reaction at the site of the bite. After 2 to 6 days, fever, weakness, and malaise develop with lymphadenopathy. The swollen, extremely tender lymph nodes (buboes) typically occur most commonly in the groin, neck (rarely), or axilla and are often unilateral (Color Plate 9-52). Bacteremia is common. Without treatment, bubonic plague can progress to sepsis, shock, and death.
- Primary *septicemic plague* may develop without buboes. This form has a higher fatality rate than bubonic plague, possibly because of delays in diagnosis. Hypotension and disseminated intravascular coagulation can occur with shock and organ failure (Color Plate 9-53).
- *Pneumonic plague* may result from secondary spread to the lungs of bubonic plague or from primary infection caused by contact with a human or cat with respiratory involvement. Most cases of primary pneumonic plague in the United States are currently related to exposure to infected cats.[8] Pneumonic plague is highly fatal and can lead to further horizontal transmission to close contacts through respiratory spread.
- *Pharyngeal plague* also results from respiratory infection and is characterized by sore throat, pharyngitis, and local lymphadenopathy.
- Meningeal plague is rare but may be a complication of bubonic plague.[5]

Disease in Animals

Although certain subpopulations of the rodent hosts of the disease are apparently resistant to developing clinical infection, other individuals are susceptible, so that high mortality rates can occur. In these latter groups, such as prairie dogs, monitoring acute mortality can help predict plague activity in an area.

Cats are known to be susceptible to plague and can exhibit bubonic, pneumonic, or septicemic forms of the disease. Bubonic plague of the head and neck is the most common form in cats following bites from infected flea or consumption of infected rodents (Color Plate 9-54).[15] Secondary septicemic or pneumonic plague can also develop in cats; this form has led to primary pneumonic plague infection of humans in close contact with such cats (Figure 9-93). Signs in cats include fever, malaise, cough, and buboes. Without treatment, feline plague can be fatal in a substantial proportion of cases. Wild felids such as bobcats and mountain lions are also susceptible to plague.

Although dogs are less likely to develop clinical illness than cats, signs of infection have been documented in three naturally infected dogs in New Mexico (Color Plate 9-55).[16] Clinical signs included fever, lethargy, submandibular lymphadenitis, a purulent intermandibular lesion, oral cavity lesions, and cough. In dogs, antibodies to plague appear by day 8, peak by day 21, and decline by day 100 after exposure. This characteristic, combined with their relative resistance to clinical illness, makes dogs potentially useful as sentinels for plague risk in enzootic areas.

Table 9-47 summarizes the clinical presentations of plague in humans and other animals.

Diagnosis

The differential diagnosis of bubonic plague in humans includes other causes of acute lymphadenopathy, including bartonellosis (cat-scratch disease), staphylococcal abscess, tuberculosis, and lymphogranuloma venereum. The rapid onset and associated symptoms should help the clinician make the diagnosis. Pneumonic plague can resemble other rapidly progressive pneumonias. A history of exposure to fleas, rodents, sick cats, or wild carnivores can be helpful, as well as any information of recent outbreaks among animals or humans where the person lives or has recently traveled.

Samples of blood and wound drainage should be sent for culture and chest x-rays films should be obtained. A national network of laboratories has been established for rapid

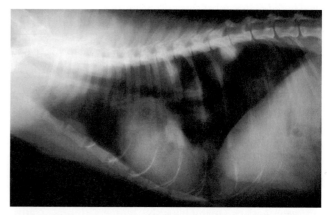

Figure 9-93 ■ Thoracic radiograph of a cat with pneumonic plague. (From Greene CE: *Infectious diseases of the dog and cat*, ed 3, St Louis, 2006, Saunders Elsevier. Courtesy Dennis Macy, Colorado State University, Fort Collins.)

Table 9-47 ■ Plague: Comparative Clinical Presentations in Humans and Other Animals

Species	Risk Factors	Incubation Period	Clinical Manifestations	Laboratory Findings
Humans				
Bubonic plague	Flea bite, contact with infected animal	2-7 days	Fever, lymphadenopathy	Elevated WBC count, abnormal liver function tests, culture of blood, DFA of LN aspirate
Septicemic plague			Fever, hypotension, DIC	
Pneumonic plague	Infectious aerosol	1-4 days[1]	Cough, hemoptysis, fever	Abnormal coagulation studies
Pharyngeal plague			Sore throat, pharyngitis, cervical lymphadenopathy	Pulmonary infiltrates on x-ray
Plague meningitis	Can result from bubonic plague		Meningeal signs	WBCs in CSF
Cats				
Bubonic plague (pneumonia may accompany)	Flea bites, ingestion of rodent	2-7 days	Lymphadenopathy with cellulitis on head and neck, abscess formation, drainage, fever, depression, dehydration, anorexia, oral ulcers	Culture of blood, lymph node biopsy or aspirate, DFA of LN aspirate Serology HI (may persist more than a year in surviving animals)
Septicemic plague			Fever, depression, vomiting	
Pneumonic plague	Inhalation of infectious aerosol		Fever, cough, bloody sputum[3]	
Dogs	Flea bites	7-10 days[17]	Often subclinical, mild fever, depression	Serology HI
Rodents, Rabbits	Flea bites	Days	May be subclinical in a minority of cases Death	

CSF, Cerebrospinal fluid; *DIC*, disseminated intravascular coagulation; *DFA*, direct immunofluorescence antibody; *HI*, hemagglutination inhibition; *LN*, lymph node; *WBC*, white blood cell.

diagnosis of plague, and consultation should be obtained regarding the appropriate testing facility to process specimens. In bubonic plague, the bubo can be aspirated and sent for Gram stain, Wayson stain, DFA, and culture.[5] PCR tests may be available. Diagnosis can be confirmed by serology obtained acutely and after several weeks showing a fourfold rise in titer, a single titer greater than 1:128,[18] or by positive bacteriophage testing from a culture isolate.

In animals, culture and DFA of tissues antibody serology testing are the mainstays of diagnosis. Diagnostic samples can include wound drainage, lymph node aspirates, blood, and necropsy specimens biopsy of liver, lung, spleen, or bone marrow. If there is evidence of respiratory involvement, a pharyngeal swab can be performed. Specimens should be kept chilled.[3]

Treatment

Treatment in Humans

Treatment in human beings with antibiotics should be begun as soon as the diagnosis is suspected. Patients should be hospitalized in an intensive care unit with wound drainage and droplet precautions until 48 hours of appropriate antibiotics with clinical improvement (including defervescence). Although streptomycin has the greatest proven efficacy, it is not widely available in the United States, and gentamicin or doxycycline may be used (Table 9-48).[19] If buboes become

large and fluctuant they may require incision and drainage. Supportive care with intravenous fluids and close hemodynamic monitoring is necessary for most patients.

Persons with close contact with a patient or animal with pneumonic plague or other potential exposures (bite from a cat with potentially infectious saliva, bubo drainage in an open wound, and so on) should receive antibiotic prophylaxis and surveillance for symptoms for 7 days after exposure ceases.

Treatment in Animals

Infected cats should be hospitalized, isolated, and have immediate flea treatment with imidacloprid or pyrethrin. Antibiotics should be begun immediately and intravenous fluids and other supportive measures used aggressively. Cats with the pneumonic form of the disease should be considered for euthanasia if adequate infection control is not available in a veterinary hospital because of the infectious nature of the respiratory droplets and the high fatality rate of primary pneumonic plague.[17] Table 9-48 lists recommendations for antibiotic treatment of plague in humans and animals.

References

1. Heymann DL, ed. *Control of communicable diseases manual.* 19th ed. Washington DC: American Public Health Association; 2008.
2. Eisen RJ, Reynolds PJ, Ettestad P, et al. Residence-linked human plague in New Mexico: a habitat-suitability model. *Am J Trop Med Hyg.* 2007;77(1):121.

Table 9-48 ■ Treatment of Plague Infection in Humans and Other Animals

Species	Primary Treatment	Alternative Treatment
Humans (adult)	Gentamicin 5 mg/kg IV q24h *or* streptomycin 15 mg/kg gm IV bid	Doxycycline 200 mg × 1, then 100 mg PO *or* IV *or* ciprofloxacin 500 mg PO bid, *or* 400 mg IV q12h, *or* gentamicin plus doxycycline
Prophylaxis (close contact with infected animal or human)	Doxycycline 100 mg PO bid × 7 days[20]	Ciprofloxacin 500 mg PO bid × 7 days[20]
Cats	Immediate flea treatment Imidacloprid	
Bubonic form	Tetracycline 25 mg/kg PO q8h × 10 days; parenteral 7.5 mg/kg q12h Chloramphenicol 30-50 mg/kg PO q8h[21]	Doxycycline
Pneumonic form	Euthanasia if infection control is inadequate	
Dogs	Flea treatment Antibiotic treatment generally not necessary	

3. Centers for Disease Control and Prevention. *Emergency preparedness and response: plague: veterinary issues: dogs and ungulates.* http://www.bt.cdc.gov/agent/plague/trainingmodule/7/04.asp.

4. Rocke TE, Mencher J, Smith SR, et al. Recombinant F1-V fusion protein protects black-footed ferrets *(Mustelae nigripes)* against virulent *Yersinia pestis* infection. *J Zoo Wildl Med.* 2004;35:142.

5. Mandell GL, Bennett JE, Dolin R. *Principles and practice of infectious diseases.* 6th ed. Philadelphia: Churchill Livingstone Elsevier; 2005.
6. Centers for Disease Control and Prevention. Biological and chemical terrorism: strategic plan for preparedness and response. Recommendations of the CDC Strategic Planning Workgroup. *MMWR.* 2000;49:1.
7. Eisen RJ, Glass GE, Eisen L, et al. A spatial model of shared risk for plague and hantavirus pulmonary syndrome in the southwestern United States. *Am J Trop Med Hyg.* 2007;77(6):999.
8. Gage KL, Dennis DT, Orloski KA, et al. Cases of human plague associated with exposure to infected domestic cats. *Clin Infect Dis.* 2000;30:893.
9. Centers for Disease Control and Prevention. *Plague fact sheet.* http://www.cdc.gov/ncidod/dvbid/plague/facts.htm.
10. Cully Jr JF, Barnes AM, Quan TJ, et al. Dynamics of plague in a Gunnison's prairie dog colony complex from New Mexico. *J Wildlife Dis.* 1997;33:706.
11. Acha PN, Szyfres B. *Zoonoses and communicable diseases common to man and animals, vol. I: bacterioses and mycoses.* 3rd ed. Washington, DC: Pan American Health Organization; 2003.
12. Webb CT, Brooks CP, Gage KL, et al. Classic flea-borne transmission does not drive plague epizootics in prairie dogs. *Proc Natl Acad Sci USA.* 2006;103(16):6236.
13. Wilder AP, Eisen RJ, Bearden SW, et al. *Oropsylla hirsuta* (Siphonaptera: Ceratophyllidae) can support plague epizootics in black-tailed prairie dogs *(Cynomys ludovicianus)* by early-phase transmission of *Yersinia pestis. Vector Borne Zoonotic Dis.* 2008;8(3):359.
14. Colville J, Berryhill D. *Handbook of zoonoses: identification and prevention.* St Louis: Mosby Elsevier; 2007.
15. Eidson M, Thilsted JP, Rollag OJ. Clinical, clinicopathologic, and pathologic features of plague in cats: 119 cases (1977–1988). *J Am Vet Med Assoc.* 1991;199(9):1191.
16. Orloski KA, Eidson M. Yersinia pestis infection in three dogs. *J Am Vet Med Assoc.* 1995;207:316.
17. Barr SC, Bowman DD. *The 5-minute veterinary consult clinical companion: canine and feline infectious diseases and parasitology.* Ames, IA: Blackwell; 2006.
18. St. Louis University School of Public Health: Institute for Biosecurity. *Bioterrorism agent fact sheet: plague/Yersinia pestis.* http://bioterrorism.slu.edu/bt/quick/plague01.pdf.
19. Boulanger L, Ettestad P, Fogarty J, et al. Gentamicin and tetracyclines for the treatment of human plague: a review of 75 cases in New Mexico, 1985–1999. *Clin Infect Dis.* 2004;38(5):663.
20. Gilbert DN, Moellering RC, Eliopoulos GM, et al. *Sanford guide to antimicrobial therapy. 2009.* 39th ed. Sperryville, VA: Antimicrobial Therapy; 2009.
21. Tilley LP, Smith FWK. *Blackwell's five-minute veterinary consult: canine and feline.* 4th ed. Ames, IA: Blackwell; 2008.

Q FEVER

Peter M. Rabinowitz and Lisa A. Conti

Q fever (ICD-10 A78)

Other names in humans: query fever, coxiellosis, abattoir fever, Australian Q fever, nine-mile fever, quadrilateral fever, Balkan influenza[1]

Other names in animals: coxiellosis

Q fever is a disease caused by *Coxiella burnetii* that has a reservoir in a number of animal species. It is spread to humans by direct contact, most commonly through inhalation of organisms but also possibly through ingestion or other intake routes. It causes potentially serious disease in a proportion of people infected, and because of its high infectiveness and environmental persistence has been considered a potential bioterrorism agent. The true impact of Q fever as a zoonotic disease is probably underrecognized because of the nonspecific nature of the illness in many cases.

Key Points for Clinicians and Public Health Professionals

Public Health Professionals

- Human disease is reportable to public health authorities.
- In the event of a case report, determine whether others are at risk and whether there is an ongoing risk of exposure (consider bioterrorism potential of this agent).

- Recommend cleaning sources of contaminated soils and dusts from the environment (understanding that the organism is highly resistant to chemical and physical agents) and disinfection with 0.05% hypochlorite, 5% peroxide, or 1:100 Lysol solution.[2]
- Educate the public, veterinarians, and human health clinicians about risk factors for transmission; organisms localize in reproductive and mammary tissues and can be also be shed in urine and feces and spread by ticks (viable organisms have been recovered from tick feces after 19 months and after 42 months in milk at 4° to 6°C).[2]
- Support the maintenance of milk pasteurization to prevent infection in the general population.

Human Health Clinicians

- Report human disease to public health authorities. http://www.cdc.gov/ncphi/disss/nndss/casedef/q_fever_2008.htm.
- Consider diagnosis in high-risk individuals such as persons with occupational exposure.
- Consider in the differential diagnosis of patients presenting with culture-negative endocarditis.
- Provide occupational preventive services to high-risk individuals, including counseling on PPE and biosafety, as well as consideration of vaccine. Persons with valvular heart disease should not work in laboratory settings with *C. burnetii*.
- Vaccine: a vaccine has been developed for high-risk individuals in Australia but is limited to those at high risk of exposure and who have no demonstrated sensitivity to Q fever antigen.[3] The vaccine is not currently available in the United States either commercially or through an investigational new drug permit.
- Person-to-person transmission is rare but has been reported through sexual contact and to health care staff during obstetrical procedures on infected patients.

Veterinary Clinicians

- Instruct owners and any others in contact with infected animals to immediately seek medical advice.
- Segregate parturient animals and destroy (burn or bury) placentas and other reproductive discharges to reduce transmission.
- Ensure veterinary staff follow proper biosafety procedures, including around parturient animals.
- Isolate infected animals and implement airborne transmission precautions for staff.
- Ensure that ruminants used for research purposes are free of *C. burnetii* through serological testing.
- A vaccine for livestock has been developed and shown to reduce infection in calves and reduce shedding in previously infected animals. However, the vaccine is not currently commercially available in the United States.

Agent

Q fever is caused by *Coxiella burnetii*, a gram-negative obligate intracellular, coccobacillus organism in the gamma subdivision of Protobacteria (along with *Legionella,*

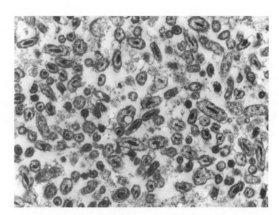

Figure 9-94 ▪ Electron photomicrograph of *Coxiella burnetii*–infected caprine placenta. (From Songer JG, Post KW: *Veterinary microbiology: bacterial and fungal agents of animal disease*, St Louis, 2005, Saunders Elsevier. Courtesy Raymond E. Reed.)

Francisella, and *Rickettsiella*) (Figure 9-94). The organism is highly infectious, with an infective dose of 1 to 10 organisms.[3] It exists in two different antigenic phases, and the human antibody response generated to each antigen phase can be used to assess progression of infection. Phase II antibodies are more predominant in humans experiencing acute infection, whereas phase I antibodies are proportionately more common in chronic disease states, such as endocarditis.[4] There are also at least two different morphologic forms of the bacteria; one is large and bacilliform, another is small and coccoid. The small, high-density form (small cell variant [SCV]) has some resemblance to a spore in terms of its hardiness; it is highly resistant to environmental degradation and therefore plays an important role in transmission.

Geographical Occurrence

C. burnetii occurs worldwide. It is probably more prevalent than recognized owing to the often subclinical nature of disease in humans and animals and the difficulty with laboratory diagnosis. In 2000, cases were reported in California, Colorado, Idaho, Kansas, Minnesota, Nebraska, Nevada, Oregon, and Utah.

Groups at Risk

Q fever often occurs as an occupational disease. Workers at risk include slaughterhouse workers; veterinarians and veterinary staff; farmers; researchers working with pregnant animals, especially sheep; and workers in diagnostic laboratories where the organism may be cultured. However, even casual contact with farm environments or farm animals can lead to infection. Also, because the agent may be spread on dust, persons living near high-risk areas may be at risk for infection through windborne spread.

Although it is less commonly reported among children than adults, Q fever does occur in children, especially among those exposed to farm animals and farm environments for even brief amounts of time.[5] Children can also be infected by drinking raw milk, although they are typically asymptomatic.

Exposure to parturient cats has caused outbreaks in humans in the past among pet owners and their families.[6]

Hosts, Reservoir Species, Vectors

Animals are the natural reservoir for *C. burnetii*. It is found worldwide in sheep (Figure 9-95), cattle, goats, birds, dogs, and cats. Serological evidence of past exposure has also been shown in a variety of wild mammals. In the United States, seroprevalence studies have shown antibodies in more than 40% of sheep, 16% of goats, and 3% of cattle.[7] A study in Colorado found that more than 8% of female cats studied had evidence of *C. burnetii* in uterine tissue, raising the issue of risk to owners during birthing. A study in Asian cats found seroprevalence rates of up to 41% in stray cats and 14% in pet cats.[8] However, the risk of pet-to-human transmission may be low, as an Austrian seroprevalence study did not find that pet ownership was a risk factor for seropositivity to *C. burnetii*.[9]

Mode of Transmission and Life Cycle

Animals infected with *C. burnetii* shed high concentrations of the organism in birth products and milk, as well as lower concentrations in feces and urine (Figure 9-96). The organism can be tickborne in animal-to-animal transmission, but transmission from animals to humans is thought to result mostly from inhalation of droplets and/or aerosols containing organisms from infected placental tissue, other parturient tissues, and dusts containing dried body fluids. The organism is found commonly in raw milk with reported prevalence of >94%.[10] Milk pasteurization has been designed specifically to destroy this heat-resistant organism. Foodborne transmission to humans may occur rarely through unpasteurized milk. Transmission in domestic animals is thought, as in humans, to occur mostly through inhalation of infectious aerosols or ingestion of contaminated tissue.

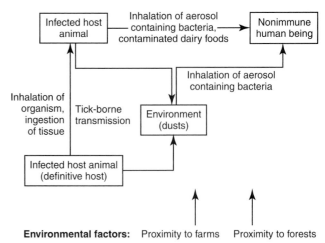

Environmental factors: Proximity to farms   Proximity to forests

Figure 9-96   ■   Life cycle, Q fever infection.

The agent can be found in a number of species of ticks, but tickborne transmission is believed to be more important in wildlife populations than in domestic animal or human infection.[1] However, the patterns of *C. burnetii* infection in wildlife remain poorly understood.

Environmental Risk Factors

Coxiella can persist for months in the environment. The SCV form of the bacteria that is shed in feces and other body fluids is similar in some ways to a spore and quite resistant to disinfectants and temperature extremes. Therefore infectious particles can persist in fomites and dusts, and aerosol transmission has occurred over long distances through windborne spread.[1] Proximity to farms is a risk factor for infection, as wind patterns appear to play a role in environmental transmission by dispersing infectious aerosols over wide areas.[11] Although the role of wildlife is not well understood, living near forested areas has been found to be a risk factor for suburban dwellers.[12]

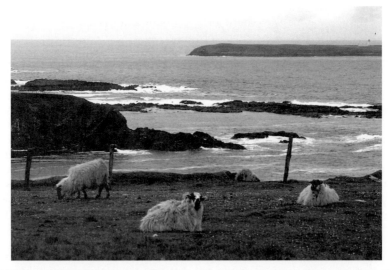

Figure 9-95   ■   Infected sheep have been associated with outbreaks of Q fever in humans. (From Centers for Disease Control and Prevention Public Health Image Library, Atlanta, Ga. Courtesy Edwin P. Ewing, Jr.)

Table 9-49 ▪ Q Fever Infection: Comparative Clinical Presentations in Humans and Other Animals

Species	Risk Factors	Incubation Period	Clinical Manifestations	Laboratory Findings
Humans	High-risk occupation	2-3 weeks (acute form)	Fever, malaise, chills, sweats, headache; hepatomegaly, abortion, placentitis	Serology, stained tissue (blood culture from endocarditis patients typically negative)
	Elderly, debilitated, underlying valvular disease	Months to years (chronic infection)	Chest pain	
Dogs	Tick exposure, contact with farm animals		Fever, neurological syndrome with vasculitis, including lethargy, anorexia, ataxia, seizures	PCR in some laboratories, serology (ELISA), and complement fixation
Cats	Tick exposure, contact with farm animals		Anorexia, lethargy, fever, abortion	
Cattle, sheep, goats	Inhalation of infectious aerosols		Anorexia, abortion	

ELISA, Enzyme-linked immunosorbent assay; *PCR*, polymerase chain reaction.

Disease in Humans

Q fever can present with acute or chronic symptoms (Table 9-49). Some cases in humans are asymptomatic or consist of sufficiently nonspecific symptoms, which results in missed diagnoses. After an incubation period of several weeks, the disease in its acute form often presents with fever, malaise, chills, weakness, headache, and sweats. Pneumonia is a predominant feature, although pulmonary symptoms may be absent even though pneumonitis may be seen on radiographs (Figure 9-97).[4] Chronic symptoms may develop over months to years. Chronic infection may include granulomatous hepatitis, meningitis, and osteomyelitis. The most serious form of chronic infection is bacterial endocarditis, which occurs particularly in persons with underlying valvular disease (Color Plate 9-56). Infection in children can often be asymptomatic but can also present acutely, with encephalitis and neurological symptoms.[13] In convalescent individuals, a postinfectious fatigue syndrome (fever fatigue syndrome) has been described.[4]

Disease in Animals

Animals typically do not manifest clinical signs with the exception of reproductive disease, especially abortion, infertility, and retained placenta (see Table 9-49; Color Plate 9-57). Because infection often goes unrecognized in animals human illness may serve as sentinel events, indicating the presence of infection in a domestic animal population.[14]

Diagnosis

The diagnosis in humans is usually made by serology. A rise in titers is seen in acute infection. Because the prevalence of antibody positivity in certain populations is relatively high, it is necessary to examine paired serological titers. Laboratories interpreting serological results need to use caution; misdiagnosis has resulted from improper interpretation.[15] IgM levels greater than 1:128 suggest acute infection.[11] A PCR test has been developed to aid in diagnosis.[14] In chronic infection, high levels of phase I antibody titers (IgG >1:800) are seen, and phase I antibody titers are usually greater than phase II titers. Blood cultures appear sterile because of the need for intracellular cultivation. Although cell culture and embryonated egg methods exist to culture the organism from blood, laboratory workers are at risk of infection through such procedures, which should not be attempted outside a specialized laboratory experienced in handling the *C. burnetii* organism. The CDC can provide assistance in isolation. *C. burnetii* is considered a "select agent," so handling of live organisms in a laboratory setting is restricted. On biopsy tissue, immunostains and electron microscopy can be diagnostic for the *C. burnetii* organism.[4]

Serological testing is also used in animals. A fourfold increase in IgG over a 4-week period is diagnostic.[16] Tissue (aborted fetus, placenta) can be submitted for immunohistochemical testing. The organism can be isolated from blood in specialized test laboratories (New Mexico Department of Agriculture, Veterinary Diagnostic Services).[16]

Treatment

Acute Q fever is treated with doxycycline as a first-line agent. Chronic infection, including infective endocarditis in humans resulting from Q fever, is treated with a combination of antibiotics for an extended time (18 months to 3 years).

Although information on the efficacy of treatment in animals is limited, prophylactic treatment of endemic herds (or asymptomatic pets) with tetracyclines may reduce the zoonotic potential (rather than eliminate infection).[17] Other control measures include segregating pregnant animals indoors and burying or burning infected reproductive tissue wastes.[7] Table 9-50 provides antibiotic treatment information for Q fever infection in humans and other animals.

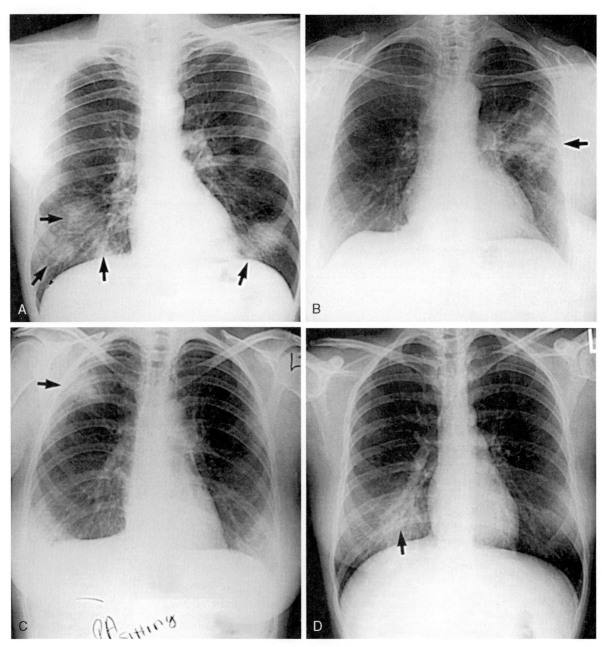

Figure 9-97 ■ Radiographic manifestations of Q fever pneumonia. All four patients are members of one family who developed Q fever after exposure to the infected products of feline conception. Their cat gave birth to kittens in their house. **A**, Multiple rounded opacities. **B**, Left upper lobe opacity. **C**, Pleural-based opacity involving the right upper lobe. **D**, Right lower lobe opacity. In an endemic area **A** is characteristic of cat-related Q fever pneumonia, and **C** is suggestive of this diagnosis. However, **B** and **D** are not at all distinctive and could be due to any pulmonary pathogen. (From Mandell GL, Bennett JE, Dolin R [eds]: *Principles and practice of infectious diseases*, ed 6, Philadelphia, 2005, Churchill Livingstone Elsevier.)

References

1. Acha PN, Szyfres B. *Zoonoses and communicable diseases common to man and animals, vol. II: chlamydioses, rickettsioses and viroses*. 3rd ed. Washington, DC: Pan American Health Organization; 2003.

2. Dvorak G, Rovid-Spickler A, Roth JA, et al. *Handbook for zoonotic diseases of companion animals*. Ames, IA: The Center for Food Security and Public Health, Iowa State University College of Veterinary Medicine; 2008.

3. U.S. Department of Health and Human Services, Centers for Disease Control and Prevention, National Institutes of Health. *Biosafety in microbiological and biomedical laboratories*. 4th ed. Washington, DC: US Government Printing Office. Available at http://www.cdc.gov/od/ohs/biosfty/bmbl4/bmbl4toc.htm, Accessed February 14, 2009.

Table 9-50 ▪ Antibiotic Treatment of Q Fever Infection in Humans and Other Animals

Species	Primary Treatment	Alternative Treatment
Humans: acute disease	Doxycycline 100 mg bid	Erythromycin
Chronic disease	Ciprofloxacin *or* doxycycline *PLUS* rifampin	Fluoroquinolone *PLUS* doxycycline × 3 yr
Endocarditis	Doxycycline 100 mg PO bid *PLUS* hydroxychloroquine 600 mg qd × 1-3 yr[18]	Pregnancy: need long-term TMP-SMX[18]
Acute disease	Doxycycline	Erythromycin
Chronic disease	Ciprofloxacin or doxycycline	Fluoroquinolone *PLUS* Doxycycline × 3 yr
Dogs	Tetracycline 22 mg/kg PO q8h × 2-6 wk	Doxycycline 20 mg/kg PO q12h × 1wk / Enrofloxacin 10 mg/kg PO q12h × 1 wk[16]
Cats	Tetracycline 10–20 mg/kg PO q8-12h × 2-3 wk	Doxycycline 5-10 mg/kg PO q12-24h × 2-4 wk
Cattle, sheep, goats	Tetracycline[7]	

4. Heymann DL, ed. *Control of communicable diseases manual.* 19th ed. Washington, DC: American Public Health Association; 2008.
5. Barralet JH, Parker NR. Q fever in children: an emerging public health issue in Queensland. *Med J Aust.* 2004;180(11):596.
6. Pinsky RL, Fishbein DB, Greene CR, et al. An outbreak of cat-associated Q fever in the United States. *J Infect Dis.* 1991;164(1):202.
7. Kahn CM, Line S, eds. *The Merck veterinary manual.* 9th ed. Whitehouse Station, NJ: Merck; 2005.
8. Komiya T, Sadamasu K, Kang MI, et al. Seroprevalence of *Coxiella burnetii* infections among cats in different living environments. *J Vet Med Sci.* 2003;65(9):1047.
9. Skerget M, Wenisch C, Daxboeck F, et al. Cat or dog ownership and seroprevalence of ehrlichiosis, Q fever, and cat-scratch disease. *Emerg Infect Dis.* 2003;9(10):1337.
10. Kim SG, Kim EH, Lafferty CJ, et al. *Coxiella burnetii* in bulk tank milk samples, United States. *Emerg Infect Dis.* 2005;11:619.
11. Tissot-Dupont H, Amadei MA, Nezri M, et al. A pedagogical farm as a source of Q fever in a French city. *Eur J Epidemiol.* 2005;20(11):957.
12. Gardon J, Heraud JM, Laventure S, et al. Suburban transmission of Q fever in French Guiana: evidence of a wild reservoir. *J Infect Dis.* 2001;184(3):278.
13. Ravid S, Shahar E, Genizi J, et al. Acute Q fever in children presenting with encephalitis. *Pediatr Neurol.* 2008;38(1):44.
14. Cutler SJ, Bouzid M, Cutler RR. Q fever. *J Infect.* 2007;54(4):313.
15. Conti LA, Belcuore TR, Nicholson WL, et al. Pseudoepidemic of Q fever at an animal research facility. *Vector Borne Zoonotic Dis.* 2004;4(4):343.
16. Barr SC, Bowman DD. *The 5-minute veterinary consult clinical companion: canine and feline infectious diseases and parasitology.* Ames, IA: Blackwell; 2006.
17. American Veterinary Medical Association. *Backgrounder: Q fever.* http://www.avma.org/public_health/biosecurity/qfever_bgnd.asp. Accessed February 14, 2009.
18. Gilbert DN, Moellering RC, Eliopoulos GM, et al. *Sanford guide to antimicrobial therapy. 2008.* 38th ed. Sperryville, VA: Antimicrobial Therapy; 2008.

RABIES

Peter M. Rabinowitz and Lisa A. Conti

Rabies (ICD-10 A82)

Other names in humans: lyssa, hydrophobia

Other names in animals: rage

Rabies is one of the most feared zoonotic diseases because it almost invariably causes fatal human encephalitis. Despite the availability of an effective vaccine for humans and domestic animals, rabies continues to be a global public health problem. The first World Rabies Day by the Alliance for Rabies Control took place in September 2007, drawing attention to the need for human health and animal health professionals to work together to reduce this disease threat.[1] This is intended to be an annual event.

Human rabies is relatively rare in North America, but exposure to potentially rabid wild or feral animals occurs frequently. Owner noncompliance with rabies vaccination protocols of their pets, especially cats, can be a source of exposure as well. Managing and preventing such exposures requires an understanding by human health and animal health professionals of the status of rabies infection in local wildlife and domestic animal populations, the judicious use of vaccination strategies, and animal control measures.

Rabies can therefore serve as a model for improved communication and cooperation among public health, animal health, and human health professionals.

Key Points for Clinicians and Public Health Professionals

Public Health Professionals

- Provide rabies control and prevention guidance to the public, veterinarians, and human health clinicians (see World Rabies Day education bank, http://www.worldrabiesday.org/EN/Education-Bank/english.html). Risk reduction measures include:
  - Animal bite avoidance, especially with children
  - Keeping cats indoors and monitoring dogs when outside
  - Avoidance of feeding or handling wildlife or unknown cats and dogs
  - Appropriate exclusion of bats from buildings
- Analyze and report trends from compulsory reports of animal and human rabies.
- Advise the public that any bite wound or potential exposure to rabies should be thoroughly washed with soap and water, and the bite reported to local health authorities.

- Work with local human and veterinary medical providers and animals control officials in the management of potential rabies exposures.
- Support the preexposure vaccination of high-risk individuals.
- Explore methods of control of viral transmission in wildlife population (such as oral vaccine).
- Discourage ownership of pet wildlife or wild/domestic hybrids.
- Support appropriate vaccination requirements and policies to reduce translocation and importation of potentially rabid animals.
- Support scientific research on which to base public health policy.
- Provide access to appropriately trained laboratorians to diagnose the disease.

Human Health Clinicians

- In evaluating any patient with an animal bite, take an accurate history of the species involved and circumstances of the bite incident (see Figure 9-105).
- Coordinate with public health and animal control authorities as PEP may not be required if the animal is able to be tested, or the dog, cat, or ferret is available for observation. Certain monkey bites may need to be evaluated for herpes B exposure potential.
- Prevention of the development of clinical disease through the use of preexposure and postexposure vaccination strategies is the mainstay of preventing rabies deaths in humans. Become familiar with *Human Rabies Prevention—United States, 2008: Recommendations of the Advisory Committee on Immunization Practices (ACIP)* (http://www.cdc.gov/mmwr/preview/mmwrhtml/rr57e507a1.htm). Ensure that candidates for PEP are rapidly evaluated and treated appropriately. Note that persons previously vaccinated with the human diploid cell vaccine (HDCV) or purified chick embryo cell (PCEC) vaccine should not receive human rabies immunoglobulin (HRIG).
- Report bite incident or use of PEP if required in the state.
- Report suspected human cases of rabies to public health authorities (consider using the Wisconsin protocol for rabies treatment: http://www.mcw.edu/FileLibrary/Groups/Pediatrics/InfectiousDiseases/Milwaukee_rabies_protocol2_1.pdf).
- Coordinate with state health authorities for collection of proper human diagnostic samples for rabies testing at CDC laboratories (http://www.cdc.gov/rabies/statehealthdept.html).
- Provide preexposure vaccinations to high-risk workers including veterinarians and staff working with rabies vector species and laboratory workers in facilities handling rabies vaccine. For persons previously unvaccinated against rabies, initial preexposure vaccination consists of a regimen of three 1-mL doses of HDCV or PCEC vaccines administered intramuscularly.
- Counsel travelers to rabies-endemic countries about the risk from exposure to dogs and other animals. Consider pretravel rabies immunization. In evaluating travelers returning from rabies-endemic countries, obtain history of any animal exposures (see Chapter 10).

Veterinary Clinicians

- Be familiar with the most recent National Association of State Public Health Veterinarians *Compendium on Animal Rabies Prevention and Control* (http://www.nasphv.org/Documents/RabiesCompendium.pdf).
- Ensure dogs, cats, ferrets, and appropriate livestock (e.g., horses) are currently vaccinated against rabies following the label use of the vaccine.[2] There is no parenteral vaccine approved for use in wolf hybrids or pet wildlife.
- Report adverse vaccine reactions, including rabies in a vaccinated animal to the USDA, APHIS, Center for Veterinary Biologics at http://www.aphis.usda.gov/animal_health/vet_biologics/vb_adverse_event.shtml.
- Work with public health officials in observing a healthy dog, cat, or ferret that has bitten a human for signs of illness within 10 days from the time of a bite. If no illness occurs, the person has not been exposed to rabies from that animal.
- Consider assisting public health officials by providing appropriate animal isolation and observation for clinical sign of rabies:
  o If a currently vaccinated dog, cat, or ferret is exposed to a known or suspect rabid animal, it should be revaccinated, confined, and observed for 45 days.
  o If the dog, cat, or ferret is not currently vaccinated, it should be isolated and observed for clinical signs of rabies for 6 months (vaccinated 1 month before release).
- Consider assisting public health officials by providing animal decapitation services for rabies testing.
- Consider rabies in the differential diagnosis of any dog, cat, ferret, horse, or livestock with behavioral changes or exhibiting unexplained neurological signs.
- Contact public health authorities immediately with suspected animal case of rabies.
- Disinfect any cage and housing of a rabid animal with soap solutions, 1% sodium hypochlorite, 2% glutaraldehyde, iodine solutions, or quaternary ammonium compounds.[3]
- Support the PEP of staff at high risk for rabies exposure.

Agent

Rabies is caused by a number of related rhabdoviruses, which are bullet-shaped RNA viruses belonging to the genus *Lyssavirus*. Lyssa viruses are unique among rhabdoviruses in their ability to replicate in a host animal's CNS.[4] Different strains of rabies virus are adapted to particular animal species and can have spillover to other species. Rabies viruses can affect any mammal.

Geographical Occurrence

Rabies viruses occur worldwide on all continents except Antarctica and Australia but in varying degrees of prevalence.

Reliable data on the prevalence in many countries are not available. Certain Pacific and Caribbean islands, including Hawaii, are considered to be free of the virus.[5] The WHO has estimated that 55,000 fatal cases occur in humans annually, with the greatest disease burden in Asia (31,000 deaths), followed by Africa (24,000 deaths).[6]

Groups at Risk

The majority of human cases occur in countries where rabies is endemic in the dog population. Travelers to such areas are therefore one group at risk of exposure and infection.

Occupational groups at risk include veterinarians, wildlife rehabilitators, wildlife management workers, zoologists, animal quarantine workers, animal control officers, and laboratory workers.

Children may be at increased risk because of their behavior of contacting wild and domestic animals. Once exposed, immunocompromised individuals may be at increased risk of contracting infection.

Unvaccinated dogs and cats with exposure to wild animals, particularly raccoons, bats, foxes, and skunks, are at increased risk of rabies exposure and infection.

Hosts, Reservoir Species, Vectors

Animals are the natural reservoir for rabies viruses. Although all mammals are considered susceptible to infection, only carnivores and bats are capable of maintaining the viral reservoir (Figure 9-98).[4] Worldwide, domestic and wild canids and other carnivores are the principal reservoir species for rabies virus. In the United States, dog rabies strain has now been eliminated largely as a result of aggressive vaccination and animal control efforts. However, the disease is now most frequently reported among wild mammals with identifiable virus variants circulating in bats, raccoons, skunks, and foxes (Table 9-51). These variants can affect other mammals including humans, cats, and dogs.[4,7] The disease is generally not reported in small rodents (e.g., squirrels, hamsters, gerbils, mice, or rats), lagomorphs (rabbits), or marsupials (opossums).

Unlike many other zoonotic diseases, animals are not believed to be subclinical carriers. Bats, canines, and other animals that develop rabies and are capable of spreading infection to other animals typically die of the disease within a short time.[8]

In the United States and Europe, oral rabies vaccine programs are used to contain and eliminate the virus from

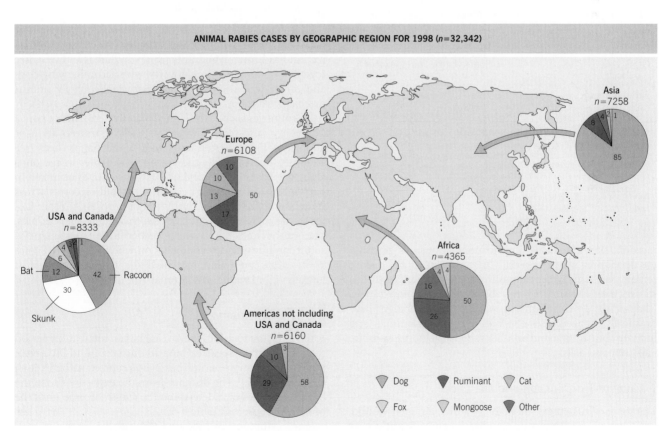

ANIMAL RABIES CASES BY GEOGRAPHIC REGION FOR 1998 (n=32,342)

Figure 9-98 ■ Animal rabies cases by geographic region for 1998. A total of 32,342 cases are displayed. According to World Health Organization sources in the 34th World Survey, which was based on data from 110 countries reporting from 193 members, wildlife rabies predominates in some regions, such as the United States and Canada, and dogs remain a significant reservoir in many other countries. Values shown are percentages. (NOTE: Rabies has been diagnosed among bats in Australia, but these cases are not represented here.) (From Cohen J, Powderly WG: *Infectious diseases*, ed 2, Philadelphia, 2004, Mosby Elsevier.)

Table 9-51 ■ Reported Animal Cases of Rabies in the United States (1998-2002)

Animal*	Average No. of Cases (1998-2002)	Geographical Focus†
Raccoon	2962	Eastern United States
Skunk	2257	California, upper and lower Midwest, eastern United States
Bat	1175	Entire United States, except Hawaii
Fox	443	Alaska, Texas, southwestern United States
Cat	276	Entire United States, except Hawaii
Cattle	106	Entire United States, except Hawaii
Dog	105	Entire United States, except Hawaii
Horse or mule	62	Entire United States, except Hawaii
Mongoose	58	Puerto Rico
Woodchuck	50	Eastern United States
Bobcat	30	Entire United States, except Hawaii
Sheep or goat	9	Entire United States, except Hawaii
Other wild animal	24	Entire United States, except Hawaii
Other domestic animal	3	Entire United States, except Hawaii

*All mammals are considered susceptible to rabies, and incidental (or spillover) infection from wild animal reservoirs may occur in any species.

†Rabies may occur in an exposed animal in any location; the geographical foci listed here are based on current epidemiological trends. No cases of rabies have been reported in Hawaii or in American Samoa, the Commonwealth of the Northern Mariana Islands, Guam, or the U.S. Virgin Islands.

From Rupprecht CE, Gibbons RV: Clinical practice. Prophylaxis against rabies, *N Engl J Med* 351(25):2626-35, 2004.

raccoon, skunk, fox, and coyote populations.[9] In parts of the developing world, especially Asia and Africa, the disease remains endemic in the domestic dog populations and constitutes a risk to travelers to rabies endemic countries (see Chapter 10). In Latin America, vaccination campaigns have drastically reduced cases of rabies in domestic animals and humans, but canine and wildlife rabies (including vampire bats) remains a risk.

Mode of Transmission and Life Cycle

The rabies virus enters the body by a bite, an open wound, or by contact with mucous membranes and replicates near the site of exposure (Figures 9-99 and 9-100). It then travels slowly through sensory and motor nerves to the CNS, where it causes encephalitis. Finally, it spreads centrifugally to the salivary glands and other organs through peripheral nerves. Blood, urine, and feces are not considered infectious.

Humans are usually exposed through a bite from a rabid animal. Not all humans bitten by rabid animals become infected, even in the absence of prophylactic immunization. The likelihood of transmission depends in part on the amount of virus in the saliva. Therefore very minor bites and bites through clothing may be less likely to transmit infection.[8] Transmission by contact of saliva with mucous membranes and conjunctiva is possible but less common than bite-related transmission. Both humoral and cell-mediated immunity appear to play an important role in susceptibility to infection. Immunocompromised individuals are therefore at higher risk of infection from exposure to a rabid animal.

Aerosol transmission has been reported in humans entering caves frequented by bats and in laboratory settings, but this route of exposure is considered rare. Human infection through ingestion of infected meat or milk has not been reported.[8] Person-to-person transmission has rarely been reported through corneal or organ donation.[10]

Transmission between animals results from direct contact such as bites. Dogs and other infected animals are infectious for several days (as long as 13 days has been reported with some rabies virus strains) before symptoms appear and then continue to shed virus in saliva until death; the total period of infectiousness may vary among species.[8]

Environmental Risk Factors

Worldwide, factors affecting the density of dog populations have been drivers of rabies infection risk. Increasing urbanization has brought migrants from rural areas to live closer together, often in extreme poverty, with accompanying dogs and other domestic animals that are inadequately immunized against rabies.

In countries such as the United States where wildlife populations are reservoirs, key factors include translocation of animals from a rabies-endemic area to one that has been free of rabies. For example, the epizootic of rabies in raccoons along the Eastern Seaboard of the United States occurred in part because of the transportation of rabid raccoons across state lines to be released for hunting purposes. Another factor is the increasing contact between wildlife such as bats, raccoons, skunks, and coyotes related to encroachment of suburban housing developments on wildlife habitat (Figure 9-101). Cats could play a potential role in increasing contact between rabid wildlife and human populations.

Disease in Humans

After exposure to rabies the disease has an incubation period that varies from weeks to months (usually 20 to 90 days),[8] but the incubation period has been reported to be as long as several years.[11] The distance from the exposure site to the head and neck helps determine the length of time until the onset of symptoms (Table 9-52).

Early symptoms include anxiety, headache, fever, and malaise. There may be pain, irritation, and other sensory changes around the bite. The patient often becomes excitable with sensitivity to light and sound and demonstrates aerophobia (fear of flying)[12] as well as pupil dilation and increased salivation. Over a short period (2 to 6 days), the disease progresses inexorably

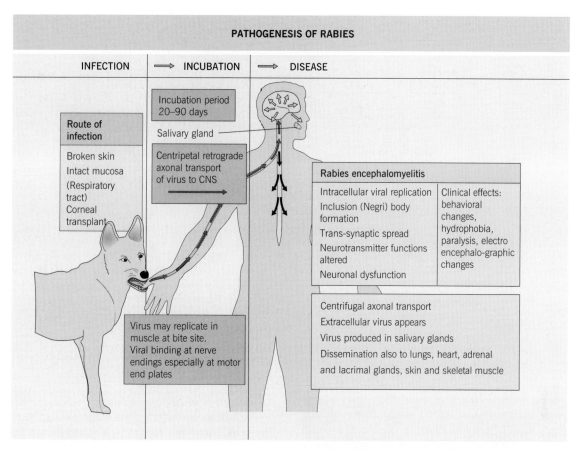

PATHOGENESIS OF RABIES

INFECTION ⟹ INCUBATION ⟹ DISEASE

Incubation period
20–90 days

Salivary gland

Route of
infection

Broken skin
Intact mucosa
(Respiratory
tract)
Corneal
transplant

Centripetal retrograde
axonal transport
of virus to CNS

Rabies encephalomyelitis

Intracellular viral replication
Inclusion (Negri) body
formation
Trans-synaptic spread
Neurotransmitter functions
altered
Neuronal dysfunction

Clinical effects:
behavioral
changes,
hydrophobia,
paralysis, electro
encephalo-graphic
changes

Centrifugal axonal transport
Extracellular virus appears
Virus produced in salivary glands
Dissemination also to lungs, heart, adrenal
and lacrimal glands, skin and skeletal muscle

Virus may replicate in
muscle at bite site.
Viral binding at nerve
endings especially at motor
end plates

Figure 9-99 ■ Pathogenesis of rabies. (From Cohen J, Powderly WG: *Infectious diseases*, ed 2, Philadelphia, 2004, Mosby Elsevier.)

to weakness; paralysis, including spasm of the swallowing muscles, leading to inability to swallow even liquids; and fear of water (hydrophobia). Delirium and seizures can follow, as well as generalized paralysis, with death usually to the result of respiratory arrest.

In the United States, most autochthonous human rabies cases have been identified as bat rabies variants among people who did not recognize their exposure or who did not seek postexposure treatment.

Disease in Animals

The incubation period appears to vary among species (see Table 9-52) but usually last weeks to months. Once clinical signs develop, there are two major manifestations of rabies infection in animals, termed *furious rabies* and *dumb (paralytic) rabies.* Either or both forms may occur during the course of infection in a single infected animal.

Furious rabies is characterized by agitation, aggression (including unprovoked biting attacks on other animals, humans, and itself), sexual stimulation and priapism, roaming behavior, excess salivation and drooling, and abnormal vocalizations (Figure 9-102). Convulsions often develop.

Dumb rabies is marked by lethargy and paralysis. The muscle paralysis begins in the head and neck, with difficulty swallowing that may lead a dog owner to become exposed

by trying to help the animal swallow. The paralysis spreads to the extremities, leading to generalized paralysis and death (Figures 9-103 and 9-104).

Management of Rabies Exposures in Humans

Management of potential rabies exposure consists of three components: (1) wound first aid, (2) risk assessment, and (3) administration of PEP if indicated.

First-Aid

Any bite or scratch from a potentially infected animal should be cleaned immediately with soap and water and irrigated copiously with water and/or a dilute solution of povidone-iodine and water. A tetanus booster should be administered if more than 10 years have elapsed since the last vaccination (see Chapter 10).

Risk Assessment

Risk assessment and decisions regarding PEP are crucial steps in the management of rabies exposures. This requires the clinician to gather an accurate history of the exposure, including the following information that should be included in the clinical chart:

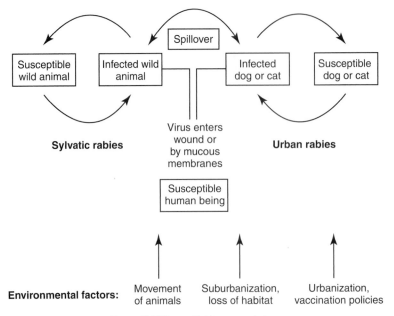

Figure 9-100 ■ Rabies transmission.

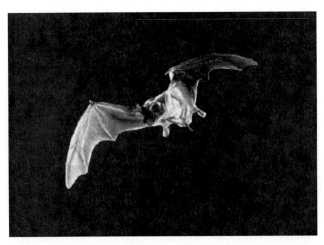

Figure 9-101 ■ The brown bat *Eptesicus fuscus* ranges from southern Canada through North and Central America to extreme northern South America. (From Centers for Disease Control and Prevention Public Health Image Library, Atlanta, Ga. Courtesy Ivan Kuzmin.)

- Current location of animal, and whether animal control or other authority is aware of incident and is going to quarantine/observe or euthanize the animal (in which case PEP can be reserved unless the test results for rabies are positive)
- Type of exposure (e.g., bite to exposed skin, bite through clothing, scratch, lick, contact with intact skin only)
- The exact location of all bites or scratches
- When exposure occurred
- Rabies immunization history of the individual
- Whether the individual is immunocompromised
- The species of animal involved, if known
- Whether the animal showed any signs of illness (including the signs of rabies listed in Table 9-52)

- Whether a bite or scratch occurred or whether the circumstances suggest an unrecognized exposure (such as a bat found in a room where someone was sleeping)
- If the animals is a domestic animal, record of immunization and name/contact information of veterinarian caring for animal

Using this information, the clinician can then assess the risk of rabies transmission and the need for PEP. Public health officials can be consulted to assist in determining the need for rabies PEP.

Figure 9-105 shows an algorithm for making this decision. The risk assessment process often requires close cooperation among the treating clinician, the public health department, animal control or veterinarian evaluating the animal, and the public health or other laboratory performing tests on the brain of the animal (if available).

Postexposure Prophylaxis

If the biting animal is tested for rabies or is a dog, cat, or ferret that can be monitored for 10 days, PEP is not necessary unless the animal shows clinical signs and subsequent test results are positive for rabies. However, if it is determined that PEP is indicated, it should be initiated as soon as possible after rabies exposure. The CDC posts updated recommendations for PEP on its Web site.[14] PEP should be started even if a prolonged time has elapsed since exposure because the incubation of human rabies can be many months. Table 9-53 lists the vaccines and antibody preparations available in the United States.

For persons who have never been vaccinated against rabies, PEP should include administration of both passive antibody (rabies immune globulin) and vaccine. For previously unvaccinated persons, the vaccine regimen consists of HDCV or PCECV, 1.0 mL IM (deltoid area), one each on days 0, 3, 7, and 14. The deltoid area should be used in adults and the anterior

Table 9-52 ▪ Rabies Infection: Comparative Clinical Presentations in Humans and Other Animals

Species	Risk Factors	Incubation Period	Clinical Manifestations	Signs that May Increase Risk of Human Exposure
Humans	Handling rabies vector species	Usually 2-12 weeks, but can be years	*Prodrome:* malaise, fever, pain or pruritus at the site of bite Increasing agitation, anxiety, confusion, difficulty swallowing Hyperexcitability or paralysis Death within 2-10 days of onset of clinical signs	
Dogs	Unvaccinated, allowed unsupervised outdoors	Usually 10-60 days[8]	All species: *Furious rabies:* Irritable, attacking, biting, scratching, swallow objects, chewing, salivation	Furious rabies more common than paralytic form[8]
Cats	Unvaccinated, allowed unsupervised outdoors			
Bats	Reservoir species	Variable		Flying in daytime, resting on ground, attacking animals, fighting, roosting in buildings, carried into the house by pet
Raccoons	Reservoir species	Variable	*Dumb (paralytic) rabies:* Paralysis of throat and masseter muscles, inability to swallow, profuse salivation, paralysis extending to rest of body[13]	Loss of fear of humans, aggression, active during the day
Skunks	Reservoir species	Variable	Phonation may be altered or animal may exhibit signs of choking	Abnormal aggression (such as attacking a porcupine)
Cattle	Unvaccinated Rabies-endemic area	25-150 days		Cessation of lactation, abnormal bellowing, signs of choking
Horses	Unvaccinated Rabies-endemic area	14-60 days		Rolling on ground, resembling colic

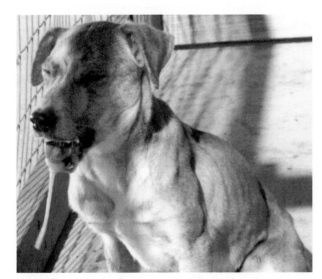

Figure 9-102 ▪ Dog with rabies. Note open jaw and visible tongue with excessive salivary secretions resulting from the inability to swallow. (From Greene CE: *Infectious diseases of the dog and cat*, ed 3, St Louis, 2006, Saunders Elsevier. Courtesy Centers for Disease Control and Prevention, Atlanta, Ga.)

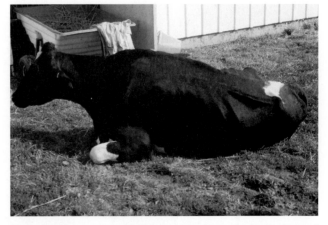

Figure 9-103 ▪ A 4-year-old Holstein was first noticed to be abnormal when she buckled on both hind limbs coming into the parlor. Within 2 hours, she was recumbent, would not eat, and began bellowing. Cerebrospinal fluid had a lymphocytic pleocytosis. She tested positive for rabies. (From Divers T: *Rebhun's diseases of dairy cattle*, ed 2, St Louis, 2008, Saunders Elsevier.)

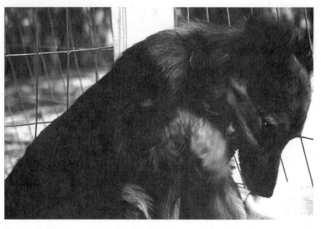

Figure 9-104 ■ Dog with dumb rabies, manifested as depression, lethargy, and a seemingly overly tame disposition. Domesticated animals with dumb rabies may become increasingly depressed and try to hide in isolated places, whereas wild animals seem to lose their fear of humans, often appearing unusually friendly. (From Centers for Disease Control and Prevention Public Health Image Library, Atlanta, Ga.)

thigh can be used in children. The gluteal area should not be used for rabies immunization. Hema rabies immune globulin (HRIG, 20 international units/kg body weight) should be given just once, at the beginning of antirabies prophylaxis, and infiltrated directly around the wound site if possible.

Do not administer HRIG to a person who previously received any of the rabies vaccinations from Table 9-53 either for preexposure or postexposure purposes. Previously immunized individuals should receive only vaccine (HDCV or PCECV, 1.0 mL IM [deltoid area]), one each on days 0 and 3 after exposure.

Management of Rabies Exposure in Animals

Vaccinated dogs, cats, ferrets, and livestock that have been exposed to a known or suspected rabid animal should be revaccinated and observed in the home or farm for 45 days for signs of rabies.[15] If an unvaccinated dog, cat, ferret, or livestock animal is bitten by a rabid or potentially rabid animal, it should be euthanized or maintained in strict quarantine and monitored

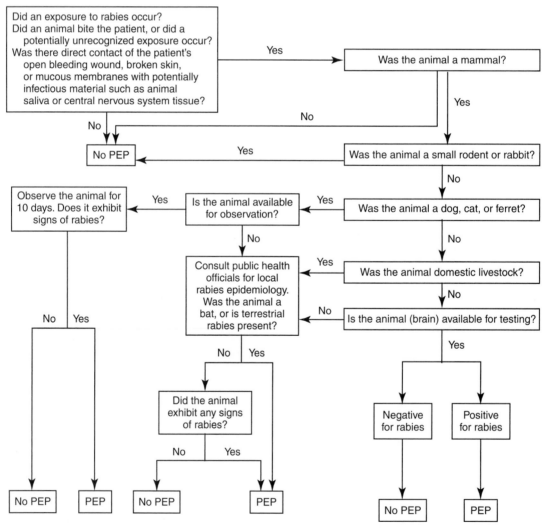

Figure 9-105 ■ Decision tree for rabies postexposure prophylaxis. (Modified from Rupprecht CE, Gibbons RV: Clinical practice. Prophylaxis against rabies, *N Engl J Med* 351[25]:2626-35, 2004.)

Type	Name	Route	Indications
Human diploid cell vaccine (HDCV)	Imovax Rabies	Intramuscular	Preexposure or postexposure
Purified Chick Embryo Cell Vaccine (PCEC)	RabAvert	Intramuscular	Preexposure or postexposure
Human rabies immune globulin	Imogam Rabies-HT	Local infusion at wound site, with additional amount IM at site distant from vaccine	Postexposure
Human rabies immune globulin	HyperRAB TM S/D	Local infusion at wound site, with additional amount IM at site distant from vaccine	Postexposure

Table 9-53 ■ **Rabies Vaccines and Immunoglobulin Available in the United States**

From Centers for Disease Control and Prevention: *Rabies post-exposure*. http://www.cdc.gov/rabies/exposure/postexposure.html.

closely for signs of rabies for 6 months. Quarantine should be under the supervision of local animal control or public health authorities at an approved boarding site. If the animal victim is a valuable specimen (e.g., zoo animal), contact public health professionals to determine possible management.

Diagnosis

The diagnosis in humans can be made by biopsy of the skin at the nape of the neck (at the hairline) and by using DFA staining of frozen skin sections. Serology is also used to detect viral neutralizing antibody in serum and CSF,[12] and a PCR test is available to detect *Lyssavirus* RNA. Clinicians must work with their state public health officials to submit specimens to the CDC laboratory.

In animals, the brain of euthanized animals is examined using DFA staining (Color Plate 9-58).[2] A rapid immunohistochemical test has recently been developed and provides high sensitivity and specificity.[16]

Treatment

Treatment in Humans

Although a number of aggressive attempts to treat symptomatic rabies infection with antiviral therapy have reported survival success in an isolated case (see Milwaukee Protocol at http://www.chw.org/display/PPF/DocID/33223/router.asp),[17] clinical rabies infection in humans remains an almost invariably fatal disease, with the principal treatment supportive intensive care.

Therefore prevention of the development of clinical disease through the use of preexposure and postexposure vaccination strategies is the mainstay of preventing rabies deaths in humans. (See *Human Rabies Prevention—United States, 2008 Recommendations of the Advisory Committee on Immunization Practices* (ACIP) at http://www.cdc.gov/mmwr/preview/mmwrhtml/rr57e507a1.htm.)

Treatment in Animals

Treatment is not attempted in animals. Rabid animals are euthanized. Disinfection of the cage area should be accom-

plished with disinfectants such as a 1% solution of household bleach.[2]

References

1. Alliance for Rabies Control. *World Rabies Day*. http://www.worldrabiesday.org. Accessed August 23, 2008.
2. Barr SC, Bowman DD. *The 5-minute veterinary consult clinical companion: canine and feline infectious disease and parasitology*. Ames, IA: Blackwell; 2006.
3. Dvorak G, Rovid-Spickler A, Roth JA, et al. *Handbook for zoonotic diseases of companion animals*. Ames, IA: The Center for Food Security and Public Health, Iowa State University College of Veterinary Medicine; 2008.
4. Nel LH, Markotter W. Lyssaviruses. *Crit Rev Microbiol*. 2007; 33(4):301.
5. Kansas State University College of Veterinarian Medicine: Kansas State Veterinary Diagnostic Laboratory: Rabies Laboratory. Rabies serology and animal transport to rabies-free areas. http://www.vet.ksu.edu/depts/dmp/service/rabies/table.htm. Accessed August 23, 2008.
6. World Health Organization. *Fact sheets: rabies*. http://www.who.int/mediacentre/factsheets/fs099/en/. Accessed August 23, 2008.
7. Rupprecht CE, Gibbons RV. Clinical practice. Prophylaxis against rabies. *N Engl J Med*. 2004;351(25):2626.
8. Acha PN, Szyfres B *Zoonoses and communicable diseases common to man and animals, vol. II: chlamydioses, rickettsioses, and viroses*. 3rd ed. Washington, DC: Pan American Health Organization; 2003.
9. Slate D, Rupprecht CE, Rooney JA, et al. Status of oral rabies vaccination in wild carnivores in the United States. *Virus Res*. 2005; 111(1):68.
10. Srinivasan A, Burton EC, Kuehnert MJ, et al. Rabies in transplant recipients investigation team. Transmission of rabies virus from an organ donor to four transplant recipients. *N Engl J Med*. 2005; 352(11):1103.
11. Smith JS, Fishbein DB, Rupprecht CE, et al. Unexplained rabies in three immigrants in the United States: a virologic investigation. *N Engl J Med*. 1991;324(4):205.
12. Heymann DL, ed. *Control of communicable diseases manual*. 19th ed. Washington, DC: American Public Health Association; 2008.
13. Kahn CM, Line S, eds. *The Merck veterinary manual*. 9th ed. Whitehouse Station, NJ: Merck; 2005.
14. Centers for Disease Control and Prevention. Rabies post-exposure. http://www.cdc.gov/rabies/exposure/postexposure.html. Accessed August 23, 2008.
15. Centers for Disease Control and Prevention. Human Rabies Prevention—United States, 2008: Recommendations of the Advisory Committee on Immunization Practices. *MMWR*. 2008;57(RR-3):1.
16. Lembo T, Niezgoda M, Velasco-Villa A, et al. Evaluation of a direct, rapid immunohistochemical test for rabies diagnosis. *Emerg Infect Dis*. 2006;12(2):310.
17. Hemachudha T, Wilde H. Survival after treatment of rabies. *N Engl J Med*. 2005;8; 353(10):1068.

ROCKY MOUNTAIN SPOTTED FEVER AND OTHER RICKETTSIAL INFECTIONS

Peter M. Rabinowitz and Lisa A. Conti

Rocky Mountain spotted fever (ICD-10 A77.0)

Other names in humans: North American tick typhus, New World spotted fever, tickborne typhus fever, São Paolo fever

Other names in animals: none

Rocky Mountain spotted fever (RMSF) and other named diseases caused by *Rickettsia rickettsii*, refer to a severe tickborne infection occurring in the Americas that is one of the deadliest known infectious diseases. In the preantibiotic era, case fatality was as high as 75%. Currently in the United States, the mortality rate is approximately 20% for untreated cases and 5% for treated cases,[1] with frequent long-term sequelae in survivors including limb amputation and neurological signs such as deafness.[2] RMSF causes similarly severe disease in dogs. The number of cases reported each year has increased since 2001, and there is evidence of expansion of host range and tick vector species. At the same time, RMSF probably remains underdiagnosed and underreported by both human health care providers and veterinarians. The diagnosis can be difficult because many patients present with nonspecific signs and may not have the classic triad of fever, rash, and tick bite. Estimation of RMSF mortality indicates that national surveillance for the disease misses some 60% of fatal cases.[3] In numerous instances, there have been temporal relationships between RMSF cases in dogs and human infection in members of the same households, demonstrating that dogs can serve as sentinels for human environmental infection risk.[4] Tragically, lack of communication between veterinarians and human health care providers has contributed to delays in diagnosis, sometimes with fatal consequences. In other cases, however, detection of RMSF in dogs has alerted human health care providers to initiate timely treatment of an infected person.[5] In addition to tick bites, a risk factor for human infection is exposure to infectious tick feces, tissues, or fluids when removing ticks from dogs. RMSF is therefore a grim reminder to human and animal health professionals of the importance of considering the diagnosis, sharing information about animal and human cases, and educating patients and clients about proper measures to prevent tickborne disease.

Key Points for Clinicians and Public Health Professionals

Public Health Professionals

- Characterize the risk of rickettsial disease in the community.
- Educate the public to prevent tick exposure through the following measures:
  - Avoid tick-infested areas, but if not possible, wear appropriate clothing (long sleeves, long pants, tuck pants legs into socks, and wear light-colored clothing to visualize ticks). Wash clothes with hot water.[6]
  - Use CDC-recommended tick repellents such as DEET or permethrin (apply to clothes, not skin). Be sure to follow label instructions before using any repellent.
  - Do frequent tick checks to remove even tiny immature-stage ticks. Inspect children at least once daily for ticks. When in heavily infested areas, inspect children every 3 to 4 hours.
  - Use appropriate technique to remove ticks, such as a tick removal "spoon," or wear gloves or grasp tick with tweezers as close to the skin as possible and pull gently. Applying matches, diesel fuel, nail polish, or petroleum jelly on the tick is not recommended and could lead to additional exposure to infectious material from the tick.[7]
  - Disinfect tick bites with household 70% isopropyl alcohol or 2% iodine solution. Follow up by cleaning the area, applying antibiotic topical on the tick bite site, and washing hands.
  - Implement integrated pest management techniques including landscape management (see Box 9-3) to reduce tick exposures.
- Advocate for tick prevention in dogs to reduce human exposure of the infection.

Human Health Clinicians

- Instruct patients on tick exposure prevention (see above).
- Consider the diagnosis in all patients with animal contact and/or travel to endemic countries.
- Report suspicion of disease immediately to public health authorities. See http://www.cdc.gov/ncidod/dvrd/rmsf/Case_Rep_Fm.pdf for the CDC case report form.

Veterinary Clinicians

- Recommend preventive acaricide treatment for pets.
- Notify health care professional if cases are diagnosed in dogs. Such cases could both pose a risk to humans and serve as a sentinel warning of environmental exposure risk.

Agent

The causative agent of RMSF, *Rickettsia rickettsii*, is a member of a family of closely related spotted fever Rickettsiae that are found worldwide. Rickettsiae are obligate intracellular coccobacilli with one of the smallest bacterial genomes.[8]

Because of a history of laboratory-acquired infections, many of which have proven fatal,[9] handling of *R. rickettsii* cultures requires biosafety level 3 containment. Because this bacterium was added to the select agent list, only approved laboratories can maintain cultured *R. rickettsii*.

Table 9-54 shows diseases caused by Rickettsiae in the spotted fever group. Several of these agents in addition to

Table 9-54 ■ RMSF: Diseases Worldwide Caused by Rickettsiae of the Spotted Fever Group

Agent	Disease	Geographical Distribution
Rickettsia rickettsii	Rocky Mountain spotted fever	North Central and South America
Rickettsia conorii	Mediterranean spotted fever, boutonneuse fever, Israeli spotted fever, Astrakhan fever, Indian tick typhus	Europe, Asia, Africa, India, Israel, Sicily, Russia
Rickettsia parkeri[10]	American boutonneuse fever[11]	United States, possibly South America
Rickettsia akari	Rickettsialpox	Worldwide
Rickettsia sibirica	Siberian tick typhus, North Asian tick typhus	Siberia, People's Republic of China, Mongolia, Europe
Rickettsia australis	Queensland tick typhus	Australia
Rickettsia honei	Flinders Island spotted fever, Thai tick typhus	Australia, South Eastern Asia
Rickettsia africae	African tick-bite fever	Sub-Saharan Africa, Caribbean
Rickettsia japonica	Japanese or Oriental spotted fever	Japan
Rickettsia felis	Cat-flea rickettsiosis, flea-borne typhus	Worldwide
Rickettsia slovaca	Necrosis, erythema, lymphadenopathy	Europe
Rickettsia heilongjiangensis	Mild spotted fever	China, Asian region of Russia

Adapted from Centers for Disease Control and Prevention: *Rocky Mountain spotted fever: epidemiology.* http://www.cdc.gov/ncidod/dvrd/rmsf/Epidemiology.htm.

R. rickettsii are found in the United States. *Rickettsia akari* causes rickettsialpox, a disease transmitted from mice to humans via mites that causes a vesicular skin rash, fever, and adenopathy and has been reported in urban dwellers in the eastern United States.[12] *Rickettsia parkeri* can cause a mild form of spotted fever with eschar formation at the site of a tick bite.[10,13] *Rickettsia felis* is transmitted by cat fleas to other animals, including humans, and is one of the causes of flea-borne (murine) typhus, a mild rickettsial disease.[12]

Geographical Occurrence

Despite its name, human cases of RMSF occur throughout the United States with higher incidence in the south Atlantic and western-central regions (Color Plate 9-59).[12] Even in endemic areas, infection rates of ticks with *R. rickettsii* are low. Outside the United States, RMSF occurs throughout the Western Hemisphere, with cases reported from Canada to Brazil and Argentina.

Groups at Risk

Since 1920, the disease has gone through three major cycles of emergence and has been increasing in incidence since 2000. The reasons for this are unclear.[14] The majority of reported cases in the United States occur in children younger than 15 years with a peak incidence between ages 5 and 9 years. This is believed to be due to behaviors that expose children to ticks.[15] Living near dogs carrying ticks is a reported risk factor. Laboratory workers are at risk and should use caution when handling infected material and cultures because infection can occur by accidental parenteral exposure or through aerosols.

Hosts, Reservoir Species, Vectors

Ixodid (hard) ticks are both a disease reservoir and the vectors for RMSF, although *R. rickettsii* appears to cause mortality in ticks. At present, the two principal tick species associated with RMSF in the United States are the American dog tick (*Dermacentor variabilis*) (Figure 9-106) found east of the Great Plains, and the Rocky Mountain wood tick (*Dermacentor andersoni*) (Figure 9-107) found between the Cascade and Rocky Mountains of the west.

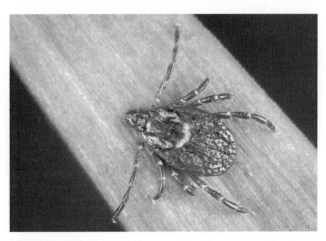

Figure 9-106 ■ American dog tick (*Dermacentor variabilis*). (From Centers for Disease Control and Prevention: *Rocky Mountain spotted fever: natural history.* http://www.cdc.gov/ncidod/dvrd/rmsf/natural_hx.htm.)

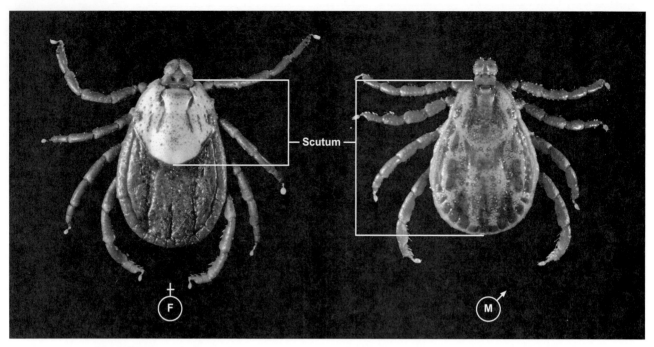

Figure 9-107 ■ Rocky Mountain wood tick *(Dermacentor andersoni)*. (From Centers for Disease Control and Prevention: *Rocky Mountain spotted fever: natural history.* http://www.cdc.gov/ncidod/dvrd/rmsf/ natural_hx.htm.)

Immature ticks of these two species feed predominantly on small rodents in rural and suburban environments, including the rice rat, golden mouse, white-footed mouse, and pine vole.[16] The brown dog tick *(Rhipicephalus sanguineus)*, by contrast, feeds mainly on dogs and has been associated with recent human infections in the southwestern United States and is the principal vector of RMSF in Mexico (Figure 9-108).[17] In South America, the major tick vector is *Amblyomma cajennense.*

In addition to ticks, dogs and rodents can also serve as disease reservoirs for RMSF as well as infected hosts that may develop clinical disease.[18]

Mode of Transmission and Life Cycle

Once infected with *R. rickettsii*, many ticks die.[14] Those that survive remain infected for life, and female ticks can pass the infection to their offspring through transovarial transmission. The ticks have a three-stage life cycle from larva to nymph and adult (Figure 9-109). To progress from one stage to another, the tick must have a blood meal; all three stages feed on vertebrates and can transmit infection. During blood meals, *R. rickettsii* in the salivary gland of an infected tick can be injected into the dermis of the host animal, resulting in transmission. If an uninfected tick feeds on an infected host animal, the tick can become infected with the organism. For tick-to-human transmission to occur, the tick must be attached for at least 6 hours and may remain attached for days to weeks.

In addition to tick bites, humans can become infected by exposure to tick feces, tissues, or fluids by removing and crushing an infected tick, allowing secretions to contact cuts or broken skin.[8] The rickettsial organism can also be spread human to human by blood transfusion.[19]

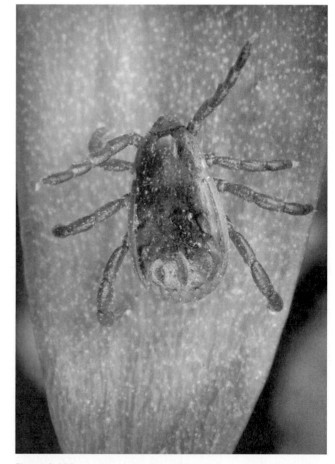

Figure 9-108 ■ Brown dog tick *(Rhipicephalus sanguineus)*, an emerging vector of Rocky Mountain spotted fever. (From Centers for Disease Control and Prevention Public Health Image Library, Atlanta, Ga. Courtesy James Gathany and William Nicholson.)

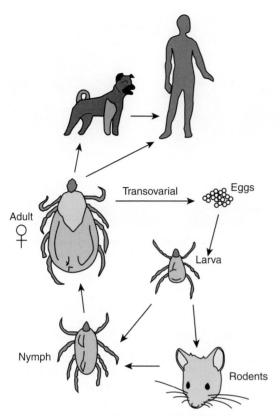

Figure 9-109 ■ Relations of tick and hosts in RMSF transmission. (From Songer JG, Post KW: *Veterinary microbiology: bacterial and fungal agents of animal disease*, St Louis, 2005, Saunders Elsevier.)

Environmental Risk Factors

Environmental factors driving the emergence of RMSF are poorly understood and are thought to vary with the ecology of the different tick reservoir species. In areas where *D. variabilis* is the principal tick reservoir, the environmental risk of RMSF has been estimated based on the density of small mammals in a particular area that serve as hosts for the tick.[16] Seasonality and climate play a strong role in human infection risk, with most cases in the United States reported between April and December when the adult ticks are more active.[15]

Disease in Humans

In the early stage of RMSF, symptoms can be nonspecific, including fever, myalgias, and headache. Only 3% to 18% of patients present at their first medical visit with the classic triad of fever, rash, and a history of a tick bite.[20] Therefore the disease should be suspected even if one of these signs is absent. Abdominal pain, nausea, and vomiting can be prominent features. The rash of RMSF occurs eventually in most cases and is often a maculopapular eruption with central petechiae that typically begins in the extremities around the wrists and ankles and spreads centripetally toward the trunk (Figure 9-110). In many, but not all, cases the rash involves the palms and soles (Color Plate 9-60).[8] Elderly and dark-skinned patients may have no visible rash (Rocky Mountain *spotless* fever).

Thrombocytopenia, elevated liver function test results, and hyponatremia are often seen. Nearly half of patients experience

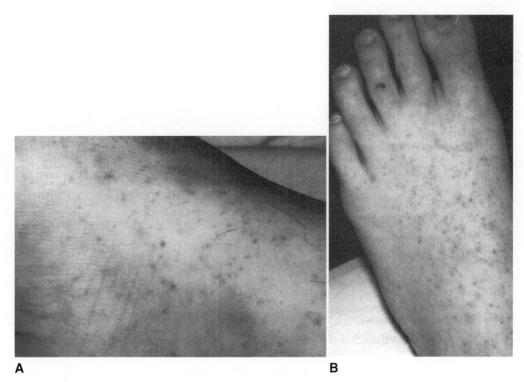

A   **B**

Figure 9-110 ■ **A,** Exanthem of Rocky Mountain spotted fever. **B,** Close-up view. (From McGinley-Smith DE, Tsao SS: Dermatoses from ticks, *J Am Acad Dermatol* 49:363, 2003.)

hemorrhages from vasculitis rather than low platelets. In severe cases, renal failure, pulmonary edema, and respiratory distress develop. The development of neurological signs, including meningismus, neurological deficits, deafness, and photophobia, is associated with a poor prognosis. Death can occur between 8 and 15 days after the onset of symptoms if antibiotic treatment has not been started early enough in the course of the disease.[8] Survivors of severe cases may have deafness, other neurological deficits, and gangrene of the extremities.[2] Male gender, advanced age, chronic alcoholism, African American race, and glucose-6-phosphate dehydrogenase deficiency have been associated with a greater risk of fulminant disease.[1]

Disease in Animals

Dogs are often infected in endemic areas, with reported seroprevalence rates ranging from 4% to 63%, some of which could be due to cross-reactivity with other Rickettsiae in the spotted fever group.[18] Infection causes a systemic vasculitis with signs resembling some of those in humans. Within several days of tick attachment, dogs may develop fever, lethargy, lameness, and anorexia. Other signs can include edema of the scrotum, face, ears, or extremities; epistaxis and other bleeding problems, including ecchymoses and petechiae; respiratory distress; ataxia, conjunctivitis; and eye pain (Figure 9-111 and Color Plate 9-61). Neurological disease is seen in about a third of cases.[21] Cases can be mild or severe with fatality as a result of arrhythmias, shock, and disseminated intravascular coagulation. The vasculitis can result in gangrene of the extremities in severely affected dogs. The case fatality rate can be as high as 10%. In recovered animals, immunity appears to be lifelong.[19]

RMSF has rarely been reported in cats, which are believed to be much less susceptible to infection than dogs.[19] The organisms have been isolated from opossums, rabbits, chipmunks, squirrels, rats, and mice, which seem to have inapparent infection. Table 9-55 summarizes the clinical presentation of RMSF in humans and other animals.

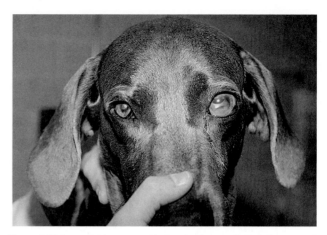

Figure 9-111 ■ Weimaraner with chronic glaucoma in the left eye secondary to bilateral uveitis from *Rickettsia rickettsii* infection. Buphthalmia is present in the left eye, with corneal edema. (From Dziezyc J, Millichamp NJ: *Color atlas of canine and feline ophthalmology*, St Louis, 2005, Saunders Elsevier.)

Diagnosis

The differential diagnosis of RMSF in humans includes a large number of other acute febrile illnesses, including viral respiratory tract infection, gastroenteritis, other tickborne diseases including ehrlichiosis (which causes fever but no rash), thrombocytopenic purpura, and mononucleosis. Clinicians must maintain a high level of suspicion for infection in endemic areas. Clues to the diagnosis include presence of fever and rash, exposure to ticks, and occurrence of RMSF in other humans or dogs in the household or area.

Findings of thrombocytopenia, hyponatremia, and elevated transaminase values support the diagnosis. Physicians should never delay treatment waiting for laboratory confirmation. Immunohistochemistry can offer timely diagnosis but is not widely available. A PCR test is available in some centers but is not 100% sensitive. Diagnostic serology can be done but is mostly useful for retrospective diagnosis of cases. Therefore the burden falls on clinicians to

Table 9-55 ■ RMSF: Clinical Presentations in Humans and Other Animals

Species	Risk Factors	Incubation Period	Clinical Manifestations	Laboratory Findings
Humans	*Children:* Exposures to ticks, dogs with ticks Elderly, African American, G6PD deficiency at risk for severe sequelae	2-14 days	Early symptoms often nonspecific; fever, myalgias, abdominal pain, nausea, centripetal rash Neurological signs, hemorrhage, respiratory and renal failure	Thrombocytopenia, elevated liver function tests, hyponatremia PCR, immunohistochemistry, positive serological titers for confirmation Fourfold rise in titer IFA, ELISA
Dogs	Tick exposure, mtost often in <3 years	2-14 days[19]	Fever, anorexia, lethargy, swelling, epistaxis, conjunctivitis, respiratory distress, ataxia, ecchymoses, petechiae, shock	Thrombocytopenia Positive serology: fourfold rise in titer by IFA, ELISA, latex agglutination immunofluorescence PCR if available

G6PD, Glucose-6 phosphate dehydrogenase.

Table 9-56 ▪ Antibiotic Treatment of RMSF in Humans and Other Animals		
Species	**Primary Treatment**	**Alternative Treatment**
Humans	Doxycycline 100 mg PO/IV bid × 7 days or 2 days after normalization of temperature[22]	
Dogs[23]	Doxycycline 10 mg/kg PO or IV q12h × 10 days	Enrofloxacin 3 mg/kg PO, SC q12h × 10 days[19]

suspect the diagnosis and initiate antibiotics often on clinical grounds.

In dogs, the disease can be confused with canine ehrlichiosis, which responds to the same treatment. The scrotal edema may resemble that seen in brucellosis. Helpful laboratory diagnostic findings in dogs include thrombocytopenia and serology using immunofluorescence (micro-IF or direct), ELISA, or latex agglutination. PCR is available in some centers.[19]

Treatment

The treatment of choice for RMSF in adults and children is doxycycline (Table 9-56).[1] In pregnant women, the benefit may also outweigh the risk, but an infectious disease specialist and/or the patient's obstetrician should be consulted. Antibiotic treatment should never be delayed while awaiting results of diagnostic testing, because delay in treatment can lead to fatal outcomes.[20] Patients may require supportive care in intensive care settings if necessary if complications develop. Treatment in dogs usually involves inpatient care with early administration of antibiotics and supportive treatment with intravenous fluids and blood transfusion if necessary.

References

1. Chapman AS, Bakken JS, Folk SM, et al. Diagnosis and management of tickborne rickettsial diseases: Rocky Mountain spotted fever, ehrlichioses, and anaplasmosis—United States: a practical guide for physicians and other health-care and public health professionals. *MMWR.* 2006;55(RR-4):1.
2. Archibald LK, Sexton DJ. Long-term sequelae of Rocky Mountain spotted fever. *Clin Infect Dis.* 1995;20(5):1122.
3. Paddock CD, Holman RC, Krebs JW, et al. Assessing the magnitude of fatal Rocky Mountain spotted fever in the United States: comparison of two national data sources. *Am J Trop Med Hyg.* 2002;67(4):349.
4. Elchos BN, Goddard J. Implications of presumptive fatal Rocky Mountain spotted fever in two dogs and their owner. *J Am Vet Med Assoc.* 2003;223(10):1450–1452, 1433.
5. Paddock CD, Brenner O, Vaid C, et al. Short report: concurrent Rocky Mountain spotted fever in a dog and its owner. *Am J Trop Med Hyg.* 2002;66(2):197.
6. Centers for Disease Control and Prevention. *Lyme disease prevention: protect yourself from tick bites.* http://www.cdc.gov/ncidod/dvbid/lyme/Prevention/ld_Prevention_Avoid.htm. Accessed September 28, 2008.
7. Needham GR. Evaluation of five popular methods for tick removal. *Pediatrics.* 1985;75(6):997.
8. Mandell GL, Bennett JE, Dolin R, eds. *Principles and practice of infectious diseases.* 6th ed. New York: Churchill Livingstone Elsevier; 2005.
9. Pike RM. Laboratory-associated infections: summary and analysis of 3921 cases. *Health Lab Sci.* 1976;13(2):105.
10. Paddock CD, Sumner JW, Comer JA, et al. *Rickettsia parkeri*: a newly recognized cause of spotted fever rickettsiosis in the United States. *Clin Infect Dis.* 2004;38(6):805.
11. Goddard J. American boutonneuse fever: a new spotted fever rickettsiosis. *Infect Med.* 2004;21:207.
12. Heymann DL, ed. *Control of communicable diseases manual.* 18th ed. Washington, DC: American Public Health Association; 2004.
13. Whitman TJ, Richards AL, Paddock CD, et al. *Rickettsia parkeri* infection after tick bite, Virginia. *Emerg Infect Dis.* 2007;13(2):334.
14. Dumler JS, Walker DH. Rocky Mountain spotted fever—changing ecology and persisting virulence. *N Engl J Med.* 2005;353(6):551.
15. Centers for Disease Control and Prevention. *Rocky Mountain spotted fever: epidemiology.* http://www.cdc.gov/ncidod/dvrd/rmsf/Epidemiology.htm. Accessed August 2, 2008.
16. Kollars Jr TM. Interspecific differences between small mammals as hosts of immature *Dermacentor variabilis* (Acari: Ixodidae) and a model for detection of high risk areas of Rocky Mountain spotted fever. *J Parasitol.* 1996;82(5):707.
17. Demma LJ, Traeger MS, Nicholson WL, et al. Rocky Mountain spotted fever from an unexpected tick vector in Arizona. *N Engl J Med.* 2005;353(6):587.
18. Kahn CM, Line S, eds. *The Merck veterinary manual.* 9th ed. Whitehouse Station, NJ: Merck; 2005.
19. Barr SC, Bowman DD. *The 5-minute veterinary consult clinical companion: canine and feline infectious diseases and parasitology.* Ames, IA: Blackwell; 2006.
20. Centers for Disease Control and Prevention. Consequences of delayed diagnosis of Rocky Mountain spotted fever in children—West Virginia, Michigan, Tennessee, and Oklahoma. *MMWR.* 2000;49(39):885.
21. Dvorak G, Rovid-Spickler A, Roth JA, et al. *Handbook for zoonotic diseases of companion animals.* Ames, IA: The Center for Food Security and Public Health, Iowa State University College of Veterinary Medicine; 2008.
22. Gilbert DN, Moellering RC, Eliopoulos GM, et al. *Sanford guide to antimicrobial therapy 2009.* 39th ed. Sperryville, VA: Antimicrobial Therapy; 2009.
23. Langston C. Postexposure management and treatment of anthrax in dogs—Executive Councils of the American Academy of Veterinary Pharmacology and Therapeutics and the American College of Veterinary Clinical Pharmacology. *AAPS Journal.* 2005;07(02):E272.

RIFT VALLEY FEVER*

Tracy DuVernoy

Rift Valley fever (ICD–9 066.3)

Other names in humans: none

Other names in animals: enzootic hepatitis

Rift Valley fever (RVF) is a zoonotic arboviral disease that primarily affects ruminant livestock (cattle, sheep, and goats) and camels, but the disease can also occur in humans. Cattle, sheep, and goats appear to be particularly susceptible to infection. Animal infection is characterized by acute hepatic necrosis; increased abortions among pregnant animals; and high mortality rates in young, neonatal livestock populations. Most human infections are asymptomatic or may present as an uncomplicated influenza-like illness. However, a small percentage of human infections may result in significant neurological illness, retinitis, hepatitis, or hemorrhage progressing to death. RVF virus could potentially be introduced into the United States by an infected person or animal, especially during their viremic phase, or by an infected vector. Although RVF is currently found in Africa and the Arabian Peninsula, the virus has the potential to become established in other geographical areas owing to the abundant range of competent vectors capable of transmitting infection, the high level of viremia that develops in both infected animals and humans that allows sustainability of the virus, and the ability of the virus to adapt to different ecological conditions. However, for the virus to become established in the United States, climatic conditions must be favorable to ensure survivability of the mosquito vector, and appropriate numbers of livestock are necessary for adequate amplification of the virus. A recent publication evaluated potential pathways of RVF introduction into the United States and concluded that air transportation of a viremic civilian or mechanical transportation via aircraft or ship of an RVF-infected vector were likely pathways for introduction of RVF virus into the United States.[1] Therefore it is essential that communication among animal and human health officials be coordinated to detect this potentially devastating zoonotic infectious disease. Fortunately, a multiagency working group has been formed to discuss a research agenda, modeling efforts, and surveillance and response capabilities, among other activities, to develop a comprehensive national RVF prevention and response plan.[2]

*The opinions and assertions contained in this chapter are the private views of the author and are not to be construed as official or reflecting true views of the Department of the Army or the Department of Defense, to whom the author was contracted during the writing of this chapter.

The author is grateful for the contributions of Dr. Kenneth Linthicum to this section.

Key Points for Clinicians and Public Health Professionals

Public Health Professionals

- Be alert to the possibility of RVF introduction into the Western hemisphere and the subsequent spread by mosquito vectors.
- The irregular interval between RVF epizootics/epidemics adds to the challenge of preventing and controlling this virus. Consider increased use of techniques such as satellite remote sensing to predict global outbreaks of RVF. Environmental criteria in west and south Africa may require further evaluation to determine the validity and applicability of remote sensing imagery in these areas.
- Ensure that populations that work with livestock in endemic areas use proper precautions when butchering and processing meat.
- Use of mosquito control techniques may be highly effective in either preventing the introduction of the virus in domestic animal populations by killing immature stages of vectors[3] or control of adults during epizootic/epidemic conditions.

Human Health Clinicians

- Generally, the risk of infection in travelers is low. However, travelers to RVF-affected areas during an epizootic or epidemic should take appropriate precautions, such as using bed nets during sleep periods, using mosquito repellents, and avoiding contact with infected livestock.
- Due to the zoonotic nature of this virus, it is critical that individuals take appropriate precautions when (1) performing necropsies on suspect animals, (2) performing laboratory procedures, (3) assisting with livestock parturitions, (4) butchering possibly infected animals, or (5) performing other procedures that may place them at high risk of exposure to RVF virus.
- Report any suspected case of RVF to the appropriate local and state public health authorities. RVF cases suspected or confirmed in active duty U.S. military personnel are reportable to their respective services per the Tri-Service Reportable Events guidelines.[4]
- Use appropriate precautions especially when handling acute-phase blood products from suspect patients.
- No commercially available preventive vaccine exists for use in humans. An experimental inactivated vaccine has been used to protect laboratory and veterinary workers at high risk of RVF infection.

Veterinary Clinicians

- Consider RVF infection with increased abortions in ruminants; high mortality rates in neonatal and young lambs, kids, and calves; and human illness particularly after heavy rains.

- In the United States, RVF is a foreign animal disease; therefore for any suspected case of RVF, it is critical to promptly notify the appropriate state and federal veterinary regulatory authorities.
- Ensure that appropriate PPE is worn when performing a necropsy on a suspect animal, when treating an ill suspect case, or when assisting with reproductive procedures. At a minimum, consider wearing a mask (to help avoid aerosols), gloves, and goggles.
- Before submitting any specimens for diagnostic purposes, contact the appropriate reference laboratory[5] to inquire about shipping requirements, diagnostic capabilities, and required specimens for submission.
- Animal disease prevention in enzootic areas may be accomplished by vaccination of susceptible livestock. The administration to small ruminants of one dose of a live attenuated virus vaccine (Smithburn strain) may confer long-term immunity and will minimize animal disease before the onset of an epizootic. However, live vaccine use may induce abortions or fetal abnormalities in pregnant animals. For disease prevention in pregnant ruminants in nonzoonotic areas, an initial dose and booster dose of a formalin-inactivated vaccine may be administered to cattle, sheep, and goats; annual revaccination is required. In addition, animal movement control is essential to prevent introduction of infected animals into new geographical locations that can support maintenance of the virus.

Agent

RVF is a mosquito-borne virus of the genus *Phlebovirus* in the family Bunyaviridae[6] (Figure 9-112). Vector transmission may occur by mechanical or biological means. It is a single-stranded enveloped RNA virus with three segments—

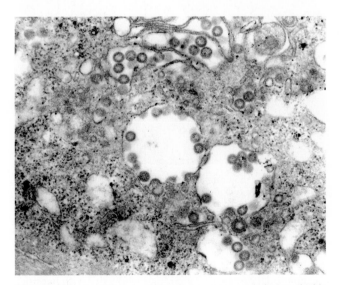

Figure 9-112 ■ This transmission electron micrograph depicts a highly magnified view of a tissue that had been infected with RVF virus. (From Centers for Disease Control and Prevention Public Health Image Library, Atlanta, Ga. Courtesy F.A. Murphy and J. Dalrymple.)

S (small), M (medium), and L (large)—that is readily inactivated by a pH below 6.8, lipid solvents, or strong solutions of sodium hypochlorite.[7] There is only one serotype of RVF virus. However, there are three distinct lineages: Egyptian, West African, and Central East-African.[8]

Geographical Occurrence

RVF is a disease that occurs primarily in Africa and the Arabian Peninsula. RVF was first identified in 1930 in Merino sheep along the shores of Lake Naivasha in the Rift Valley of Kenya[9] when a total of 3500 lambs and 1200 ewes died of acute hepatic necrosis after a period of excessive rainfall. Herdsmen who managed the flocks on the farm also complained of fever and arthralgia.[9] Animal epizootics, along with human epidemics, have occurred periodically since then, primarily in sub-Saharan Africa. Significant RVF outbreaks were reported in 1950-1951 (South Africa); 1997-1998 (Kenya, Tanzania, Somalia); 2006-2007 (Kenya, Tanzania, Somalia); 2007 (Sudan), and recently in 2008 (South Africa, Madagascar). The 1997-1998 outbreak in east Africa was the largest to date in terms of human disease, with approximately 89,000 human cases and 478 fatalities.[10] During the past three decades, human and animal disease has also been confirmed in western Africa and Egypt, associated with the construction of dams and subsequent flooding or irrigation projects that favor mosquito production. In 1977-1978 an outbreak that affected both humans and animals was confirmed in Egypt, the first time the virus had been identified outside sub-Saharan Africa.[11] A second occurrence of RVF occurred in Egypt in 1993. In 2000, RVF infection was reported in southern Saudi Arabia and northern Yemen along the Red Sea, the first time this virus was confirmed outside the African continent. The appearance of the virus in this new geographical location was likely due to the importation of viremic livestock from eastern Africa into the Arabian Peninsula.[12] In Saudi Arabia, 882 human cases were reported that resulted in 124 deaths,[13] and Yemen reported 1087 suspected case patients and 121 deaths.[14] Abortions in small ruminants and increased mortality in young susceptible livestock were reported concurrent with human illness.

Groups at Risk

Human groups at increased risk of RVF infection include veterinarians, abattoir workers, livestock herdsmen, and virology laboratorians as a result of occupational exposures. During epidemics, the general human population is at risk as a result of direct contact with infected livestock or animal products (including unpasteurized milk) or exposure to mosquito vectors. During epidemics, the risk of infection to travelers, soldiers, relief workers, or other individuals may be high if exposed to infected mosquitoes or to infected animals, their blood, or infected tissues.

Within animal populations, newborn ruminants (sheep, goats, and cattle) are particularly susceptible to RVF virus, resulting in a fatal infection; followed by pregnant ruminants; and then young sheep and cattle. Adult ruminants are less susceptible to infection; however, exotic breeds are more susceptible and exhibit more pathology. Horses and swine are even less susceptible.

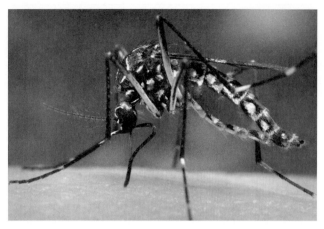

Figure 9-113 ■ Female *Aedes* mosquito in the process of acquiring a blood meal from her human host. (From Centers for Disease Control and Prevention Public Health Image Library, Atlanta, Ga. Courtesy Frank Hadley Collins, University of Notre Dame).

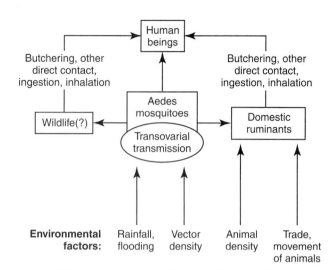

Figure 9-114 ■ Transmission and life cycle of Rift Valley fever infection, including the ecological drivers for outbreaks.

Hosts, Reservoir Species, Vectors

Many different species of mosquitoes are involved in the transmission of RVF; the virus has been isolated from more than 30 species among six genera of mosquitoes (Figure 9-113).[15] Additionally, RVF virus has been isolated from flies and *Culicoides*, biting midges. However, a few arthropod species play key roles in the transmission during epidemics/epizootics and during the period between these disease-occurring events. The reservoir of RVF in sub-Saharan Africa is thought to be *Aedes* mosquitoes (*Ae. vexans*, *Ae. mcintoshi*, and *Ae. dalzieli* primarily) that can transovarially transmit RVF virus to their drought-resistant eggs,[16] thereby allowing the virus to remain dormant and survive for long periods in soil depressions pending significant rainfall.[17] This vertical transmission is critical in maintaining RVF in endemic/enzootic areas.

The natural reservoir of RVF virus is currently unknown. The role of wildlife in the perpetuation, maintenance, and circulation of virus during the interepizootic period is also not clearly understood.[18] Experimentally, rhesus macaques[19] and inbred laboratory mice[20] have been shown to demonstrate clinical signs of disease once infected with RVF virus.

Mode of Transmission and Life Cycle

Once appropriate levels of rainfall occur and land depressions fill with water, dormant RVF-infected *Aedes* mosquito eggs hatch and adults emerge (Figure 9-114) and, acting as primary vectors, feed on susceptible livestock (Figure 9-115). Infected livestock amplify the virus, developing significant viremias—up to $10^{8.0}$ plaque-forming units (PFUs)/mL[1]— and contribute to epizootic maintenance, circulation, and spread of the virus via secondary vectors (*Culex* mosquitoes) that feed on livestock and perpetuate the infection. Intense virus activity may last for 6 to 12 weeks.[21]

Human infection can occur after a bite from an infected mosquito or by mechanical transmission from other insects. However, most infections occur as a result of direct or indirect exposure to infected blood, tissues, or body fluids of infected animals; by the butchering or slaughtering of infected animals; or by performing veterinary or obstetrical procedures

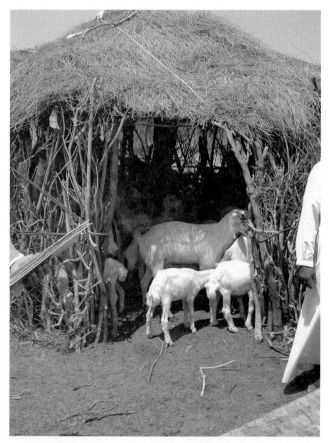

Figure 9-115 ■ Epidemiological investigation in Saudi Arabia that had been initiated as a response to a Rift Valley fever outbreak in the region. These goats were penned in a village that was within the geographical parameters of the investigation. (From Centers for Disease Control and Prevention Public Health Image Library, Atlanta, Ga. Courtesy Abbigail Tumpey.)

on infected animals. In this way, RVF can be considered an occupational disease of individuals who work with livestock (see Chapter 12). Infection occurs by way of inoculation or aerosolization and inhalation of virus. Infection may also occur subsequent to consuming unpasteurized milk from infected animals. Direct human-to-human transmission has not been documented; however, two recent articles describe case reports of vertical transmission of RVF infection from pregnant mother to fetus.[22,23] Direct animal-to-animal transmission has not been reported.

Environmental Risk Factors

Epizootics and epidemics occur at irregular internals (ranging from 3 to 15 years)[21,24] and typically follow significant rainfall that floods areas of sub-Saharan eastern and southern Africa, subsequently hatching dormant floodwater *Aedes* mosquito eggs.[25] However, in more arid areas of Africa, the interval may approach every 15 to 35 years. The frequency depends on rainfall and other climatic conditions that favor large vector populations, susceptible animal species populations, and the existence or introduction of virus in the geographical area. For these reasons, satellite imagery may offer an early warning of environmental conditions that favor disease occurrence, allowing a few months' lead time to mitigate disease impacts in both animals and humans. The National Aeronautical and Space Agency (NASA) and other agencies have used satellite imagery remote sensing to create predictive risk maps for RVF outbreaks. This remote sensing approach incorporates measures such as the normalized difference vegetation index (an indicator of recent rainfall and green vegetation), sea surface temperature, and rainfall.[26] In October 2006, this technology assessed such environmental conditions and accurately forecasted an outbreak of RVF in Kenya before an actual confirmed outbreak in December 2006. Figure 9-116 shows an example of an environmental risk map for RVF produced by NASA.

The outbreak in Egypt along the Nile Delta in 1977-1978 was a concern because the virus had not been previously identified north of the Sahara Desert. However, conditions that favored an outbreak included construction of the Aswan High Dam and flooding of the Nile River delta[24] and a concurrent large outbreak in East Africa. Another incident following a change to the environment occurred in western Africa in Mauritania and Senegal in 1987. One year after the construction of the Diama Dam and subsequent flooding of the Senegal River basin, an outbreak of RVF affected both humans and other animals.[24,27] Despite the linkages between recent flooding and rainfall to many RVF outbreaks,

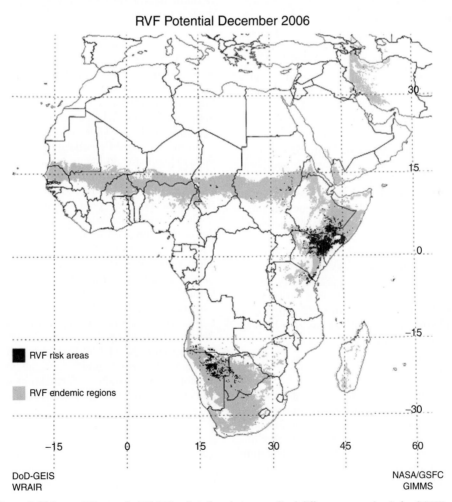

Figure 9-116 ▪ Risk map for Rift Valley fever based on normalized difference vegetation index (NVDI, an indicator of green vegetation). (From U.S. Department of Defense, Global Emerging Infections Surveillance and Response System: *Rift Valley fever (RVF): monthly updates: state of climate and environmental conditions.* http://www.geis.fhp.osd.mil/GEIS/SurveillanceActivities/RVFWeb/monthlypages/0612.htm.)

not all follow this pattern because some outbreaks appear to be related to the trade and movement of infected viremic domestic animals across borders.[11,12,24]

Disease in Humans

In humans, the incubation period of RVF is 2 to 6 days; RVF produces an influenza-like illness with fever, headache, arthralgia, and myalgia.[28] Viremic titers are high after infection and can persist for more than 1 week. Recovery is usually complete; however, complications or a more serious form of the disease can manifest as three different syndromes.

Retinitis

Between 0.5% and 2% of human RVF infections result in retinitis; onset occurs 1 to 3 weeks after the initial symptoms. The disease may resolve within 10 to 12 weeks; however, permanent vision loss may occur in 1% to 10% of those with this syndrome. Death is uncommon in those infected with the ocular form of RVF.

Meningoencephalitis

Meningoencephalitis occurs in 1% of those infected with RVF, generally 1 to 4 weeks subsequent to the initial symptoms. Patients may report an intense headache, photophobia, memory loss, and confusion; convulsions and coma may ensue. The death rate is low; however, neurological sequelae are common in individuals with this form of RFV infection.

Hemorrhagic Fever

Fewer than 1% of those infected have hemorrhagic fever, which typically develops 2 to 4 days after illness onset; jaundice is generally observed first. Additional hepatic involvement manifests as hemorrhage, hematemesis, melena, ecchymoses, and persistent bleeding from other sites. Death occurs 3 to 6 days after onset of these symptoms; the case fatality rate may approach 50%.

The overall case fatality rate of RVF infection in humans typically ranges from 0.5% to 1.0%. However, during a recent outbreak in Kenya, the case fatality rate was 29% among 404 confirmed or probable cases during a 3-month period from November 30, 2006, to January 25, 2007.[29] The high case fatality rate was likely due to severe illness and the hemorrhagic fever presentation of many of those infected.

Disease in Animals

RVF causes morbidity and mortality in many different livestock species. In Africa, exotic livestock breeds are more susceptible to infection than indigenous breeds such as *Bos indicus*.[21] In pregnant ungulates, abortion is the most common clinical sign. Abortion may occur at any time during the gestation period and the rate may approach 100% in infected pregnant ewes. In newborn lambs, kids, and calves after an incubation period as short as 12 hours, the most prevalent clinical sign is death, preceded by fever. Mortality rates can approach close to 100% in some species. Older animals may demonstrate weakness, anorexia, listlessness, and a nasal discharge. Infection in adult cattle and small ruminants is often subclinical; however, some animals may develop fever, anorexia, bloody diarrhea, and a mucopurulent nasal discharge. Adult camels do not demonstrate clinical signs of illness; however, they do abort. The mortality rate in adult livestock may range from 10% in cattle to 20% in sheep. Infection and disease in domestic animals causes considerable economic losses because of the significant number of abortions, the high rate of mortality in young ruminants, and the disruption in trade and exports that are associated with epizootics.

Although some species of wildlife have detectable antibody levels against RVF, such infections are generally subclinical. One recent publication reported that of 16 different wildlife species sampled during 1999-2006 in Kenya, seven had detectable neutralizing antibodies against RVF. These data suggest that native wildlife are indeed infected with RVF[30]; however, additional studies are needed to determine their role as reservoirs or amplifiers of the virus. Table 9-57 shows the comparative presentation of disease in humans and other animals.

Diagnosis

In humans, RVF should be suspected in the differential diagnosis when the following conditions are observed: influenza-like illness, retinitis, and/or meningoencephalitis and hemorrhagic fever in individuals with livestock contact, especially in the setting of high mosquito vectors associated with recent flooding or after significant rainfall. Cases of abortion in ruminants also support the diagnosis in humans. Recent human infection is determined by serology to detect IgM antibodies by ELISA; by virus isolation during the acute, viremic phase; or by RT-PCR to detect viral antigen.[28]

In animals, the differential diagnoses for a "storm" of abortions in pregnant ruminants and a high mortality rate among young/neonatal ruminants includes a number of diseases such as brucellosis, ovine enzootic abortion, Nairobi sheep disease, rinderpest, peste de petit ruminants, vibriosis, ephemeral fever, Wesselsbron disease, trichomonas, and heartwater. To detect RVF infection in animals, heparinized blood may be analyzed for virus isolation, especially during the acute phase when virus levels are elevated. Acute and convalescent sera can be used to detect a rise in antibody levels by ELISA or hemagglutination inhibition; antibody is present within 6 to 7 days after infection.[31] Tissue specimens may also be submitted for virus isolation as long as they are not formalinized. Electron microscopy may be used to detect viral particles in tissue specimens or RT-PCR can be used to detect viral antigen. For histopathological review, the best necropsy samples to submit in 10% buffered formalin include the spleen, liver, and brain (particularly from aborted fetuses).

Treatment

Asymptomatic human infections typically do not warrant treatment. For individuals with more significant illness, treatment is supportive. Although there are no specific antivirals that are effective once symptoms occur, antivirals such as ribavirin and interferon-alpha have shown some promise in treatment trials involving nonhuman primates. There is no treatment available for infected animals.

Table 9-57 ▪ Clinical Presentation of Rift Valley Fever in Humans and Other Animals

Species	Risk Factors	Incubation Period	Clinical Manifestations	Diagnostic Findings
Humans	Direct or indirect contact with infected livestock/products, aerosolization via slaughtering, mosquito bites	2-6 days	Asymptomatic or mild influenza-like illness. More severe disease (<2% of cases): retinitis, meningoencephalitis, or hemorrhagic fever	IgM serology (ELISA), RT-PCR, virus isolation
Neonatal and young domestic ruminants	Exposure to infected mosquitoes	12 hours-3 days	Fever, anorexia, weakness, listlessness, diarrhea, mucopurulent nasal discharge, high mortality rate	Virus isolation, RT-PCR, histopathology
Adult domestic ruminants		1-3 days	Abortions. Subclinical in nonpregnant animals; however, some develop fever, anorexia, ptyalism, diarrhea	ELISA to detect IgG and IgM, virus isolation, RT-PCR
Wild ruminants		Unknown	Subclinical; however, may abort (African buffalo)	Serological evidence of antibodies

References

1. Kasari TR, Carr DA, Lynn TV, et al. Evaluation of pathways for release of Rift Valley fever virus into domestic ruminant livestock, ruminant wildlife, and human populations in the continental United States. *J Am Vet Med Assoc*. 2008;232(4):514.

2. Britch SC, Linthicum KJ. Rift Valley Fever Working Group: Developing a research agenda and a comprehensive national prevention and response plan for Rift Valley fever in the United States. *Emerg Infect Dis*. http://www.cdc.gov/eid/content/13/8/e1.htm. Accessed July 2, 2008.

3. Linthicum KJ, Logan TM, Thande PC, et al. Efficacy of a sustained release methoprene formulation on vectors of Rift Valley fever in field studies in Kenya. *J Am Mosq Control Assoc*. 1989;5(4):603.

4. Armed Forces Health Surveillance Center. *Tri-Service reportable events: guidelines and case definitions, June 2009*. http://www.afhsc.mil/Documents/TriService_CaseDefDocs/June09/TriServeGuide.pdf. Accessed October 31, 2009.

5. Davies FG, Martin V. *Recognizing Rift Valley fever (FAO Animal Health Manual 17)*. Rome: Food and Agriculture Organization of the United Nations; 2003.

6. Mahy BWJ, ter Meulen V. *Topley & Wilson's microbiology and microbial infections, Virology*. 10th ed. London: Hodder Arnold/American Society of Microbiology Press.

7. Metwally S. Rift Valley fever. In: Brown C, Torres A, eds. *Foreign animal diseases*. 7th ed. Boca Raton, FL: Boca Publications Group, 2008.

8. Sall AA, de A Zanotto PM, Vialat P, et al. Origin of 1997–98 Rift Valley fever outbreak in East Africa. *Lancet*. 1998;352(9140):1596.

9. Daubney R, Hudson JR, Garnham PC. Enzootic hepatitis or Rift Valley fever: an undescribed virus disease of sheep, cattle and man from East Africa. *J Pathol Bacteriol*. 1931;34:545.

10. Centers for Disease Control and Prevention. Rift Valley fever—East Africa, 1997–1998. *MMWR*. 1998;47(13):261.

11. Gad AM, Feinsod FM, Allam IH, et al. A possible route for the introduction of Rift Valley fever virus into Egypt during 1977. *J Trop Med Hyg*. 1986;89(5):233.

12. Shoemaker T, Boulianne C, Vincent MJ, et al. Genetic analysis of viruses associated with emergence of Rift Valley fever in Saudi Arabia and Yemen, 2001–01. *Emerg Infect Dis*. 2002;8(12):1415.

13. Balkhy HH, Memish ZA. Rift Valley fever: an uninvited zoonosis in the Arabian peninsula. *Int J Antimicrob Agents*. 2003;21(2):153.

14. Centers for Disease Control and Prevention. Outbreak of Rift Valley fever—Yemen, August-October 2000. *MMWR*. 2000;49(47):1065.

15. House JA, Turell MJ, Mebus CA. Rift Valley fever: present status and risk to the Western hemisphere. *Ann N Y Acad Sci*. 1992;653:233.

16. Peters CJ, Linthicum KJ. Rift Valley Fever. In: Beran GW, Steele JH, eds. *Handbook of zoonoses*. 2nd ed. Boca Raton, FL: CRC Press; 1994.

17. Linthicum KJ, Davies FG, Kairo A, et al. Rift Valley fever virus (family Bunyaviridae, genus *Phlebovirus*). Isolations from *Diptera* collected during an inter-epizootic period in Kenya. *J Hyg (Lond)*. 1985;95(1):197.

18. LaBeaud AD, Muchiri EM, Ndzovu M, et al. Interepidemic Rift Valley fever virus seropositivity, northeastern Kenya. *Emerg Infect Dis*. 2008;14(8):1240.

19. Peters CJ, Jones D, Trotter R, et al. Experimental Rift Valley fever in rhesus macaques. *Arch Virol*. 1988;99(1–2):31.

20. Ritter M, Bouloy M, Vialat P, et al. Resistance to Rift Valley fever virus in *Rattus norvegicus*: genetic variability within certain "inbred" strains. *J Gen Virol*. 2000;81(Pt 11):2683.

21. Geering WA, Davies FG. *Preparation of Rift Valley fever contingency plans (FAO Animal Health Manual 15)*. Rome: Food and Agriculture Organization of the United Nations; 2002.

22. Adam I, Karsany MS. Case report: Rift Valley fever with vertical transmission in a pregnant Sudanese woman. *J Med Virol*. 2008;80(5):929.

23. Arishi HM, Aqeel AY, Al Hazmi MM. Vertical transmission of fatal Rift Valley fever in a newborn. *Ann Trop Paediatr*. 2006;26(3):251.

24. Gerdes GH. Rift Valley fever. *Rev Sci Tech*. 2004;23:613.

25. Davies FG, Linthicum KJ, James AD. Rainfall and epizootic Rift Valley fever. *B World Health Org*. 1985;63(5):941.

26. Linthicum KJ, Anyamba A, Tucker CJ, et al. Climate and satellite indicators to forecast Rift Valley fever epidemics in Kenya. *Science*. 1999;285(5426):397.

27. Flick R, Bouloy M. Rift Valley fever virus. *Curr Mol Med*. 2005;5(8):827.

28. World Health Organization. Rift Valley fever fact sheet. *Wkly Epidemiol Rec*. 2008;83(2):17.

29. Centers for Disease Control and Prevention. Rift Valley fever outbreak—Kenya, November 2006–January 2007. *MMWR*. 2007;56(4):73.

30. Evans A, Gakuya F, Paweska JT, et al. Prevalence of antibodies against Rift Valley fever in Kenyan wildlife. *Epidemiol Infect*. 2008;136(9):1261.

31. World Organisation for Animal Health. *Manual of diagnostic tests and vaccines for terrestrial animals (OIE terrestrial manual)*. 6th ed. Paris: World Organisation for Animal Health; 2008.

SALMONELLOSIS

Peter M. Rabinowitz and Lisa A. Conti

Salmonellosis (ICD-10 A02)

Other names in humans: Salmonella *infection*

Other names in animals: salmonellosis, songbird fever, fowl typhoid

The genus *Salmonella* was named after Dr. Daniel Salmon, a noted veterinary pathologist. As an infectious disease challenge, it epitomizes the importance of human health and animal health clinicians working collaboratively. It is one of the most common causes of infectious diarrhea and gastroenteritis. At the same time, its true importance is probably underestimated; it is thought that fewer than 1% of cases in industrialized countries, and even fewer in developing countries, are reported.

Key Points for Clinicians and Public Health Professionals

Public Health Professionals

- Educate clinicians that *Salmonella* infection is reportable to public health authorities.
- Educate the public about the risk to children and others of *Salmonella* poisoning from food.
- Use good kitchen hygiene; be particularly careful with foods prepared for children, the elderly, or immunocompromized individuals.
- Thoroughly wash raw vegetables and fruits.
- Do not eat foods made with raw eggs or unpasteurized milk products.
- Cook poultry, ground beef, and eggs thoroughly.
- Breastfeeding prevents salmonellosis and many other health problems in infants.[1]
- Educate the public, veterinarians, and human health clinicians on CDC guidelines for prevention of reptile and other animal associated salmonellosis; such educational messages have proven effective[2] (Box 9-6; see also http://www.cdc.gov/healthypets/spotlight_an_turtles.htm).[3]
- Ensure that local petting zoos and other areas where the public has contact with animals have policies and procedures for reduction of infection risk such as handwashing stations.
- Ensure that local pet stores are not selling small turtles.
- Disinfect with 1% sodium hypochlorite, 70% ethanol, 2% glutaraldehyde, or iodine solutions.

Human Health Clinicians

- The disease is reportable to public health authorities.
- Ask about a history of pet and other animal contact in all patients presenting with gastroenteritis and other *Salmonella* infections.

BOX 9-6   *RECOMMENDATIONS FOR PREVENTING TRANSMISSION OF SALMONELLA FROM REPTILES AND AMPHIBIANS TO HUMANS*

- Pet store owners, health care providers, and veterinarians should provide information to owners and potential purchasers of reptiles and amphibians about the risks for and prevention of salmonellosis from these pets.
- Persons at increased risk for infection or serious complications from salmonellosis (e.g., children younger than 5 years and immunocompromised persons) should avoid contact with reptiles and amphibians and any items that have been in contact with reptiles and amphibians.
- Reptiles and amphibians should not be allowed in households that include children younger than 5 years or immunocompromised persons. A family expecting a child should remove any pet reptile from the home before the infant arrives.
- Reptiles and amphibians should not be allowed in child care centers.
- Persons always should wash their hands thoroughly with soap and water after handling reptiles and amphibians or their cages.
- Reptiles and amphibians should not be allowed to roam freely throughout a home or living area.
- Pet reptiles and amphibians should be kept out of kitchens and other food-preparation areas. Kitchen sinks should not be used to bathe reptiles and amphibians or to wash their dishes, cages, or aquariums. If bathtubs are used for these purposes, they should be cleaned thoroughly and disinfected with bleach.
- Reptiles and amphibians in public settings (e.g., zoos and exhibits) should be kept from direct or indirect contact with patrons except in designated animal-contact areas equipped with adequate handwashing facilities. Food and drink should not be allowed in animal contact areas.

From Centers for Disease Control and Prevention: *Diseases from reptiles.* http://www.cdc.gov/healthypets/animals/reptiles.htm. Accessed January 16, 2009.

- Counsel pregnant women to remove any reptiles kept as pets in the house.[4]
- Counsel immunocompromised patients, young children, older adults, and patients with sickle cell anemia to avoid contact with puppies and kittens that have diarrhea and with any reptiles, baby chicks, or ducklings.

Veterinary Clinicians

- Counsel pet owners not to feed dogs and cats raw meat diets and to wash hands after handling animals, feces, and animal food treats.
- Counsel owners to practice good sanitation of cages, runs, feed and water dishes; proper storage of feed and feed utensils; reduce overcrowding situations; isolate and screen for illness in new animals.
- Ensure that appropriate infection control procedures are being followed by staff in veterinary care facilities.
- Counsel clients that immunocompromised individuals, infants, and older adults should avoid contact with reptiles, baby chicks, and ducklings.

- Counsel owners who want to give antibiotics prophylactically to their pets that that practice is ill advised due to the possibility of selecting for antibiotic-resistant strains.
- Be aware of CDC recommendations about reptiles and pets; see http://www.cdc.gov/healthypets/spotlight_an_turtles.htm.
- Counsel reptile owners on proper handwashing after pet handling and not bathing reptiles in bathtubs or sinks (Figure 9-117).[5]

Agent

Salmonella are gram-negative, facultative anaerobic rod-shaped bacteria belonging to the family Enterobacteriaceae that colonize the small intestine. There are thousands of distinct serovars, many adapted to particular animal species. In humans, the most common agents are *S. typhimurium* and *S. Enteritidis*. *Salmonella* Typhi, the causative agent of typhoid fever, and *S. Enteritidis* serotype Paratyphi are found only in humans. Most *Salmonella* serovars have animal reservoirs and are potentially zoonotic. β-Lactamase–mediated antimicrobial resistance is common. Antibiotic resistance in *Salmonella* species has been linked to the use of antibiotics in animal agriculture.[6]

Geographical Occurrence

Salmonella occur commonly worldwide in both animals and humans. *S. Enteritidis* is the most common species, followed by *S. typhimurium*.

Groups at Risk

Young children appear to be at increased risk of significant infection. Playing in sandboxes has been linked to risk in children.[7] Older adults and immunocompromised individuals are also considered high-risk groups. Individuals with HIV infection are at risk of recurrent septicemia. Patients with sickle cell disease can develop focal infections such as osteomyelitis. Other risk factors include achlorhydria, antacid treatment, antibiotic therapy, and malnutrition.

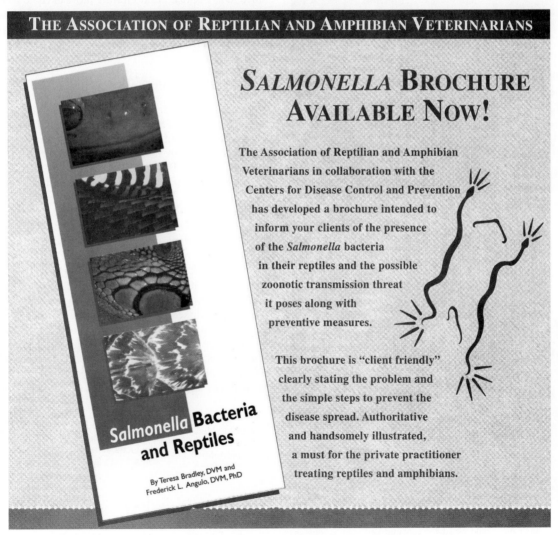

THE ASSOCIATION OF REPTILIAN AND AMPHIBIAN VETERINARIANS

SALMONELLA BROCHURE AVAILABLE NOW!

The Association of Reptilian and Amphibian Veterinarians in collaboration with the Centers for Disease Control and Prevention has developed a brochure intended to inform your clients of the presence of the *Salmonella* bacteria in their reptiles and the possible zoonotic transmission threat it poses along with preventive measures.

This brochure is "client friendly" clearly stating the problem and the simple steps to prevent the disease spread. Authoritative and handsomely illustrated, a must for the private practitioner treating reptiles and amphibians.

Salmonella **Bacteria and Reptiles**

By Teresa Bradley, DVM and Frederick L. Angulo, DVM, PhD

Figure 9-117 ■ Association of Reptilian and Amphibian Veterinarians *Salmonella* brochure. Clients must be warned of potential risks of reptile ownership. (From Mader DR: *Reptile medicine and surgery*, ed 2, St Louis, 2006, Saunders Elsevier.)

Ownership of reptiles and other pets (including rodents) is a risk factor for infection (Figures 9-118 and 9-119). An estimated 4% of the U.S. population owns reptiles, and a FoodNet study estimated that 6% of reported salmonellosis cases in the United States were attributable to reptile and amphibian ownership.[8]

Salmonellosis can also be an occupational disease. An outbreak occurred among 45 workers in companion animal veterinary medical facilities, and lack of proper biosafety precautions was considered the cause.[9] Other cases have occurred among veterinary pathologists performing necropsies,[10] workers producing poultry vaccines,[11] and workers exposed to raw meat.[7]

Newborns and debilitated animals are at risk of more severe disease. Crowding, boarding, mixing, and malnutrition are stressors that predispose many animals to infection. Group housing is associated with higher rates of infection in cats. Feeding dogs and cats raw meat has been found to increase the risk of infection.[12] Dry pet food and pig ear dog treats have been found to be contaminated and pose a risk to pets and their owners.

Hosts, Reservoir Species, Vectors

Animals are the natural reservoir for all *Salmonella* species except *S.* Typhi and *S.* Paratyphi. A wide range of species may be asymptomatic carriers of *Salmonella*, including dogs, cats, birds (including poultry), cattle, swine, horses, reptiles and amphibians, wildlife (including rodents), carnivores, and even crustaceans. Poultry are considered one of the principal reservoirs for *Salmonella* organisms and have harbored hundreds of different serovars.

Prevalence rates of subclinical infection in dogs is between 1% and 35%.[13] A recent survey found infection rates as high as 50% in group-housed cats.[14] Infected migrating songbirds can result in epidemics in bird-hunting cats.

Reptiles have rates of subclinical infection as high as 90% and pose a significant risk of transmission to pet owners and animal handlers in zoos and pet stores. The sale or distribution of small turtles has been illegal in the United States since 1975 because children were more likely to treat smaller turtles as toys and put them in their mouths.[15] However, pet turtles continue to be sold illegally and have caused recent outbreaks of salmonella infection.

Mode of Transmission and Life Cycle

Salmonella is considered primarily a foodborne disease, usually of animal origin. Food or water that is contaminated with feces from an infected animal is then ingested by a susceptible human host (Figure 9-120). Person-to-person spread can occur by the fecal-oral route or by food handlers who are shedding organisms and contaminate ready-to-eat food items.

Infection can occur sporadically or in large outbreaks involving thousands of individuals with a common exposure.[16] Contaminated peanut butter and peanut paste was the source of a multistate outbreak of *S.* Typhimurium infection for people and pets through contamination of processed foods and pet treats.[17]

An outbreak in humans and dogs in the United States and Canada was linked to contaminated raw food pet treats; presumably the owners did not wash their hands adequately after handling the treats.[18] Coprophagia and scavenging spreads the bacteria. Zoonotic transmission can also occur by direct contact with the feces of an infected animal. Animals with acute illness shed copious numbers of *Salmonella* in feces.

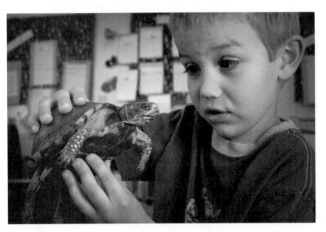

Figure 9-118 ■ Young boy holding a box turtle. Turtles and other reptiles and amphibians are sources of *Salmonella* infection, which is potentially dangerous to children. (From Centers for Disease Control and Prevention Public Health Image Library, Atlanta, Ga. Photo courtesy James Gathany.)

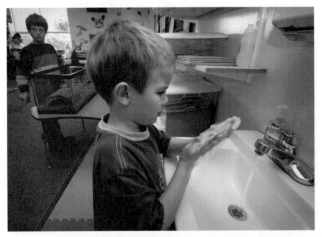

Figure 9-119 ■ A young child appropriately washing his hands after handling a turtle, which could have been contaminated with *Salmonella*. (From Centers for Disease Control and Prevention Public Health Image Library, Atlanta, Ga. Photo courtesy James Gathany.)

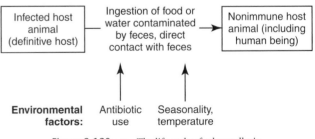

Figure 9-120 ■ The life cycle of salmonellosis.

Environmental Risk Factors

Salmonella can persist for months in food, feces, soil, and water given appropriate environmental conditions. The bacteria are resistant to dehydration and salinity. Survival in composted manure is as short as a week, and pasteurization kills *Salmonella* organisms.[19] Seasonality appears to affect the occurrence of disease, with more cases reported in the spring and summer.[20]

Disease in Humans

Human infection with non-typhi *Salmonella* can take a number of forms, including gastroenteritis, bacteremia and vascular infection, localized infection, and chronic carrier state (Figure 9-121).[21] Gastroenteritis in an immunocompetent adult often manifests as self-limited diarrhea. The incubation period is 6 to 72 hours. The principal symptoms are acute onset of diarrhea, often accompanied by nausea, abdominal pain, headache, fever, myalgias, vomiting, and malaise. Dehydration, sometimes severe, may occur, especially among the young and elderly. In most cases, symptoms resolve within 3 to 7 days. Diarrhea lasting longer than 10 days should suggest another diagnosis. However, convalescent patients may shed bacteria for weeks or months, and a chronic carrier state can occur in adults.[21]

Certain strains of *Salmonella* are particularly pathogenic in humans, such as *S. choleraesuis* and *S. dublin*, which can cause prolonged bacteremia, invasive disease, and death.[6,22] However, other *Salmonella* serotypes can also cause bacteremia, which can be accompanied by endovascular infection.

Localized infection can occur in 5% to 10% of cases of bacteremia. Specific infections include osteomyelitis, septic arthritis, endocarditis, meningitis, and pneumonia. Patients with sickle cell anemia are more susceptible to some of these conditions.[21]

In patients with AIDS and other immunocompromised individuals, bacteremia is common and often includes severe complications including localized infections, fulminant diarrhea, and death.

Disease in Animals

In adult cattle, sheep, pigs, and horses the disease takes three forms: subclinical carriage, mild clinical disease, or acute onset of fever and diarrhea, often with dehydration, abdominal pain, and sometimes bacteremia and death (Color Plates 9-62 to 9-64). Abortion may be the presenting sign of infection. Malabsorption and pneumonia may be part of the clinical syndrome. Newborn calves, lambs, piglets, and foals are more likely to develop septicemia (Figure 9-122). Outbreaks occur on farms, often precipitated by crowding, stress, calving, and mixing in feedlots.[19] Outbreaks also occur in equine hospitals.[19]

In dogs and cats, the disease is often subclinical. In puppies, kittens, or adults stressed by hospitalization, boarding, or concurrent disease, acute diarrhea with fever and septicemia can occur. Complications can include development of chronic infection and recurrence of disease under stressful conditions.

In caged birds, clinical salmonellosis is rare but may be seen in immunocompromised or stressed animals (songbird fever) (Color Plate 9-65). Although poultry often do not manifest disease, two serovars adapted to poultry, *S.* Pullorum and *S.* Gallinarum, cause serious losses on farms worldwide. Pullorum disease causes anorexia and diarrhea in chicks and has a high mortality rate. Fowl typhoid due to *S.* Gallinarum is a disease of adult birds (Figure 9-123).

Reptiles can shed *Salmonella* without clinical signs; however they may develop abscesses (Figure 9-124). Infection in wildlife is common, and clinical cases have been seen even in manatees and beluga whales.[19] Table 9-58 provides clinical presentations of salmonellosis in humans and other animals.

Non-typhoid *Salmonella* gastroenteritis

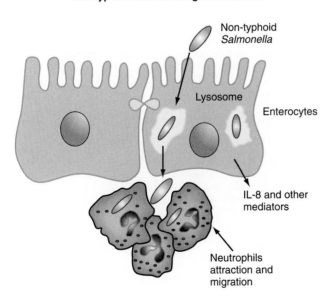

Figure 9-121 ▪ Pathogenesis of *Salmonella* gastroenteritis. (Adapted from Kliegman RM, Behrman RE, Jenson HB et al: *Nelson textbook of pediatrics*, ed 18, Philadelphia, 2007, Saunders Elsevier.)

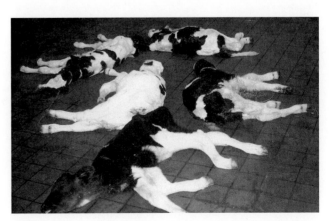

Figure 9-122 ▪ One day's death toll of neonatal calves from a dairy farm with high mortality rates in cattle of all ages during an epidemic caused by a highly virulent *Salmonella typhimurium* strain. (From Divers TJ, Peek SF: *Rebhun's diseases of dairy cattle*, ed 2, St Louis, 2008, Saunders Elsevier.)

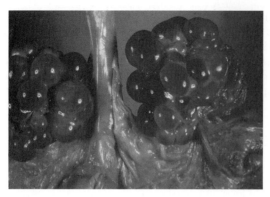

Figure 9-123 ■ Avian salpingitis as a result of *Salmonella* infection. (From Songer JG, Post KW: *Veterinary microbiology: bacterial and fungal agents of animal disease*, St Louis, 2005, Saunders Elsevier. Courtesy Raymond E. Reed.)

Diagnosis

Gastroenteritis in humans due to *Salmonella* can resemble other bacterial, viral, and protozoal forms of diarrhea. The incubation period and the presence of fever and often bloody stools can help narrow the differential diagnosis, and definitive diagnosis is made by bacterial culture

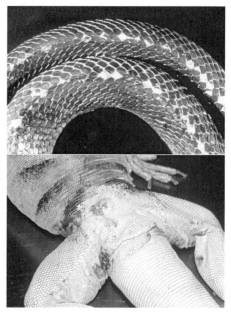

Figure 9-124 ■ *Salmonella* species dermatitis in an Eastern Indigo snake (*Drymarchon cooperi*, *top*) and green iguana (*Iguana iguana*, *bottom*). (From Mader DR: *Reptile medicine and surgery*, ed 2, St Louis, 2006, Saunders Elsevier. Photograph courtesy D. Mader.)

Table 9-58 ■ *Salmonella* Infection: Comparative Clinical Presentations in Humans and Other Animals

Species	Risk Factors	Incubation Period	Clinical Manifestations	Laboratory Findings
Humans (*S.* Typhimurium, *S.* Enteritidis, others)				
Gastroenteritis	Contaminated food, immunocompromised status, children at increased risk, prior antibiotic treatment, contact with animals	6-72 hours	Diarrhea, often with mucus or blood; abdominal cramping, fever	Fecal leukocytes, organisms seen on Gram stain, dark-field, or phase-contrast microscopy of feces, stool culture
Bacteremia	HIV/AIDS, other immuno-compromised status, sickle cell anemia, older age		Fever, localized infection (bone, joint vascular, CNS, other)	Blood culture, culture of localized infection
Dogs, cats	Puppies and kittens at increased risk; raw meat diets; recent hospitalization, concurrent disease/immunocompromised status, pregnant dogs	3 days[19]	Acute diarrhea with septicemia, pneumonia, abortion, chronic febrile illness, conjunctivitis (cats)	Leukopenia with left shift, fecal culture, fecal leukocytes, blood culture
Cattle, sheep, swine, horses	Young animals at increased risk, crowding, malnutrition, mixing, stress, rodents, Infected feed, contact with sick animals	Variable, 6-24 hours in horses	Acute septicemia in newborns[19] Acute or subacute enteritis in adults and young animals with fever, watery diarrhea, decreased milk production, abdominal pain, abortion Chronic enteritis (pigs and cattle)	Leukopenia (horses)
Caged birds	Clinical disease with stress, immunocompromised status			
Poultry	Chicks at increased risk for *S.* Pullorum	<2 weeks	Anorexia, diarrhea, death	Serology for *S.* Pullorum, *S.* Gallinarum

CNS, Central nervous system.

Table 9-59 ▪ Antibiotic Treatment of *Salmonella* Infection in Humans and Other Animals

Species	Primary Treatment	Alternative Treatment
Humans (gastroenteritis)	Ciprofloxacin 500 mg PO BID × 5-7 days (14 days if immunocompromised status)[23]	Azithromycin 1 gm PO once, then 500 mg PO q24h × 6 days
Dogs, cats (neonate, geriatric, or debilitated animal)	Follow culture and sensitivity results: trimethoprim-sulfamethoxazole 15 mg/kg PO or SC q12h, chloramphenicol dogs 50 mg/kg PO, IV, IM, or SC q8h; cats 50 mg/kg PO, IV, IM, SC q12h[24] Amoxicillin 10-20 mg/kg PO q8h × 10 days (use trimethoprim-sulfamethoxazole and chloramphenicol with caution in neonates and pregnant animals)	Enrofloxacin 5 mg/kg PO or SC q12h × 7 days[25] (avoid in neonates, pregnant or growing animals)
Cattle, sheep, swine, horses	Septicemia: broad-spectrum antibiotics initially, consider trimethoprim-sulfamethoxazole	Ampicillin, fluoroquinolones, third-generation cephalosporins; check local antimicrobial resistance patterns[19]

of feces, blood, or other localized infections (such as joint fluid or CSF) from ill individuals. Serology is not useful in humans.

In animals, fecal analysis and culture are used to diagnose infection. In poultry, serology is used to identify and eliminate flocks that have carriers of *S. pullorum* and *S. gallinarum*.

Treatment

Treatment in Humans

The mainstay of treatment for enteritis caused by *Salmonella* in immunocompetent adults is fluid and electrolyte replacement. Mild and asymptomatic infection does not require antibiotic treatment. Indications for the use of antibiotics include age younger than 1 year or older than 50 years, compromised immune status, and presence of vascular grafts or prosthetic joints.

When antibiotics are used, their use should be guided by the culture and sensitivity results because some *Salmonella* organisms are resistant to ciprofloxacin and other antibiotics. Evidence of localized infection is an indication for longer courses of treatment. Antimicrobial treatment may also prolong the carrier state, which may affect the ability of some food workers to return to work.

Treatment in Animals

Subclinical carriage in animals is not treated with antibiotics. If an adult dog or cat has uncomplicated gastroenteritis, it also can be treated without antibiotics with isolation, supportive care, and gastrointestinal protectants. Infected neonates, aged, and immunocompromised animals are candidates for isolation, possible plasma transfusions, supportive care, and glucocorticoid (for endotoxic shock) and antibiotic therapy. Fecal cultures should be monitored on a monthly basis to determine whether an animal is a carrier. Table 9-59 shows recommend antibiotics for treatment of *Salmonella* infection in humans and other animals when antibiotic treatment is appropriate.

References

1. Centers for Disease Control and Prevention. *Division of Foodborne, Bacterial and Mycotic Diseases: Salmonellosis: general information.* http://www.cdc.gov/nczved/dfbmd/disease_listing/salmonellosis_gi.html. Accessed August 15, 2008.
2. de Jong B, Andersson Y, Ekdahl K. Effect of regulation and education on reptile-associated salmonellosis. *Emerg Infect Dis.* 2005;11(3):398.
3. Centers for Disease Control and Prevention. Reptile-associated salmonellosis—selected states, 1998–2002. *MMWR.* 2003;52(49):1206.
4. Milstone AM, Agwu AG, Angulo FJ. Alerting pregnant women to the risk of reptile-associated salmonellosis. *Obstet Gynecol.* 2006;107(2 Pt 2):516.
5. Bender JB, Minicucci L. Diseases pets and people share. *Minn Med.* 2007;90(4):43.
6. Acha PN, Szyfres B. *Zoonoses and communicable diseases common to man and animals, vol. I: bacterioses and mycoses.* 3rd ed. Washington, DC: Pan American Health Organization; 2003.
7. Doorduyn Y, Van Den Brandhof WE, Van Duynhoven YT, et al. Risk factors for *Salmonella enteritidis* and *typhimurium* (DT104 and non-DT104) infections in The Netherlands: predominant roles for raw eggs in *Enteritidis* and sandboxes in *typhimurium* infections. *Epidemiol Infect.* 2006;134(3):617.
8. Mermin J, Hutwagner L, Vugia D, et al. Reptiles, amphibians, and human *Salmonella* infection: a population-based, case-control study. *Clin Infect Dis.* 2004;38(suppl 3):S253.
9. Wright JG, Tengelsen LA, Smith KE, et al. Multidrug-resistant *Salmonella typhimurium* in four animal facilities. *Emerg Infect Dis.* 2005;11(8):1235.
10. Bemis DA, Craig LE, Dunn JR. *Salmonella* transmission through splash exposure during a bovine necropsy. *Foodborne Pathog Dis.* 2007;4(3):387.
11. Centers for Disease Control and Prevention. *Salmonella* serotype *enteritidis* infections among workers producing poultry vaccine—Maine, November–December 2006. *MMWR.* 2007;56(34):877.
12. Stiver SL, Frazier KS, Mauel MJ, et al. Septicemic salmonellosis in two cats fed a raw-meat diet. *J Am Anim Hosp Assoc.* 2003;39(6):538.
13. Finley R, Ribble C, Aramini J, et al. The risk of salmonellae shedding by dogs fed *Salmonella*-contaminated commercial raw food diets. *Can Vet J.* 2007;48(1):69.
14. van Immerseel F, Pasmans F, De Buck J, et al. Cats as a risk for transmission of antimicrobial drug-resistant *Salmonella*. *Emerg Infect Dis.* 2004;10(12):2169.
15. Centers for Disease Control and Prevention. *Reptiles and Salmonella.* http://www.cdc.gov/Features/ReptilesSalmonella. Accessed August 15, 2008.
16. Centers for Disease Control and Prevention. *Salmonella.* http://www.cdc.gov/nczved/dfbmd/disease_listing/salmonellosis_gi.html. Accessed August 15, 2008.
17. Centers for Disease Control and Prevention (CDC). Multistate outbreak of *Salmonella* infections associated with peanut butter and peanut butter-containing products—United States, 2008–2009. *MMWR.* 2009;58(4):85.

18. Centers for Disease Control and Prevention. Human salmonellosis associated with animal-derived pet treats—United States and Canada, 2005. *MMWR.* 2006;55(25):702.
19. Kahn CM, Line S, eds. *The Merck veterinary manual.* 9th ed. Whitehouse Station, NJ: Merck; 2005.
20. Oloya J, Theis M, Doetkott D, et al. Evaluation of *Salmonella* occurrence in domestic animals and humans in North Dakota (2000–2005). *Foodborne Pathog Dis.* 2007;4(4):551.
21. Mandell GL, Bennett JE, Dolin R, eds. *Principles and practice of infectious diseases.* 6th ed. New York: Churchill Livingstone Elsevier; 2005.
22. Jones TF, Ingram LA, Cieslak PR. Salmonellosis outcomes differ substantially by serotype. *J Infect Dis.* 2008;198(1):109.
23. Gilbert DN, Moellering RC, Eliopoulos GM, et al. *Sanford guide to antimicrobial therapy 2009.* 39th ed. Sperryville, VA: Antimicrobial Therapy; 2009.
24. Tilley LP, Smith FWK. *Blackwell's five-minute veterinary consult: canine and feline.* 3rd ed. Ames, IA: Blackwell; 2004.
25. Barr SC, Bowman DD. *The 5-minute veterinary consult clinical companion: canine and feline infectious diseases and parasitology.* Ames, IA: Blackwell; 2006.

SCABIES

Russell W. Currier and Roger I. Ceilley

Sarcoptic itch (ICD-10 B86) Other acariasis (ICD-10 B88.0)

Other names in humans: sarcoptic itch, acariasis, crusted scabies, Norwegian scabies, pseudoscabies, cavalryman's itch, pig-handler's itch

Other names in animals: sarcoptic mange, cutaneous acariasis

Scabies is a skin infestation caused by the mite *Sarcoptes scabiei*. Reports of scabies in humans date back to antiquity, and it was the first infectious disease linked to a specific etiology with the use of a microscope. In 1834 the mite was conclusively demonstrated on a young female patient in a Paris clinic, establishing the association between the mite and its dermatological manifestations.[1] This little-appreciated historical event represented the first etiological diagnosis in medicine. In human medicine, scabies continues to cause both sporadic cases and outbreaks in industrial countries, and immunocompromised persons can experience severe infection. Dogs and many other animals also experience significant infections with variants of *S. scabiei* that are adapted to particular host species. With close contact such as occupational exposure, transmission of animal scabies variants from animals to humans can occur. Although such zoonotic infestations (pseudoscabies) are usually self-limited, they underscore the importance of communication between human and animal health professionals about cases of skin rashes occurring concurrently in humans and animals. This section focuses on scabies, but there are a number of other mite species that infest animals and are capable of causing self-limited skin infections in humans that may be misdiagnosed or missed by medical providers.

Key Points for Clinicians and Public Health Professionals

Public Health Professionals

- Be alert for outbreaks of skin disease caused by scabies in situations of human crowding.
- Consider zoonotic mite infestation as a cause of outbreaks of skin rashes in the community; consult with local veterinarians.
- Educate veterinarians about the zoonotic potential of scabies and other mites and encourage voluntary reporting of cases of sarcoptic mange in animals.

Human Health Clinicians

- Disease usually not reportable but public health authorities should be notified in outbreak settings such as among institutionalized persons and day care centers.
- In evaluating cases of pruritic skin rash, consider possibility of zoonotic transmission of scabies or other mites (pseudoscabies); ask about contact with animals or fomites that could contain mites. Consider consulting a veterinarian.
- Immunocompromised patients may present with heavier scabies mite burdens, requiring extended treatment regimens.
- Delusions of parasitosis can be an underlying condition in the absence of scabies or following diagnosis and treatment of actual infestations.

Veterinary Clinicians

- Counsel owners of a pet with scabies about the risk of human transmission and that it could be self-limiting or persistent, requiring treatment after the pet has been treated.
- Advise health care providers and public health professionals about the risk to humans of animal scabies and other mite infestations.
- Companion animals should be carefully screened for scabies and other mite infestations.
- Animal scabies may be reportable to agriculture/public health authorities if history is linked with a pet store or facility that permits contact with animals in public settings (e.g., petting zoo).
- Some states require reporting of sarcoptic mange in sheep and cattle.

Agent

Sarcoptes scabiei is a species of mite in the family Sarcoptidae that lives parasitically on or in the skin of mammals. Adult mites are 0.3 to 0.5 mm long and roughly circular with four pairs of legs (Figure 9-125). Variants of *S. scabiei* are found in a variety of animal species but are taxonomically

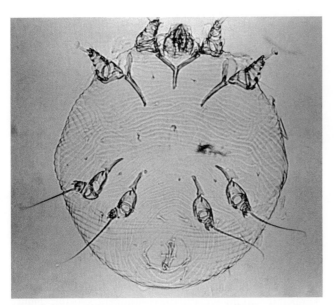

Figure 9-125 ▪ Ventral view of a cleared and mounted *Sarcoptes scabiei* mite. (From Centers for Disease Control and Prevention Public Health Image Library, Atlanta, Ga.)

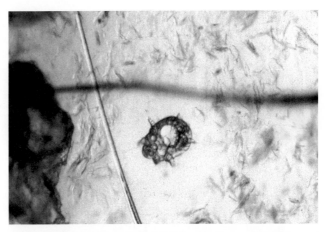

Figure 9-126 ▪ Feline scabies. Microscopic image of *Notoedres cati* mite from a skin scraping as seen with a ×10 objective. (From Medleau L, Hnilica KA: *Small animal dermatology: a color atlas and therapeutic guide,* ed 2, St Louis, 2006, Saunders Elsevier. Courtesy G. Norsworthy.)

indistinguishable between human and animal species. For example, scabies in dogs is caused by *S. scabiei* var *canis*.[2] In addition to *S. scabiei*, a number of other mites that infest animals are able to also cause skin rashes in humans. Table 9-60 lists some of these mite species with zoonotic potential.

Dermanyssus gallinae, the red poultry mite, is a nocturnal blood-sucking mite that is the most common mite found in pigeons. Close contact with poultry, wild birds, or nesting material can lead to human infection, which presents as a nonspecific dermatitis that is intensely pruritic and often misdiagnosed.[3,4]

Cheyletiella species, the walking dandruff mite, may be present as a subclinical infection in dogs and cats but can cause an erythematous, papular rash in humans in contact with infected animals. The papules are usually on the arms, trunk, and buttocks and develop into yellow crusted lesions that can be intensely pruritic. Rarely, bullous eruptions and systemic reactions have been reported.[5,6]

Otodectes cynotis is a common mite found in the ears of dogs and cats, where it causes local irritation. It can migrate to other parts of the pet's body, and because it is not host

specific, it is capable of infecting humans as well, causing a papular skin rash or an external otitis.[6]

Notoedres cati (feline scabies) is a rare but highly contagious disease of cats that can also infect humans,[7] causing a pruritic rash within hours without visible skin burrows (Figure 9-126 and Color Plate 9-66).

Geographical Occurrence

Scabies is a global problem with widespread distribution in human populations of all ages. It is also found in animal populations worldwide. Outbreaks of often fatal sarcoptic mange in animals have occurred in wildlife populations such as foxes, leading to fluctuations in population size.

Groups at Risk

Human scabies can occur in outbreaks among institutionalized patients[8] or in other situations of crowding such as refugee camps. The presence of immunocompromised patients in such settings may facilitate transmission, and immunocompromised individuals are at risk of more severe infection. Sexual contact is another major risk factor for disease transmission.

Persons at risk for zoonotic transmission of scabies include farmers, veterinarians, wildlife rehabilitators, and pet owners who have close contact with potentially infected animals.

In industrialized nations, scabies often presents as a sexually transmitted parasitic infection with secondary transmission to household members, especially children, who are easily infected when parents or caretakers are infested.[9]

Patients with HIV-AIDS and other immunocompromising states are easily infected and sustain heavy mite burdens leading to crusted or hyperkeratotic scabies.[10]

In animal populations, contact with infected animals is the major risk factor for scabies infection. Puppies, especially those from a pound or animal shelter or whelped in a large breeding kennel, may be at increased risk. Dogs that are allowed to roam freely and contact wildlife or other dogs, including at dog parks, may be at higher risk of infestation.[6]

Table 9-60 ▪ Mites With Zoonotic Potential		
Mite Species	**Name**	**Host Species**
Sarcoptes scabiei	Scabies	Humans, dogs, cattle, foxes, horses, pigs
Dermanyssus gallinae	Red poultry mite	Chickens, pigeons, other birds
Cheyletiella species	Fur mite, walking dandruff mite	Cat, dog, rabbit, small mammals
Otodectes cynotis	Ear mite	Dogs, cats
Notoedres cati	Feline scabies	Cats

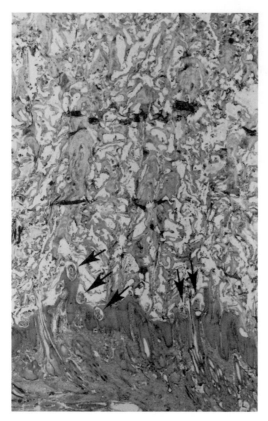

Figure 9-127 ■ Hyperkeratosis caused by *Sarcoptes scabiei* in the fox (×22). The mites *(arrows)* are found in the deeper layers of the greatly thickened epidermis. (From Bowman DD: *Georgis' parasitology for veterinarians,* ed 9, St Louis, 2009, Saunders Elsevier.)

Debilitated animals may be at increased risk of severe cases of sarcoptic mange.

Wildlife also can sustain scabies; foxes are particularly susceptible to heavy mite infestations (Figure 9-127). In one case report, a wild red fox *(Vulpes vulpes)* infected a wildlife rehabilitator and a veterinarian who were treating the animal, as well as several dogs residing near a golf course where the affected fox was originally found.[11]

Hosts, Reservoir Species, Vectors

Only one distinct genus and species of *S. scabiei* exists but variants are somewhat host adapted to humans and various specific animal populations. Species affected include dogs, cattle, sheep, pigs, horses, and foxes. Variants adapted to one species may infect another species, but in such instances sustained transmission does not occur.

The *S. scabiei* mite is not considered a vector for other infectious agents, although cases of infestation may become superinfected with *Staphylococcus, Streptococcus,* or other bacteria.

Mode of Transmission and Life Cycle

Scabies is transmitted through sustained direct skin-to-skin contact[12] during activities such as sexual contact, holding infants and animals, or while performing hands-on care. Casual contact such as handshaking is unlikely to lead to transmission. Sustained person-to-person and other intraspecies transmission requires adult female mites. After impregnation, the female burrows quickly into the epidermis of the host animal, forming a tunnel in the stratum corneum at the boundary with the stratum granulosum (Figure 9-128). Two to three large eggs are laid daily and these hatch in 4-6 days, giving rise to nymphal mites that molt to adult forms. Eggs develop into adult mites within 10 to 14 days.

Because many variants of the scabies mite cannot live long outside the body, indirect transmission via fomites is generally less important than direct transmission. However, in the case of crusted (hyperkeratotic) scabies, infected individuals have enormous quantities of mites on their person and shed mites on clothing, bed linen, and even furniture.[13] These mites can persist for days on particles of sloughed epidermis. In such situations, contact with fomites can easily lead to further disease transmission.

When an animal strain of *S. scabiei* infects a human, the mite is able to penetrate the skin and rapidly cause a pruritic rash but is unable to successfully reproduce and persist. The result is the self-limited condition termed *pseudoscabies.* Reverse zoonotic transmission can also occur.

Environmental Risk Factors

Mites in the environment are highly susceptible to temperature and humidity conditions and rarely survive beyond 2 to 3 days. Higher ambient temperatures lead to lower survival times.[7] Environmental conditions that predispose human to scabies transmission include crowding and institutionalization. Similarly, environments with animal crowding and

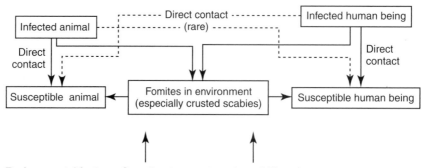

Environmental factors: Crowding, temperature, dog-wildlife contact

Figure 9-128 ■ Scabies transmission.

extensive animal-to-animal contact, such as animal shelters, breeding colonies, dog parks, and crowded kennels, may encourage animal-to-animal transmission of scabies. Areas where wildlife such as foxes contact domestic animals also represent environmental risks.

Disease in Humans

Scabies in humans is manifested about 20 to 35 days after transmission and results in pruritus that is particularly evident in the evening hours while the affected person is trying to sleep. This hypersensitivity is incompletely understood and results from some metabolite of the mites. Skin lesions commonly appear on the webbing of the fingers, genitalia, breasts, flexor surface of the wrists, elbows, and later the abdomen. The burrow or track is diagnostic (Color Plate 9-67) but is not always visible. More commonly papules and vesicles are the most typical skin lesions. Feet and legs are commonly affected areas in children. Rarely do lesions appear on the face and neck except in infants and immunocompromised patients, in whom face and neck lesions are more common.

Elderly patients such as residents of long-term care facilities frequently have extensive lesions on the shoulders and upper back as well as the usual areas noted. Secondary eczematization or thickening of the skin is common in this population, as well as low-grade bacterial infections such as *Staphylococus aureus* and *Streptococcus pyogenes*. Although these cases are fairly easy to diagnose, they also are more challenging to treat.

Crusted or hyperkeratotic (Norwegian) scabies occurs usually in immunocompromised patients and has a distinctive appearance of grey-green crustiness on the hands and feet, occasionally elbows and arms. Pruritus may be absent. This condition is also easy to diagnose but very difficult to treat. Color Plate 9-68 shows a patient with crusted scabies. In cases of pseudoscabies, intense pruritus and an erythematous rash are often present, but burrows may be absent.

Disease in Animals

The presentation of disease in animals is variable as shown in Table 9-61. The hallmark of animal scabies is pruritus

Table 9-61 ▪ Clinical Presentation of Scabies in Humans and Other Animals

Species	*Sarcoptes scabiei* Variant	Risk Factors	Incubation Period	Clinical Manifestations	Diagnostic Findings
Humans					
Scabies	Variant *hominis*	Crowding	2-6 weeks (1-4 days if previously infested)[18]	Papular rash, vesicles, pruritus	Skin scraping may reveal mites
Crusted scabies	Variant *hominis*	Immunocompromised status, fomites	2-6 weeks[18]	Diffuse crusting lesions, pruritus may be absent	Skin scraping reveals high mite burden
Pseudoscabies (zoonotic)	Animal variants	Direct contact with infected animal	2-6 weeks[18]	Self-limited rash, pruritus	Skin scraping often negative
Dogs	Variant *canis*	Kennels, animal shelters, dog parks, contact with infected wildlife; puppies at increased risk	2-6 weeks[18]	Pruritic papules with thick crusts; abdomen, chest, ears, elbows, and legs affected; alopecia minimal early in disease with more hair loss later	Skin scraping, fecal flotation may reveal mites or eggs; ELISA antibody test can show specific antibodies[7]
Cattle	Variant *bovis*	Rare in United States; contact with infected animals	2-6 weeks[18]	Head, neck, shoulders with later spread to entire body	
Sheep	Variant *ovis*	Rare in United States; contact with infected animals	2-6 weeks[18]	Lesions on nonwooly skin	
Goat	Variant *caprae*	Rare in United States	2-6 weeks[18]	Generalized hyperkeratosis	Skin scrapings showing either mites, eggs, or scybala
Horses	Variant *equi*	Rare in United States; contact with infected animals	2-6 weeks[18]	Intense pruritus Head, neck, shoulders affected; alopecia and crusting; later lichenified with skin folds	
Pigs	Variant *suis*	Contact with infected animals or bedding	2 to 11 weeks	Generalized pruritus; crusting of luminal surface of ears	
Foxes	Variant *vulpes*	Contact with infected animal or bedding	2-6 weeks[18]	Diffuse alopecia, crusting, wasting	

that may not represent location of mites; this is also true for humans (Figures 9-129 and 9-130). Generally longer duration infestations result in thickening of skin with secondary bacterial infections.[7]

In clinical veterinary practice, sarcoptic mange is a common presentation in dogs. The infestation has no age, breed, or sex predilection, occurs with no seasonality, and presents as an intensely pruritic, papular crusting dermatosis affecting the periocular skin, pinnal margins, elbows, and hocks, which may later progress to more generalized involvement, especially of the ventral areas (Figure 9-131). There may be very little to moderate hair loss in contradistinction to demodicosis (eyelash mites) or red mange, which shows little pruritus and extensive alopecia.

In horses, sarcoptic mange is the most severe type of mange, with intensely pruritic lesions on the head, neck, and shoulders. Swine historically have suffered extensive involve-

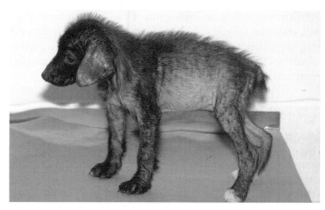

Figure 9-131 ■ Canine scabies. Generalized alopecia and crusts affecting a pruritic puppy. The alopecic ear pinnae are characteristic of scabies. (From Medleau L, Hnilica KA: *Small animal dermatology: a color atlas and therapeutic guide*, ed 2, St Louis, 2006, Saunders Elsevier.)

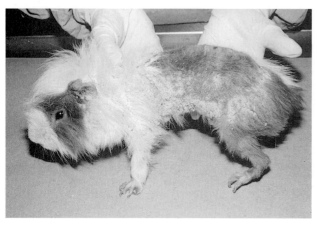

Figure 9-129 ■ Sarcoptic mange in a guinea pig caused by *Trixacarus caviae.* (From Quesenberry K, Carpenter JW: *Ferrets, rabbits, and rodents: clinical medicine and surgery*, ed 2, St Louis, 2004, Saunders Elsevier.)

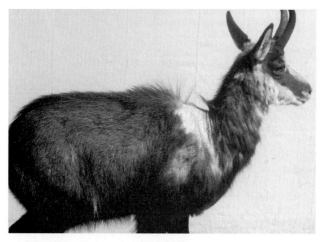

Figure 9-130 ■ Chamois with clinical scabies. The typical lesions begin at the head and neck and then spread over the back. (From Fowler M, Miller RE: *Zoo and wild animal medicine current therapy*, ed 6, St Louis, 2008, Saunders Elsevier. Courtesy T. Steineck, Research Institute of Wildlife Ecology, VMU, Vienna.)

ment, calling for routine mass treatment of most herds. Modern antihelmintic treatment of swine with broad-spectrum parasiticides has successfully eliminated this problem. Foxes may develop severe sarcoptic mange that can be fatal.

Diagnosis

Skin scrapings are the most common and reliable method to demonstrate the presence of mites, eggs, and scybala (discrete fecal pellets) in both humans and other animals. This procedure is as simple as it is essential and could be performed by technicians, nursing staff, physicians, and veterinarians. Standard references[14] call for applying mineral oil (some clinicians prefer to use type B microscopic immersion oil because it is more viscous and easier to work with) to a lesion or placing oil on a sterile scalpel blade (disposable #10 or #20), which is held at a right angle to the skin surface and used to scrape the area in a manner to remove visible skin debris until the superficial skin or stratum corneum is removed, leaving the scraped area pink but not necessarily hemorrhaging. The material adhering to the blade from two to three postage stamp–sized areas is then transferred to a microscope slide, diluted with more oil if necessary, with a cover slip applied after using it to scrape excess oil adhering to the scalpel blade, and the wet mount specimen is examined under ×4 and ×10 low power. The slide should be methodically examined as follows: Sweep left to right, move down one field, and right to left until the entire slide area is examined for mites (adults, nymphs, or larval mites) or distinctive eggs and the smaller scybala (fecal pellets that are numerous and distinct brown-gold/orange in color). Occasionally some skin lesions may be due to the *Demodex folliculorum* mite (eyelash mite) that has widespread distribution in human populations. These distinctive cigar-shaped mites have an elongated tail structure, whereas *Sarcoptes* mites have a distinctive turtle-like shape with four pairs of legs (Figure 9-132).

The scraping procedure not only enables diagnosis within minutes, but also helps to classify patients for mite load. A human patient's scraping with only a mite or two prob-

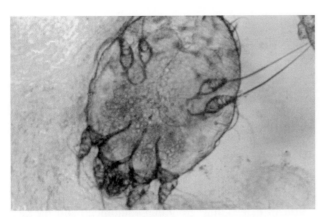

Figure 9-132 ■ Scabies organism in a wet mount preparation. (From Mandell GL, Bennett JE, Dolin R (eds): *Principles and practice of infectious diseases*, ed 6, Philadelphia, 2005, Churchill Livingstone Elsevier.)

ably is not highly infectious for others (average of 10 adult female mites on a patient) and needs only minimal treatment and simple contact precautions for a brief period of a day or two. However, patients with crusted or hyperkeratotic scabies demonstrate an extraordinary number of mites on each slide. Patients, especially the elderly with a history of extensive home care or long-term care residency, may have a large number of mites from skin with

red, raised, pruritic lesions and evidence of secondary eczematization. Although these lesions are not specifically crusted scabies, these cases are classified as "atypical crusted scabies" or "aggressive scabies" and require more intense treatment and oversight.[15]

In dogs and humans, skin scrapings may not always produce mites or their effects but call for thorough attempts at recovery nonetheless. After scraping and in the absence of mites, a diagnosis can be made based on exclusion of other diseases, epidemiological links, clinical impression (degree of pruritus, history, distribution pattern), and response to treatment.

Other techniques for diagnosis include epidermal shave biopsy, needle biopsy, and burrow ink test. In the latter technique, a blue or black felt-tip pen is rubbed over the lesions and then ink is removed with an alcohol pledget and the blue or black ink dye is pulled into the burrow by capillary action and is diagnostic. A solution of tetracycline can also be applied and examined under a Wood's light.

Treatment

Treatment in Humans

Table 9-62 outlines treatment guidelines with various scabicides. Treatment is preceded with a bath or shower in water

Table 9-62 ■ Treatment of Scabies in Humans and Other Animals

Species	Primary Treatment	Alternative
Humans		
Scabies	Permethrin 5% cream, apply entire skin chin to toes, leave on 8-14 hr, repeat in 1 wk (safe in children >2 months)	Ivermectin 200 mcg/kg PO once, second dose after 14 days *or* Crotamiton 10% cream, apply × 24 hr, rinse and reapply × 24 hr[17]
Immunocompromised, crusted (Norwegian) scabies	Permethrin 5% as above day 1, then 6% sulfur in petrolatum daily days 2-7, repeat × several weeks	Ivermectin 200 mcg/kg PO on days 1 and 14 *PLUS* permethrin 5% cream on days 1 and 14[16]
Pseudoscabies (zoonotic mite transmission)	No treatment may be necessary; veterinary consultation for treatment of animal contacts	
Dogs	Lime sulfur dip for young dogs, several dips 5 days apart Selamectin 6 mg/kg topically; repeated twice at 1-month interval[7]	Ivermectin 200 mcg/kg PO or SC, for 2 treatments 2 weeks apart (contraindicated in Collies and Collie crosses)
Cattle	Toxaphene, coumaphos, phosnet, lime sulfur dip (dairy cattle)	Injectable avermectins except dairy cattle
Sheep, Goat	Injectable ivermectin	Doramectin or moxidectin
Horses	Organophosphate insecticide or lime-sulfur solution by spraying, sponging, or dipping; repeat at 12- to 14-day intervals at least 3-4 times[7]	Ivermectin or moxidectin 200 mcg/kg PO × several treatments 2-3 weeks apart
Pigs	Ivermectin 300 mcg/kg SC, repeat in 2 weeks *or* doramectin 300 mcg/kg IM	Lindane, malathion, or chlordane sprays[7]
Foxes	Ivermectin 200 mcg/kg PO or SC, for 2 treatments 2 weeks apart	

of tepid temperature. Patients should clip fingernails and toenails, remove rings and bracelets, and wash the area under nails with a hand brush or toothbrush. Apply the scabicide according to directions behind the ears and from the neck down, paying particular attention to the hands (especially between fingers), the umbilical area, groin, the buttocks, and feet (especially between the toes). The medication should be left on for the prescribed number of hours and then thoroughly rinsed off with tepid soapy water (bath or shower). At the conclusion of therapy, intimate articles of clothing and bed linens should be laundered in hot water and dried on the hot cycle. Patients should be counseled that 24 hours after therapy, they no longer are infectious but may still experience itching for a few weeks afterward. Family members should be treated even if asymptomatic. The majority of patients respond to one treatment, and although there is a lack of well-controlled studies documenting that two applications are better than one, treatment is usually repeated, especially if there is microscopic and/or morphologic evidence of treatment failure. Patients in institutional settings may have a higher mite burden and require one to two additional treatments.

Scabies in immunocompromised individuals (crusted or Norwegian scabies) generally requires much more intense scabicidal treatment. Keratolytic agents (salicylic acid or alpha-hydroxy acid products) can be used to soften tissue, permitting better penetration of topicals, coupled with frequent reassessment and longer periods of contact isolation. Bedding and personal effects initially need special handling. Such patients have heavy mite burdens and need multiple applications of topical treatments.

Treatment of pseudoscabies due to zoonotic mite transmission often relies on treatment of the infected animal and disinfection of the environment. Consultation with a veterinarian is recommended if zoonotic transmission is suspected.

Treatment in Animals

Treatments for animals are summarized in Table 9-62. Requirements vary with species and age of the animal. It is wise to follow label directions owing to risk of toxicity. It is important to counsel animal handlers about risk of human transmission.

Treatment may be approached topically or systemically. Topical treatments include a 2.5% lime sulfur dip (Lym Dip; DVM Pharmaceutical, Inc.) that is licensed for weekly use with a wide margin of safety. Disadvantages include foul odor and staining of light-colored coats. Amitraz (Mitaban; Pharmacia & Upjohn Animal Health) is an alternative and is applied as a 0.025% sponge-on solution at 2-week intervals. Amitraz should not be used on Chihuahuas, in pregnant bitches, or puppies younger than 3 months. Clipping hair of dogs with long coats and/or dense hair coats is recommended. Amitraz vapors can induce hyperglycemia; it should not be

handled by individuals with diabetes or applied to patients with diabetes.

Systemic therapy is an attractive alternative and includes extralabel use of macrocyclic lactones—for example, ivermectin (Ivomec; Merial Animal Health), milbemycin (Interceptor; Novartis Animal Health), moxidectin (Cydectin; Fort Dodge Animal Health), and selamectin (Revolution; Pfizer Animal Health) that are licensed for treatment of canine sarcoptic mange. Ivermectin should not be used in Collies or sheep dogs and their crosses. Consult product literature for safe and proper administration.[16]

It would be prudent to also treat all dogs known to have contact with an affected animal. Concurrent environmental treatment of bedding, grooming equipment, and the general areas of habitation with an ascaricidal spray (e.g., one containing permethrin) is recommended to prevent possible reinfestation.

References

1. Friedman R. The story of scabies. *Medical Life.* 1934;41(8):381.
2. Champion RH, Burton JL, Burns DA, et al., eds. *Rook/Wilkinson/Ebling textbook of dermatology.* 6th ed. Malden MA: Blackwell; 1998.
3. Cafiero MA, Camarda A, Circella E, et al. Pseudoscabies caused by *Dermanyssus gallinae* in Italian city dwellers: a new setting for an old dermatitis. *J Eur Acad Dermatol Venereol.* 2008;22(11):1382.
4. Rosen S, Yeruham I, Braverman Y. Dermatitis in humans associated with the mites *Pyemotes tritici, Dermanyssus gallinae, Ornithonyssus bacoti* and *Androlaelaps casalis* in Israel. *Med Vet Entomol.* 2002;16(4):442.
5. Dobrosavljevic DD, Popovic ND, Radovanovic SS. Systemic manifestations of *Cheyletiella* infestation in man. *Int J Dermatol.* 2007; 46(4):397.
6. Moriello KA. Zoonotic skin diseases of dogs and cats. *Anim Health Res Rev.* 2003;4(2):157.
7. Kahn CM, Line S, eds. *The Merck veterinary manual.* 9th ed. Whitehouse Station, NJ: Merck; 2005.
8. Arlian LG. Biology, host relations, and epidemiology of *Sarcoptes scabiei. Ann Rev Entomol.* 1989;34:139.
9. Green MS. Epidemiology of scabies. *Epidemiol Rev.* 1989;11:126.
10. DePaoli RT, Marks VJ. Crusted (Norwegian) scabies: treatment of nail involvement. *J Am Acad Dermatol.* 1987;17(1):136.
11. Rabinowitz PM, Gordon Z. Outfoxing a rash: clinical example of human-wildlife interaction. *EcoHealth.* 2004;1:404.
12. Mellanby K. Scabies in 1976. *R Soc Health J.* 1977;97(1):32.
13. Carslaw RW, Dobson RM, Hood AJK, et al. Mites in the environment of Norwegian scabies. *Br J Dermatol.* 1975;92(3):333.
14. Muller G, Jacobs PH, Moore NE. Scraping for human scabies: a better method for positive preparations. *Arch Dermatol.* 1973;107(1):70.
15. Lerche NW, Currier RW, Juranek DD, et al. Atypical crusted "Norwegian" scabies: report of nosocomial transmission in a community hospital and an approach to control. *Cutis.* 1993;31(6):637.
16. van den Hoek JA, et al. A persistent problem with scabies in and outside a nursing home in Amsterdam: indications for resistance to lindane and ivermectin. *Eurosurveillance.* 2008;13(48).
17. Gilbert DN, Moellering RC, Eliopoulos GM, et al. *Sanford guide to antimicrobial therapy 2009.* 39th ed. Sperryville, VA: Antimicrobial Therapy; 2009.
18. Heymann DL, ed. *Control of communicable diseases manual.* 19th ed. Washington, DC: American Public Health Association; 2008.

TOXOCARA INFESTATION

Peter M. Rabinowitz and Lisa A. Conti

Visceral larva migrans (ICD-10 B83.0)

Other names in humans: roundworm infection, ocular larva migrans, Toxocara *infection)*

Other names in animals: roundworm infection, ascariasis

Infection with roundworms of the genus *Toxocara* is probably one of the most common infections associated with ownership of cats and dogs. Puppies and kittens often have symptomatic infections. Visceral or ocular larval migrans can occur in people. Seroprevalence studies suggest 5% to 30% of children may be infected.[1,2]

Key Points for Clinicians and Public Health Professionals

Public Health Professionals

- Provide descriptive epidemiology of the likely prevalence in animal and human populations.
- Educate the public on modes of transmission and ways to prevent infection:
  - Control stray dogs and cats.
  - Encourage dog and cat owners to have their animals regularly dewormed by a veterinarian.
  - Encourage basic handwashing awareness.
  - Discourage keeping raccoons as pets.
  - Cover sandboxes when not in use.
- Promote local measures to require that dog and cat feces are picked up by owners and do not contaminate local soils and play areas.
- Educate the local veterinary and human health clinicians in risk areas and during high-risk periods about groups at risk and the signs and symptoms of disease.

Human Health Clinicians

- Teach parents, especially pet owners, of the danger of contamination and exposure of areas by feces from untreated dogs and cats.
- Teach parents to not allow geophagia.
- Teach patients to always wash hands after handling soil and before eating.[3]
- Encourage patients with dogs and cats to ensure adequate veterinary treatment for worm infection. It is especially important for pregnant dogs and cats and young puppies and kittens to be dewormed. If a human health clinician inquires about this, it might raise awareness.
- No human vaccine is available.

Veterinary Clinicians

- Ensure pet owners bring animals for strategic deworming and prompt parasite treatment.

- Counsel pet owners about the proper disposal of animal feces and handwashing.
- See the CDC manual about toxocariasis for veterinarians that reviews specific prevention and treatment measures[4]; available online at http://www.cdc.gov/ncidod/dpd/parasites/ascaris/prevention.htm.
- Recommend keeping cats indoors.

Agent

Toxocara canis and *T. cati* are ascarid roundworms (nematodes) that are large (10 to 12 cm long) and live in the small intestine of carnivorous mammals but also migrate into tissues and cause extraintestinal pathology (Figure 9-133). *T. canis* is recognized more widely in both animals and humans than *T. cati*

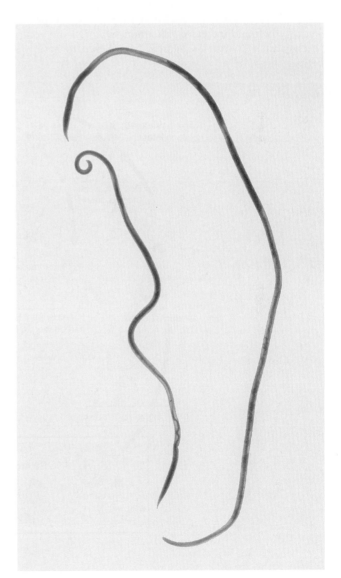

Figure 9-133 ▪ Adults of *Toxocara canis*. The male measures 6 cm and the female measures 9 cm in length. (From Long SS, Pickering LK, Prober CG: *Principles and practice of pediatric infectious diseases*, ed 3, Edinburgh, 2008, Churchill Livingstone Elsevier.)

and causes more serious infections in dogs.[5] *Toxascaris leonina* is seen in adult dogs and cats and is less well recognized as a zoonotic agent. The raccoon roundworm, *Baylisascaris procyonis*, results in rare but serious disease in humans.

Geographical Occurrence

Toxocara infections occur worldwide, with human seroprevalence rates varying widely (from 0 to more than 80%) among populations.[3] A recent CDC study estimated the seroprevalence rate in the United States at 14%.[6] In one study, more than 30% of dogs younger than 6 months sampled across the United States were shedding *T. canis* eggs, whereas rates of feline infection with *T. cati* have been reported to exceed 25%.

Groups at Risk

Although roundworms can occur in adults, disease in children is most frequently reported. A recent CDC seroprevalence study found increased risk among children and youth younger than 20 years. Children are believed to have the highest attack rates as a result of direct contact with dogs and cats and/or soil contaminated by infective eggs. Children with pica (inappropriate ingestion of soil and other substances related to nutritional deficiencies) are considered at increased risk.

Hosts, Reservoir Species, Vectors

Humans, dogs, cats, and wild carnivores can develop clinical manifestations. Humans are a terminal host, meaning that the roundworms cannot reproduce and carry on their life cycle. Rodents are paratenic hosts.[7]

Mode of Transmission and Life Cycle

In both animals and humans, infection often begins by swallowing of infective, embryonated eggs. Because the eggs take up to two weeks to embryonate, the source of eggs is usually contaminated soil or food rather than direct contact with an infected animal.[8] These eggs then hatch, the larvae penetrate the intestinal mucosa, and then migrate through the liver and bloodstream to the lungs (Figure 9-134). In humans,

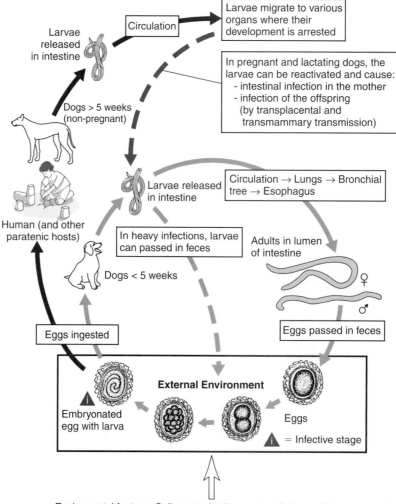

Figure 9-134 ■ Life cycle of *Toxocara canis* and *Toxocara cati*, the causal agents of toxocariasis. (Adapted from Centers for Disease Control and Prevention Public Health Image Library, Atlanta, Ga.)

they may then pass to other tissues as well, causing granulomatous lesions in the lungs and abdominal organs (visceral larva migrans) or the eye (ocular larva migrans).[3] If infective eggs are swallowed by a puppy, the larvae hatch and migrate as above; but once in the lungs, the larvae are often coughed up and swallowed to then mature into adult worms in the animal's small intestine. These adult worms then produce eggs, which are shed in the puppy's feces, and also can cause abdominal distention and obstruction.

Transplacental transmission occurs when a pregnant bitch transmits infective larvae directly to the developing fetus. Larvae that migrate to the mammary gland can also be passed to puppies during nursing.[5]

Cats are thought to be infected by eating tissue containing larvae of other infected animals, especially rodents.[7] Transplacental passage of *T. canis* is not thought to occur in cats, but transmammary transmission has been reported.[4]

Environmental Risk Factors

Because the eggs of *Toxocara* species can survive for years in soils,[7] the degree of environmental contamination of playgrounds, sandboxes, and other locations frequented by children is a significant environmental risk factor. In surveys in the United States, the United Kingdom, and Japan, 30% of playground soil samples and 75% of sampled sandboxes contained potentially infectious eggs.[3]

Disease in Humans

Toxocara infection in humans is usually asymptomatic. When disease develops, it is often chronic and mild and related to hypersensitivity response to larval invasion of tissues. The two main forms of disease are visceral larva migrans and ocular larva migrans.

Visceral larva migrans is seen particularly among preschool children. Signs and symptoms include fever, weight loss, wheezing, cough, abdominal pain, skin rashes, and hepatosplenomegaly. Laboratory findings include leukocytosis and eosinophilia.

Ocular larva migrans may develop as long as 10 years after infection with *T. canis* and is usually seen among older children who present with unilateral vision loss. Findings on examination can include a subretinal mass, leukocoria, cataracts, and retinal scarring (Color Plate 9-69).[8] When motile larvae are trapped in the eye, a diffuse unilateral subacute neuroretinitis can occur.[9]

Disease in Animals

T. canis infection in dogs usually produces more severe signs in puppies than in older dogs. In puppies infected in utero, a parasitic pneumonia may develop with a resultant high mortality rate. Development of a large parasitic load in the intestine may lead to abdominal distention, colic, anorexia, vomiting, rough hair coat, diarrhea, cachexia, coughing, and sometimes death. Neurological involvement may occur including twitching and seizures. Eosinophilia is often seen.

Cats generally have less severe disease than dogs. A potbellied appearance, diarrhea, and vomiting may develop. Eosinophilia is common.[7]

Table 9-63 compares the clinical presentations of toxocariasis in humans and other animals.

Diagnosis

In humans, clues to the diagnosis of visceral larva migrans include a history of exposure to contaminated soils or foods, the appearance of typical signs and symptoms, eosinophilia,

Table 9-63 ▪ Toxocariasis: Clinical Presentations in Humans and Other Animals

Species	Risk Factors	Incubation Period	Clinical Manifestations	Laboratory Findings
Humans: visceral larva migrans	Preschool age: ingestion of contaminated soils or food	Weeks to months (the disease is self-limited but the larvae may remain dormant in tissues for years)	Abdominal pain, fever, hepatosplenomegaly, rash, wheezing	Leukocytosis, eosinophilia, anti-*Toxocara* antibodies
Humans: ocular larva migrans	Children	Up to 10 years	Unilateral vision loss, retinal scarring/subretinal mass on examination	
Dogs (usually *Toxocara canis*)	Prenatal exposure, nursing, ingestion of contaminated soils	Weeks	Parasitic pneumonia, respiratory difficulty, death Abdominal infection: abdominal distention, vomiting, diarrhea	Eosinophilia, leukocytosis, eggs in feces
Cats (usually *T. cati*)	Ingestion of soils containing eggs, nursing or eating animal tissue containing larvae	Weeks	Abdominal distention, vomiting, diarrhea	Eosinophilia, leukocytosis, eggs in feces

and antibodies to *Toxocara*. Enzyme immunoassay with *Toxocara* excretory-secretory antigens is the preferred serological test.[8] However, it may lead to underdiagnosis if a person is infected with an unusual serovar not well covered by the standard test. Serial serology titers are required to document seroconversion; a fourfold increase in titer is considered evidence of recent infection.[10]

Ocular migrans is diagnosed clinically. Antibody titers to *Toxocara* species may be elevated in aqueous and vitreous fluid compared with serum levels, which may aid in diagnosis. The differential diagnosis includes other causes of retinal masses, including retinoblastoma.[9]

In animals, the detection of eggs in feces through a fecal flotation test is diagnostic (Figure 9-135). The spherical, pitted eggs of *T. canis* and *T. cati* can be distinguished from the smooth, ovoid eggs of *T. leonine*, which has less zoonotic potential.[5]

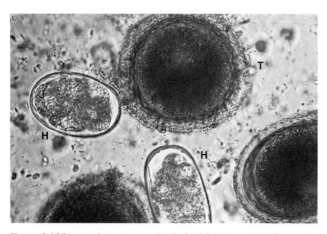

Figure 9-135 ■ Photomicrograph of a fecal flotation analysis from a dog demonstrating characteristic ova from hookworms *(H)* and *Toxocara canis (T)*. (Magnification ×400.) (From Willard MD: Disorders of the intestinal tract. In Nelson RW, Couto CG (eds): *Small animal internal medicine*, ed 4, St Louis, 2009, Mosby Elsevier. Courtesy Tom Craig, Texas A & M University.)

Treatment

Treatment in Humans

Antihelmintic treatment is directed toward relief of symptoms. Because infection is generally asymptomatic in humans, treatment is sometimes withheld. In cases of severe organ involvement, steroids may be indicated in addition to antihelmintics. Table 9-64 outlines treatment guidelines in humans and other animals.

Treatment in Animals

In dogs and cats, infection is usually treated aggressively with a number of antihelmintic agents. Because transplacental infection does not occur with *T. cati*, cats are usually treated as kittens.

Strategic deworming against roundworms (and hookworms) includes deworming the pregnant dog; treating puppies and kittens beginning at 2 weeks of age, then every 2 weeks through weaning (6 to 8 weeks); and then treating monthly until the pet is 6 months old. Nursing dogs and queens should be treated with their litters. Older animals can be monitored through at least annual fecal examinations. Many pups and kittens are not brought to the veterinarian until they are 6 to 8 weeks, so owners of pregnant animals need to work with their veterinarians to ensure earlier deworming.

References

1. Ellis Jr GS, Pakalnis VS, Worley G, et al. *Toxocara canis* infestation. Clinical and epidemiological associations with seropositivity in kindergarten children. *Ophthalmology.* 1986;93(8):1032.
2. Marmor M, Glickman L, Shofer F, et al. *Toxocara canis* infection of children: epidemiological and neuropsychologic findings. *Am J Public Health.* 1987;77(5):554.
3. Heymann DL, ed. *Control of communicable diseases manual.* 19th ed. Washington, DC: American Public Health Association; 2008.
4. Centers for Disease Control and Prevention. *CDC guidelines for veterinarians: prevention of zoonotic transmission of hookworm and ascarid infection of dogs and cats.* http://www.cdc.gov/ncidod/dpd/parasites/ascaris/prevention.pdf. Accessed February 7, 2008.

Table 9-64 ■ Toxocariasis Treatment in Humans and Other Animals		
Species	**Primary Treatment**	**Alternative**
Humans: visceral larva migrans	Albendazole 400 mg PO BID × 5 days	Mebendazole 100-200 mg PO bid × 5 days[11]
Humans: ocular migrans	First 4 weeks of symptoms: prednisone 30-60 mg PO qd, *PLUS* subtenon triamcinolone 40 mg/week × 2 weeks[11]	
Dogs: treatment in pregnancy	Fenbendazole 50 mg/kg PO q24h from day 40 of gestation to 2 weeks after birth Milbemycin oxime 0.5 mg/kg PO Pyrantel pamoate 5-10 mg/kg PO	Ivermectin 1 mg/kg PO q24 on days 20 and 42, or 0.5 mg/kg PO on days 38, 41, 44, and 47[7]
Dogs: pups at 2 weeks of age then every 2 weeks until 8 weeks, then monthly thereafter	Pyrantel pamoate 5 mg/kg PO Fenbendazole 50 mg/kg PO q24h × 3 days Milbemycin oxime 0.5 mg/kg PO	Praziquantel/pyrantel/febantel (praziquantel 5-12 mg/kg) PO once
Cats	Fenbendazole 50 mg/kg PO q24h × 3 days Pyrantel pamoate 5 mg/kg PO	Selamectin 6/mg/kg topically

5. Kahn CM, Line S, eds. *The Merck veterinary manual.* 9th ed. Whitehouse Station, NJ: Merck; 2005.
6. Won K, Kruszon-Moran D, Schantz P, et al. National seroprevalence and risk factors for zoonotic *Toxocara* spp. infection. *Am J Trop Med Hyg.* 2008;79(4):552.
7. Barr SC, Bowman DD. *The 5-minute veterinary consult clinical companion: canine and feline infectious diseases and parasitology.* Ames, IA: Blackwell; 2006.
8. Kwan-Gett TS, Kemp C, Kovarik C. *Infectious and tropical diseases: a handbook for primary care.* St Louis: Mosby Elsevier; 2005.
9. Mandell GE, Bennett JE, Dolin R, eds. *Principles and practice of infectious diseases.* 6th ed. Philadelphia: Churchill Livingstone Elsevier; 2005.
10. Acha PN, Szyfres B. *Zoonoses and communicable diseases common to man and animals: vol. 1: bacterioses and mycoses.* 3rd ed. Washington, DC: Pan American Health Organization;
11. Gilbert DN, Moellering RC, Eliopoulos GM, et al. *Sanford guide to antimicrobial therapy 2009.* 39th ed. Sperryville, VA: Antimicrobial Therapy; 2009.

TOXOPLASMOSIS

Peter M. Rabinowitz and Lisa A. Conti

Toxoplasmosis (ICD-10 B58) Congenital toxoplasmosis (P37.1)

Other names in humans: *Toxoplasma* infection

Other names in animals: *Toxoplasma* infection

Toxoplasmosis is a common zoonotic infection in nearly all mammals and some birds caused by the obligate, intracellular organism *Toxoplasma gondii.* Cats are the definitive host, shedding oocysts in their feces. Toxoplasmosis can cause severe and fatal disease in fetuses and immunocompromised patients. Ingestion of oocysts following contact with cat feces or contaminated soil is a pathway for human infection. However, a number of human infections are believed to result from eating raw or undercooked meat containing infectious cysts.[1] Toxoplasmosis is a disease that underscores the importance of communication between veterinarians and human health clinicians; studies have found that many physicians provide inappropriate advice to their pregnant patients regarding the risk of disease from cats.

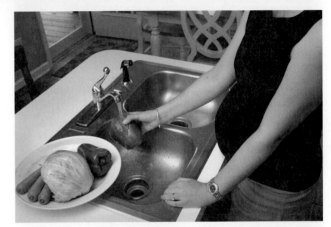

Figure 9-136 ▪ A pregnant woman in the process of washing a batch of assorted produce before the preparation of a salad. Note that the food preparation area around the sink is also kept clean and free of unclean kitchen implements either inside or outside the sink. (From Centers for Disease Control and Prevention Public Health Image Library, Atlanta, Ga. Courtesy James Gathany.)

Key Points for Clinicians and Public Health Professionals

Public Health Professionals

- Educate the public on reducing risk of infection by:
  - Proper food handling (fruits and vegetables thoroughly washed or peeled) and cooking (145° F for beef or lamb; 160° F for pork, ground meat, or wild game; 180° F for poultry).
  - Appropriate kitchen hygiene (washing items in hot soapy water after they come in contact with raw meats or unwashed fruits and vegetables) (Figure 9-136).
  - Appropriate hand hygiene: washing hands after handling raw meats, soil, or sand.
  - Pregnant women and immunocompromised persons should wear gloves when handling soil, sand, and avoid handling soil. They should avoid handling cat feces by having someone else change the cat litter or by wearing gloves to do so. They should not have to give up their cat (Figure 9-137).
  - Keeping sandboxes covered and vegetable gardens fenced.

- Educate local veterinary and human health clinicians about the signs and symptoms of the disease.
- Work with local animal control agencies to encourage control of stray cat populations.

Human Health Clinicians

- Educate patients (particularly seronegative pregnant patients and immunocompromised patients) about risk reduction (avoidance). With such measures, pregnant and immunocompromised individuals should not have to give up a cat.
- No human vaccine is available.

Veterinary Clinicians

- Counsel pet owners about the following additional preventive steps:
  - Do not feed bones, viscera, unpasteurized milk (especially goat's milk), or raw or undercooked meat to cats.
  - Wash your hands after handling cats and cat litter.
  - Dispose of cat litter on a daily basis to reduce the risk of exposure to infectious oocysts.
  - Disinfect cat litter box with boiling water on a weekly basis.
  - Keep cats indoors.

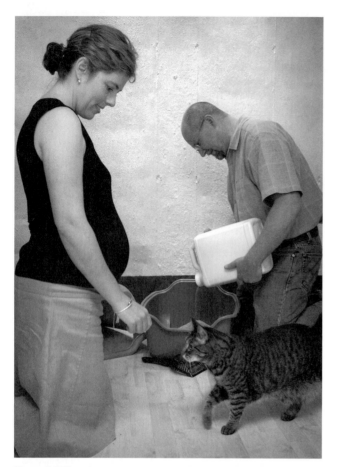

Figure 9-137 ■ A pregnant woman is about to pet her cat while her husband is in the process of changing the cat's litter so that the woman can avoid contact with possible pathogens such as *Toxoplasma gondii*, the etiologic agent responsible for the disease toxoplasmosis. (From Centers for Disease Control and Prevention Public Health Image Library, Atlanta, Ga. Courtesy James Gathany.)

- Counsel owners that healthy seropositive cats are little danger to owners. Seronegative cats that have the potential to become infected and shed oocysts are more of a human risk.
- A modified live vaccine is available in Europe and New Zealand for sheep.

Agent

Toxoplasma gondii is a protozoan that has three infectious stages: oocysts (shed in the feces, containing sporozoites), tachyzoites (rapidly multiplying form found in tissues), and bradyzoites (slowly multiplying form found in tissues; Figure 9-138).[2] In addition, tissue cysts (found in muscle or CNS tissue) contain dormant bradyzoites.

Geographical Occurrence

The disease is found worldwide. The U.S. National Health and Nutrition Examination Survey (NHANES 1999-2004) found an age-adjusted *T. gondii* seroprevalence among persons 6 to 49 years old of 10.8% (95% confidence limits [CL] 9.6%, 11.9%), and a rate among women of childbearing age (15 to 44 years) of

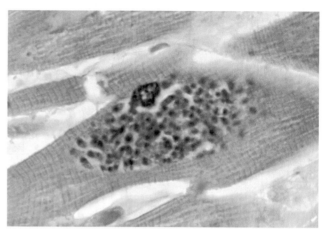

Figure 9-138 ■ Histopathology of active toxoplasmosis of myocardium. Numerous tachyzoites of *Toxoplasma gondii* are visible within a pseudocyst in a myocyte. (From Centers for Disease Control and Prevention Public Health Image Library, Atlanta, Ga. Courtesy Edwin P. Ewing, Jr.)

11.0% (95% CL 9.5%, 12.4%).[3] Higher rates have been reported in other parts of the world, including European countries where undercooked meat consumption is common, and sub-Saharan Africa where extensive contact with cats can occur.[1]

Groups at Risk

Analysis of NHANES data has suggested that individuals in occupations with soil contact, lower educational level, living in crowded conditions, and foreign-born individuals are at increased risk.[1] Other studies have reported increased risk with cat ownership, soil contact, eating unwashed vegetables, and eating undercooked or raw meat. In a number of studies, however, current ownership of a cat has not been associated with increased risk of seropositivity.[1] Fetuses and immunocompromised persons are particularly vulnerable to severe sequelae from infection.

Hosts, Reservoir Species, Vectors

Cats and other felids are the only hosts in which *T. gondii* can reproduce sexually. Infection is most commonly seen in intermediate hosts such as humans, sheep, goats, swine, dogs, and horses, although most mammals and some birds are infected. Game animals such as deer can be infected with tissue cysts, posing a risk for human consumption.

Mechanical vectors include contaminated vegetables and other food products, soil, and sand.

Mode of Transmission and Life Cycle

When naïve cats ingest viable *Toxoplasma* organisms, the parasite is able to reproduce in the cat's intestinal lining and results in the shedding of immature oocysts in the feces. After a period of 2 to 3 weeks, the cat develops immunity and no longer sheds oocysts. The immature oocysts shed in cat feces are not immediately infectious but take 1 to 5 days to sporulate into mature oocysts with viable sporozoites (Figure 9-139). These infectious oocysts can persist in the environment for

Toxoplasmosis
(Toxoplasma gondii)

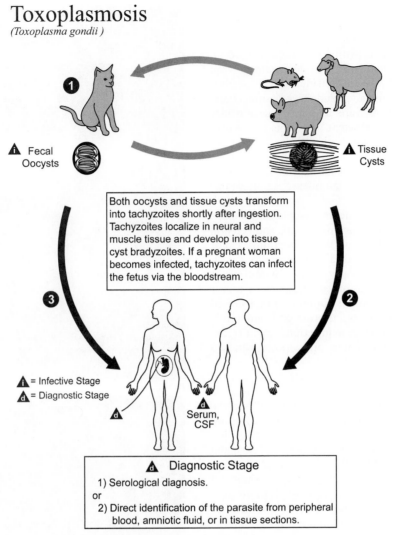

Figure 9-139 ▪ Life cycle of toxoplasmosis. (From Centers for Disease Control and Prevention Public Health Image Library, Atlanta, Ga. Courtesy Alexander J. DaSilva and Melanie Mosher.)

several months. If they are ingested by an intermediate host either directly or through contaminated soil, they begin to asexually multiply in the host's intestinal epithelium and produce tachyzoites. The tachyzoites disseminate in the intermediate host's bloodstream and lymph system both freely and intracellularly within monocytes and macrophages.[4] After several weeks of rapid multiplication, the intermediate host may develop immunity. Once the host is immune, the life cycle shifts to the production of bradyzoites, which multiply less rapidly and tend to form tissue cysts in brain, myocardial, and nervous tissue where they may persist for life.

If an intermediate host ingests raw or undercooked meat containing these cysts, the bradyzoites may be released and develop into tachyzoites. The first time cats are infected, the parasite's life cycle is completed when some of the bradyzoites initiate a sexual cycle to produce unsporulated oocysts that are shed in the feces for 1 to 2 weeks. Cats are typically resistant to reinfection.[5]

The primary routes of toxoplasmosis transmission to humans are the ingestion of raw or undercooked meat that contains viable cysts, the ingestion of infectious oocysts due to contact with cat feces or contaminated soil or fomites, and congenital infection. The relative importance of these different routes of transmission is poorly understood and probably varies by geographical region. A survey of more than 6000 commercial samples of beef, chicken, and pork from retail stores in the United States found a low incidence of infectious cysts, with viable *T. gondii* detected only in samples of pork.[6] Transplacental transmission occurs during active infection of the mother with the tachyzoite phase. The risk of transmission from an infected pregnant woman to her fetus is considered lower in early pregnancy (although the consequences to the fetus are greater) than in subsequent weeks.[7] Other transmission pathways include organ transplants and blood transfusions.

Environmental Risk Factors

A number of factors, such as humidity and temperature, determine how long it takes for immature oocysts to develop into mature infectious oocysts and how long such oocysts can persist in soil and water and on environmental surfaces.

Disease in Humans

Most cases of toxoplasmosis in immunocompetent children and adults are asymptomatic. Symptoms, when they occur, are usually self-limited and can include significant cervical or other lymphadenopathy and fever with atypical lymphocytosis. Rarer complications can include toxoplasmic chorioretinitis, myocarditis, and myositis. The incidence of ocular toxoplasmosis in immunocompetent persons is believed to be more common than previously thought, and toxoplasmosis is one of the most common causes of uveitis in the general population, leading to vision loss in some cases.[8,9] Encephalitis and even death can occur but are rare in immunocompetent hosts.[9]

In immunocompromised patients, toxoplasmosis often produces severe disease, including encephalitis and cerebral abscesses (Figure 9-140), pneumonitis, chorioretinitis (Color Plate 9-70), and myocarditis with a high mortality rate if the disease is not treated in a timely fashion. Symptoms of encephalitis can include confusion, seizures, sensorimotor deficits, and ataxia.[10] Infection in immunocompromised humans may be the result of reactivation of latent infection but can also result from acute infection. Organ transplants can be a source of infection in immunocompromised persons.[9]

One of the most significant complications of human toxoplasmosis infection occurs when a pregnant woman is in the acute phase of the illness (tachyzoite phase) and the organism passes to a fetus, resulting in congenital infection. Congenital toxoplasmosis can present as mild to severe disease, with complications including hydrops fetalis, perinatal death, prematurity, decreased birth weight, retinal scarring, and a classical triad of chorioretinitis, hydrocephalus, and cerebral calcifications (Figure 9-141). Although more than half of infected newborns are considered normal shortly after birth, most will develop ocular and/or other complications if not treated.[11]

Disease in Animals

Evidence of past infections in cats and many other animal species is common, but clinical cases are rarely recognized because most infections are subclinical (Figure 9-142). In cats, the disease is most commonly seen in congenitally infected kittens, leading to stillbirth, neonatal fever, respiratory distress, uveitis, and neurological involvement (Color Plate 9-71).[12] It is also seen in immunocompromised animals with lethargy, fever, neurological signs, or generalized retinitis (Color Plate 9-72).

Dogs, especially puppies, may develop acute signs of infection including fever, respiratory signs (Color Plate 9-73), and diarrhea. Immunosuppressed older dogs may manifest neurological involvement (Figure 9-143).

In sheep, goats, and swine, toxoplasmosis can cause abortion and neonatal mortality (Figure 9-144). Birds, including poultry, are commonly infected but generally do not manifest clinical signs. Table 9-65 compares clinical presentations of toxoplasmosis in humans and other animals.

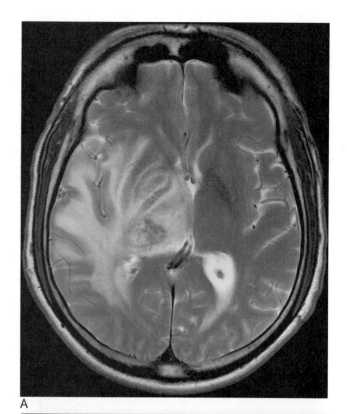

A

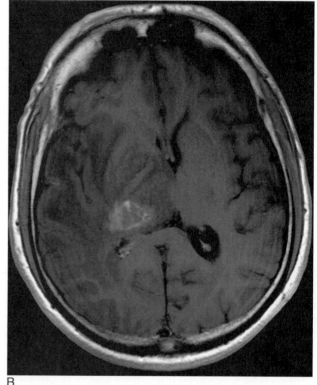

B

Figure 9-140 ■ MRI images of *Toxoplasma* abscess in the right thalamus with extensive surrounding vasogenic edema and irregular peripheral enhancement. **A**, Axial T_2-weighted and (**B**) gadolinium-enhanced T_1-weighted images. (From Adam A, Dixon AK (eds): *Grainger & Allison's diagnostic radiology*, ed 5, Edinburgh, 2008, Churchill Livingstone Elsevier.)

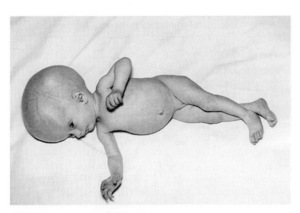

Figure 9-141 ▪ Congenital toxoplasmosis with hydrocephalus. (Courtesy Peter Rabinowitz.)

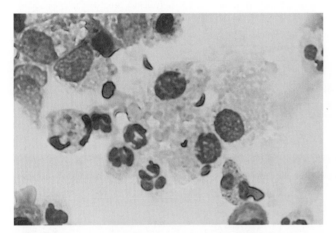

Figure 9-142 ▪ Photomicrograph of *Toxoplasma gondii* tachyzoites from the lungs of a cat with acute toxoplasmosis. The extracellular tachyzoites are crescent shaped with a centrally placed nucleus. They are approximately 6 microns in length (bronchoalveolar lavage fluid, Wright stain). (From Hawkins EC: Diagnostic tests for the lower respiratory tract. In Nelson RW, Couto CG (eds): *Small animal internal medicine*, ed 4, St Louis, 2009, Mosby Elsevier.)

Diagnosis

In humans, the cornerstone of diagnosis is serology.[13] High titer of anti-*Toxoplasma* IgM suggests an acute infection (IgM titers can persist for 18 months), whereas IgG antibodies may indicate past infection. Elevated IgM titers can be verified at a *Toxoplasma* reference laboratory such as the CDC or Toxoplasmosis Serology Lab (Palo Alto Medical Foundation Research Institute).[5] When congenital toxoplasmosis is suspected, diagnostic studies include maternal seroconversion detected via the immunosorbent agglutination assay (ISAGA), fetal ultrasound findings, and amniocentesis with PCR detection of *T. gondii*.

In animals, the serological testing for IgG, IgM, and antigen with follow-up tests in 3 weeks helps differentiate acute from chronic infection. The IgM antibodies rise 2 weeks after infection and may persist for a maximum of 3 months. A fourfold increase in IgG titers between samples is also suggestive of a recent infection.[12]

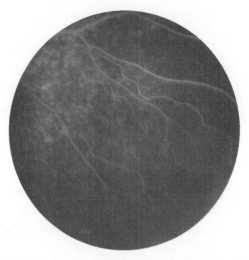

Figure 9-143 ▪ Lipemia retinalis in a Dachshund with toxoplasmosis. Lipemia retinalis makes blood vessels look pink (red blood with white lipid added). There are multifocal gray opacities indicative of active chorioretinitis. (From Dziezyc J, Millichamp NJ: *Color atlas of canine and feline ophthalmology*, St Louis, 2005, Saunders Elsevier.)

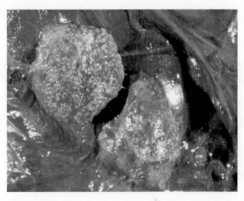

Figure 9-144 ▪ Ovine protozoal placentitis, toxoplasmosis, abortion, placenta, sheep. The cotyledons have hundreds of white foci of necrosis, a lesion that is characteristic of *Toxoplasma gondii*–induced abortion in sheep and goats. (From McGavin MD, Zachary JF: *Pathologic basis of veterinary disease*, ed 4, St Louis, 2007, Mosby Elsevier. Courtesy Ontario Veterinary College, University of Guelph.)

Treatment

Treatment in immunocompetent humans is usually not indicated because of the mild and self-limited nature of the disease. If significant organ involvement occurs or in particular clinical situations such as immunocompromise, pregnancy, and congenital infection, antimicrobial treatment is necessary (Table 9-66). In addition to antimicrobials, prednisone is added to the treatment regimens for congenital toxoplasmosis, chorioretinitis, and toxoplasma meningitis. The recommended treatment regimens are complex, and consultation with an infectious disease specialist is advisable.

Antibiotics can be used in animals but they may not clear infection.

Table 9-65 ▪ Toxoplasmosis: Comparative Clinical Presentations in Humans and Other Animals

Species	Risk Factors	Incubation Period	Clinical Manifestations	Laboratory Findings
Human beings		10-23 days		
Immunocompetent	Ingestion of raw or undercooked meat or direct exposure to oocysts from cat feces		Usually asymptomatic in immunocompetent host, or lymphadenopathy, chorioretinitis can occur	Immunohistochemical staining, PCR, serology (IFA, ELISA)
Immunocompromised	Reactivation of latent disease or new infection (see above), organ transplants		Encephalitis, pneumonitis, chorioretinitis, other	Abnormal CT, MRI, CSF findings
Congenital	Maternal infection		Fetal death, prematurity; triad of chorioretinitis, hydrocephalus, cerebral calcifications; delayed ocular disease	Maternal seroconversion detected via ISAGA; fetal ultrasound findings, amniocentesis with PCR detection of *Toxoplasma gondii*
Cats	Hunting, immunodeficiency, congenital	3-21 days	Usually subclinical Neurological involvement Fever, respiratory distress, ocular involvement	Serology (ELISA, IFA, CF), fecal flotation for active infection (oocysts are 10-12 mcm)
Dogs	Ingestion of undercooked meat, immunodeficiency, congenital	Weeks	Usually subclinical, varies with organ system involvement, including encephalitis, myositis, hepatitis, and retinitis	As with cats
Sheep, goats	Ingestion of oocysts from contaminated soil	Weeks	Abortion, neonatal death	As with cats

CF, Complement fixation; *CSF*, cerebrospinal fluid; *CT*, computed tomography, *ISAGA*, immunosorbent agglutination assay; *MRI*, magnetic resonance imaging.

Table 9-66 ▪ Toxoplasmosis Treatment in Humans[14] and Other Animals[15]

Species	Primary Treatment	Alternative
Humans: Immunocompetent		
Acute illness with lymphadenopathy	No treatment unless severe symptoms or significant organ involvement	
Active chorioretinitis, meningitis, transfusion related	Pyrimethamine 200 mg PO on day 1, then 50-75 mg q24h *PLUS* sulfadiazine 1-1.5 gm PO qid *PLUS* leukovorin (folinic acid) 5-20 mg 3×/wk, treat 1-2 week beyond resolution of signs/symptoms; continue leukovorin 1 week after stopping pyrimethamine, *PLUS* prednisone 1 mg/kg/day in 2 divided doses for acute inflammation[16]	
Acute infection in pregnancy	*<18 wk gestation:* spiramycin 1 gm PO q8h until delivery if amniotic fluid PCR negative *>18 wk gestation and documented infection:* pyramethamine 50 mg PO q12h × 2 days then 50 mg/day *PLUS* sulfadiazine 75 mg/kg PO × 1 dose then 50 mg/kg q12h (max. 4 gm/day) *PLUS* folinic acid 10-21 mg PO daily	
Congenital	Management complex; consultation with specialist advisable; pyrimethamine *PLUS* sulfadiazine *PLUS* leucovorin[16]	
Patients With AIDS		
Cerebral toxoplasmosis	Pyrimethamine 200 mg PO, then 75 mg/day PO *PLUS* sulfadiazine 1-1.5 gm PO qd *PLUS* folinic acid 10-20 mg/day PO × 4-6 weeks after signs/symptoms resolve; then suppressive treatment *or* TMP-SMX 10/50 mg/kg/day PO/IV divided q12h × 30 days	Pyrimethamine PLUS folinic acid PLUS either clindamycin, clarithromycin, azithromycin, or atovaquone[16]
Suppression after treatment of cerebral toxoplasmosis	Sulfadiazine 500-1000 mg PO 4×/day *PLUS* pyrimethamine 25-50 mg PO q24h *PLUS* folinic acid 10-25 mg PO q24h	Clindamycin PLUS pyrimethamine PLUS folinic acid *or* atovaquone[16]
Primary prophylaxis: patients with AIDS with CD4 <100 and positive IgG *Toxoplasma* antibody	TMP-SMX DS 1 tab PO q24h *or* TMP-SMX-SS 1 tab PO q24h	Dapsone PLUS pyrimethamine PLUS folinic acid *or* atovaquone[16]
Cats	Clindamycin 10-12.5 mg/kg PO/IM q12h × 2-4 wk	Trimethoprim-sulfadiazine 15 mg/kg PO/IV q12h × 2 wk
Dogs (Rare)	Clindamycin 10-12.5 mg/kg PO/IM q12h × 2-4 wk	Trimethoprim-sulfadiazine 15 mg/kg PO/IV q12h × 2 wk[13]

TMP-SMX, Trimethoprim-sulfamethoxazole.

References

1. Jones JL, Kruszon-Moran D, Wilson M, et al. *Toxoplasma gondii* infection in the United States: seroprevalence and risk factors. *Am J Epidemiol.* 2001;154(4):357.

2. Kahn CM, Line S, eds. *The Merck veterinary manual.* 9th ed. Merck; 2005.

3. Jones JL, Kruszon-Moran D, Sanders-Lewis K, et al. *Toxoplasma gondii* infection in the United States, 1999–2004, decline from the prior decade. *Am J Trop Med Hyg.* 2007;77(3):405.

4. Acha PN, Szyfres B. *Zoonoses and communicable diseases common to man and animals: vol. III: chlamydioses, parasitoses.* 3rd ed. Washington, DC: Pan American Health Organization; 2003.

5. Dvorak G, Rovid-Spickler A, Roth JA, et al. *Handbook for zoonotic diseases of companion animals.* Ames, IA: The Center for Food Security and Public Health, Iowa State University College of Veterinary Medicine; 2008.

6. Dubey JP, Hill DE, Jones JL, et al. Prevalence of viable *Toxoplasma gondii* in beef, chicken, and pork from retail meat stores in the United States: risk assessment to consumers. *J Parasitol.* 2005;91(5):1082.

7. Dunn D, Wallon M, Peyron F, et al. Mother-to-child transmission of toxoplasmosis: risk estimates for clinical counseling. *Lancet.* 1999;353(9167):1829.

8. Holland GN. Reconsidering the pathogenesis of ocular toxoplasmosis. *Am J Ophthalmol.* 1999;128(4):502.

9. Mandell GL, Bennett JE, Dolin R, eds. *Principles and practice of infectious diseases.* 6th ed. New York: Churchill Livingstone Elsevier; 2005.

10. Sax PE, Cohen CJ, Kuritzkes DR. *HIV essentials.* Royal Oak, MI: Physicians Press; 2007.

11. Kliegman RM, Behrman RE, Jenson HB, et al. *Nelson textbook of pediatrics.* 18th ed. Philadelphia: Saunders Elsevier; 2007.

12. Barr SC, Bowman DD. *The 5-minute veterinary consult clinical companion: canine and feline infectious diseases and parasitology.* Ames, IA: Blackwell; 2006.

13. Remington JS, Thulliez P, Montoya JG. Recent developments for diagnosis of toxoplasmosis. *J Clin Microbiol.* 2004;42(3):941.

14. Gilbert DN, Moellering RC, Eliopoulos GM, et al. *Sanford guide to antimicrobial therapy 2009.* 39th ed. Sperryville, VA: Antimicrobial Therapy; 2009.

15. Giguere S, Prescott JF, Baggot JD, et al. *Antimicrobial therapy in veterinary medicine.* 4th ed. Ames, IA: Blackwell; 2006.

TRANSMISSIBLE SPONGIFORM ENCEPHALOPATHIES

Peter M. Rabinowitz and Lisa A. Conti

Subacute spongiform encephalopathy, Creutzfeldt-Jakob disease (CJD) (ICD-10 A81.0)

Other names in humans: variant CJD, fatal familial insomnia (FFI), and Gerstmann-Sträussler-Scheinker disease (GSS), prion disease, TSE, kuru

Other names in animals: bovine spongiform encephalopathy (BSE), mad cow disease, feline spongiform encephalopathy (FSE), chronic wasting disease of elk and deer (CWD), transmissible mink encephalopathy (TME), exotic ungulate encephalopathy, scrapie

In 1986, an outbreak of bovine spongiform encephalopathy (BSE) occurred in the United Kingdom that was eventually linked to the use of livestock feed containing meat and bone from animals infected with a prion disease (*prion* is short for *proteinaceous infectious particle*). Shortly afterward, outbreaks of transmissible spongiform encephalopathies (TSEs) were reported in zoo animals and domestic cats that had consumed BSE-contaminated meat products. In retrospect, this unusual occurrence of prion diseases in animals was a sentinel event for human health risk. In 1996, the emergence in humans of a variant form of Creutzfeldt-Jakob disease (vCJD), a progressive dementia, was attributed to consumption of contaminated beef from BSE-infected cattle. As a result of the implementation of a number of feed bans, such as a prohibition against feeding mammalian protein to any farmed animals in the United Kingdom, the incidence of reported cases of both BSE and vCJD has dropped dramatically in recent years. Outbreaks in cats and other animals also declined related to similar feed bans.

Despite the success in controlling BSE and vCJD, prion diseases continue to be a public health concern. Sporadic Creutzfeldt-Jakob disease (CJD), which has no known link to animal prion diseases, occurs worldwide at a case rate of approximately 1 case per 1 million persons.[1] Other variations of human prion disease are reported worldwide at lower rates (see "Disease in Humans" section on the following page). Chronic wasting disease (CWD), a prion disease of wildlife such as deer and elk, is extending its range in the United States and Canada. Scrapie, a prion disease of sheep, continues to affect sheep and goat populations in some parts of the world. The origin, transmissibility, and ability for cross-species infection of these diseases remain poorly understood. Therefore ongoing vigilance for the emergence of TSE-related disease in humans and other animals by human and veterinary clinicians and public health authorities is warranted.

Key Points for Clinicians and Public Health Professionals

Public Health Professionals

- Encourage reporting of human prion disease to public health authorities. CJD is reportable in some states. If it is not reportable in your region, consider adding it to the list of reportable diseases.
- Ensure safety of the blood supply (leukodepletion, screening of donors to exclude those who have resided in high-risk areas).[2]
- Ensure that steps are being taken to reduce the possibility of transmission of prion diseases through organ transplant and infected surgical instruments; see guidelines at http://www.who.int/csr/resources/publications/bse/WHO_CDS_CSR_APH_2000_3/en/.
- In areas where CWD has been reported, educate hunters about measures to reduce the risk of exposure to the CWD agent, including not harvesting deer or elk that appear sick or abnormal; wearing puncture-resistant rubber, vinyl, or latex gloves while dressing carcasses; avoiding contact with brain, spinal cord, and lymphoid tissues; deboning meat; disinfecting knives, saws, and tables with 50% bleach; and having animals tested for CWD.[3]
- Investigate clusters of human cases of neurodegenerative disease.

Human Health Clinicians

- Report suspected cases of iatrogenic CJD, vCJD, or human CWD cases to local and state health departments.
- Conduct an autopsy on suspected human cases and submit tissues for diagnosis to the National Prion Disease Pathology Surveillance Center; see http://www.cjdsurveillance.com/.
- Remove or institute enhanced sterilization procedures on contaminated surgical or dental instruments from practice.[4,5]

Veterinary Clinicians

- Consider the diagnosis of a TSE in cattle, sheep, cats, and other animals with abnormal behavior and progressive neurological deterioration consistent with prion disease.
- Counsel owners and farmers about federal feed restrictions and proper feeding practices to reduce risk of disease transmission.

Agent

TSEs are believed to be caused by abnormal forms (PrP^{sc}) of naturally occurring (PrP^C) cellular prion proteins.[6] These misshapen prion proteins are capable of self-replication and transmissibility and form protease-resistant deposits in the brains of infected animals. For many years, TSEs were referred to as *slow virus infections* because of their transmissibility, resistance to filtration, and long latent periods. Most pathologic features of prion diseases involve the CNS. TSE agents, such as the agent of scrapie, are remarkably resistant to disinfection and inactivation by heat, radiation, or chemicals,[7] although more robust disinfection strategies are effective.[8] Strains differ between abnormal prions infecting different species, possibly related to variations in the three-dimensional protein structure or length and sequence of the amino acid chain. The BSE agent has been transmitted experimentally, using a variety of techniques and doses, to other species, including cats, mice, pigs, sheep, goats, cattle, mink, macaque monkeys, and marmosets.[9]

Geographical Occurrence

vCJD has been reported mostly in the United Kingdom, with smaller numbers of cases reported elsewhere in Europe and in Japan. Three cases reported in the United States and one case reported in Canada are believed to be the result of exposure to the BSE agent overseas. In addition to the United Kingdom, BSE has been reported in smaller numbers in most other European countries and in Japan, Israel, Canada, and the United States.

Cases of feline spongiform encephalopathy (FSE) were reported in captive felids in zoos in the United Kingdom and domestic cats in the United Kingdom and Europe. Cases have declined greatly since a ban on bovine spleen and CNS tissue in cat foods.[2]

CWD of deer and elk occurs primarily in an endemic area of Colorado and Wyoming. In recent years, CWD has been detected in neighboring states, as well as in Wisconsin, Illinois, West Virginia, New York, and in the provinces of Alberta and Saskatchewan in Canada.

The prevalence of scrapie among sheep in the United States has been estimated at approximately 0.2%, based on voluntary surveillance.[10] Scrapie is considered eradicated from Australia and New Zealand.

Transmissible mink encephalopathy (TME), first described in 1947, has occurred sporadically in the United States, Canada, Finland, Germany, and Russia.

Groups at Risk

Groups at increased risk for vCJD include those who resided in the United Kingdom during the BSE epidemic and consumed beef products. Hunters are at risk of exposure to CWD in deer and elk through dressing carcasses and meat consumption. Similarly, persons working with sheep and goat carcasses may have some exposure to the scrapie agent, and mink farmers may have exposure to TME. To date, no cases of TSEs related to CWD, FSE, or TME exposure have been described in humans.[11]

Hosts, Reservoir Species, Vectors

BSE is a disease of cattle, but concurrent with the BSE outbreak in the United Kingdom, a similar disease tied to BSE-contaminated feed consumption appeared in other bovids kept in zoos, including kudu, eland, oryx, gemsbok, bison, nyala, and Ankole (exotic ungulate encephalopathy).

FSE has been found in fewer than 100 domestic cats and captive felids, including cheetahs, pumas, ocelots, and a tiger.[9]

CWD occurs in captive and free-ranging Cervidae, including mule deer, white-tailed deer, and elk, and has been detected in a moose.

Scrapie occurs in sheep and goats.

Mode of Transmission and Life Cycle

Transmission of BSE, vCJD, FSE, and TME is believed to be due to ingestion of contaminated animal products (Figure 9-145). Scrapie can be transmitted horizontally in flocks. In addition, maternal transmission appears to play a role in scrapie infection.[12] Person-to-person transmission of vCJD has been reported through contaminated blood products, possibly due to the persistence of the agent in lymphocytes. CWD transmission appears related to both direct contact between animals and indirect contact with contaminated environments.

Environmental Risk Factors

Transmission of iatrogenic CJD involves contaminated articles such as surgical instruments. For other TSEs, the role of environmental contamination is less clear. CWD is spread horizontally between deer and elk, and such transmission is believed to be due in part to environmental contamination, leading to ingestion of the agent.[3] Research is focusing on the role of saliva in the environmental spread of disease. Scrapie may also be transmitted through pastures contaminated with birth products from an infected animal.[3]

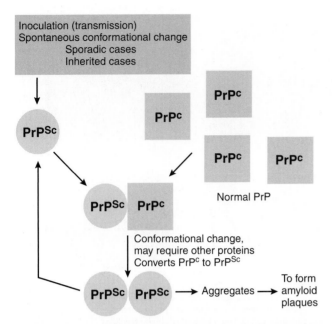

Figure 9-145 ▪ Prion protein. In prion diseases (spongiform encephalopathies), PrP *(PrPᶜ)*, a normal neuronal protein, is converted to an abnormal β-pleated sheet isoform *(PrPˢᶜ)* through the interaction of PrPˢᶜ with PrPᶜ. (From McGavin MD, Zachary JF: *Pathologic basis of veterinary disease*, ed 4, St Louis, 2007, Mosby Elsevier.)

Disease in Humans

At least four different prion-related diseases have been reported in humans, all chronic and invariably fatal neurodegenerative conditions. These include CJD, Gerstmann-Sträussler-Sheinker syndrome (GSS), fatal familial insomnia (FFI), and kuru. Of these, CJD is the most common.[2] GSS and FFI are genetically mediated diseases, whereas kuru transmission has been linked to cannibalism among islanders in the South Pacific.

CJD has three main variants: sporadic CJD (sCJD), iatrogenic CJD, and variant CJD (vCJD). vCJD is associated with BSE. Recently a new type of CJD has been described, known as *proteinase-sensitive prionopathy* (PSPr).[13]

Iatrogenic CJD is a rare form of CJD that has been linked to corneal transplants, growth hormone derived from pituitary extracts, dura matter grafts, and contaminated neurosurgical instruments.[7]

sCJD is characterized by a rapidly progressive dementia with confusion and often associated movement disorders such as ataxia and myoclonus. It is typically a disease of older individuals (median age, 68 years). In sCJD the electroencephalogram (EEG) may show periodic high-voltage complexes. Samples of CSF are acellular with normal glucose but may show elevation of protein including a protein known as 14-3-3.[14]

vCJD differs from sCJD in a number of ways, including the younger age of patients (median age, 28 years), the prominent symptoms of paresthesias, the lack of specific EEG findings, specific MRI findings of an increased signal in the posterior thalamus, and the ready detection of the agent in lymphoid tissue. Patients with vCJD also have a prolonged clinical course compared with patients with sCJD (median illness duration of 13 to 14 months vs. 4 to 5 months for sCJD).[7]

Disease in Animals

BSE initially presents with subtle locomotive and behavioral abnormalities that progress over a period of months. Cattle spend decreased time ruminating and demonstrate increased nose licking, sneezing, nose wrinkling, head tossing, and teeth grinding. An increased startle response can develop, but undisturbed animals may develop paresis, ataxia, and falling episodes. Weight loss and decreased lactation can occur. Recumbency (downer cow), coma, and death occur weeks to months later (Figure 9-146).

An atypical form of BSE has been reported to be due to a variant prion causing a disease termed *bovine amyloidal spongiform encephalopathy* (BASE). The molecular form of this new bovine PrPsc resembles that found in a particular form of human sporadic CJD.[6]

CWD of elk and deer produces subtle changes in behavior and weight loss (Figure 9-147). A spectrum of symptoms including loss of fear of humans, somnolence, and hyperexcitability may occur. Late disease manifests with increased water consumption, increased salivation, low head carriage, a fixed stare, and chronic weight loss despite continued feed intake.[3]

FSE produces an increase in aggressive or shy behavior, ataxia, and increased sensitivity to sound or touch. On biopsy of cases, spongiform degeneration of the neuropil of the brain and spinal cord have been described (Color Plate 9-74).[9] Death occurs within 6 to 8 weeks of onset of signs.

Scrapie also has an insidious onset, with behavioral changes including increased excitability. Tremors of the head and neck (tremblante du mouton) may occur, as can seizures. Intense pruritus develops, leading to loss of fleece over body areas (Figure 9-148).

TME produces abnormal behavior, including increased excitability, tremors, circling, and biting. The disease progresses to death within weeks or months. Table 9-67 compares clinical presentations of TSEs in humans and other animals.

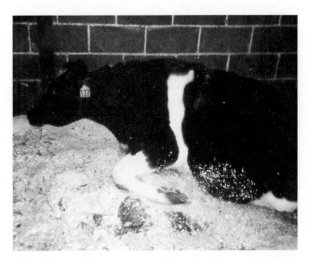

Figure 9-146 ▪ Cattle, such as the one pictured here, affected by BSE experience progressive degeneration of the nervous system. (From Centers for Disease Control and Prevention Public Health Image Library, Atlanta, Ga. Courtesy U.S. Department of Agriculture Animal and Plant Health Inspection Service, Washington, DC.)

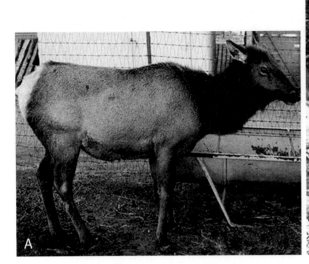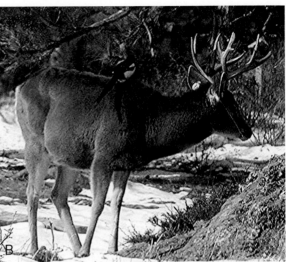

Figure 9-147 ■ Clinical chronic wasting disease (CWD) in captive female wapiti (**A**) and free-ranging male mule deer (**B**). The female wapiti had been showing subtle signs of CWD, primarily changes in response to handling and interaction with herd mates, for more than 6 months before the photo was taken. The wapiti was euthanized about 3 months later after signs progressed, although still not to classic end-stage CWD. The male mule deer showed signs that included cachexia, piloerection, diminished alertness, and vacant facial expression (all evident in photo), and mild ataxia also was appreciable when the deer moved. (From Fowler ME: *Zoo and wild animal medicine: current therapy*, ed 6, St Louis, 2008, Saunders Elsevier. *A*, Courtesy M.W. Miller; *B*, courtesy S.W. Miller.)

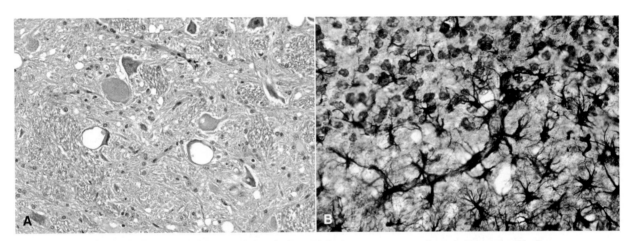

Figure 9-148 ■ Spongiform encephalopathy (scrapie), brain, motor neurons, sheep. **A**, Neuronal cell bodies contain one or more discrete and/or coalescing clear vacuoles. There are no inflammatory cells in this disease. Similar spongiosis is evident in the neuropil (hematoxylin-eosin stain). **B**, Scrapie, experimental, brain, cerebellum, mouse. The cerebellar granule cells are at the top of the figure. There is notable hypertrophy and proliferation (astrocytosis) of astrocytes and their fibers (astrogliosis) (black branching fibers). Some of the processes (running diagonally across the illustration) end, as is normal for astrocytes on the walls of capillaries. Cajal's gold sublimate stain was used for astrocytes. (From McGavin MD, Zachary JF: *Pathologic basis of veterinary disease*, ed 4, St Louis, 2007, Mosby Elsevier. *A*, Courtesy D. Gould, College of Veterinary Medicine and Biomedical Sciences, Colorado State University, and M. McAllister, College of Veterinary Medicine, University of Illinois. *B*, courtesy W.J. Hadlow.)

Diagnosis

The differential diagnosis of CJD in humans includes other causes of dementia, such as Alzheimer's disease, Lewy body dementia, normal-pressure hydrocephalus, neurosyphilis, hypothyroidism, HIV-associated dementia, and senile dementia. The diagnosis of vCJD should be suspected in any person who has resided in a BSE area who presents with behavioral abnormalities and sensory complaints accompanied by signs of dementia. Suspected cases should be referred to a qualified neurologist for definitive diagnosis.[15] MRI findings of ribbons of cortical hyperintensity or basal ganglia or thalamic hyperintensity can help suggest the diagnosis.[17]

The disease can be diagnosed by brain biopsy showing spongiform changes and the presence of the prion protein PRP^{sc} (Figure 9-149). Other tests include tonsillar biopsy for PRP^{sc} as well as CSF testing for the stress protein 14-3-3, which is elevated in some patients with CJD, although it occurs in other conditions as well.[18]

Table 9-67 ▪ Transmissible Spongiform Encephalopathies: Comparative Clinical Presentations in Humans and Other Animals				
Species/Disease	**Risk Factors**	**Incubation Period**	**Clinical Manifestations**	**Laboratory Findings**
Humans: vCJD	Linked to bovine spongiform encephalopathy	Unknown	Younger age than sCJD; confusion, progressive dementia, paresthesias, ataxia Illness duration 13-14 months	MRI increased signal in posterior thalamus Abnormal EEG Elevated CSF 14-3-3 protein Tonsil biopsy may show PrPSc[6]
Humans: sCJD	Idiopathic	Unknown	Older individuals; confusion, progressive dementia, ataxia, myoclonus Illness duration approximately 6 months[15]	EEG may show periodic high-voltage complexes
Cattle: BSE *Other bovids:* exotic ungulate encephalopathy	Linked to consumption of contaminated feed	Months to years	Abnormal behavior, abnormal movements, staring, exaggerated startle reflex, falling	ELISA or Western blot analysis on brain tissue, with confirmation by immunohistochemistry
Cats: FSE	Linked to consumption of BSE-infected foods	Weeks to months	Abnormal behavior, increased sensitivity to touch	Spongiform degeneration of neuropil on biopsy
Mink: transmissible mink encephalopathy	Thought to result from consumption of foods infected with scrapie or other TSE agent	7-12 months	Increased aggression, biting, circling	Neuropil vacuolation on brain biopsy[9]
Deer, elk: chronic wasting disease	Origin unknown, possibly scrapie	1.5-3 years	Behavior changes, weight loss, staring, low head carriage	Immunochemistry, ELISA, Western blot of brain tissue and/or lymph nodes
Sheep, goats: scrapie	Susceptible genotypes[16]	2-3 years	Excitability, tremors, pruritus with loss of fleece	ELISA or Western blot analysis of brain tissue postmortem or by biopsy of lymphoid tissue

EEG, Electroencephalogram; *MRI,* magnetic resonance imaging.

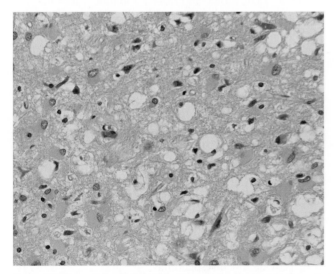

Figure 9-149 ▪ Magnified (×100) and stained with hematoxylin-eosin staining technique, this light photomicrograph of brain tissue reveals the presence of prominent spongiotic changes in the cortex and loss of neurons in a case of variant Creutzfeldt-Jakob disease. (From Centers for Disease Control and Prevention Public Health Image Library, Atlanta, Ga. Courtesy Teresa Hammett.)

In cattle, BSE is often diagnosed by ELISA or Western blot analysis on brain tissue with confirmation by immunohistochemistry.

CWD can be diagnosed by immunohistochemistry, Western blot, or ELISA on brain and/or lymph nodes.

Scrapie diagnosis is usually by ELISA or Western blot analysis of brain tissue postmortem, or by biopsy of lymphoid tissue (retropharyngeal, third eyelid, or rectal mucosa).

Treatment

At present, CJD and other prion diseases in humans are fatal neurological diseases without proven effective therapies. There is ongoing research for development of vaccines and for potential compounds with anti-prion activity.[14,19,20,21]. Current treatment of affected humans is limited to alleviating symptoms and patient comfort. Affected animals should be euthanized and removed from the food supply.

References

1. Brown P, McShane LM, Zanusso G, et al. On the question of sporadic or atypical bovine spongiform encephalopathy and Creutzfeldt-Jakob disease. *Emerg Infect Dis.* 2006;12(12):1816.
2. Heymann DL, ed. *Control of communicable diseases manual.* 19th ed.Washington, DC: American Public Health Association; 2008.
3. Kahn CM, Line S, eds. *The Merck veterinary manual.* 9th ed. Whitehouse Station, NJ: Merck; 2005.
4. Lumley JS. CJD Incidents Panel, Engineering and Scientific Advisory Committee et al: The impact of Cruetzfeldt-Jacob disease on surgical practice. *Ann R Coll Surg Engl.* 2008;90(2):91.
5. Palacios-Sánchez B, Esparza-Gómez GC, Campo-Trapero J, et al. Implications of prion disease for dentistry: an update. *Oral Surg Oral Med Oral Pathol Oral Radiol Endod.* 2008;105(3):316.
6. Casalone C, Zanusso G, Acutis P, et al. Identification of a second bovine amyloidotic spongiform encephalopathy: molecular similarities with sporadic Creutzfeldt-Jakob disease. *Proc Natl Acad Sci U S A.* 2004;101:3065.
7. Belay ED, Schonberger LB. The public health impact of prion diseases. *Ann Rev Public Health.* 2005;26:191.
8. Fichet G, Comoy E, Duval C, et al. Novel methods for disinfection of prion-contaminated medical devices. *Lancet.* 2004;364(9433):521.
9. Sigurdson CJ, Miller MW. Other animal prion diseases. *Br Med Bull.* 2003;66:199.
10. Lynn T, Grannis J, Williams M, et al. An evaluation of scrapie surveillance in the United States. *Prev Vet Med.* 2007;81(1–3):70.
11. Mawhinney S, Pape WJ, Forster JE, et al. Human prion disease and relative risk associated with chronic wasting disease. *Emerg Infect Dis.* 2006;12(10):1527.
12. Konold T, Moore SJ, Bellworthy SJ, et al. Evidence of scrapie transmission via milk. *BMC Vet Res.* 2008;8(4):14.
13. Will R, Head M. A new prionopathy. *Ann Neurol.* 2008;63(6):677.
14. Mandell GL, Bennett JE, Dolin R, eds. *Principles and practice of infectious diseases.* 6th ed. Philadelphia: Churchill Livingstone Elsevier; 2005.
15. Beisel CE, Morens DM. Variant Creutzfeldt-Jakob disease and the acquired and transmissible spongiform encephalopathies. *Clin Infect Dis.* 2004;38(5):697.
16. Baylis M, Chihota C, Stevenson E, et al. Risk of scrapie in British sheep of different prion protein genotype. *J Gen Virol.* 2004;85(Pt 9):2735.
17. Wada R, Kucharczyk W. Prion infections of the brain. *Neuroimaging Clin N Am.* 2008;18(1):183.
18. Fauci AS, Braunwald E, Kasper DL, et al. *Harrison's principles of internal medicine.* 17th ed. New York: McGraw-Hill; 2008.
19. Müller-Schiffmann A, Korth C. Vaccine approaches to prevent and treat prion infections: progress and challenges. *BioDrugs.* 2008;22(1):45.
20. Stewart LA, Rydzewaska LH, Koegh GF, et al. Systematic review of therapeutic interventions in human prion disease. *Neurology.* 2008;70(15):1272.
21. Trevitt CR, Collinge J. A systematic review of prion therapeutics in experimental models. *Brain.* 2006;129(9):2241.

TUBERCULOSIS AND OTHER MYCOBACTERIAL INFECTIONS

Elena Hollender and Peter M. Rabinowitz

Tuberculosis (ICD-10 A15-A19), Non-tuberculous mycobacterial disease (ICD-10 A31)

Other names in humans: TB; atypical mycobacterial infection, MAI, MAC, *Mycobacterium marinum*, leprosy

Other names in animals: TB; mycobacteriosis, avian tuberculosis

Tuberculosis (TB), an infectious, granulomatous disease, is one of the oldest recognized diseases in humans and animals and exemplifies the close parallels between human and animal health. *Mycobacterium tuberculosis* complex (MTBC), which includes *M. tuberculosis* and *M. bovis,* has been found in Egyptian and New World mummies[1,2] and recovered from spinal and bone lesions of Iron Age human remains in Britain and South Siberia.[3,4] In animals, there is documentation of TB in buffalo in China more than 500,000 years ago.[5] TB is believed to have been a key factor in the extinction of mammoths and mastodons around 10,000 years ago.[5]

Approximately one third of the world's human population, or about 2 billion people, are infected with TB; active cases of TB in 2006 were reported to exceed 9 million.[6] Coinfection with HIV disease accounts for more than 15 million cases of TB infection, and TB is an important cause of HIV-related deaths throughout the world. TB has now become the leading cause of death from any infectious disease worldwide, with mortality from tuberculosis in 2006 of 1.7 million.[6]

TB in livestock and wildlife is a worldwide problem and has serious socioeconomic ramifications, especially in developing nations. In the United States, recent surveillance has shown a resurgence of TB in animals among diverse species such as white-tailed deer,[7] bobcats, coyotes, opossums, raccoons, and red foxes.[8,9]

Although the public health linkage between TB in humans and other animals has been recognized for more than a century, the key issue was believed to be human infection with bovine TB through the ingestion of unpasteurized dairy products. However, recent advances in molecular diagnosis have shed light on additional human-animal TB issues including occupational and reverse zoonotic infection. This section discusses TB in humans and other animals. Infection with non-tuberculous mycobacteria (NTM) is covered in an accompanying summary.

Key Points for Clinicians and Public Health Professionals

Public Health Professionals

The control of TB in both humans and other animals relies on similar basic practices and principles:

- Identify, test, and treat/manage high-risk populations.
- Physically isolate or separate cases from other people or animals.
- Ensure appropriate medical treatment and management of the case and/or livestock and herd management.
- Provide case investigation.
  - Identify probable routes of transmission, mainly respiratory and gastrointestinal.
  - Identify close contacts of cases to prevent or control secondary cases, including companion animals

and those at high risk of infection; evaluate close contacts for active TB, perform tuberculin skin testing of contacts, treat close contacts if indicated, and work with agriculture officials to cull livestock if indicated.

o Address issues of ongoing transmission; identify potential human or animal sources of infection, shared common sources (human or animal congregate living facilities, congregate areas of potential exposure, such as waiting rooms, holding pens), and infected food or water supply (unpasteurized dairy products, especially from endemic countries).

- Encourage communication and consultation between human and veterinary public health programs and awareness of the national and local incidence and prevalence of TB in human, domestic animal, and wildlife populations.
- Encourage coordination and consultation between veterinary and human public health programs for contact investigation and recommendations for companion or household animals of active human TB cases and human contacts of veterinary TB.
- In endemic areas, encourage coordination between local agricultural and wildlife agencies regarding testing and control in domestic livestock and wildlife.
- Educate the public regarding possible means of transmission of zoonotic TB, such as consumption of unpasteurized milk and dairy products, especially from, or in, countries with endemic TB.
- Educate hunters of wildlife such as bison, deer, elk and other Cervidae and feral swine in areas of endemic zoonotic TB regarding the infection control precautions, such as gloves and protective clothing to be used when dressing and handling meat and disposing of carcasses.
- Educate medical and veterinary health clinicians regarding TB and zoonotic TB, occupational risks factors such as zookeepers and exotic animal handlers, the possibility of interspecies transmission. See veterinary guidelines at http://www.aphis.usda.gov/animal_health/animal_diseases/tuberculosis/ and at http://www.oie.int/eng/normes/mmanual/2008/pdf/2.04.07_BOVINE_TB.pdf.

Human Health Clinicians

- Immediately report cases to public health authorities: state and local public health TB programs (for a case definition, see http://www.cdc.gov/ncphi/disss/nndss/casedef/tuberculosis_current.htm; a list of state TB control offices can be found at http://www.cdc.gov/tb/pubs/tboffices.htm).
- Ensure that workers in high-risk occupations are using appropriate biosafety procedures.
- If treating a patient with active TB, determine whether pets are in the household and could have been exposed. If so, recommend veterinary evaluation.
- Inquire about occupational risk factors for zoonotic TB and ensure that workers at risk (such as zookeepers) are monitored with baseline and yearly tuberculin skin tests.

Veterinary Clinicians

- Isolate and screen herd replacements.
- Quarantine infected herds, test and slaughter to eradicate infection, and disinfect facilities where infected animals have been housed.
- Report animals with positive test results to agriculture officials and notify public health authorities.
- Ensure proper biosafety procedures are followed in the veterinary facility and that staff are aware of signs of infection in humans and other animals.
- Consider TB in animals living in a household of a human case of TB or with other close contact with a human case (if this human information is presented).
- Pulmonary or disseminated TB in a companion animal should suggest the presence of, or close contact with, active human TB. Communication with local public health officials may alert them to the possibility of an undiagnosed active TB case or provide valuable epidemiological data regarding an already known case. If applicable, contact investigation may be considered for both humans and/or other animals.
- When draining cutaneous lesions or performing a necropsy on an animal with suspected TB, use protective equipment including N-95 respirator, gloves, and eye protection.
- Disinfect surfaces with 1% sodium hypochlorite, 70% ethanol, or iodine solutions.

AGENT

Mycobacteria are nonmotile, rod-shaped, obligate aerobic bacteria classified as acid-fast because of the impermeability of their thick, waxy coats to certain dyes and stains. There are more than 120 species of mycobacteria, which are generally divided into rapidly growing (visible on culture within 7 days) and slow growing (those requiring longer periods of growth). Most mycobacteria are not considered pathogenic. The species of greatest pathogenicity to humans and other animals are those classified as *Mycobacterium tuberculosis* complex (MTBC), the etiologic agents of TB. Of all the mycobacteria, only MTBC and *M. leprae* (the agent of leprosy) are obligate intracellular organisms; the others live freely in the environment.

Because of the importance of MTBC as a pathogen to humans and other animals, other mycobacteria are generally referred to as *nontuberculous mycobacteria* (NTM) or *mycobacteria other than tuberculosis* (MOTT). However, as they are found throughout the environment, they may also be referred to as *environmental mycobacteria* (EM). These NTM are discussed below in a separate section.

Mycobacterium Tuberculosis Complex

MTBC is a highly successful clonal group pathogen of both humans and other animals that includes the species *M. tuberculosis*, *M. africanum*, *M. bovis*, *M. canettii*, *M. caprae*, *M. microti*, and *M. pinnipedii* (Table 9-68). In the past, human TB was thought to be caused solely by *M. tuberculosis*, except for zoonotic cases of *M. bovis* acquired through contact with

Table 9-68 ▪ MTBC and Common Hosts

Species	Common Hosts
M. africanum	Humans and cattle (Africa)
M. bovis	Widest host spectrum; humans, mammalian vertebrates
M. canettii	Humans (immunocompromised)
M. caprae	Goats, cattle, wild boar, pigs, humans
M. microti	Rodents, humans (immunocompromised)
M. pinnipedii	Seals
M. tuberculosis	Humans, vertebrates (e.g., cattle, primates, elephants)

unpasteurized dairy products. Similarly, TB in cattle (bovine TB) was believed to be caused only by *M. bovis*. However, recent breakthroughs in molecular analysis and mapping of the genomic sequence of *M. tuberculosis* have led to a new understanding of the pathogenesis, host range, evolution, and phenotypic differences within the MTBC, including the discovery of interspecies disease by most members of the MTBC, that challenge previous assumptions.

TB was traditionally thought to be a zoonotic disease transferred to humans during the neolithic ages through contact between humans and animals domesticated for livestock. It was therefore believed that *M. tuberculosis* had evolved from *M. bovis*. There is now evidence that all members of the MTBC evolved from a TB progenitor, *M. prototuberculosis*, estimated to be as old as 3 million years (Color Plate 9-75). In addition, researchers have shown that tubercle bacilli are able to exchange parts of their genome with other strains, a process that is crucial to the adaptation of pathogens to different host species.[10,11]

Geographical Occurrence

Mycobacteria of the MTBC group are found worldwide. Zoonotic TB due to foodborne and occupational exposures occurs more commonly in developing countries.

Groups at Risk

Certain occupational groups are at an increased risk of exposure to TB, including health care workers, exposure livestock workers, workers in zoos and animal parks, and animal care workers in primate facilities (see Chapter 12). For example, there has been zoonotic transmission of *M. bovis* from a diseased white rhinoceros to seven zookeepers.[12]

Along with zoo workers, zoo animals appear to be at an increased risk of potential infection. A multispecies epizootic transmission of *M. tuberculosis* occurred in a metropolitan zoo among Asian elephants, Rocky Mountain goats, a black rhinoceros, and humans.[13] There has also been documented transmission in an exotic animal farm among four elephants with *M. tuberculosis* and 11 of 22 handlers, one of whom subsequently had active disease. The isolates for all active cases were identical.[14]

Hosts, Reservoir Species, Vectors

As Table 9-68 shows, different members of the MTBC group are adapted to different host species, although interspecies transmission can occur. TB in wildlife has become a major problem in many parts of the world, and transmission of disease is increasingly bidirectional at the livestock-wildlife interface in industrialized and developing countries. Wildlife reservoirs such as badgers, opossums, ferrets, deer and other cervids, feral pigs, African buffalo, and bison serve as sylvatic reservoirs and ongoing sources of infection to pastured animals primarily through contamination of water and food sources within their shared environment. The presence of multiple maintenance hosts favors the long-term persistence of infection and disease among differing populations.[15,16]

Conversely, infection in wildlife species such as kudu, baboons, lions, and hyenas may represent a sporadic spillover from a livestock reservoir. Therefore TB in livestock and pastured animals will no longer be able to be eradicated or controlled by traditional livestock control programs that do not take into account the wildlife disease reservoirs. In addition to the risks of transmission between wildlife and livestock, wildlife TB can pose a zoonotic threat to game hunters who butcher carcasses (respiratory and cutaneous exposure) and who consume undercooked meat.[17,18] In addition, TB in peridomestic wildlife such as nonhuman primate populations in Asia may pose a risk of direct zoonotic transmission to humans via close contact.

Mode of Transmission and Life Cycle

Infection with TB begins when the organism is introduced into the body, usually by inhaled droplet nuclei containing tubercle bacilli, which when <5 microns reach the pulmonary alveoli (Figure 9-151). The bacilli are then phagocytized by the pulmonary alveolar macrophages and destroyed or contained. The alveolar macrophages are an important part in the initiation of the host's immune response to the mycobacteria. Antigen of the tubercle bacilli then stimulates the host's cellular immune response and the immune cascade is triggered. Immunologic control or containment of the infection is achieved through a potent cell-mediated immune response beginning with helper T-lymphocytes and, later, a delayed hypersensitivity response. This immune response also involves the production of proinflammatory cytokines, especially interferon-gamma (IFN-γ), tumor necrosis factor (TNF), and interleukin-1.

The spread of the infection may be halted by the immune system at the local lymph node level. However, because cellular immune response usually takes between 4 and 12 weeks to be elicited, it may not, or only partially, be stopped there. The MTBC bacillus may then spread systemically via the regional lymph nodes and lymphatic system and enter the bloodstream (primary disease). Hematogenous circulation of the tubercle bacilli is generalized but may affect mainly organs and tissues that are more densely vascularized, such as bone, liver, spleen, central nervous system, kidneys, and genital tract, where the bacilli are then targeted by local mononuclear phagocytes. These organs, along with lymph nodes, are therefore the most common sites of extrapulmonary disease. Studies of tissue from infected asymptomatic individuals have shown viable

M. tuberculosis in primary lesions in the lung and in lesion-free areas of lung and lymph nodes. Although primary lesions can occur anywhere in the lung, postprimary disease most commonly develops in the apical regions.[19] The immune system continues to attempt to isolate the bacillus, forming granulomas or *tubercles* (Color Plate 9-76) The granuloma may become thick walled and dense, effectively encapsulating the organism and preventing further spread. The bacilli then become latent within the granulomas. These granulomas may eventually calcify.

The major route of transmission for humans (and one of the main routes for animals) is through respiratory aerosolization. When there is active TB in the lungs, the bacillus is expelled and aerosolized in the form of droplet nuclei through coughing (or any explosive respiratory action such as singing, shouting, sneezing, or talking). For these droplet nuclei to be inhaled and reach the alveoli in humans, they must be 3 to 5 microns or less in size. In animals, the exact sizes of infecting droplet nuclei may vary depending on the species.

Other risk of exposure to infectious aerosols includes opening an infected chest cavity such as during autopsy, necropsy, or slaughter of livestock, as well as hosing down an area where an infected animal has been housed. The efficiency of transmission of TB depends on a number of factors, as shown in Box 9-7.[20]

The second most common route of transmission is through the gastrointestinal tract by the ingestion of infected material. Drinking or eating unpasteurized milk products traditionally has been the principal means by which humans have acquired zoonotic TB.[21] In industrialized countries pasteurization and strict herd testing and management have made such gastrointestinal transmission rare, but zoonotic TB caused by *M. bovis* acquired through ingestion may be seen in immigrants from countries with a continuing prevalence of *M. bovis* infection in cattle or livestock.[22,23]

Of note are the recent documented human-to-human transmissions of *M. bovis*, including an epidemiologically linked cluster of six cases identified in the United Kingdom. Five of the patients had pulmonary TB disease and one had TB meningitis[24]; only one was known to be HIV infected. The index case had a history of occupational exposure and consumption of unpasteurized milk and cheese both as a young adult and recently in a country not free from bovine TB. In another cluster, human nosocomial transmission of *M. bovis* among HIV-infected individuals occurred in a Spanish hospital, resulting in 30 deaths.[25] Humans may also serve as a source of TB infection for animals, including nonhuman primates, cattle, dogs, and macaws.[26-31]

Animal-to-animal transmission of TB occurs through respiratory and gastrointestinal routes.[32] Respiratory infection can occur in herds or closely quartered animals through pulmonary disease or draining lymphadenopathy. Infection is also acquired by ingestion of infected meat, sharing of infected water and food sources, grooming, and exposure to secretions.

Environmental Risk Factors

Because a major influence on the aerosol transmission of TB in humans and other animals is the closeness and duration of contact with the infected individual, population density can be a key environmental factor driving TB transmission. Although being outdoors significantly decreases the risk of transmission, the close or sheltered outdoor housing of animals and humans may decrease that advantage. Contaminated water can be another environmental risk for disease transmission in animals.

Disease in Humans

During primary and latent infection, the person does not exhibit signs of disease and is not considered infectious. Immunocompetent individuals will develop a balance between host and mycobacteria, and the infection will remain latent. However, if there is a breakdown of the host's immune function and the infection is no longer able to be effectively contained, active disease may develop (Figure 9-150).

More than 90% of humans infected with MTBC maintain control of the infection through immune mechanisms during their lifetime. These individuals have an approximately 10% chance of developing active TB disease during their lifetime: 5% within the first few years of infection (progressive primary TB disease) and 5% at a later stage in their lives (reactivation TB disease). However, that probability of progressing to active disease is significantly increased in the presence of comorbid conditions that compromise immune function. Factors associated with this increased risk are outlined in Box 9-8.

HIV exerts a significant adverse affect on the pathogenesis of TB. With a suppressed or poorly functioning immune system, the host will release an immature response to the tubercle bacillus. The decrease in the number and function of T-cell lymphocytes as a result of HIV disease weakens the immune reaction and the host cannot, or only poorly, contain the TB organisms that are present. There is a greater chance of rapid progression from infection to disease after recent TB infection. There is also a question of whether an individual with HIV has an increased chance of infection with TB from the loss of innate resistance. People with HIV have an 8% to

---

BOX 9-7 FACTORS DETERMINING TRANSMISSION OF TUBERCULOSIS

Characteristics of the Source Case
- Concentration of organisms in sputum
- Presence of cavitary disease
- Frequency and strength of cough

Characteristics of the Exposed Individual
- Previous tuberculosis infection
- Innate resistance to tuberculosis infection
- Genetic susceptibility to tuberculosis infection/disease

Characteristics of the Exposure
- Frequency and duration of exposure
- Dilution effect (volume of air containing infectious droplet nuclei)
- Ventilation (turnover of air in a space)
- Exposure to ultraviolet light, including sunlight

Virulence of the Infecting Strain of *Mycobacterium Tuberculosis* Complex

Adapted from CDC "Guidelines for preventing the transmission of *Mycobacterium tuberculosis* in health-care settings, 2005. http://www.cdc.gov/mmwr/pdf/rr/rr5417.pdf.

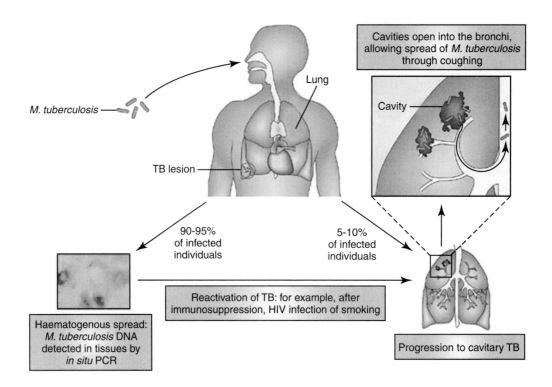

Figure 9-150 ▪ Phases of infection with tuberculosis. (From Rook GA, Dheda K, Zumla A: Immune responses to tuberculosis in developing countries: implications for new vaccines, *Nat Rev Immunol* 5(8):661-7, 2005.)

BOX 9-8	*RISK FACTORS FOR DEVELOPING TUBERCULOSIS DISEASE*

- Recent TB infection (within past 2 years)
- HIV infection
- Chest radiographic findings suggestive of previous TB
- Contact with a recent case of active TB
- Recent immigration from tuberculosis-endemic country within 5 years of immigration
- Malnutrition
- 10% below ideal body weight
- Alcohol and drug abuse (especially IV drugs)
- Newborn, infants <2 years
- Comorbid medical conditions:
  - o Diabetes
  - o Gastrectomy or jejunoileal bypass (total or partial)
  - o Silicosis (affects pulmonary macrophage function)
  - o Cancer (especially head and neck tumors)
  - o Hematologic malignancies (leukemia, lymphoma)
  - o Chronic renal failure
  - o Solid organ transplant (chronic immunosuppressive therapy)
- Immunosuppressive conditions, including:
  - o Cancer chemotherapy
  - o Prolonged treatment with corticosteroids
  - o Treatment with anti-TNFα agents

10% chance per year to progress from infection to active TB. The 1-year mortality rate for treated, HIV related TB is 4 times the rate of non-HIV related TB, around 35%. TB also worsens HIV disease by inducing stimulation and replication of T-cell lymphocytes. These T cells are then targeted by the virus, resulting in increased HIV replication. If the tuberculous infection is initially contained by the immune system, which then subsequently experiences a significant deterioration in the quantity and function of T-helper cells, the bacillus may no longer be contained and the TB reactivates. In addition, the cytokines produced in response to TB infection stimulate the production of HIV in vitro.[33]

Active TB is usually a slowly progressive disease characterized by systemic symptoms of weight loss, fatigue, anorexia, fevers, chills, night sweats, and wasting. The severe weight loss and wasting associated with the disease led to its former name of *consumption*. When the disease is pulmonary, presenting symptoms may also include a persistent cough (with or without sputum production), chest pain, and hemoptysis. Although TB is generally a chronic, debilitating disease, it may present with an acute, rapidly progressing course. Disease is generally pulmonary, followed by lymphatic drainage and local lymphadenopathy, or disseminated (especially in immunocompromised hosts; Color Plate 9-77). Manifestations may vary depending on the extrapulmonary site of disseminated disease. Central nervous system involvement may present as either meningeal or parenchymal disease. Meningitis more commonly affects the basilar meninges, and the cranial nerves may also be involved. Parenchymal lesions may be single or multiple and present as solid tuberculomas or TB abscesses. Symptoms will depend on the location of the lesion and/or mass effect from surrounding edema (Figure 9-151). TB may also present in the spinal vertebrae (Pott's disease) (Figure 9-152).

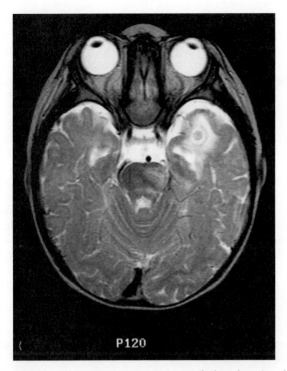

Figure 9-151 ▪ A magnetic resonance image of tuberculoma in a child with culture-positive tuberculous meningitis. The child's presenting signs and symptoms included fever, altered mental status, and hemiparesis. (From Gershon AA, Hotez PJ, Katz S: *Krugman's infectious diseases of children*, ed 11, St Louis, 2004, Mosby Elsevier.)

Disease in Animals

As in humans, TB can be either a chronic or rapidly progressive disease, with the clinical signs varying greatly according to the species involved. As with humans, it is believed that many animals infected with MTBC remain in a latent phase, although the natural history is less well understood.

In cattle, TB is often not apparent, and therefore not diagnosed, until terminal stages of the disease; it is often found only at necropsy or in abattoirs (Color Plate 9-78). This, unfortunately, allows for a prolonged period of transmission. The initial presentation, besides cachexia, progressive weakness, and anorexia, may also include cough, lymphadenitis, and draining sinus tracts, especially around the neck, face, and chest. In later stages, lymph nodes may be enlarged to the point of impingement on airways, gastrointestinal (GI) tract, or blood vessels.[34] GI tract involvement may be manifested by diarrhea or constipation. The female genital tract may be involved. At necropsy, both tuberculous granulomas and abscesses may be present.

In Cervidae, which include deer, antelope, moose, elk, and reindeer, TB has been found in both farmed and free-living animals. The course may be chronic and progressive or acute. The presentation is similar to that found in cattle with granulomas, but thin-walled abscesses are also common.

In nonhuman primates, as in humans, there is a broad clinical spectrum of disease, including latent TB, chronic

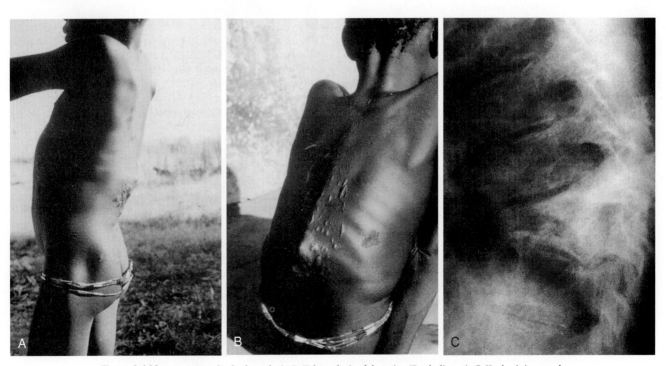

Figure 9-152 ▪ **A,** Vertebral tuberculosis. **B,** Tuberculosis of the spine (Pott's disease). **C,** Kyphosis is secondary to anterior destruction of vertebral bodies resulting in wedging of adjacent vertebrae and loss of disk space clearly seen by radiography. (From Cohen J, Powderly WG: *Infectious diseases*, ed 2, Philadelphia, 2004, Mosby Elsevier. *A* and *B*, Courtesy J. Cohen, Brighton, U.K. *C*, Courtesy A. Wightman.)

primary TB, rapidly progressing and fulminant disease, and reactivation TB.[35] Old World species appear to be more susceptible than New World species.

Culture-confirmed cases of TB have been diagnosed in at least 36 elephants in the United States from 1994 to 2006.[36] It has been reported in captive elephants, primarily Asian, although the potential for transmission to wild elephants is increasing. Clinical disease in elephants usually has a chronic, debilitating presentation. Signs may not be present until the disease is advanced and include weakness, weight loss, and coughing, although they may also be specific to the organ system involved, such as chronic vaginal discharge or conjunctivitis.

TB also occurs in domestic and companion animals. Dogs and cats may present with a typical clinical picture of wasting, anorexia, and progressive decline. If the MTBC was acquired through the respiratory tract, signs may also include cough and shortness of breath; if acquired through the ingestion of infected meat or milk, GI signs may be present.

Diagnosis

Active Disease

The key factor in the diagnosis of active TB is that of clinical suspicion based on the presenting history, signs or symptoms, chest radiograph, and/or laboratory testing. Microscopy looks for the presence of acid-fast bacilli (AFB) on direct smears of clinical specimens. The finding of AFB indicates the presence of mycobacteria but not the specific species.

Identification of the mycobacterial species is through culture or molecular testing such as polymerase chain reaction. A tissue biopsy specimen may show characteristic histological findings, such as granuloma, caseation, necrosis, calcification, and typical cellular immune response. The presumptive diagnosis of TB (mycobacteriosis) may be made on this basis, especially in animals.

Cultures may use liquid media, such as the mycobacteria growth indicator tube (MGIT, BBL Becton Dickinson Microbiology Systems, Cockeysville, Md.) and/or solid agar media, such as Bactec (Becton-Dickinson Diagnostic Instrument Systems, Sparks, Md.) Lowenstein-Jensen, or Middlebrook 7H10. MTBC is a slow-growing organism that replicates approximately every 24 hours. Growth in liquid media usually occurs within 1 to 3 weeks, whereas growth on solid media may be 6 to 8 weeks. Drug susceptibility testing is performed on isolates of MTBC routinely for isoniazid, rifampin, pyrazinamide, and ethambutol.

Since the genetic mapping of MTBC, molecular testing has been used in the diagnosis of TB. Nucleic acid amplification (NAA) tests, such as the *Mycobacterium tuberculosis* Direct (MTD) test (Gen-Probe, Inc., San Diego, Calif.) are performed on direct specimen smears based on the presence of MTBC RNA. The sensitivity and specificity of the NAA test on a positive AFB smear are greater than 95% and 99.6%, respectively. PCR is a species-specific DNA-based test used to identify MTBC. Further genotyping on positive TB cultures often may be done, usually by one of two methods:

mycobacterial interspersed repetitive units (MIRU) or spoligotyping. Genotyping is used to assist TB control programs in identifying outbreaks and recent transmission in a more real-time manner so that appropriate secondary testing and management can be performed sooner. Molecular testing of the TB isolate for genetic resistance mutations is beginning to be used.

Thoracic radiographs may be part, or the initial finding, of the clinical presentation of TB in humans and other animals (Figures 9-153 and 9-154). Classically, TB is an upper lobe disease, either unilateral or bilateral. Abnormalities typically are seen in the apical and posterior segments of the upper lobe or the superior segments of the lower lobe; however, lesions may appear in any part of the lungs. Radiographic abnormalities may present as infiltrates, nodules, cavitary lesions, pleural thickening, or a diffuse miliary pattern. Hilar and mediastinal lymphadenopathy may be present, with or without accompanying infiltrates or cavities. Immunosuppressed individuals may present with only hilar or mediastinal adenopathy, or the chest radiograph may appear normal.

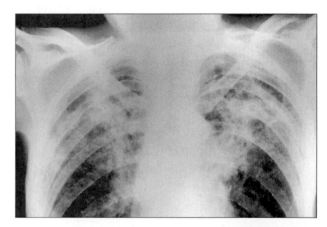

Figure 9-153 ■ Chest radiograph of a patient with pulmonary tuberculosis. There is extensive parenchymal streaking, predominantly in the upper fields of the lungs. These changes are typical of chronic bilateral pulmonary tuberculosis. Some enlargement of the heart is also evident. (From Male D, Brostoff J, Roth D et al: *Immunology*, ed 7, Philadelphia, 2006, Mosby Elsevier.)

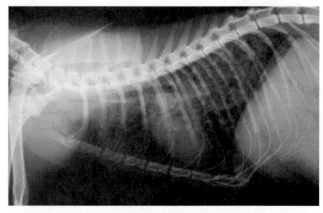

Figure 9-154 ■ Lateral thoracic radiograph of a cat with disseminated *M. bovis* infection. (From Greene CE: *Infectious diseases of the dog and cat*, ed 3, St Louis, 2006, Saunders Elsevier. Courtesy D. Gunn-Moore, University of Edinburgh, Scotland.)

Latent Infection

The tuberculin skin test (TST) has been the standard screening tool for TB infection in humans and other animals (Figure 9-155). It produces a delayed-type hypersensitivity reaction in those with tuberculous infection. It is useful for determining how many individuals in a group are

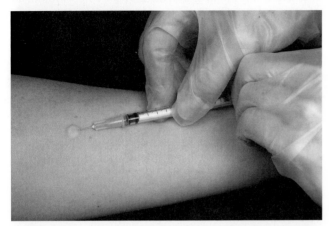

Figure 9-155 ■ This technician is in the process of correctly placing a tuberculin skin test in this recipient's forearm, which will cause a 6-mm to 10-mm wheal (i.e., a raised area of skin surface) to form at the injection site. The tuberculin skin test is used to evaluate people for latent tuberculosis infection. In the United States, this skin test consists of an intradermal injection of exactly one tenth of a milliliter of tuberculin, which contains 5 tuberculin units. Correct placement of this intradermal injection involves inserting the needle bevel slowly at a 5- to 15-degree angle. The needle bevel is advanced through the epidermis, the superficial layer of skin, approximately 3 mm so that the entire bevel is covered and lies just under the skin surface. A tense, pale wheal that is 6 mm to 10 mm in diameter appears over the needle bevel. (From Centers for Disease Control and Prevention Public Health Image Library, Atlanta, Ga. Courtesy Gabrielle Benenson.)

infected (e.g., contact investigation) and in the evaluation of those with signs or symptoms or those who are suspected of having TB.

The TST is administered by subcutaneously injecting a preparation of (inactive) mycobacterial antigens. In humans, 0.1 mL of purified protein derivative (PPD) is placed on the inner surface of the forearm. More complete information on TB skin test placement, reading, and interpretation is available at http://www.cdc.gov/TB/pubs/slidesets/core/html/trans4_slides.htm. The TST is usually read after 48 to 72 hours. The induration (not the erythema) is measured and should be recorded in millimeters, not simply as negative or positive. In humans, a positive TST reaction may be measured for up to 7 days, although a negative reaction can only be read until 72 hours. The TST, however, has limited sensitivity and specificity. In humans, there is an overall false-positive rate of 20% and a false-negative rate of 20%. False-positive results may be seen in NTM infection, recent Bacillus Calmette-Guérin (BCG) vaccination, or incorrect administration. False-negative results may occur in overwhelming TB disease, anergy, recent TB infection, newborns, recent live-virus vaccinations, some viral illnesses, incorrect administration, or waning immune response (usually due to age or prolonged time since infection). Because of the possibility of a waning immune response, in some instances a two-step TST is performed. In those situations, an initial TST may serve to stimulate, or boost, subsequent TSTs. A two-step TST is therefore currently recommended for baseline testing in those who will undergo periodic testing, such as health care workers.[37] This helps to differentiate between a boosted reaction and one due to recent infection. The criteria for determining whether a human TST is positive depends on the risk group of the individual. Table 9-69 defines the size of the induration per risk group.

Table 9-69 ■ Criteria for Tuberculin Positivity, by Risk Group

Reaction ≥5 mm of Induration	Reaction ≥10 mm of Induration	Reaction ≥15 mm of Induration
HIV positive status Recent contacts of TB case patients Fibrotic changes on chest radiograph consistent with prior TB Patients with organ transplants and other immunosuppressed patients (receiving the equivalent of 15 mg/day of prednisone for ≥1 month)*	Recent immigrants (i.e., within the past 5 years) from high-prevalence countries Injection drug users Residents and employees† of the following high-risk congregate settings: prisons and jails, nursing homes, and other long-term facilities for the elderly; hospitals and other health care facilities; residential facilities for patients with acquired AIDS; and homeless shelters Mycobacteriology laboratory personnel Persons with the following clinical conditions that place them at high risk: diabetes mellitus, chronic renal failure, some hematological disorders (e.g., leukemias and lymphomas), and other specific malignancies (e.g., carcinoma of the head or neck and lung), weight loss of ≥10% of ideal body weight, gastrectomy, and jejunoileal bypass Children younger than 4 years or infants, children, and adolescents exposed to adults at high risk	Persons with no risk factors for TB

*Risk of TB in patients treated with corticosteroids increases with higher dose and longer duration.
†For persons who are otherwise at low risk and are tested at the start of employment, a reaction of ≥15 mm induration is considered positive.
From American Thoracic Society (ATS) and the Centers for Disease Control and Prevention (CDC): Targeted tuberculin testing and treatment of latent tuberculosis infection, *MMWR Morb Mortal Wkly Rep* 49(RR-6):1–51, 2000.

Recently IFN-γ–releasing assays (IGRAs) are being used to detect latent TB infection. Generally these are whole blood assays that measure and compare the amount of IFN-γ released by white blood cells in response to antigens of MTBC. In humans, QuantiFERON-Gold (Cellestic, Inc., Valencia, Calif.) and T-SPOT.TB (Oxford Immunotec, Oxford, U.K.) are examples of assays used.[38]

In other animals, the TST is the only skin test for use in cattle prescribed by the World Organisation for Animal Health.[39] However, there is no standardization of TST testing in animals, as individual protocols are established by each country. In cattle, testing may use *M. bovis* antigen alone (caudal fold test [CFT], cervical test [CT]) or along with *M. avium* (comparative cervical test [CCT]).[8] Test results are read at 72 hours ± 6 hours. The preferred TST placement sites in animals differs by species and include the caudal fold in bovids, ear in pigs, and eyelid in primates.

Skin testing in animals produces high rates of false-positive and false-negative results. These are often from the same interference: mycobacterial species, such as *M. avium* or *M. avium* subsp. *paratuberculosis*, overwhelming or advanced disease, in the face of comorbidity that prevents an appropriate immune response, early infection, or improper test administration.

In cattle, buffalo, bison, and other bovids, several serological tests based on *M. bovis* have been developed and are in use, such as SeraLyte-Mbv (PriTest, Redmond, Wash.) and Chembio Bovid TB STAT-PAK (Chembio Diagnostic Systems, Inc., Medford, NY).[36] There are also assays for use in cervids, primates, badgers, camelids, elephants, and other exotic wildlife, among others.[40]

Treatment

Primary prevention remains the optimum course of disease control. It has proven extremely difficult, if not impossible, to eradicate any public health disease such as TB without an effective vaccine. Currently numerous studies are assessing vaccines for human and differing veterinary populations to prevent infection.

Treatment in Humans

Treatment of active TB uses a combination of antibiotics for a prolonged period of time. The exact regimen is based on or modified according to the organism's susceptibilities. For drug-susceptible isolates, treatment usually is with three or four drugs (isoniazid [INH], rifampin [RIF], pyrazinamide [PZA] with or without ethambutol [EMB]) for the first 2 months, then INH and RIF to complete 6 months' total treatment. Table 9-70 shows drug treatment regimens for pan-susceptible TB.[42] Multidrug-resistant tuberculosis (MDR-TB) is resistant to at least INH and RIF, the two best first-line TB medications. Extensively drug-resistant tuberculosis (XDR-TB) in addition to INH and RIF is also resistant to the best second-line drugs, the fluoroquinolones and an injectable such as kanamycin or capreomycin. The treatment of TB with drug-resistant organisms is more complicated and difficult and should be done by or in consultation with experts. Regimens for resistant TB

Table 9-70 ■ Drug Regimens for Culture-Positive Pulmonary Tuberculosis Caused by Drug-Susceptible Organisms								
Initial Phase			**Continuation Phase**			**Range of Total Doses** *(minimal duration)*	**Rating* (Evidence)†**	
Regimen	Drugs	Interval and Doses‡ *(minimal duration)*	Regimen	Drugs	Interval and Doses‡,§ *(minimal duration)*		HIVneg	HIVpos
1	INH RIF PZA EMB	7 days/wk for 56 doses (8 wk) *or* 5 days/wk for 40 doses (8 wk)¶	1a	INH/RIF	7 days/wk for 126 doses (18 wk) *or* 5 days/wk for 90 doses (18 wk)¶	182-130 (26 wk)	A (I)	A (II)
			1b	INH/RIF	Twice weekly for 36 doses (18 wk)	92-76 (25 wk)	A (I)	A (II)¶
			1c#	INH/RPT	Once weekly for 18 doses (18 wk)	74-58 (26 wk)	B (I)	E (I)
2	INH RIF PZA EMB	7 days/wk for 14 doses (2 wk), *then* twice weekly for 12 doses (6 wk) *or* 5 days/wk for 10 doses (2 wk),¶ *then* twice weekly for 12 doses (6 wk)	2a	INH/RIF	Twice weekly for 36 doses (18 wk)	62-58 (26 wk)	A (II)	B (II)**
			2b#	INH/RPT	Once weekly for 18 doses (18 wk)	44-40 (26 wk)	B (I)	E (I)
3	INH RIF PZA EMB	Three times weekly for 24 doses (8 wk)	3a	INH/RIF	Three times weekly for 54 doses (18 wk)	78 (26 wk)	B (I)	B (II)

Table 9-70 ▪ Drug Regimens for Culture-Positive Pulmonary Tuberculosis Caused by Drug-Susceptible Organisms—*(Continued)*								
Initial Phase			**Continuation Phase**			**Range of Total Doses** *(minimal duration)*	**Rating* (Evidence)†**	
Regimen	**Drugs**	**Interval and Doses‡** *(minimal duration)*	**Regimen**	**Drugs**	**Interval and Doses‡,§** *(minimal duration)*		**HIVneg**	**HIVpos**
4	INH	7 days/wk for 56 doses (8 wk) *or*	4a	INH/RIF	Seven days/wk for 217 doses (31 wk) *or*	273-195 (39 wk)	C (I)	C (II)
	RIF							
	EMB	5 days/wk for 40 doses (8 wk)¶			5 days/wk for 155 doses (31 wk)¶			
			4b	INH/RIF	Twice weekly for 62 doses (31 wk)	118-102 (39 wk)	C (I)	C (II)

From Blumberg HM, Burman WJ, Chaisson RE et al: American Thoracic Society/Centers for Disease Control and Prevention/Infectious Diseases Society of America: treatment of tuberculosis, *Am J Respir Crit Care Med* 167(4):603–62, 2003.
EMB, Ethambutol; *INH,* isoniazid; *PZA,* pyrazinamide; *RIF,* rifampin; *RPT,* rifapentine.
*Definitions of evidence ratings: A = preferred; B = acceptable alternative; C = offer when A and B cannot be given; E = should never be given.
†Definitions of evidence ratings: I = randomized clinical trial; II = data from clinical trials that were not randomized or were conducted in other populations; III = expert opinion.
‡When directly observed therapy (DOT) is used, drugs may be given 5 days/wk and the necessary number of doses adjusted accordingly. Although there are no studies that compare 5 with 7 daily doses, extensive experience indicates this would be an effective practice.
§Patients with cavitation on initial chest radiograph and positive cultures at completion of 2 months of therapy should receive a 7-month (31-week; either 217 doses [daily] or 62 doses [twice weekly]) continuation phase.
¶Five-day-a-week administration is always given by DOT. Rating for 5 day/wk regimens is AIII.
¶Not recommended for patients with HIV infection with CD4+ cell counts <100 cells/mL.
#Options 1c and 2b should be used only in HIV negative patients who have negative sputum smears at the time of completion of 2 months of therapy and who do not have cavitation on the initial chest radiograph. For patients who start this regimen and are found to have a positive culture from the 2-month specimen, treatment should be extended an extra 3 months.

generally use a combination of first- and/or second-line drugs for an extended period of time—between 9 and 24 months depending on the resistance pattern.

Treatment of latent TB infection (LTBI) in humans, previously referred to as *prophylaxis,* is based on the TST risk groups previously discussed. Because current skin test recommendations target high-risk groups, the intent to test is generally the intent to treat. The first-line medication for the treatment of LTBI remains INH, currently recommended for 9 months. An alternative treatment is INH for 6 months. INH regimens may be daily or intermittent. Table 9-71 shows recommended regimens for the treatment of LTBI.

Treatment in Animals

Until recently, the approach to treatment of TB in animals has not included the use of medications to treat until cure, and it is still the rare exception. The overwhelming majority of animals with suspected or confirmed TB are culled or euthanized, such as with cattle. This has been done for several reasons: an effort to halt the spread of the disease to other animals or herds and mitigate the economic loss of herd and trade; the lack of practical alternatives; the difficulty of testing methods to distinguish MTBC disease from infection or from nontuberculous mycobacterial disease; the cost of TB medication regimens; problems with drug administration and monitoring; and the inability or unreliability of monitoring response to disease or LTBI treatment. In non-herd situations or where the animal is of significant economic or species value, such as zoo animals and rare or endangered species, pharmacotherapy has been used. Treatment of elephants with multidrug regimens has been documented, including for MDR-TB.

Due to a paucity of data, the medication dosing for TB in animals has been based loosely on data from human pharmacokinetic studies and dosages. However, the increased use of pharmacotherapy for veterinary TB may result in more species-specific recommendations. For example, a number of pharmacokinetic studies have been done on TB drug levels in elephants.[41-45] Expert consultation is suggested in the treatment of veterinary TB.

The first-line TB medications used in animals are the same as humans: INH, RIF, EMB, and PZA (which is not used in the treatment of *M. bovis* as this organism is usually resistant). Other antituberculous medications also include quinolones and systemic aminoglycosides. Veterinary quinolones used for TB include enrofloxacin and marbofloxacin, and aminoglycosides include amikacin and streptomycin. Nevertheless, much more investigation is needed in the area of veterinary antituberculous pharmacotherapy.

Companion animals rarely are treated for TB, either because of the advanced condition of the animal, belief that TB cannot be treated, or concerns regarding public health. It is probable that many, if not most, cases of TB in these animals have gone undiagnosed as a result of a combination of lack of awareness of the disease, lack of information regarding diagnostics and testing, and the impression that, regardless, treatment is not feasible. That TB in companion animals is an issue of public health concern has been cited as another reason for not considering pharmacotherapy. However, it may be possible in these situations to consider some of the same principles of TB disease control as used in other human and veterinary settings, such as housing the animal separately and/or outdoors while awaiting test results or a response to therapy. Nonetheless, the logistics and feasibility

Table 9-71 ▪ Recommended Drug Regimens for the Treatment of LTBI in Adults

Drug	Interval and Duration	Comments*	Rating† HIV Negative	(Evidence)‡ HIV Infected
Isoniazid	Daily for 9 months§‖	In persons with HIV infection, isoniazid may be administered concurrently with NRTIs, protease inhibitors, or NNRTIs.	A (II)	A (II)
	Twice weekly for 9 months§‖	DOT must be used with twice-weekly dosing.	B (II)	B (II)
Isoniazid	Daily for 6 months‖	Not indicated for persons with HIV infection, those with fibrotic lesions on chest radiographs, or children.	B (I)	C (I)
	Twice weekly for 6 months‖	DOT must be used with twice-weekly dosing.	B (II)	C (I)
Rifampin¶	Daily for 4 months	Used for persons who are contacts of patients with isoniazid-resistant, rifampin-susceptible TB.	B (II)	B (III)
		In persons with HIV infection, most protease inhibitors or delavirdine should not be administered concurrently with rifampin. Rifabutin with appropriate dose adjustments can be used with protease inhibitors (saquinavir should be augmented with ritonavir) and NNRTIs (except delavirdine). Clinicians should consult Internet updates for the latest specific recommendations.		
RZ	Daily for 2 months	RZ generally should not be offered for treatment of latent tuberculosis infection for persons with or without HIV infection.	D (II)	D (II)
	Twice weekly for 2-3 months		D (III)	D (III)

Adapted from CDC: Targeted tuberculin testing and treatment of latent tuberculosis infection, *MMWR Morb Mortal Wkly Rep* 49(RR-6):1-51, 2000.

*Interactions with human immunodeficiency virus (HIV)-related drugs are updated frequently and are available at http://www.aidsinfo.nih.gov/guidelines.

†Strength of recommendation: A = Both strong evidence of efficacy and substantial clinical benefit support recommendation for use. Should always be offered. B = Moderate evidence for efficacy or strong evidence for efficacy but only limited clinical benefit supports recommendation for use. Should generally be offered. C = Evidence for efficacy is insufficient to support a recommendation for or against use, or evidence for efficacy might not outweigh adverse consequences (e.g., drug toxicity, drug interactions) or cost of the treatment or alternative approaches. Optional. D = Moderate evidence for lack of efficacy or for adverse outcome supports a recommendation against use. Should generally not be offered. E = Good evidence for lack of efficacy or for adverse outcome support a recommendation against use. Should never be offered.

‡Quality of evidence supporting the recommendation: I = Evidence from at least one properly randomized controlled trial. II = Evidence from at least one well-designed clinical trial without randomization from cohort or case-controlled analytic studies (preferably from more than one center), from multiple time-series studies, or from dramatic results from uncontrolled experiments. III. = Evidence from opinions of respected authorities based on clinical experience, descriptive studies, or reports of expert committees.

§Recommended regimen for persons aged <18 years.

‖Recommended regimens for pregnant women.

¶The substitution of rifapentine for rifampin is not recommended because rifapentine's safety and effectiveness have not been established for patients with latent tuberculosis infection.

NRTIs, Nucleoside reverse-transcriptase inhibitors; *NNRTIs,* non–nucleoside reverse-transcriptase inhibitors; *DOT,* directly observed therapy; *RZ,* rifampin plus pyrazinamide.

of this approach depend on each individual situation, and discussion with TB experts is advisable.

Nontuberculous Mycobacteria

NTM are environmental opportunistic pathogens that differ from the members of MTBC (and *M. leprae*) in that they are not obligate pathogens but rather are found in the environment and environmental reservoirs that serve as the source of infection.[46] Although most NTM do not cause human or animal disease, some may be pathogenic with potential for interspecies and zoonotic transmission. Table 9-72 shows common potentially pathogenic mycobacteria, classified according to growth rate as either rapid growing (less than 1 week) or slow growing (more than 1 week).

Transmission of NTM is achieved through inhalation or ingestion of water, particulate matter or aerosols, or through trauma.[47] NTMs are not generally considered communicable between humans and animals or as zoonotic infections and as such are not reportable diseases. Consequently, epidemiological data on the prevalence of NTM disease are not well established

and surveillance information is limited. The clinical and epidemiological presentation of NTM infection has changed dramatically in recent years. This is thought to be due, in part, to the ability of these organisms to survive and flourish in habitats shared with humans and other animals, such as drinking water. In addition, an increase in the proportion of HIV-infected and other immunosuppressed hosts suggest a continuing and increasing prevalence of NTM infections in the future. Human risk factors associated with NTM disease include comorbid lung conditions such as prior TB disease, silicosis, and bronchiectasis, and host immunosuppression such as HIV infection. With the rise of HIV infection in the 1980s came increasing reports of disseminated human NTM infections, such as *M. avium* complex (MAC).

The most common sites of NTM disease in humans are pulmonary, lymphatic, skin, and soft tissue and disseminated disease. Pulmonary disease, commonly from *M. avium, M. intracellulare, M. kansasii,* or *M. abscessus,* generally presents as a chronic condition with a persistent or varying cough; additionally, there may be fatigue, malaise, sputum production, fever, weight loss, dyspnea, and hemoptysis.

Table 9-72 ■ Potentially Pathogenic Nontuberculous Mycobacteria		
Mycobacterial Species	**Growth Classification***	**Disease Presentation**
M. abscessus	Rapid	Pulmonary, skin, soft tissue, bone
M. avium complex: M. avium, M. intracellulare, M. paratuberculosis	Slow	Pulmonary, lymphadenitis, gastrointestinal, wasting
M. chelonae	Rapid	Skin, soft tissue, bone
M. fortuitum	Rapid	Skin, soft tissue, bone
M. kansasii	Slow	Pulmonary
M. leprae	Slow	Skin, peripheral nerve
M. malmoense	Slow	Pulmonary, lymphadenitis, skin and soft tissue
M. marinum	Slow	Skin, soft tissue, bone
M. scrofulaceum	Slow	Lymphadenitis, skin
M. xenopi	Slow	Pulmonary, lymphadenitis
M. ulcerans	Slow	Skin, soft tissue (Buruli's ulcer)

*Rapid = growth <1 week; slow = growth >1 week.

In HIV unaffected individuals, pulmonary infections with NTM traditionally had been found in older males. However, it has been found that bronchiectatic MAC disease may also present in older, thin females without prior pulmonary disease (Lady Windermere syndrome), sometimes in the presence of pectus excavatum, mitral valve prolapse, or scoliosis.[48]

In HIV-infected individuals, NTM disease usually manifests when the host's CD4/T-lymphocyte cell counts are less than 50 cells/mL and often presents as a disseminated, multiorgan infection, commonly from *M. avium*. Acquisition of the NTM is usually through the GI or respiratory tracts; symptoms are nonspecific and include fever, night sweats, weight loss, anorexia, and diarrhea. Disseminated disease has also been reported with *M. intracellulare*, *M. simiae*, *M. marinum*, *M. xenopi*, and *M. abscessus*.

The diagnosis of pulmonary NTM disease is based on a combination of clinical and laboratory criteria[48]:

1. Symptoms and findings on imaging studies (chest radiograph or high-resolution CT scan) consistent with the diagnosis,
2. Exclusion of other conditions with a similar presentation, such as TB, and
3. Either multiple positive sputum cultures of the NTM species, a positive culture from a bronchial wash or lavage, or a biopsy specimen with typical histological features and a positive culture result from either the biopsy specimen or sputum.

Lymphatic disease is the most common NTM presentation in children and rarely affects immunocompetent adults. The majority of cases are due to MAC, and sites are usually unilateral in cervical, submandibular, submaxillary, or preauricular lymph nodes. The diagnosis may be made by lymph node biopsy and specimen culture. A negative skin test response (<10 mm) may be helpful. Treatment may depend on the particular species of NTM, but localized disease in immunocompetent individuals may include surgical excision of the lymph node.

Skin, soft tissue, and bone disease, most commonly caused by *M. fortuitum*, *M. abscessus*, *M. chelonae*, *M. marinum*, or *M. ulcerans*, usually occurs through penetration, such as in puncture wounds, traumatic injuries, surgical wounds or injection, or skin trauma. For example, tenosynovitis of the hand, commonly from *M. marinum*, may occur in those cleaning aquariums (Color Plate 9-79). Chronic infections may occur in tendons, joints, and bones. In addition to antibiotics, surgical intervention may be indicated.

M. ulcerans is the agent causing Buruli's ulcer, which is an increasing cause of morbidity and disability in many parts of the world, especially West Africa.[49] In animals, natural infections with *M. ulcerans* have been observed in koalas, ringtail possums, and an alpaca.[50]

In animals, *M. paratuberculosis* is the causative agent of Johne's disease (Figure 9-156). This is a progressive infection affecting ruminants, causing GI symptoms such as diarrhea and wasting, and is an important cause of economic losses in cattle. *M. paratuberculosis* also has been postulated as a cause of Crohn's disease in humans.

Avian mycobacteriosis (avian TB) in birds may be caused by several species of NTM, usually of the MAC or *M. genavense*, which are environmentally ubiquitous. These organisms may infect any bird (though uncommon in grey-cheeked parakeets), but is more common in older or immunosuppressed birds (Color Plate 9-80 and Figure 9-157).

Avian TB usually presents as a chronic disease involving the GI tract and liver; signs include wasting despite a good appetite and loose droppings. Primary respiratory signs are uncommon. Rarely, tubercles may be seen on the face and oral cavity of infected birds.[51] The diagnosis of avian TB usually has been made by culture of the organism, although adequate culture specimens may be difficult to obtain. The

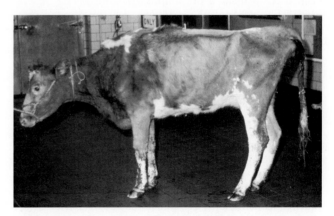

Figure 9-156 ■ Granulomatous enteritis, Johne's disease (*Mycobacterium avium* spp. paratuberculosis) in a cow. There is chronic wasting and diarrhea in this 18-month-old heifer. The age at which this cow showed clinical signs is not typical of the disease. Signs usually occur 2 or more years after initial infection. (From McGavin MD, Zachary JF: *Pathologic basis of veterinary disease*, ed 4, St Louis, 2007, Mosby Elsevier. Courtesy College of Veterinary Medicine, Cornell University.)

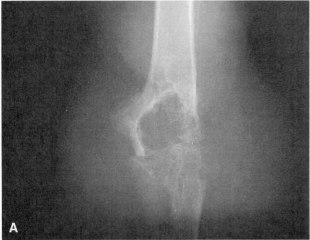

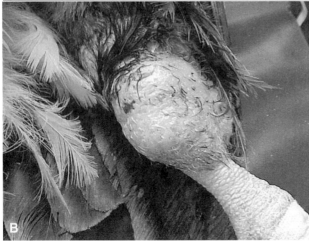

Figure 9-157 ■ **A**, *Mycobacterium avium* is an important pathogen of wild birds. This bald eagle presented with systemic lesions. **B**, The most notable sign was the classic distal tibiotarsal osteomyelitis. (From Mitchell M, Tully TN Jr: *Manual of exotic pet practice*, St Louis, 2008, Saunders Elsevier.)

finding of mycobacterial organisms in histology associated with inflammatory cells and the clinical presentation have been used to make a presumptive diagnosis. PCR testing is available, although the results must be interpreted carefully.[52] A positive result means that there are mycobacteria present but does not necessarily mean that it is the cause of disease. Most birds with avian TB either succumb to the disease or are euthanized. In some areas it is a reportable avian disease.

Other than in birds, MAC infection in mammals is sporadic and not considered transmissible. However, disseminated disease has been reported in captive, nondomestic hoofed animals and in immunosuppressed dogs and cats.[53]

M. marinum may commonly be found in marine animals and water. It can be transmitted directly from fish or marine animals to humans; it may indirectly be transmitted through water or contaminated equipment, such as aquariums (see above). Infection in ecothermic fish may present as a systemic disease with internal tuberculomas, anorexia, weight loss, skin defects, spinal deformities, abdominal distention, and exophthalmia. The prognosis in fish is poor; those affected are usually killed and removed from the environment, as infection may be transmitted if the fish are cannibalized.

M. leprae is the causative agent of leprosy (Hansen's disease) in humans, a chronic, granulomatous disease primarily affecting the skin and peripheral nerves. Leprosy has also been reported in wild armadillos and nonhuman primates. *M. lepraemurium* is the etiologic agent of murine leprosy, a disease primarily affecting the skin and viscera of rats and mice.[54]

References

1. Zink AR, Sola C, Reischl U, et al. Characterization of *Mycobacterium tuberculosis* complex DNAs from Egyptian mummies by spoligotyping. *J Clin Microbiol*. 2003;41(1):359.
2. Konomi N, Lebwohl E, Mowbray K, et al. Detection of mycobacterial DNA in Andean mummies. *J Clin Microbiol*. 2002;40(12):4738.
3. Taylor GM, Murphy E, Hopkins R, et al. First report of *Mycobacterium bovis* DNA in human remains from the Iron Age. *Microbiology*. 2007;153(Pt 4):1243.
4. Taylor GM, Young D, Mays S. Genotyping analysis of the earliest known prehistoric case of tuberculosis in Britain. *J Clin Microbiol*. 2005;43(5):2236.
5. Rothschild BM, Martin LD. Did ice-age bovids spread tuberculosis? *Naturwissenschaften*. 2006;93(11):565.
6. World Health Organization (WHO). *Global tuberculosis control 2008: surveillance, planning, financing*. Geneva: WHO Press; 2008.
7. Schmitt S, Fitzgerald S, Cooley T, et al. Bovine tuberculosis in free-ranging white-tailed deer from Michigan. *J Wildl Dis*. 1997; 33(4):749.
8. Norby B, Bartlett PC, Fitzgerald SD, et al. The sensitivity of gross necropsy, caudal fold and comparative cervical tests for the diagnosis of bovine tuberculosis. *J Vet Diagn Invest*. 2004;16(2):126.
9. Bruning-Fann CS, Schmitt SM, Fitzgerald SD, et al. Bovine tuberculosis in free-ranging carnivores from Michigan. *J Wildl Dis*. 2001;37(1):58.
10. Brosch R, Pym AS, Gordon SV, et al. The evolution of mycobacterial pathogenicity: clues from comparative genomics. *Trends Microbiol*. 2001; 9(9):452.
11. Cole ST. Comparative and functional genomics of the *Mycobacterium tuberculosis* complex. *Microbiology*. 2002;148(Pt 10):2919.
12. Oh P, Granich R, Scott J, et al. Human exposure following *Mycobacterium tuberculosis* infection of multiple animal species in a metropolitan zoo. *Emerg Infect Dis*. 2002;8(11):1290.
13. Dalovisio JR, Stetter M, Mikota-Wells S. Rhinoceros' rhinorrhea: cause of an outbreak of infection due to airborne *Mycobacterium bovis* in zoo-keepers. *Clin Infect Dis*. 1992;15(4):598.
14. Michalak K, Austin C, Diesel S, et al. *Mycobacterium tuberculosis* infection as a zoonotic disease: transmission between humans and elephants. *Emerg Infect Dis*. 1998;4(2):283.
15. Michel AL. Implications of tuberculosis in African wildlife and livestock. *Ann N Y Acad Sci*. 2002;969:251.
16. Palmer MV. Tuberculosis: a reemerging disease at the interface of domestic animals and wildlife. *Curr Top Microbiol Immunol*. 2007;315:195.
17. Wilkins MJ, Bartlett PC, Frawley B, et al. *Mycobacterium bovis* (bovine TB) exposure as a recreational risk for hunters: results of a Michigan hunter survey. *Int J Tuberc Lung Dis*. 2003;7(10):1001.
18. Wilkins MJ, Meyerson J, Bartlett PC, et al. Human *Mycobacterium bovis* infection and bovine tuberculosis outbreak, Michigan, 1994–2007. *Emerg Infect Dis*. 2008;14(4):657.
19. Stewart GR, Robertson BD, Young DB. Tuberculosis: a problem with persistence. *Nat Rev Microbiol*. 2003;1(2):97.
20. Taylor Z, Nolan CM, Blumberg HM. Controlling tuberculosis in the United States: Recommendations from the American Thoracic Society, CDC, and the Infectious Diseases Society of America. *MMWR*. 2005;54(R-12):1.
21. Gutiérrez García JM. Milk as a vector of transmission of bovine tuberculosis to humans in Spain: a historical perspective. *Vet Herit*. 2006;29(2):41.
22. Hlavsa MC, Moonan PK, Cowan LS, et al. Human tuberculosis due to *Mycobacterium bovis* in the United States, 1995–2005. *Clin Infect Dis*. 2008;47(2):168.
23. O'Reilly LM, Daborn CJ. The epidemiology of *Mycobacterium bovis* infections in animals and man: a review. *Tuber Lung Dis*. 1995; 76(suppl 1):1.

24. Evans JT, Smith EG, Banerjee A, et al. Cluster of human tuberculosis caused by *Mycobacterium bovis:* evidence for person-to-person transmission in the UK. *Lancet.* 2007;369(9569):1270.

25. Rivero A, Márquez M, Santos J, et al. High rate of tuberculosis reinfection during a nosocomial outbreak of multidrug-resistant tuberculosis caused by *Mycobacterium bovis* strain B. *Clin Infect Dis.* 2001;32(1):159.

26. Michel AL, Huchzermeyer HF. The zoonotic importance of Mycobacterium tuberculosis: transmission from human to monkey. *J S Afr Vet Assoc.* 1998;69(2):64.

27. Ocepek M, Pate M, Zolnir-Dovc M, et al. Transmission of *Mycobacterium tuberculosis* from human to cattle. *J Clin Microbiol.* 2005;43(7):3555.

28. Hackendahl NC, Mawby DI, Bemis DA, et al. Putative transmission of *Mycobacterium tuberculosis* infection from a human to a dog. *J Am Vet Med Assoc.* 2004;225(10):1573–1577. 1548.

29. Erwin PC, Bemis DA, McCombs SB, et al. *Mycobacterium tuberculosis* transmission from human to canine. *Emerg Infect Dis.* 2004;10(12):2258.

30. Steinmetz HW, Rutz C, Hoop RK, et al. Possible human-avian transmission of *Mycobacterium tuberculosis* in a green-winged macaw *(Ara chloroptera). Avian Dis.* 2006;50(4):641.

31. Washko RM, Hoefer H, Kiehn TE, et al. *Mycobacterium tuberculosis* infection in a green-winged macaw *(Ara chloroptera)*: report with public health implications. *J Clin Microbiol.* 1998;36(4):1101.

32. Menzies FD, Neill SD. Cattle-to-cattle transmission of bovine tuberculosis. *Vet J.* 2000;160(2):92.

33. DeFranco AL, Locksley RM, Roberston M. *Immunity: the immune response to infectious and inflammatory disease.* New York: Oxford University Press; 2007.

34. World Organisation for Animal Health (OIE). *Manual of diagnostic tests and vaccines for terrestrial animals (OIE terrestrial manual).* 6th ed. Paris: World Organisation for Animal Health; 2008.

35. Lin PL, Yee J, Klein E, et al. Immunological concepts in tuberculosis diagnostics for non-human primates: a review. *J Med Primatol.* 2008;37(suppl 1):44.

36. United States Animal Health Association. *Report of the Committee on Tuberculosis,* 2007.

37. Jensen PA, Lambert LA, Iademarco MF, et al. Guidelines for preventing the transmission of *Mycobacterium tuberculosis* in health-care settings, 2005. *MMWR.* 2005;54(RR-17):1.

38. Mazurek GH, Jereb J, LoBue P, et al. Guidelines for using the QuantiFERON-TB Gold Test for detecting *Mycobacterium tuberculosis* infection, United States. *MMWR.* 2005;54(RR-15):49.

39. World Organisation for Animal Health (OIE). *Terrestrial animal health code.* 17th ed. Paris: World Organisation for Animal Health; 2008.

40. Cousins DV, Florisson N. A review of tests available for use in the diagnosis of tuberculosis in non-bovine species. *Rev Sci Tech.* 2005;24(3):1039.

41. Blumberg HM, Leonard Jr MK, Jasmer RM. Update on the treatment of tuberculosis and latent tuberculosis infection. *JAMA.* 2005;293(22):2776.

42. Maslow JN, Mikota SK, Zhu M, et al. Population pharmacokinetics of isoniazid in the treatment of *Mycobacterium tuberculosis* among Asian and African elephants (*Elephas maximus* and *Loxodonta africana*). *J Vet Pharmacol Ther.* 2005;28(1):1.

43. Maslow JN, Mikota SK, Zhu M, et al. Pharmacokinetics of ethambutol (EMB) in elephants. *J Vet Pharmacol Ther.* 2005;28(3):321.

44. Zhu M, Maslow JN, Mikota SK, et al. Population pharmacokinetics of pyrazinamide in elephants. *J Vet Pharmacol Ther.* 2005;28(5):403.

45. Peloquin CA, Maslow JN, Mikota SK, et al. Dose selection and pharmacokinetics of rifampin in elephants for the treatment of tuberculosis. *J Vet Pharmacol Ther.* 2006;29(6):1.

46. Primm TP, Lucero CA, Falkinham 3rd JO. Health impacts of environmental mycobacteria. *Clin Microbiol Rev.* 2004;17(1):98.

47. Falkinham JO. The changing pattern of nontuberculous mycobacterial disease. *Can J Infect Dis.* 2003;14(5):281.

48. Griffith DE, Aksamit T, Brown-Elliott BA, et al. An official ATS/IDSA statement: diagnosis, treatment, and prevention of nontuberculous mycobacterial diseases. *Am J Respir Crit Care Med.* 2007;175(4):367.

49. Katoch VM. Infections due to non-tuberculous mycobacteria (NTM). *Indian J Med Res.* 2004;120(4):290.

50. Portaels F, Chemlal K, Elsen P, et al. *Mycobacterium ulcerans* in wild animals. *Rev Sci Tech.* 2001;20(1):252.

51. Rosenthal KL. *Aspergillus* and mycobacteria diagnostics. In: *Small animal and exotics. Proceedings of the North American Veterinary Conference, volume 20,* Orlando, Florida, USA, 7–11 January, 2006. 1580.

52. Tell LA, Foley J, Needham ML. Diagnosis of avian mycobacteriosis: comparison of culture, acid-fast stains, and polymerase chain reaction for the identification of *Mycobacterium avium* in experimentally inoculated Japanese quail (*Coturnix coturnix japonica*). *Avian Dis.* 2003;47(2): 444.

53. Thorel MF, Huchzermeyer HF, Michel AL. *Mycobacterium avium* and *Mycobacterium intracellulare* infection in mammals. *Rev Sci Tech.* 2001;20(1):204.

54. Rojas-Espinosa O, Løvik M. *Mycobacterium leprae* and *Mycobacterium lepraemurium* infections in domestic and wild animals. *Rev Sci Tech.* 2001;20(1):219.

TULAREMIA

Peter M. Rabinowitz and Lisa A. Conti

Tularemia (ICD-10 A21)

Other names in humans: rabbit fever, Francis disease, deer-fly fever, Ohara's disease, market men's disease

Other names in animals: rabbit fever, deerfly fever

Francisella tularensis causes an acute febrile illness in humans and other animals that can be fatal. The incidence of tularemia has decreased in the United States since the first half of the twentieth century.[1] However, sporadic outbreaks continue to occur, and the disease has emerged in regions where it previously had not been recognized. Moreover, its widespread occurrence in wildlife and arthropod vectors, its ability to persist in water and soils, and its high infectiousness for both humans and domestic animals make it both a high-priority biological terrorism agent as well as a zoonotic pathogen with potential to cause significant health effects in human and animal populations.

Key Points for Clinicians and Public Health Professionals

Public Health Professionals

- Provide epidemiological analysis of this reportable disease.
- Educate the public to avoid tick, fly, and mosquito bites by using appropriate clothing and repellents.
- Educate hunters to use puncture-resistant gloves when skinning or handling game, especially rabbits, and to cook wild meat thoroughly.
- The CDC recommends that laboratory personnel be alerted when tularemia is suspected. Diagnostic

procedures involving tularemia should be performed in at least biosafety level 2 conditions. Examining suspected cultures should be done in a biological safety cabinet. Procedures that could produce aerosols or droplets require biosafety level 3 conditions.[2]

- Disinfect with 1% sodium hypochlorite, 70% ethanol, and glutaraldehyde.
- Consider the possibility of bioterrorism in the event of a cluster of unexplained cases.

Human Health Clinicians

- Report disease to public health authorities using the case definition; see http://www.cdc.gov/ncphi/disss/nndss/casedef/tularemia_current.htm.
- Consider the diagnosis in persons presenting with acute onset of fever and exposure to ticks or animals.
- Inquire about occupational risk factors for infection and ensure that workers at risk take precautions.
- Ensure that any laboratory workers handling strains of tularemia virulent to humans are using biosafety level 3 precautions.[3]
- Provide PEP following aerosol exposure.
- A vaccine for tularemia is under review by the FDA but is not currently available in the United States.[4]

Veterinary Clinicians

- In many states tularemia in horses is a reportable disease to the state veterinarian. Disease in cats and dogs may be reportable to public health authorities.
- In endemic areas, counsel owners to neuter cats to prevent roaming and keep cats indoors.
- Treat dogs, cats, and horses for ectoparasites.
- Ensure policies are in place to isolate suspected cases and for veterinary staff to use protective equipment and extreme care in handling infected animals, carcasses, or tissues.
- Treat early if tularemia is suspected; otherwise, prognosis is poor.

Agent

Francisella tularensis is a small, gram-negative intracellular coccobacillus. Two major subspecies are recognized with different biochemical and pathological characteristics: *F. tularensis tularensis* and *F. tularensis holarctica*. *F. tularensis* subspecies *tularensis* (Jellison type A) is considered to have higher virulence, with human case fatality rates between 5% and 15% without treatment and a median lethal dose (LD_{50}) in rabbits of 1 to 10 organisms. *F. tularensis* subspecies *holarctica* (Jellison type B) has a lower infectivity (LD_{50} >10^6 organisms in rabbits) and rarely causes human fatalities.[5] Recently type A isolates in the United States have been further divided, using molecular techniques, into type A-East and type A-West, with type A-West less virulent than either type A-East or type B.[6] Viable organisms can be found for months in fomites or the carcasses or hides of infected animals and years in frozen infected meat. The organism can be disinfected with 1% hypochlorite, 70% ethanol, glutaraldehyde, or formaldehyde or inactivated by moist heat (121°C for at least 15 minutes) and dry heat (160-170°C for at least 1 hour).[7]

Geographical Occurrence

Tularemia is a disease of the Northern Hemisphere. Historically, the highest prevalence has been recorded in the United States and Russia. However, in both countries the prevalence has declined significantly since World War II. In the United States, the incidence peaked in 1939 with 2291 reported cases; in recent decades the average number of U.S. cases has been less than 200 annually.[1] Most cases occur in the south-central and western states, including Missouri, Alaska, Oklahoma, South Dakota, Tennessee, Kansas, Colorado, Illinois, Utah, and Montana.[8] The two major pathogenic strains vary in their geographical distribution. *F.* subspecies *tularensis* is primarily confined to North America, although isolation of strains resembling *F. tularensis* subspecies *tularensis* has recently been reported in Europe.[9] *F. tularensis holarctica* is also found in North America but to a lesser extent. By contrast, it is the predominant strain in Europe and Northern Asia. A third strain, *F. tularensis* subspecies *mediasiatica*, is found in central Asia.

Groups at Risk

In the United States, higher attack rates occur in children aged 5 to 9 years and individuals 75 years or older. Native Americans/Alaskan natives have an incidence of 0.5 per 100,000, 10 times the rate in whites (0.04/100,000). It is thought that the higher rates in children reflect exposure risk due to tick and other insect bites, whereas the increased risk in Native Americans may be related to increased exposure. High rates of infection in ticks and dogs have been found in reservations reporting human outbreaks.[1]

Other risk groups include farmers, landscapers (especially those engaged in mowing lawns[10]), and hunters who may encounter carcasses of infected rabbits or other animals. Cat ownership has been reported as a risk factor for infection in areas experiencing outbreaks.[11] Veterinarians and wildlife rehabilitators may be at risk through handling sick animals. Laboratory workers are also at risk because of the infectiousness of the organism.

Hosts, Reservoir Species, Vectors

Tularemia is found in more than 250 species of mammal, birds, reptiles, and fish.[8] Aquatic animals have developed tularemia after being immersed in contaminated water Different species vary in their susceptibility to the disease. In the United States, cottontail rabbits (*Sylvilagus* species) as well as jackrabbits, beaver, moles, squirrels, muskrat, meadow voles, and sheep are prone to the disease, which is often fatal.

Cats are at increased risk because of their predatory habits. A serological survey found evidence of past infection in 24% of cats tested in Connecticut and New York, suggesting that the disease in cats may be more common than often recognized.[12]

Tularemia is found in a number of vector species, including several species of tick, deer flies, mites, lice, midges, fleas, bedbugs, and mosquitoes. Vector-transmitted infections are believed to account for the majority of human and other animal cases in the United States. Recognized vectors in the United States include the wood tick *(Dermacentor andersoni),* dog tick *(D. variabilis),* lone star tick *(Amblystoma americanum),* and the deer fly *(Chrysops discalis).*[8] Flies can carry *Francisella* for 2 weeks and ticks may be infected throughout their lifespan.

Mode of Transmission and Life Cycle

Animal-to-animal and animal-to-human transmission of tularemia appears to take place through a variety of mechanisms, including direct inoculation through a bite from an infected arthropod vector, a bite or scratch or conjunctival contact from an infected animal, inhalation of aerosols containing organisms, and ingestion of contaminated food or water (Figure 9-158). Human-to-human transmission has not been reported. The mode of transmission helps determine the clinical form of the disease.

In the United States, the most common form of the disease is the ulceroglandular type, which develops after a vector bite (usually a tick or fly) and consists of an ulcer at the site of the bite with associated lymphadenopathy and fever. Direct handling of infected carcasses (especially rabbits) can also result in this form of infection. Less commonly, the inhalation of organisms results in primary pneumonic tularemia. Contact with mucous membranes of a susceptible host causes the oculoglandular form of the disease. Ingestion of contaminated meat or water can cause a typhoidal form of the disease characterized by fever and nonspecific GI symptoms, including diarrhea.[13]

Although rare, there are cases of humans developing infection from contact with infected cats and dogs. Exposure risk factors include cat bites[14] and being licked by an infected dog.[15]

Environmental Risk Factors

F. tularensis can survive for months in water and sediment. A number of human outbreaks have occurred next to bodies of water, including one associated with crayfish fishing.[16]

In an outbreak of pneumonic tularemia in Martha's Vineyard, skunks and raccoons were found to frequently be seroreactive, raising the possibility of peridomestic environmental contamination by feces; however, this has not been confirmed as the source of illness.[17] Another environmental factor is the changing conditions that can lead to increases in rodent populations; outbreaks have been associated with increases in populations of rodents. Intentional introduction of game animals such as hares into new geographical areas for hunting has lead to outbreaks in Spain, where it had not been previously reported.[18]

Disease in Humans

Tularemia causes an acute febrile disease that usually begins 3 to 5 days after exposure. Although most cases are charac-

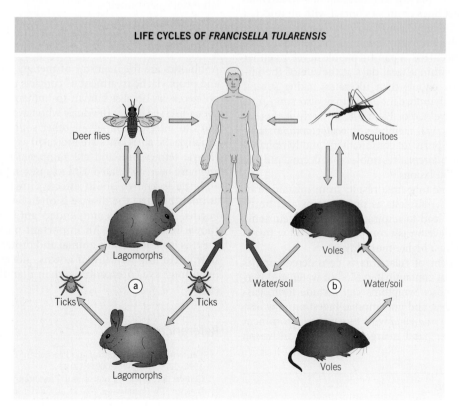

Figure 9-158 ■ Life cycles of *Francisella tularensis.* (From Cohen J, Powderly WG: *Infectious diseases,* ed 2, Philadelphia, 2004, Mosby Elsevier.)

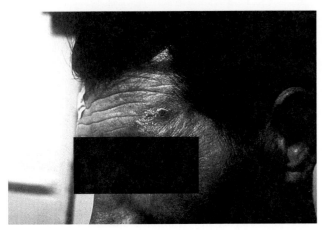

Figure 9-159 ■ This Vermont muskrat trapper contracted tularemia, which manifested as a cutaneous lesion on his left lateral forehead. (From Centers for Disease Control and Prevention Public Health Image Library, Atlanta, Ga.)

terized by the abrupt onset of fever, chills, fatigue, myalgia, headache, and nausea, several distinct forms of the disease are related to the mode of transmission and the virulence of the organism. Infection caused *F. tularensis* subspecies *tularensis* may progress to septicemia, with disseminated intravascular coagulation, acute respiratory distress syndrome, CNS involvement, and multiorgan failure. Disease related to *F. tularensis* subspecies *holarctica* is more likely to produce mild symptoms with a low case fatality rate.

Most cases (87%)[19] present as *ulceroglandular tularemia*, resulting from insect bites or direct contact with an infected carcass (Figure 9-159 and Color Plate 9-81). One of the first symptoms is lymphadenopathy localized in the area where the bite or scratch occurred. A painful papule develops either simultaneously or within several days at the site of the initial skin entry. This papule then ulcerates, taking several weeks to heal.[5] The lymphadenopathy may also suppurate and become ulcerative (Color Plate 9-82). Rarely, if there is contact with conjunctival membranes, *oculoglandular tularemia* develops, with purulent conjunctivitis and lymphadenopathy. *Glandular tularemia* resembles the ulceroglandular form but without skin lesions.[19]

Primary pneumonic tularemia results from inhalation of infected aerosols and manifests as pneumonitis and bronchiolitis, which may lead to respiratory failure. Pneumonic tularemia may also develop as a complication of other forms and is associated with a higher mortality rate.[19]

The *typhoidal* form of tularemia is considered rare, is caused by ingestion of contaminated food or water, and may be difficult to diagnose. Symptoms can include fever, gastroenteritis, septicemia, and pneumonia. Ingestion may also lead to *oropharyngeal tularemia* with throat pain, prominent pharyngitis, oral ulcers, and enlargement of cervical lymph nodes.

Disease in Animals

Susceptibility to *F. tularensis* infection varies among animal species. Rabbits and many rodents develop fatal disease. Sheep also have high mortality rates.

Cats can develop an acute febrile syndrome caused by tularemia that can be fatal (Color Plate 9-83). Ulceroglandular disease in cats has also been reported.[20] Dogs appear to be more resistant and likely to develop asymptomatic infection. However, fever, anorexia, and lethargy have been reported in a dog that ate an infected rabbit.[21]

Horses can develop a febrile infection associated with impaired coordination and depression.[22] Cattle appear to be resistant. Table 9-73 compares clinical presentations of tularemia in humans and other animals.

Diagnosis

Diagnosis in humans is usually based on clinical signs and confirmed by serological studies showing at least a fourfold rise in titer that occurs 2 weeks after the onset of illness. A direct immunofluorescence test and/or PCR test may be available for rapid diagnosis.

Culture of body fluids should be performed only in reference laboratories because of risk of infection to laboratory personnel. Lymph nodes should not be biopsied unless antibiotics have already been started because of the risk of inducing bacteremia.[5]

In other animals, a direct antibody or IFA assay (Color Plate 9-84) is considered the most rapid and accurate means of diagnosis[15]; an immunohistochemical analysis for formalin-fixed tissue has also been developed. Serology is used if the animal survives, with a fourfold titer difference between acute and convalescent titers confirming infection. Culture of the bacterium can be performed but poses a health risk for laboratory personnel.

Treatment

Antibiotics are the mainstay of therapy. Isolation of patients and prophylactic treatment of contacts of human patient are not necessary because human-to-human transmission has not been observed. For individuals who have had high-risk exposures to infected animals or other sources of the organism, prophylactic antibiotics are indicated as shown in Table 9-74. (NOTE: tetracycline and chloramphenicol are bacteriostatic and have been associated with relapses in humans).

Little is known about effective treatment regimens in animals because the disease is often fatal before treatment begins. However, recommended antibiotic regimens are shown in Table 9-74. An important part of animal treatment is isolation of the animal and protection of veterinary staff, including wearing of gowns, gloves, and face masks, including eye protection, when handling a suspected case.[15]

References

1. Centers for Disease Control and Prevention. Tularemia—United States, 1990–2000. *MMWR.* 2002;51(9):182.
2. Centers for Disease Control and Prevention: Abstract of Dennis DT, Inglesby TV, Henderson DA, et al. Consensus statement: tularemia as a biological weapon: medical and public health management. *JAMA.* 2001;285(21):2763.
3. Titball RW, Sjostedt A, Pavelka Jr MS, et al. Biosafety and selectable markers. *Ann N Y Acad Sci.* 2007;1105:405.

Table 9-73 ▪ Tularemia: Comparative Clinical Presentations in Humans and Other Animals

Species	Risk Factors	Incubation Period	Clinical Manifestations	Laboratory Findings
Humans	Children, Native Americans, hunters, landscapers, others with wildlife contact	Usually 3-5 days (range, 1-14)[5]	Fever, lymphadenopathy, fatigue, pneumonia Ulceroglandular form: ulcer at site of entry Glandular form Primary pneumonic form Oropharyngeal form Typhoidal form	Positive serology, direct immunofluorescence
Cats, dogs	Outdoor/hunting cats Tick and other insect bites Dogs more resistant than cats	2-7 days[15]	Fever, anorexia, lethargy, lymphadenopathy, hepatosplenomegaly Ulcers in mouth, pseudomembrane on tongue[15] Mucous membranes icteric	Pan leukopenia, leukocytosis, elevated liver function tests DFA of tissues, serology, blood culture
Sheep	Tick exposures	1-10 days[8]	Fever, septicemia, rigid gait, diarrhea, urination, respiratory distress, death[22]	
Swine	Tick exposures	1-10 days[8]	*Adults fairly resistant:* fever, shortness of breath, depression[22] *Young animals:* lack of coordination, depression, anorexia, neurological signs	
Rabbits	Very susceptible	1-10 days[8]	Depression, anorexia, ataxia, roughened coat, tendency to huddle, weakness, fever, ulcers, abscesses at site of infection, dyspnea, swelling of regional lymph nodes, sudden death Usually not recognized until dead or dying	
Horses	Tick exposure (rare)	1-10 days[8]	Lack of coordination, fever, depression, dyspnea	

DFA, Direct immunofluorescence antibody.

Table 9-74 ▪ Antibiotic Treatment of Tularemia Infection in Humans and Other Animals

Species	Primary Treatment	Alternative Treatment
Humans (adult)		
Inhalational	Streptomycin 15 mg/kg IV bid *or* gentamicin 5 mg/kg IV qd × 10 days	Doxycycline 100 mg PO or IV bid × 14-21 days *or* ciprofloxacin 400 mg IV (or 750 mg PO) bid × 14-21 days[24]
Typhoidal	Gentamicin or tobramycin 5 mg/kg/day divided q8h IV × 7-14 days	Add chloramphenicol if evidence of meningitis[24]
Postexposure prophylaxis: adult	Doxycycline 100 mg PO bid × 14 days	Ciprofloxacin 500 mg PO bid × 14 days
Cats, dogs (early treatment is critical)	Amoxicillin 20 mg/kg IM or SC q12h or PO q8h *PLUS* gentamicin 4.4 mg/kg IM or SC q12h once, then q24h thereafter until clinical response or until 7 days	Enrofloxacin 10-15 mg/kg PO, IM, IV, or SC q12h[15]
Sheep	Streptomycin or gentamicin	Chloramphenicol 25 mg/kg IV qid *or* tetracyclines[8]

4. Centers for Disease Control and Prevention. *Key facts about tularemia.* http://www.cdc.gov/ncidod/dvbid/tularemia.htm.

5. Heymann DL, ed. *Control of communicable diseases manual.* 19th ed. Washington, DC: American Public Health Association; 2008.

6. Staples JE, Kubota KA, Chalcraft LG, et al. Epidemiologic and molecular analysis of human tularemia, United States, 1964–2004. *Emerg Infect Dis.* 2006;12(7):1113.

7. Center for Food Security and Public Health, Iowa State University. *Tularemia.* http://www.cfsph.iastate.edu/Factsheets/pdfs/Tularemia.pdf. Accessed April 6, 2009.

8. Kahn CM, Line S, eds. *The Merck veterinary manual.* 9th ed. Whitehouse Station, NJ: Merck; 2005.

9. Gurycova D. First isolation of *Francisella tularensis* subsp. *tularensis* in Europe. *Eur J Epidemiol.* 1998;14(8):797.

10. Feldman KA, Stiles-Enos D, Julian K, et al. Tularemia on Martha's Vineyard: seroprevalence and occupational risk. *Emerg Infect Dis.* 2003; 9(3):350.

11. Eliasson H, Lindback J, Nuorti JP, et al. The 2000 tularemia outbreak: a case-control study of risk factors in disease-endemic and emergent areas, Sweden. *Emerg Infect Dis.* 2002;8(9):956.

12. Magnarelli L, Levy S, Koski R. Detection of antibodies to *Francisella* tularensis in cats. *Res Vet Sci.* 2007;82(1):22.

13. Greco D, Allegrini G, Tizzi T, et al. A waterborne tularemia outbreak. *Eur J Epidemiol.* 1987;3(1):35.

14. Arav-Boger R. Cat-bite tularemia in a seventeen-year-old girl treated with ciprofloxacin. *Pediatr Infect Dis J.* 2000;19(6):583.

15. Barr SC, Bowman DD. *The 5-minute veterinary consult clinical companion: canine and feline infectious diseases and parasitology.* Ames, IA: Blackwell; 2006.

16. Anda P, Segura del Pozo J, Diaz Garcia JM, et al. Waterborne outbreak of tularemia associated with crayfish fishing. *Emerg Infect Dis.* 2001;7(suppl 3):575.

17. Matyas BT, Nieder HS, Telford SR 3rd. Pneumonic tularemia on Martha's Vineyard: clinical, epidemiologic, and ecological characteristics. *Ann N Y Acad Sci.* 2007;1105:351.

18. Andres Puertas C, Mateos Baruque ML, Buron Lobo I, et al. Epidemic outbreak of tularemia in Palencia [in Spanish]. *Rev Clin Esp.* 1999;199(11):711.

19. Mandell GL, Bennett JE, Dolin R, eds. *Principles and practice of infectious diseases.* 6th ed. New York: Churchill Livingstone Elsevier; 2005.

20. Valentine BA, DeBey BM, Sonn RJ, et al. Localized cutaneous infection with *Francisella tularensis* resembling ulceroglandular tularemia in a cat. *J Vet Diagn Invest.* 2004;16(1):83.

21. Meinkoth KR, Morton RJ, Meinkoth JH. Naturally occurring tularemia in a dog. *J Am Vet Med Assoc.* 2004;225(4):545–547 538.

22. Acha PN, Szyfres B. *Zoonoses and communicable diseases common to man and animals: vol. I: bacterioses and mycoses.* 3rd ed. Washington, DC: Pan American Health Organization; 2001.

23. Kwan-Gett TS, Kemp C, Kovarik C. *Infectious and tropical diseases: a handbook for primary care.* St Louis: Mosby Elsevier; 2005.

24. Gilbert DN, Moellering RC, Eliopoulos GM, et al. *Sanford guide to antimicrobial therapy 2009.* 39th ed. Sperryville, VA: Antimicrobial Therapy; 2009.

WEST NILE VIRUS AND OTHER ARBOVIRUS INFECTIONS

Carina Blackmore

West Nile virus infection (ICD-10 A92.3)

Other names in humans: West Nile fever, West Nile meningitis, West Nile encephalitis, West Nile poliomyelitis

Other names in animals: West Nile virus infection

West Nile virus (WNV) was first isolated from a febrile woman in Uganda in 1937.[1] The first human disease outbreak occurred 20 years later in Israel. The virus was first detected in the Americas in 1999 by a veterinary pathologist when a flavivirus was identified as the cause of an apparent zoonotic encephalitis outbreak in humans and corvid birds (e.g., crows and jays) in Queens, New York. WNV has since become the most important cause of mosquito-borne disease in North America. It spread across the 48 continental United States in 6 years, and more than 27,000 human cases and 25,000 horse cases of WNV disease were reported during the period 1999 to 2007. Outbreaks of human or equine WNV encephalitis have also occurred in southern Europe, Israel, the Democratic Republic of the Congo, and Russia. WNV is an example of a disease where tracking sentinel cases in birds,[2] horses, dogs,[3] and other animals, as well as WNV positive pools of mosquitoes, has proved useful for efforts aimed at early detection and prevention of human cases.

Several zoonotic arthropod-borne (arboviral) diseases are known to circulate within the United States, including St. Louis encephalitis (SLE), Eastern equine encephalitis (EEE), La Crosse encephalitis (LAC) and Western equine encephalitis (WEE). These arboviruses may have different vector and vertebrate hosts than WNV but many of the guidances discussed below are relevant for prevention of and control of them all. They are also relevant for potentially emerging zoonotic arboviruses such as Rift Valley Fever virus.

Key Points for Clinicians and Public Health Professionals

Public Health Professionals

- Recommend to the public:
  - Do not go outdoors at dusk and dawn when mosquitoes are most active.
  - Empty containers and drain stagnant waters where mosquitoes lay their eggs.
  - Install or repair window and door screens.
  - Dress so skin is covered with clothing.
  - Stock ornamental ponds with mosquito-eating fish.
  - Maintain pools.
  - Protect bare skin and clothing with a mosquito repellent. Make certain the repellent is used according to its label. Do not use repellents over cuts, wounds, or irritated skin. Do not use repellent under clothing.
- DEET (*N,N*-diethyl-3-methylbenzamide)[4] and picaridin[5] are effective repellents registered for skin application by the EPA. Depending on the duration of protection desired, products containing 4.75% DEET provide roughly 90 minutes' effectiveness; products containing 23.8% DEET provide an average of 5 hours of protection.[6]
- Among plant-based repellents registered with the EPA, oil of lemon eucalyptus provides longer-lasting protection than others, with an efficacy similar to a

repellent with low concentrations of DEET. Repellents can be reapplied according to the manufacturer's instructions.

- Sunscreen and insect repellent can be applied simultaneously. However, it is not recommended to use a product combining sunscreen and repellents as sunscreen often needs to be applied more frequently and repeated application may increase the toxic effects of the repellent.
- Permethrin, a pyrethroid product, is an effective repellent registered for application on clothing, camping gear, or mosquito nets.
- Safety precautions when using repellents on children:
  o Keep repellents out of the reach of children.
  o Do not allow young children to apply insect repellent to themselves; have an adult do it for them.
  o Apply the repellent to your own hands and then rub them on the child. Avoid children's eyes and mouth and use it sparingly around their ears.
  o Do not apply repellent to children's hands as children may tend to put their hands in their mouths.
  o Wash treated skin with soap and water after returning indoors and wash treated clothing.
  o The American Academy of Pediatrics does not recommend repellents be used on children younger than 2 months. Instead, they recommend the use of mosquito netting over infant carriers. Oil of lemon eucalyptus products should not be used on children younger than 3 years.
- Determine and implement the most appropriate surveillance methods for WNV risk in your region, considering possible use of mosquito, bird, or mammal sentinel information, as well as climate tracking (Color Plates 9-85 and 9-86).

Human Health Clinicians

- In suspected cases, submit serum and/or CSF for WNV antibody testing.
- Monitor public health surveillance on human WNV disease in the local area, including surveillance of sentinel animals, to estimate current human health risk.
- Counsel all patients, especially adults older than 50 years and families with infants, to avoid being bitten by mosquitoes, including the appropriate use of repellents and mosquito netting.
- Report cases to the health department if required in the state per recommended case definition.

Veterinary Clinicians

- Advise horse owners on how to prevent equine WNV disease. Horses should be protected from mosquito bites. This can be done by eliminating mosquito breeding sites, providing screened housing, and applying insect repellents.
- Vaccinate horses against WNV disease. There are three licensed WNV vaccines currently available: an inactivated whole virus vaccine, a live recombinant canary pox vector vaccine, and a modified live chimera vaccine. The American Association of Equine Practitioners

provides the following guidance on WNV vaccination of horses[7]: Primary vaccination of previously unvaccinated horses with either the inactivated or canary pox vector vaccine involves administration of 2 doses of vaccine 4 to 6 weeks apart followed by revaccination at a 12-month interval. Label instructions for the modified live chimera vaccine recommend a single injection followed by a 12-month revaccination interval. More frequent boosters may be warranted for juvenile (<5 years) or geriatric (>15 years) horses. Although the licensed WNV vaccines are currently not labeled for administration to pregnant mares, many veterinary practitioners do administer them to pregnant mares. Booster vaccination of pregnant mares 4 to 6 weeks before foaling provides passive, colostral protection to their foals. To avoid interference from colostral antibodies, primary vaccination of foals from vaccinated mares should be started at 4 to 6 months of age. Foals should receive a third dose in the spring of the year following their birth. Foals of unvaccinated mares should ideally receive two doses of vaccine before the mosquito-borne disease season starting at 3 months of age. The modified live flavivirus chimera vaccine is labeled for foals 5 months or older. A single dose should be administered followed by a second dose at 10 to 12 months of age (before the next WNV season).
- Prevent dogs and cats from eating birds and other wildlife.
- Maintain barrier precautions when performing necropsies, particularly on birds.
- Related flaviviruses are destroyed by 1% sodium hypochlorite, 2% glutaraldehyde, and 70% ethanol.[8]

▌ Agent

WNV is part of the Flaviviridae family in the genus *Flavivirus* (Figure 9-160). Flaviviruses are small (40 to 60 nm), lipid-enveloped RNA viruses containing a single positive-strand genomic RNA. The lipid surface contains the viral envelope (E) and membrane (M) "spike" proteins. WNV and SLE virus are closely related and both are members of the

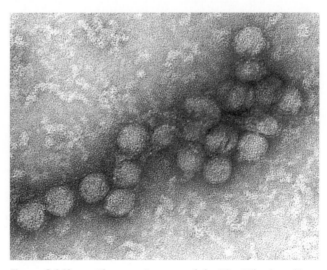

Figure 9-160 ▪ Electron microscopy of the West Nile virus. (From Auerbach PS: *Wilderness medicine*, ed 5, Philadelphia, 2007, Mosby Elsevier.)

Japanese encephalitis antigenic serocomplex.[1] More distantly related mosquito-borne flaviviruses in the Americas include yellow fever and Dengue virus.

Geographical Occurrence

WNV was first identified in Uganda in 1937. It is now endemic in parts of Africa, Europe, Australia, and Asia as well as North, Central, and South America.[9,10]

Groups at Risk

WNV is transmitted by mosquito bite, and persons in all age groups are at risk of infection. In areas where WNV is hyperendemic, it is a mild, common childhood illness.[11] In industrialized temperate areas the incidence of neuroinvasive WNV disease and death increases in those who are immunosuppressed or 50 years and older.[11,12] The risk for WNV meningitis and encephalitis is also slightly higher among males than females.

Hosts, Reservoir Species, Vectors

WNV is a mosquito-borne virus. The enzootic cycle involves transmission of the virus among infected *Culex* mosquitoes and wild birds (Figure 9-161). Many bird species can become infected by WNV, although only a small proportion are likely to be important reservoir hosts. Passerine birds (crows, jays, finches, grackles, sparrows) are thought to play a role in the WNV transmission cycle. They are common, widespread, and develop a high and prolonged viremia,[13] all important features for a vertebrate reservoir host. Humans, horses, and other mammals are incidental hosts of the virus.

Mode of Transmission and Life Cycle

WNV is maintained in nature by mosquitoes and wild birds (Figure 9-162). The overwintering mechanisms of the virus are not fully understood; however, overwintering adult mosquitoes are thought to play a role.[14] Human and other mammals are incidental hosts of the virus. Non-mosquito-borne transmission such as transplacental infection, breastfeeding, blood transfusion, and organ transplantation have also been documented.[15] Fecal-oral transmission has been reported among animals including alligators, cats, some raptors, hamsters, and golden crows.[16]

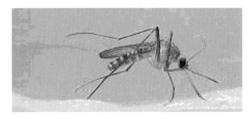

Figure 9-161 ■ *Culex* mosquito. (From Florida Medical Entomology Laboratory, Michelle Cutwa-Francis, photographer.)

West Nile Virus Transmission Cycle

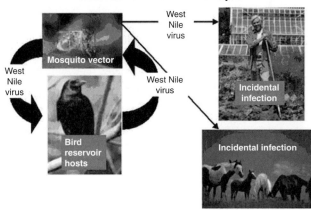

Figure 9-162 ■ West Nile virus transmission cycle. (From Centers for Disease Control and Prevention: *Flowchart: West Nile virus transmission cycle.* http://www.cdc.gov/ncidod/dvbid/westnile/cycle.htm.)

Environmental Risk Factors

Virus amplification and transmission are favored by warm temperatures, and the peak virus activity occurs in the late summer months. Different vectors prefer different breeding habitats. The *Culex pipiens* species breed in stagnant pools of groundwater, artificial containers, catch basins, or sewage seepage. They prefer to breed in highly organic (polluted) water. *Culex tarsalis*, the most important WNV vector in the western United States, tolerates a wide range of habitats but prefers permanent or semipermanent seepage areas and surface pools associated with irrigated pastures. *Culex nigripalpus,* a principle WNV vector in the Southeast, is a floodwater mosquito.

Disease in Humans

Most individuals infected with WNV (80%) remain asymptomatic.[17] The clinical presentation ranges from a mild nonneuroinvasive fever illness to encephalitis, coma, and death (Table 9-75). It is estimated that fewer than 1% of infected persons develop severe neurological disease. Typical symptoms of West Nile fever include fatigue, fever, headache, and muscle weakness. Half of the persons interviewed in a survey among West Nile fever patients in Chicago also had difficulty concentrating.[18] More severe clinical syndromes include aseptic meningitis, myelitis, polyradiculitis, and encephalitis. Patients often present with a prodrome of fever, headache, and other nonspecific symptoms. Many develop movement disorders such as severe tremors and parkinsonism.[19]

Disease in Animals

Horses infected with WNV may develop fever, depression or apprehension, stupor, behavioral changes, intermittent lameness, ataxia, caudal paralysis, droopy lip, teeth grinding, muscle twitching, tremors, difficulty rising, recumbency, convulsions, and death.[20,21] In one study, approximately 33% of horses with clinical signs of WNV infection died from the disease.

Clinical signs of WNV infection in birds vary greatly among species. Many avian species develop clinically

Table 9-75 ▪ West Nile Virus Infection: Comparative Clinical Presentations in Humans and Other Animals

Species	Risk Factors	Incubation Period	Clinical Manifestations	Laboratory Findings
Humans	Mosquito exposure, age, immunosuppression after organ transplantation, and male gender are risk factors for severe illness[19] Other risk factors include receiving blood transfusions or organ donations, and occupational exposure Infants may become infected by maternal infection during pregnancy or breastfeeding	3-14 days[18]	Fever, headache, muscle pain, weakness, fatigue, ocular pain, malaise, anorexia, maculopapular or morbilliform rash on neck, trunk, and extremities 5-12 days after onset[18,19] *Neuroinvasive disease:* ataxia and extrapyramidal signs, optic neuritis, seizures, tremor, myoclonus, parkinsonism and altered mental status[12,27] Rash, polyradiculitis, and acute asymmetric poliomyelitis like flaccid paralysis are seen in a small number of patients.[19,28]	*CSF:* Specific WNV IgM antibodies, lymphocytic pleocytosis, elevated protein, normal glucose *Blood:* Specific WNV IgM or IgM and IgG antibodies in serum Peripheral blood total leukocyte count normal or elevated, anemia, and lymphocytopenia Brain magnetic resonance imaging results often normal Signal abnormalities may be detected in the basal ganglia, thalamus, and brainstem of patients with encephalitis and in the anterior spinal cord in patients with flaccid paralysis[19] Virus detection in CSF or tissues is also possible
Horses	Mosquito exposure	3-15 days	Fever, depression or apprehension, stupor, behavioral changes, intermittent lameness, knuckling over at the metacarpo- or metatarsophalangeal joints, ataxia, caudal paralysis, droopy lip, teeth grinding, muscle twitching, fasciculations and tremors, difficulty rising, recumbency, convulsions, blindness, and colic or death[16,20,21]	Fourfold rise in WNV serum antibody, positive IgM ELISA antibody test in serum or CSF Antigen detection in brain tissue using viral culture, PCR, or immunohistochemistry
Birds	Mosquito exposure Possible contact with other birds or their excretions Possible exposure from predation on other infected birds/mammals	Unknown	Signs of WNV neurological disease include sudden onset of mild ataxia, abnormal head posture, circling, reclining, quadriparesis, and tremors; nystagmus, seizures, disorientation, signs of depression, anorexia, weight loss, impaired vision, and sudden death may also be present.[16,23]	WNV detection in brain, heart, kidney or liver tissue Fourfold rise in WNV antibody titer Rapid screening tests on oral or cloacal swabs, swabs of organ tissue, or feather pulp
Dogs, cats	Allowed to roam outdoors, stray animals	Unknown[22]	Usually asymptomatic, fever, lethargy reported in cats, encephalitis, arthritis, myocarditis in dogs	Serology, PCR

CSF, Cerebrospinal fluid.

inapparent infections, whereas others become severely ill and succumb to the virus. Signs of WNV neurological disease include sudden onset of mild ataxia, abnormal head posture, circling, reclination, quadriparesis, and tremors. Nystagmus, seizures, disorientation, signs of depression, weight loss, impaired vision, and sudden death may also be present.[9,23] Birds shed virus orally and in their feces, and bird-to-bird transmission has been reported.[9,24] Gross pathology often includes an enlarged, necrotic, and hem-

orrhaging liver and spleen, myocardial degeneration and inflammation, pericardial lesions, pancreatitis, and chronic adrenalitis.

Dogs and cats appear to be relatively resistant to WNV and generally develop subclinical disease after exposure. Acute encephalitis, polyarthritis, and myocarditis have been reported in dogs.[22] Fever and lethargy have been reported in cats. In addition, WNV has been isolated from the brain of a cat with neurological disease.[25]

Outbreaks of WNV disease with high mortality rates have been seen among farm-raised alligators. The virus appears to spread via fecal-oral transmission in the alligator pens (Color Plates 9-87 and 9-88).

WNV infection has also been documented in bats, a skunk, and a few rodent species.

Diagnosis

Serological tests used to diagnose WNV infection include ELISA and antigen (IgM and IgG) capture ELISA, hemagglutination inhibition, plaque reduction neutralization, and virus neutralization. Virus can also be identified in the CNS and other tissues using virus isolation, PCR, and immunohistochemistry.

For surveillance of WNV in dead birds, public health and partner agencies have used the VecTest antigen-capture assay (Medical Analysis Systems, Camarillo, Calif.),[29] Rapid Analyte Measurement Platform (RAMP) assay (Response Biomedical Corp, Burnaby, British Columbia, Canada),[30] and real-time RT-PCR.

Treatment

There is no specific treatment for WNV infection in either humans or animals. In more severe human cases, intensive supportive care is indicated, such as hospitalization, intravenous fluids, airway management, respiratory support (ventilator), prevention of secondary infections (pneumonia, urinary tract, etc.), and good nursing care. Research trials are under way to identify effective antiviral treatment and vaccines.

Nonspecific immunoglobulin and plasmapheresis should be considered for patients with Guillain-Barré syndrome. The treatment is not indicated for patients with paralysis due to damage of anterior horn cells.[28]

References

1. Hayes CG. West Nile virus: Uganda, 1937, to New York City, 1999. *Ann N Y Acad Sci.* 2001;951:25.
2. Komar N. West Nile virus surveillance using sentinel birds. *Ann N Y Acad Sci.* 2001;951:58.
3. Resnick MP, Grunenwald P, Blackmar D, et al. Juvenile dogs as potential sentinels for West Nile virus surveillance. *Zoonoses Public Health.* 2008;55(8–10):443.
4. US Environmental Protection Agency. *The insect repellent DEET.* http://www.epa.gov/pesticides/factsheets/chemicals/deet.htm. Accessed September 8, 2008.
5. US Environmental Protection Agency. *New pesticide fact sheet: picaridin.* http://www.epa.gov/opprd001/factsheets/picaridin.pdf. Accessed September 8, 2008.
6. Centers for Disease Control and Prevention. *West Nile virus: questions and answers: insect repellent use and safety.* http://www.cdc.gov/ncidod/dvbid/westnile/qa/insect_repellent.htm. Accessed September 8, 2008.
7. American Association of Equine Practitioners. *West Nile virus.* http://www.aaep.org/wnv.htm. Accessed September 8, 2008.
8. Dvorak G, Rovid-Spickler A, Roth JA, et al. *Handbook for zoonotic diseases of companion animals.* Ames, IA: The Center for Food Security and Public Health, Iowa State University College of Veterinary Medicine; 2008.
9. Petersen LR, Marfin AA. West Nile virus: a primer for the clinician. *Ann Intern Med.* 2002;137(3):173.
10. Diaz LA, Komar N, Visintin A, et al. West Nile virus in birds, Argentina. *Emerg Infect Dis.* 2008;14(4):689.
11. Campbell GL, Marfin AA, Lanciotti RS, et al. West Nile virus. *Lancet Infect Dis.* 2002;2(9):519.
12. Centers for Disease Control and Prevention. *West Nile virus: clinical description.* www.cdc.gov/ncidod/dvbid/westnile/clinicians/clindesc.htm. Accessed September 8, 2008.
13. Komar N, Langevin S, Hinten S, et al. Experimental infection of North American birds with the New York 1999 strain of West Nile virus. *Emerg Infect Dis.* 2003;9(3):311.
14. Nasci RS, Savage HM, White DJ, et al. West Nile virus in overwintering Culex mosquitoes, New York City, 2000. *Emerg Infect Dis.* 2001;7(4):742.
15. Hayes EB, Komar N, Nasci RS, et al. Epidemiology and transmission dynamics of West Nile virus disease. *Emerg Infect Dis.* 2005;11(8):1167.
16. Trevejo RT, Eidson M. West Nile virus. *J Am Vet Med Assoc.* 2008;232(9):1302.
17. Mostashari F, Bunning ML, Kitsutani PT, et al. Epidemic West Nile encephalitis, New York, 1999: results of a household-based seroepidemiological survey. *Lancet.* 2001;358:261.
18. Watson JT, Pertel PE, Jones RC, et al. Clinical characteristics and functional outcomes of West Nile fever. *Ann Intern Med.* 2004;141(5):360.
19. Hayes EB, Seyvar JJ, Zaki SR, et al. Virology, pathology and clinical manifestations of West Nile virus disease. *Emerg Infect Dis.* 2005;11(8):1174.
20. Schuler LA, Khaitsa ML, Dyer NW, et al. Evaluation of an outbreak of West Nile virus infection in horses: 569 cases. *J Am Vet Med Assoc.* 2002;225(7):1084.
21. Ward MP, Levy M, Thacker HL, et al. Investigation of an outbreak of encephalomyelitis caused by West Nile virus in 136 horses. *J Am Vet Med Assoc.* 2002;225(7):84.
22. Austgen LE, Bowen RA, Bunning ML, et al. Experimental infection of dogs and cats with West Nile virus. *Emerg Infect Dis.* 2004;10(1):82.
23. D'Agostino JJ, Isaza R. Clinical signs and results of specific diagnostic testing among captive birds housed at zoological institutions and infected with West Nile virus. *J Am Vet Med Assoc.* 2004;224(10):1640.
24. McLean RG, Ubico SR. Arboviruses in birds. In: Thomas NJ, Hunter DB, Atkinson CT, eds. *Infectious diseases of wild birds.* Ames, IA: Blackwell; 2007.
25. Komar N. West Nile virus: epidemiology and ecology in North America. *Adv Virus Res.* 2003;61:185.
26. Deubel V, Fiette L, Gounon P, et al. Variations in biological features of West Nile viruses. *Ann N Y Sci.* 2001;951:195.
27. Sejvar JJ, Haddad MB, Tierney BC, et al. Neurologic manifestations and outcome of West Nile virus infection. *J Am Med Assoc.* 2003;390(4):511.
28. Sejvar JJ, Leis AA, Stokic DS, et al. Acute flaccid paralysis and West Nile virus infection. *Emerg Infect Dis.* 2003;9(7):788.
29. Stone WB, Okoniewski JC, Therrien JE, et al. VecTest as diagnostic and surveillance tool for West Nile virus in dead birds. *Emerg Infect Dis.* 2004;10(12):2175.
30. Stone WB, Therrien JE, Benson R, et al. Assays to detect West Nile virus in dead birds. *Emerg Infect Dis.* 2004;11(11):1770.

Infectious Disease Scenarios

10

Peter M. Rabinowitz and Lisa A. Conti

TRAVEL AND ANIMAL CONTACT

The U.S. Department of Commerce estimates that at least 30 to 40 million Americans visit other countries each year.[1] Some of these travelers contract diseases while overseas and may return home still symptomatic. Some of these travel-related diseases are zoonoses resulting from contact with domestic or wild animals.

Many international travelers restrict their stays to hotels in urban or other well-developed areas that involve reduced risk of animal contact. Yet the growing popularity of eco-tourism, religious pilgrimages, wildlife safaris, and other forms of adventure travel may increase the chances of travelers contracting an animal-related infectious disease during their trips. Animal contacts are possible even in cities and elsewhere on the beaten path; for example, high levels of pet allergens have been found in vacation hotels in some countries.[1]

Animal travel across borders is increasing as well. In 2006, more than 287,000 dogs were estimated to have entered the United States from foreign countries (including Mexico and Canada), 25% of which were unvaccinated.[2] Many of these dogs were imports, accompanying their owners. The increasing popularity of traveling with one's pet may result in a wide range of exposure risks for both the pet and owner. In addition, some individuals may acquire a pet overseas and return home with it.

Key Points for Clinicians and Public Health Professionals

Public Health Professionals

- Consider recent foreign travel in human beings or other animals as a risk factor for unexplained cases or outbreaks of infectious disease in the community.
- Collaborate with agriculture officials on the regulation of animal movement of public health importance.

Human Health Clinicians

- When providing pretravel screening and counseling, inquire about whether the person is traveling with pets and provide counseling about health risks from animal contacts while traveling. See the CDC's "Your Survival Guide to Safe and Healthy Travel," available online at http://wwwn.cdc.gov/travel/contentSurvivalGuide.aspx.
- If a patient is planning to travel with a pet, advise him or her to consult a veterinarian for pretravel risk assessment and preventive care.
- When evaluating the returning traveler with illness, inquire about animal contacts as well as the health of any pets that have accompanied the traveler or that the traveler has acquired overseas.

Veterinary Clinicians

- Provide appropriate pretravel risk assessment and vaccination of pets and documentation of animal health status.
- Counsel owner about signs of illness to monitor in his or her pet and quarantine regulations.
- In the evaluation of an ill animal after travel, consider risks of imported diseases.
- Advise clients regarding the health risks of adopting a pet overseas (e.g., documented cases of rabies, leishmaniasis, and leptospirosis have been reported in imported pets).

TRAVEL MEDICINE

Travel medicine is a medical discipline that deals with prevention of infectious diseases during international travel as well as the personal safety of travelers and the avoidance of environmental risks during travel.[3] Medical providers who care for human beings traveling to other countries need to be aware of the principles of travel medicine and be able to perform the functions of pretravel risk assessment and

Table 10-1 ▪ Elements of Travel Medicine Practice

Category	Elements
Assessing the health of the traveler*	Assessment of underlying medical conditions, medications, and allergies Assessment of immunization history
Assessing the health risk of travel	Itinerary Season of travel Duration Reason for travel Style of travel Planned activities
Preventative advice[†]	Vaccine-preventable illness Traveler's diarrhea prevention and self-treatment Insect avoidance measures Vector-borne and waterborne illness prevention (e.g., malaria) Personal safety, behavior, and sexual health Environmental illness (related to altitude, heat, cold, swimming, and diving) Motion sickness and jet lag Animal bites and rabies avoidance Long-term travelers, expatriates, and business travelers Special needs travelers (e.g., pregnant women, patients with diabetes, immunocompromised patients, transplant recipients) Travel health resources (e.g., traveler-oriented Web sites) Travel medical kits Travel health and medical evacuation insurance Access to medical care overseas
Vaccination	
Posttravel assessment	

From Hill DR, Ericsson CD, Pearson RD et al: The practice of travel medicine: guidelines by the Infectious Diseases Society of America, *Clin Infect Dis* 43:1499, 2006.
*Permanent records should be maintained.
[†]Advice should be given both verbally and in writing.

preventive counseling, vaccination, and posttravel evaluation of illness. A complete discussion of the many travel-related health risks is beyond the scope of this book. However, Table 10-1 shows the key elements of travel medicine practice.

Veterinary providers who care for animals that are either traveling internationally or arriving from another country also need to be aware of the principles of travel medicine and be able to perform similar functions of pretravel risk assessment and counseling, vaccination, and posttravel assessment on animals.

PRETRAVEL RISK ASSESSMENT AND ANIMAL CONTACT COUNSELING

In a pretravel risk assessment, clinicians consider both the medical status of the traveler as well as the infectious and other environmental risks related to the countries they plan to visit and the activities they plan to undertake (see Table 10-1). Risks of travel-related animal contact may be overlooked during such visits. Table 10-2 summarizes these risks and provides the basics of counseling on risk reduction for particular animal contact situations.

HUMAN HEALTH RISKS OF ANIMAL CONTACT WHILE TRAVELING

Injuries From Animals

Animal bites and other animal-related injuries can be a significant hazard during travel (Color Plate 10-1). Although an attack from a wild animal, including snakes, crocodiles, large felids, and elephants, can cause dramatic injuries, falls from horseback or attacks by bulls or other large domestic animals can also maim and kill (Figures 10-1 and 10-2; Color Plates 10-2 and 10-3). A review of animal-associated injuries reported to the GeoSentinel Surveillance Network found that dog bites were the most common animal-associated injury to travelers, followed by bites from monkeys and cats. Three-quarters of the exposures occurred in countries where rabies is endemic, with the majority occurring in Asia. Fifty percent of bitten travelers had a travel duration of 1 month or less, and traveling for tourism was associated with an increased risk of an animal injury. Males were more likely to receive a dog bite, whereas monkey exposures were more common for females. Children were also at increased risk of exposure.[4] Despite the risk of rabies from such exposures (fatal cases of human rabies have occurred in U.S. travelers from dog bites received during international travel[5]), a study of returning travelers with animal injuries found that most had not had pretravel rabies vaccine[6] and two thirds of persons with injuries did not receive postexposure prophylaxis (which may not be routinely available in some countries). Rabies vaccine should be considered for all travel to rabies-endemic countries, especially for children, although a minimum travel duration of 6 weeks in an endemic area is recommended by some experts as an indication for vaccine. The strength of that recommendation should be influenced by the availability of medical care and rabies immunization products locally.

Other reported diseases related to bite and scratch exposures in travelers include bacterial infection from *Pasteurella* or other agents, rat-bite fever from rodents (see Animal and Human Bites below), and *Bartonella* infection from cats, the most common animal-associated infection reported in the GeoSentinel study.

Exposure to nonhuman primates can occur during travel; monkey temples are a popular tourist site in Asia. Simian foamy virus infection has been reported in a visitor to a monkey temple.[7] Bites from Old World monkeys also carry a risk of herpes B infection that can cause fatal disease in human beings (see Animal and Human Bites later in this chapter). Herpes B infections in human beings have been mostly observed in occupational settings (see Chapter 12), and to date no known cases have been reported in travelers.[8]

Travelers should never try to pet, handle, or feed unfamiliar animals, domestic or wild, particularly in areas of endemic rabies. Because children are at greatest risk of animal bites, including severe injuries, and may be less likely to report a bite incident,[8] they need to be counseled to avoid petting or handling dogs, cats, or other animals and should be supervised

Table 10-2 ▪ Prevention of Human Health Risks Associated With Travel and Animal Contact

Activity	Types of Contact	Pathogens	Preventive Steps
Bites, scratches from direct contact with animal	Contact with dogs, cats, monkeys	*Pasteurella*, rabies virus, *Bartonella*, other	Avoid animal contact in rabies-endemic countries, supervise children around animals
		Simian immunodeficiency viruses, herpes B	Consider pretravel rabies vaccine for visits to rabies-endemic countries Avoid contact with monkeys Wash wound immediately and seek medical care immediately if bitten or scratched
Farm visits, agricultural tourism	Contact with goats, sheep, cattle, poultry, hogs, contaminated dusts	Q fever, brucellosis, *E. coli*, Nipah, avian influenza, anthrax	Avoid close contact with animals or confined spaces with dust, handwashing after contact
Religious pilgrimages, festivals (e.g., Hajj/Eid al-Adha, Lunar New Year)	Slaughter and consumption of animals	Anthrax (cattle, camels, goats) Avian influenza (poultry)	Avoid contact with slaughter activities Avoid live animal markets, bird farms; avoid contact with sick or dead birds Handwashing
Live animal markets	Slaughter of animals; fecal contamination of surfaces, air	Avian influenza, SARS, *E. coli*, other	Avoid visiting live animal markets
Safaris, wilderness travel	Mosquito-borne infections	Malaria, yellow fever, dengue, Chikungunya fever	Use DEET and/or Picaridin insect repellents; other mosquito, tick, and fly precautions
	Tickborne infections	Rickettsial infection (scrub typhus), tick paralysis	
	Fly-borne	Trypanosomiasis, leishmaniasis	
	Rodent-infested buildings	Hantavirus	Avoid rodent areas (see Chapter 9)
	Infected fresh water	Leptospirosis, *E. coli*, other pathogens	Avoid swimming in or drinking untreated fresh water
	Exposures to bats or bat guano	Rabies, other viral pathogens, histoplasmosis	Use caution visiting caves and sleeping outdoors to avoid bats and bat guano
Local delicacies, bushmeat	Undercooked meat, raw milk	*Campylobacter, Salmonella,* bovine tuberculosis, brucellosis, listeriosis, anthrax	Avoid uncooked meats, fish, raw/unpasteurized dairy products, soft cheeses
	Primate meat	Simian viruses, Ebola	Avoid bushmeat consumption
	Bear	*Trichinella*	
	Raw fish, shellfish	Cholera, hepatitis, gnathostomiasis, paragonimiasis, rat lungworm	
Souvenirs	Animal skins drums	Anthrax	Avoid purchasing unprocessed animal hide souvenirs
Beaches, sandboxes	Walking barefoot, swimming	Hookworm infection, tungiasis, marine envenomations	Do not walk barefoot on beaches, use caution when swimming
Travel with pet	Pet can come in contact with local domestic and wildlife species, may also develop vector-borne disease and/or toxic exposures	Zoonotic infections Allergy from pet	Use of pet insecticide, periodic deworming of pet, avoid feeding uncooked meat, do not allow pet to roam free outdoors, pretravel and posttravel vet visits (see Boxes 10-2 and 10-3)

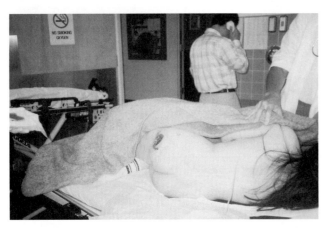

Figure 10-1 ■ Wound from bison goring. (From Auerbach PS: *Wilderness medicine,* ed 5, Philadelphia, 2007, Mosby Elsevier. Photo courtesy Karen Hansen.)

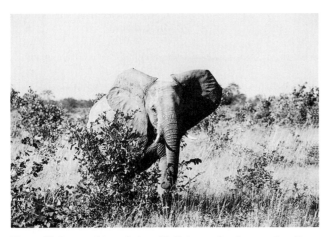

Figure 10-2 ■ African elephant bluff-charges the photographer. (From Auerbach PS: *Wilderness medicine,* ed 5, Philadelphia, 2007, Mosby Elsevier. Photo courtesy Cary Breidenthal.)

around animals at all times. If an exposure occurs, clean the wound thoroughly and immediately seek medical care for possible rabies postexposure prophylaxis (see Chapter 9). Tetanus prophylaxis is also indicated if the traveler is not up to date with tetanus vaccination. In the case of an Old World monkey bite, medical care should be sought as soon as possible for prophylactic treatment against herpes B infection.

Envenomations from snakes, scorpions, and spiders represent another animal-associated injury risk to travelers; medical care should be sought immediately. The treatment of snakebites and other venomous animal bites usually depends on the species of animal responsible (see Chapter 8).

Farm Visits

Agricultural tourism is the experience of visiting a working farm or related operation for enjoyment and is a growing type of tourism both nationally and internationally (Figure 10-3).[9] Specialized tour operators offer package tours to farms in a number of countries. During such visits tourists may come in contact with both farm animals and contaminated soils and dusts that may contain infectious pathogens. Q fever is considered to be underdiagnosed in travelers, who can acquire it by exposure to farm animals or contaminated

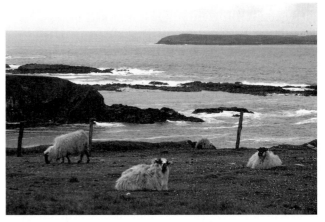

Figure 10-3 ■ Farm contact may expose the traveler to diseases such as Q fever and brucellosis. (From Centers for Disease Control and Prevention Public Health Image Library, Atlanta, Ga. Photo courtesy Edwin P. Ewing Jr.)

aerosols.[10] Travel to a farm in Guyana was associated with a cluster of human cases of Q fever, presumably from contact with a parturient goat and dog on a farm.[11] If the farm contains poultry, risks include exposure to *Chlamydophila, Campylobacter, Salmonella,* and avian influenza virus. Brucellosis is another potential farm-related exposure, either through direct contact with animals or consumption of unpasteurized dairy products. Brucellosis has been termed a "travel-associated foodborne zoonosis" in Germany, where a recent rise in cases has been traced to consumption of unpasteurized cheese from brucellosis-endemic countries.[12] In a series of brucellosis cases in San Diego, travel to Mexico was a risk factor for infection.[13]

Festivals Involving Animal Contact

An increasing amount of international travel is related to religious and cultural festivals. Each year several million Muslims participate in the Hajj pilgrimage to Mecca. Although local agricultural authorities have taken steps to reduce animal contact risks to pilgrims,[14] the end of the Hajj is marked by the festival of Eid al-Adha, which may involve increased exposure to animal slaughtering activities. For example, a suspected outbreak of anthrax was linked to slaughter and distribution of infected meat from a camel during the festival.[15]

Similarly, the Lunar New Year festivals in Asia often involve increased slaughtering and consumption of poultry, with an attendant increased risk of avian influenza. The CDC has issued travel advisories for U.S. travelers visiting Asia during the Lunar New Year festival. These recommendations include handwashing; avoidance of bird farms or live bird markets; not touching live or dead birds, including chickens, ducks, and wild birds, even if they do not seem sick; and not touching surfaces contaminated with bird feces, blood, or other body fluids.[16]

Live Animal Markets

At any time of year visits to live animal markets, present in many cities and villages in a large number of countries, carry a risk of infection with zoonotic agents. In such markets numerous species of wildlife and domestic animals may be housed in close proximity, creating an increased opportunity for disease transmission. Color Plate 10-4 shows a typical scene from a live animal market in Asia. Human infection with the H5N1 avian influenza virus has been linked to visits to live bird markets, even for individuals who denied direct contact with sick or healthy-appearing poultry.[17] Avian influenza has been found on surfaces and dusts in such markets, and exposure may occur by touching contaminated surfaces as well as breathing contaminated dusts. Severe acute respiratory syndrome (SARS) is another infection linked to live animal markets in Asia. Travelers wishing to reduce risk of zoonotic diseases while traveling should avoid visiting live animal markets, especially if a country is experiencing an outbreak of highly pathogenic avian influenza.[18] A current list of countries is maintained at http://www.cdc.gov/flu/avian/outbreaks/current.htm.

Safaris and Wilderness Travel

Wilderness travel overseas increases the risk of exposure to a number of pathogens as well as injuries from snakes, crocodiles, and other wildlife. Visitors on safari to game parks in Africa have become infected with African tick fever and other rickettsial infections that may have a reservoir in the local wildlife populations.[19] Although most forms of malaria, one of the most common causes of fever in returning travelers, are not zoonotic, certain monkey malaria species such as *Plasmodium knowlesi* have been described in human beings and may be underdiagnosed.[20] Other zoonotic arthropod-borne infections such as trypanosomiasis, yellow fever, and Chikungunya fever have been reported in safari and wilderness travelers.[21,22] Sleeping in huts and shelters that may also be home to local rodent populations can increase risk of infection with hantaviruses and various hemorrhagic fevers, including Lassa fever.[23] Swimming in fresh water in areas frequented by wildlife has led to outbreaks of leptospirosis in adventure travelers.[24] Wilderness travelers may be exposed to bats when visiting caves or sleeping outside in areas frequented by bats, where they could come in contact

with bat droppings or sustain bat bites. In addition to rabies risk, bats are reservoirs for a wide range of other viral pathogens, including other lyssa viruses, Nipah virus, SARS-like coronavirus, and Marburg virus.[25] Exposure to aerosolized bat guano has also been associated with the development of acute pulmonary histoplasmosis in travelers.[26]

Local Delicacies Involving Animal Products and Bushmeat Consumption

Many local delicacies that travelers encounter may involve animal products from domestic or wild animals. Meat and dairy products may be served raw or undercooked and may be a source for zoonotic infections such as brucellosis, trichinosis, and salmonellosis in returning travelers.[27] Raw chicken sashimi from an island in Japan is known to be contaminated with *Campylobacter*. However, local residents do not appear to become ill, suggesting a role for acquired protective immunity that a traveler would presumably not enjoy.[28] Travelers to Southeast Asia and Africa have become infected with parasites, including *Paragonimus*, trematodes *Clonorchis sinensis* or *Haplorchis pumilio*, and gnathostomes. Paragonimiasis is acquired by eating raw freshwater crabs or crayfish. Gnathostomiasis is a nematode infection acquired by ingestion of various intermediate hosts in addition to fish.[29,30] Eating unwashed produce and undercooked foods such as mollusks in some countries poses risks of numerous infectious diseases, including viral hepatitis, bacterial enteritis, and eosinophilic meningitis from rat lungworm.[31] There is increasing awareness of the infectious risks of improperly cooked poultry products. Such practices have been linked to cases of avian influenza.[32] Bovine tuberculosis transmission to human beings can involve consumption of uncooked meat as well as raw milk (see Chapter 9).[33]

Bushmeat (wild game killed for food) is an important source of animal protein for communities in many parts of the world. It has been estimated that in Central Africa alone more than 1 billion kilograms of meat from wild animals are consumed each year (Figure 10-4).[34] Table 10-3 shows the diversity of

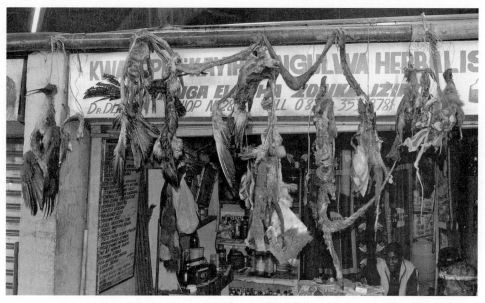

Figure 10-4 ▪ South African market with bushmeat for sale. (From Fowler ME: *Zoo and wild animal medicine: current therapy,* ed 6, St Louis, 2008, Saunders Elsevier. Photo courtesy R. A. Cook.)

Table 10-3 ■ Protected and Unprotected Species Sold in Village and Urban Bushmeat Markets in Northeastern Democratic Republic of Congo During Peacetime and Wartime*

Taxon†	Village (Kiliwa) Market Day Sales			Urban (Dungu) Market Day Sales		
	Peace (kg)	War (kg)	P	Peace (kg)	War (kg)	P
Protected Species						
Elephant, *Loxodonta africana*	0.0 ± 0.0	0.0 ± 0.0	NS	23.5 ± 1.5	120.3 ± 10.3	<.05
Hippo, *Hippopotamus amphibius*	0.0 ± 0.0	0.0 ± 0.0	NS	9.3 ± 0.6	48.0 ± 4.2	<.05
Buffalo, *Syncerus caffer*	0.1 ± 0.1	0.0 ± 0.0	NS	19.6 ± 1.2	98.2 ± 8.4	<.05
Bongo, *Tragelaphus euryceros*	0.0 ± 0.0	0.0 ± 0.0	NS	0.5 ± 0.1	2.2 ± 0.5	<.05
Large antelope, multiple species‡	0.2 ± 0.1	0.3 ± 0.3	NS	3.7 ± 0.3	23.7 ± 2.1	<.05
Pigs, multiple species§	0.4 ± 0.1	0.4 ± 0.2	NS	5.6 ± 0.3	9.5 ± 1.1	<.05
Chimpanzee, *Pan troglodytes*	0.0 ± 0.0	0.0 ± 0.0	NS	0.6 ± 0.1	0.5 ± 0.2	NS
Aardvark, *Orycteropus afer*	0.1 ± 0.1	0.0 ± 0.0	NS	0.7 ± 0.1	0.8 ± 0.2	NS
All protected species	0.8 ± 0.2	0.8 ± 0.4	NS	63.6 ± 3.7	303.1 ± 25.5	<.05
Unprotected Species						
Duikers, multiple species‖	1.0 ± 0.2	1.7 ± 0.7	NS	16.7 ± 0.5	15.7 ± 0.9	NS
Monkeys, multiple species¶	1.5 ± 0.3	1.8 ± 0.6	NS	8.7 ± 0.3	8.4 ± 0.5	NS
Crested porcupine, *Hystrix cristata*	0.2 ± 0.1	0.2 ± 0.1	NS	1.0 ± 0.0	1.0 ± 0.1	NS
Uganda grass hare, *Poelagus marjorita*	0.3 ± 0.1	0.7 ± 0.3	NS	2.5 ± 0.1	2.6 ± 0.1	NS
Cane rat, *Thryonomys swinderianus*	0.2 ± 0.1	0.1 ± 0.1	NS	0.7 ± 0.0	0.7 ± 0.0	NS
All unprotected species	3.1 ± 0.6	4.5 ± 1.5	NS	29.7 ± 0.8	28.3 ± 1.4	NS

From De Merode E, Cowlishaw G: Species protection, the changing informal economy, and the politics of access to the bushmeat trade in the Democratic Republic of Congo, *Conserv Biol* 20:1262, 2006.

*Mean and standard error of kilograms of fresh meat sold per market day. Tests for statistical significance (*P*) indicate whether the difference between peacetime and wartime is significant (*P* < .05) or not significant (NS). Sample sizes (market days) in peacetime and wartime are 96 and 341 for the rural markets and 336 and 120 for the urban markets, respectively. To calculate daily sales (incorporating both market days and nonmarket days), multiply all rural figures by 0.29 (i.e., 2 market days/week) and multiply all urban figures by 2.71 (i.e., 19 market days/weeks).

†Taxa are grouped according to protected and unprotected status, although all species are protected within the boundaries of Garamba National Park and ordered by decreasing body size within these groups. Where several species are incorporated into a single taxon, the median species weight is used, with all body size data taken from Rowcliffe JM, de Merode E, Cowlishaw G: Do wildlife laws work? Species protection and the application of a prey choice model to poaching decisions, *Proc Biol Sci* 271:2631-2636, 2004. Where a taxon is composed of multiple species, allocation of that taxon to either one of these groups depends on the relative proportion of protected and unprotected species; if at least half of the species is protected, the taxon is placed in the protected group. Taxonomy follows Kingdon J: *The Kingdon field guide to African mammals*, San Francisco, 1997, Academic Press.

‡Hartebeest (*Alcelaphus buselaphus*), kob (*Kobus kob*), waterbuck (*Kobus ellipsiprymnus*), bohor reedbuck (*Redunca redunca*), bushbuck (*Tragelaphus scriptus*), and sitatunga (*Tragelaphus spekii*). Hartebeest, waterbuck, and sitatunga are protected.

§Giant forest hog (*Hylochoerus meinertzhageni*), common warthog (*Phacochoerus africanus*), and red river hog (*Potamochoerus porcus*). Giant forest hog and red river hog are protected.

‖Bay duiker (*Cephalophus dorsalis*), red-flanked duiker (*Cephalophus rufilatus*), blue duiker (*Cephalophus monticola*), and bush duiker (*Sylvicapra grimmia*). None of these species is protected.

¶Agile mangabey (*Cercocebus agilis*), tantalus monkey (*Cercopithecus [aethiops] tantalus*), red-tailed monkey (*Cercopithecus [cephus] ascanius*), patas monkey (*Cercopithecus [erythrocebus] patas*), Dent's monkey (*Cercopithecus [mona] denti*), de Brazza's monkey (*Cercopithecus neglectus*), guereza colobus (*Colobus guereza*), and olive baboon (*Papio anubis*). None of these species is protected.

species that may end up being sold for human consumption, especially during times of civil unrest.[35] Emerging pathogens linked to bushmeat consumption include simian immunodeficiency viruses, anthrax, and hemorrhagic fever viruses.[36] Although the risk of infection from bushmeat exposure may be greatest to persons who butcher carcasses, travelers to areas where bushmeat is an important part of local diets may be at risk if they consume improperly cooked bushmeat.

Beaches and Sandboxes

Travelers should avoid going barefoot on beaches frequented by animals. Many beaches that travelers visit during international vacations are frequented by dogs and cats. Walking barefoot on beaches contaminated with their feces is a risk factor

for acquiring zoonotic hookworm infection (cutaneous larva migrans, also known as *creeping eruption* (see Chapter 9 and Color Plate 9-33).[37] Another beach-related zoonosis is tungiasis, a skin infestation caused by the sand flea *Tunga penetrans* (jiggers). Walking barefoot on beaches also carries risks of stings from jellyfish and other marine organisms (see Chapter 8). Sandboxes and play areas are another source of contact for hookworms, roundworms (*Toxocara*), and *Toxoplasma*.

Souvenirs

Persons purchasing souvenirs while traveling should be aware that improperly processed hides used for drums and other souvenirs may be a source of exposure for cutaneous anthrax (see Chapter 9).[38] However, this risk is considered to be low.

POSTTRAVEL ASSESSMENT

In the returning traveler with illness, a careful history of animal-related exposures should be obtained in addition to the standard questions (Box 10-1). If the response to any of these questions is affirmative, further evaluation is warranted.

TRAVELING WITH A PET AND OTHER ANIMAL TRAVEL MEDICINE ISSUES

Traveling with pets is becoming increasingly popular. There are a number of reasons why people travel with a pet. These include emotional, economic, gene transfer, and seeking specialized veterinary care.[39] Emotional reasons include companionship, treating an animal as a member of the family, and reluctance to leave an animal behind. Economic factors can include the cost of arranging care for the animal while traveling. Gene transfer involves activities such as taking a pedigreed animal to another location to breed with another animal. Finally, owners may take an ill animal to another location for specialized veterinary care.[39]

Veterinarians should go through similar steps as their human health counterparts in evaluating animals that are traveling. These include pretravel risk assessment and owner counseling, vaccines and other preventive care as necessary, and evaluation of returning and newly imported animals after travel.

Infectious Disease Risks and Pets That Travel

Many of the infectious disease risks to traveling companion animals are shared with human beings. Even travel to different regions in the same country can expose an animal to new health risks. Pets that travel also face potential exposure to animal diseases that are not zoonotic in nature, such as canine parvovirus, canine viral hepatitis, and feline panleukopenia virus.

Particular zoonoses associated with dog travel include rabies, leishmaniasis, and roundworm infection.[40-43] A case of a rabid puppy imported illegally from Morocco to France by a traveling couple resulted in the prophylactic treatment

of 21 persons, the euthanasia of a contact animal, and legal action against the travelers.[44] In 2007, a puppy rescued from an animal shelter in India by a veterinarian who brought the animal into the United States at 11 weeks of age was found to be positive for rabies by the Alaska Department of Health and Social Services.[45] Such introduction of rabies from animal travel can involve foreign rabies virus variants. As a result, the CDC is considering strengthening federal regulations regarding the importation of companion animals.[2]

Vector-borne diseases are a documented risk to traveling dogs. For example, leishmaniasis has been reported in dogs traveling in high-incidence countries, leading to the introduction of disease upon returning home.

Other Risks Associated With Traveling Animals

Animals may cause allergic reactions if they come into contact with sensitized travelers or airline, train, or other transportation personnel. Animals with allergy may also be exposed to a variety of allergens during travel.

Toxic risks to traveling animals include contaminated pet food,[46] water, pesticides, and accidental ingestion of rodenticides (see Chapter 8).

Animals risk physical injury from being shipped in containers or otherwise restrained, heat stress and cold exposures, and fights with other animals. Other potential stressors include unfamiliar surroundings, disruption of circadian schedules, noise, and other noxious stimuli.

Logistics

Travelers wishing to travel with pets will need to identify the logistic requirements for transporting and housing the animal during travel. Airlines may vary in their rules regarding whether an animal can be carried in a pet container that can be placed under a seat, or whether all animals need to be placed in cargo. There have been instances of companion animals dying from heat and cold stress and other trauma while being shipped in cargo, and owners should be aware of the risks to animals undergoing air travel.[47] There may be restrictions on the number of animals allowed. Rental car companies, trains, buses, and hotels may also have restrictive policies about pets. These policies should be clarified in advance of travel.

Documentation and Regulation of Animal Travel and Importation

Animals that travel often need documentation of vaccination status, tick or other prophylactic treatments, and a statement from a veterinarian that they are free of communicable disease and able to travel safely. Such documentation may be necessary for the animal to enter another country. Owners should contact the embassies of countries they plan to visit to go through the required entry processes as well as determine the U.S. clearance processes upon return.[48] Policies of some countries may require an animal to be quarantined or destroyed without proper documentation. Additional information is available at http://www.aphis.usda.gov/import_export/animals/animal_exports.shtml.

BOX 10-1   *EVALUATION OF THE RETURNING TRAVELER REGARDING ANIMAL-RELATED RISKS*

- Were you in the vicinity of live animals, either on a farm, in a house, or in a market? If so, what types of animals and environments? Did you touch any animals or notice any sickness in the animals?
- Were you bitten, scratched, or licked by dogs, cats, monkeys, or other animals?
- Did you eat uncooked or undercooked meat, fish, or shellfish?
- Did you consume bushmeat?
- Did you eat or drink unpasteurized dairy products?
- Did you walk barefoot on beaches or swim in fresh water?
- Did you travel in the wilderness?
- Did you visit caves or sleep outdoors in areas frequented by bats?
- Did you receive bites from ticks, flies, or mosquitoes?

Many countries limit movement of dogs and other animals based on rabies status. Dogs and cats generally cannot pass from a rabies-endemic country to a rabies-free country without a process of quarantine and/or vaccination documentation. Table 10-4 lists countries reporting no indigenous rabies in 2005.

A number of federal agencies are involved with regulation of animals entering the United States. The CDC regulates the importation into the United States of dogs, cats, turtles, bats, monkeys, and other animals as well as animal products capable of causing human disease (see http://wwwn.cdc.gov/travel/yellowBookCh7-AnimalImport.aspx).[48] Pets taken out of the United States are subject to the same regulations when returning to the country as are newly imported animals. The U.S. Department of Agriculture (USDA) regulates a number of species being imported based on their disease risk to plants and animals of agricultural concern.

No single agency regulates entry of dogs into the United States. Although the CDC does not require a general certificate of health for dogs, dogs with evidence of illness may not be allowed entry. Documentation of rabies vaccination at least 30 days before entry is required, although dogs younger than 3 months and dogs without proof of rabies vaccination may be allowed to enter if the owner completes a confinement agreement and certifies the animal will be vaccinated and kept confined at least 30 days after vaccination. Unvaccinated dogs from countries considered rabies free (see Table 10-4) may also be allowed entry.[49] In addition to CDC regulations, the USDA regulates the importation of dogs potentially carrying diseases of agricultural importance, including screwworms or some *Taenia* species of tapeworm.[2]

For cats, a general certificate of health is not required to enter the United States, but some states and air carriers may require such documentation. Rabies vaccination is also not required, but some states may require proof of rabies vaccine documentation. All pet cats entering Hawaii and Guam are subject to local quarantine requirements.[49]

Importation of birds is regulated by the USDA Animal and Plant Health Inspection Service.[50] The USDA currently restricts importation of pet birds from countries where highly pathogenic avian influenza H5N1 is present in poultry. To import a pet bird of non-U.S. origin, the importer or owner must obtain a USDA import permit,[51] have a certificate of health from a veterinarian in the exporting country, and allow the bird to be quarantined for 30 days in a USDA animal import center at the owner's expense. Pet birds arriving from Canada are not required to be quarantined.[52] Entry into the United States of birds that are covered by endangered species conventions is regulated by the U.S. Fish and Wildlife Service.

The CDC periodically issues embargoes on specific animals associated with disease risk, including civets (SARS), birds from specific countries (avian influenza), and African rodents (monkeypox).

CDC regulations do not apply to horses not known to be carrying diseases infectious to human beings, but the USDA may regulate horse import due to risks of diseases of agricultural importance such as screwworm.

Importation of fish into the United States is not regulated by the CDC, but U.S. Fish and Wildlife Service regulations may apply.

Finally, importation of certain animals and animal products is regulated by other federal agencies such as the U.S. Customs Service.[53]

If animals are traveling, they should have a veterinary evaluation for pretravel risk assessment and administration of necessary vaccines and other preventive treatments. Box 10-2 outlines the elements of such a visit.

The veterinarian should determine whether travel is medically advisable for the animal. Travel is riskier for immunocompromised animals, including young animals and animals with underlying illness. Certain species, such as snakes, may not be allowed entry by other countries. Animals with behavioral problems may attack other animals or people or present other travel risks.

The veterinarian should ensure that animals with ongoing illnesses have an adequate supply of medications and that plans for emergency veterinary medical care while traveling are discussed with the owner.

Table 10-4 ▪ Countries and Political Units Reporting No Indigenous Cases of Rabies During 2005*

Region	Countries
Africa	Cape Verde, Libya, Mauritius, Réunion, São Tome and Principe, Seychelles
Americas	*North*: Bermuda, St. Pierre et Miquelon *Caribbean*: Antigua and Barbuda, Aruba, Bahamas, Barbados, Cayman Islands, Dominica, Guadeloupe, Jamaica, Martinique, Montserrat, Netherlands Antilles, Saint Kitts (Saint Christopher) and Nevis, Saint Lucia, Saint Martin, Saint Vincent and Grenadines, Turks and Caicos, Virgin Islands (U.K. and U.S.) *South*: Uruguay
Asia	Hong Kong, Japan, Kuwait, Lebanon, Malaysia (Sabah), Qatar, Singapore, United Arab Emirates
Europe	Austria, Belgium, Cyprus, Czech Republic†, Denmark†, Finland, France†, Gibraltar, Greece, Iceland, Ireland, Isle of Man, Italy, Luxemburg, Netherlands†, Norway, Portugal, Spain† (except Ceuta/Melilla), Sweden, Switzerland, United Kingdom†
Oceania‡	Australia†, Northern Mariana Islands, Cook Islands, Fiji, French Polynesia, Guam, Hawaii, Kiribati, Micronesia, New Caledonia, New Zealand, Palau, Papua New Guinea, Samoa, Vanuatu

*Bat rabies may exist in some areas that are reportedly free of rabies in other animals.
†Bat lyssa viruses are known to exist in these areas that are reportedly free of rabies in other animals.
‡Most of Pacific Oceania is reportedly rabies free.
From Centers for Disease Control and Prevention: *CDC health information for international travel 2008: prevention of specific infectious diseases: rabies.* http://wwwn.cdc.gov/travel/yellowBookCh4-Rabies.aspx#653.

Evaluation of Illness in an Animal After Travel

Animals imported into the United States are required to be healthy. However, if illness develops, evaluation should involve the steps outlined in Box 10-3. If infectious conditions are identified, the possibility of zoonotic transmission to the animal's owner should be considered, and there should be rapid communication to either a human health care provider, public health department, or both.

Further steps should be based on the results of this preliminary evaluation.

References

1. Office of Travel & Tourism Industries. *U.S. citizen air traffic to overseas regions, Canada and Mexico.* 2007. http://tinet.ita.doc.gov/view/m-2007-O-001/index.html. Accessed February 28, 2008.
2. McQuiston JH, Wilson T, Harris S, et al. Importation of dogs into the United States: risks from rabies and other zoonotic diseases. *Zoonoses and Public Health.* 2008;55(8–10):421–426.
3. Hill DR, Ericsson CD, Pearson RD, et al. Infectious Diseases Society of America: The practice of travel medicine: guidelines by the Infectious Diseases Society of America. *Clin Infect Dis.* 2006;43(12):1499–1539.
4. Gautret P, Schwartz E, Shaw M, et al. GeoSentinel Surveillance Network Animal-associated injuries and related diseases among returned travelers: a review of the GeoSentinel Surveillance Network. *Vaccine.* 2007;25(14):2656–2663.
5. Schmiedel S, Panning M, Lohse A, et al. Case report on fatal human rabies infection in Hamburg, Germany, March 2007. *Euro Surveill.* 2007;12(5):E070531.5.
6. Gautret P, Shaw M, Gazin P, et al. Rabies postexposure prophylaxis in returned injured travelers from France, Australia, and New Zealand: a retrospective study. *Travel Med.* 2008;15(1):25–30.
7. Jones-Engel L, Engel GA, Schillaci MA, et al. Primate-to-human retroviral transmission in Asia. *Emerg Infect Dis.* 2005;11(7):1028–1035.
8. Centers for Disease Control and Prevention. *CDC health information for international travel 2008: animal associated hazards.* http://wwwn.cdc.gov/travel/yellowBookCh6-Animal.aspx. Accessed October 16, 2008.
9. Lobo R, Small Farm Center, University of California-Davis. *Helpful agricultural tourism (agritourism) definitions.* http://www.sfc.ucdavis.edu/agritourism/definition.html. Accessed May 29, 2008.
10. Terheggen U, Leggat PA. Clinical manifestations of Q fever in adults and children. *Travel Med Infect Dis.* 2007;5(3):159–164.
11. Baret M, Klement E, Dos Santos G, et al. *Coxiella burnetii* pneumopathy on return from French Guiana [in French]. *Bulletin de la Societe de Pathologie Exotique.* 93(5):325–327, 2000.
12. Dahouk SA, Neubauer H, Hensel A, et al. Changing epidemiology of human brucellosis, Germany, 1962–2005. *Emerg Infect Dis.* 2007;13(12):1895–1900.
13. Troy SB, Rickman LS, Davis CE. Brucellosis in San Diego: epidemiology and species-related differences in acute clinical presentations. *Medicine.* 2005;84(3):174–187.
14. Ahmed QA, Arabi YM, Memish ZA. Health risks at the Hajj. *Lancet.* 2006;367(9515):1008–1015.
15. International Society for Infectious Diseases: *Dengue/DHF update 2008.* http://promedmail.org.
16. Centers for Disease Control and Prevention. *In the news: keeping yourself safe from bird flu: an important message for people traveling to Asia to celebrate the Lunar New Year.* 2008. http://wwwn.cdc.gov/travel/content AvianFluLunarNewYear08.aspx. Accessed February 28, 2008.
17. Yu H, Feng Z, Zhang X, et al. Avian influenza H5N1 study group. Human influenza A (H5N1) cases, urban areas of People's Republic of China, 2005–2006. *Emerg Infect Dis.* 2007;13(7):1061–1064.
18. Hurtado TR. Human influenza A (H5N1): a brief review and recommendations for travelers. *Wilderness Environ Med.* 2006;17(4):276–281.
19. Buchau AS, Wurthner JU, Reifenberger J, et al. Fever, episcleritis, epistaxis, and rash after safari holiday in Swaziland. *Arch Dermatol.* 2006;142(10):1365–1366.
20. Ng OT, Ooi EE, Lee CC, et al. Naturally acquired human *Plasmodium knowlesi* infection, Singapore. *Emerg Infect Dis.* 2008;14(5):814–816.
21. Jelinek T, Bisoffi Z, Bonazzi L, et al. European Network on Imported Infectious Disease Surveillance. Cluster of African trypanosomiasis in travelers to Tanzanian national parks. *Emerg Infect Dis.* 2002; 8(6): 634–635.
22. Centers for Disease Control and Prevention. Chikungunya fever diagnosed among international travelers—United States, 2005–2006. *MMWR Morb Mortal Wkly Rep.* 2006;55(38):1040–1042.
23. Castillo C, Nicklas C, Mardones J, et al. Andes hantavirus as possible cause of disease in travellers to South America. *Travel Med Infect Dis.* 2007;5(1):30–34.
24. Centers for Disease Control and Prevention. Outbreak of acute febrile illness among participants in EcoChallenge Sabah 2000-Malaysia, 2000. *JAMA.* 2000;284(13):1646.
25. Wong S, Lau S, Woo P, et al. Bats as a continuing source of emerging infections in humans. *Rev Med Virol.* 2007;17(2):67–91.
26. de Vries PJ, Koolen MG, Mulder MM, et al. Acute pulmonary histoplasmosis from Ghana. *Travel Med Infect Dis.* 2006;4(5):286–289.

27. Dore K, Buxton J, Henry B, et al. Multi-provincial *Salmonella Typhimurium* case-control study steering committee. Risk factors for *Salmonella typhimurium* DT104 and non-DT104 infection: a Canadian multi-provincial case-control study. *Epidemiol Infect.* 2004;132(3):485–493.

28. Moore JE, Matsuda M. Consumption of raw chicken sashimi, Kyushu Island, Japan—risk of campylobacteriosis or not. *Travel Med Infect Dis.* 2007;5(1):64–65.

29. Del Giudice P, Cua E, Le Fichoux Y, et al. Gnathostomiasis: an emerging parasitic disease [in French]? *Ann Dermatol Venereol.* 2005;132(12 Pt 1):983–985.

30. Hale DC, Blumberg L, Frean J. Case report: gnathostomiasis in two travelers to Zambia. *Am J Trop Med Hyg.* 2003;68(6):707–709.

31. Weir E. Travel warning: eosinophilic meningitis caused by rat lungworm. *CMAJ.* 2002;166(9):1184.

32. Centers for Disease Control and Prevention. *Guidelines and recommendations: interim guidance about avian influenza (H5N1) for U.S. citizens living abroad.* http://wwwn.cdc.gov/travel/contentAvianFluAmericansAbroad.aspx. Accessed February 28, 2008.

33. Etter E, Donado P, Jori F, et al. Risk analysis and bovine tuberculosis, a re-emerging zoonosis. *Ann N Y Acad Sci.* 2006;1081:61–73.

34. Karesh WB, Cook RA. The human-animal link. *Foreign Affairs.* 2005;84:38–50.

35. De Merode E, Cowlishaw G. Species protection, the changing informal economy, and the politics of access to the bushmeat trade in the Democratic Republic of Congo. *Conserv Biol.* 2006;20(4):1262–1271.

36. Wolfe ND, Daszak P, Kilpatrick AM, et al. Bushmeat hunting, deforestation, and prediction of zoonoses emergence. *Emerg Infect Dis.* 2005;11(12):1822–1827.

37. van Nispen tot Pannerden C, van Gompel F, Rijnders BJ, et al. An itchy holiday. *Neth J Med.* 2007;65(5):188–190.

38. Centers for Disease Control and Prevention. *Anthrax Q&A: anthrax and animal hides.* http://www.bt.cdc.gov/agent/anthrax/faq/pelt.asp. Accessed March 29, 2008.

39. Leggat PA, Speare R. Travel with pets. *J Travel Med.* 2000;7:325–329.

40. Deplazes P, Staebler S, Gottstein B. Travel medicine of parasitic diseases in the dog [in German]. *Schweiz Arch Tierheilkd.* 2006;148(9):447–461.

41. Barr F, British Small Animal Veterinary Association Scientific Committee. Checklist of infections that may be imported into the UK by the travelling pet. *J Small Anim Pract.* 2001;42(2):95–97.

42. Teske E, van Knapen F, Beijer EG, et al. Risk of infection with *Leishmania* spp. in the canine population in The Netherlands. *Acta Vet Scand.* 2002;43(4):195–201.

43. Impact of pet travel on animal and public health. *Vet Rec.* 2008;162(14):429–430.

44. Galperine T, Neau D, Moiton MP, et al. The risk of rabies in France and the illegal importation of animals from rabid endemic countries [in French]. *Presse Med.* 2004;33(12 Pt 1):791–792.

45. Castrodale L, Walker V, Baldwin J, et al. Rabies in a puppy imported from India to the USA March 2007. *Zoonoses and Public Health.* 2008;55(8–10):427–430.

46. Brown CA, Jeong KS, Poppenga RH, et al. Outbreaks of renal failure associated with melamine and cyanuric acid in dogs and cats in 2004 and 2007. *J Vet Diagn Invest.* 2007;19(5):525–531.

47. Humane Society of the United States. *Tips for safe pet air travel.* http://www.hsus.org/pets/pet_care/caring_for_pets_when_you_travel/traveling_by_air_with_pets/. Accessed October 21, 2008.

48. Centers for Disease Control and Prevention. *Importation of pets, other animals, and animal products into the United States.* http://www.cdc.gov/ncidod/dq/animal/index.htm. Accessed February 28, 2008.

49. Centers for Disease Control and Prevention. *Bringing an animal into the United States.* http://www.cdc.gov/ncidod/dq/animal/dogs.htm. Accessed October 21, 2008.

50. U.S. Department of Agriculture. *Pet travel: tips, facts, and scam information—for you and your pet.* http://www.aphis.usda.gov/animal_welfare/pet_travel/content/wp_c_pet_travel_tips.shtml. Accessed May 29, 2008.

51. U.S. Department of Agriculture. *Animal health permits.* http://www.aphis.usda.gov/permits/index.shtml. Accessed October 15, 2008.

52. U.S. Department of Agriculture. *Animal and animal product import: non-US origin pet birds.* http://www.aphis.usda.gov/import_export/animals/nonus_pet_bird.shtml. Accessed October 10, 2008.

53. U.S. Customs Service. *Pets and wildlife.* http://www.cbp.gov/linkhandler/cgov/newsroom/publications/travel/pets_wild.ctt/pets.pdf. Accessed May 29, 2008.

EXOTIC AND WILDLIFE PETS

Animal and human health clinicians need to understand the scope of the exotic and wildlife pet trade, the related health risks, and ways to reduce such risks. Driven by popular demand, trade in live animals for pets has been increasing both in the United States and worldwide.[1] More than 200 million animals, representing thousands of individual species, are estimated to be legally imported into the United States from more than 160 countries. The majority of these imports were for the pet and aquarium trade.[2] The number of animals illegally imported each year is unknown but is also believed to be considerable.[3] As a result, the United States is the world's largest importer of live animals.[2] At the same time, many potential pet owners are unaware of the health risks of such nontraditional pets.[4]

Key Points for Clinicians and Public Health Professionals

Public Health Professionals

- Support efforts of the National Association of State Public Health Veterinarians (NASPHV) and Council of State and Territorial Epidemiologists (CSTE) to do the following:
  - Develop comprehensive federal regulations with enforcement that provide oversight to the private ownership of exotic and wild animals.
  - Develop and maintain a list of approved species for interstate distribution and importation.
  - Limit ports of entry.
  - Improve regulation and inspection of exotic animal breeders, dealers, auctions, swap meets, Internet sales, pet outlets, and animal imports.
  - Develop a system to track imported and captive-bred exotic animals in the pet trade.
- Support the USDA and local agencies to ensure that individuals and events selling or bartering exotic animals, including pet stores, are properly licensed and that exotic, wild, and imported animals are screened for known zoonoses, quarantined and observed for signs of disease, and have limited opportunities for ecological release into the nonnative environment.
- Educate the public and health care providers about the risks of ownership and contact with wildlife and exotic pets, including zoonotic infections, injury, and

(depending on species) envenomation. Discourage exotic or wild pet ownership among immunocompromised persons and families with children younger than 5 years. Discourage contact with mammals at high risk of transmitting rabies (e.g., bats, raccoons, skunks, foxes, and coyotes).

- Ensure that local pet stores, pet swap meets, petting zoos, schools, and other venues with human-animal contact are aware of the recommendations of the NASPHV for reducing risk of transmission in such settings, including adequate handwashing facilities, separation of animal and nonanimal areas, and avoidance of high-risk species.[5]
- If a human health clinician reports a zoonotic disease associated with an exotic or wildlife pet, coordinate a response with agricultural and wildlife veterinarians.
- Form interdisciplinary networks and working groups to address exotic and wild animal pet issues that arise locally and regionally. Groups should consist of veterinarians, public health professionals, wildlife agencies and rehabilitators, zoologic park staff, university representatives, physicians, and environmental health professionals.

Human Health Clinicians

- Ask patients about ownership and contact with exotic or wild animals. If they report such contact, list the species, origin, and types of interactions. Consider consulting the patient's veterinarian about the health risks (zoonotic and injury potential) of particular species.
- Discourage acquisition, contact with, and maintenance of exotic and wildlife pets, particularly for families with children or immunocompromised persons.
- If patients report ownership of venomous animals, ensure they are aware of the steps to take if envenomation occurs and that local emergency treatment (such as appropriate antivenin) is available locally (see Chapter 8).
- If zoonotic disease is suspected or identified in a person in contact with exotic or wild animals (pets, recreational or occupational exposure) or works in a pet shop or other animal handling facility, notify the local and state public health department.

Veterinary Clinicians

- Support efforts of state and national agencies to regulate or license ownership of exotic or wild pets.
- Counsel clients to refrain from owning wild-caught animals, about disease transmission routes, and the risks of ownership and contact with wildlife and exotic animals as pets.[6]
- Assist prospective pet owners in appropriate pet selection.
- Counsel owners on techniques to avoid high-risk contact with exotic or wild animals.

SCOPE OF THE PROBLEM

Much of the pet trade involves traditional pets, species that have been bred and maintained over multiple generations for human companionship and have acknowledged popularity as pets. Examples include dogs, cats, and horses. Caged birds such as parakeets and canaries and pocket pets such as gerbils and hamsters are also popular and are bred for the pet trade. Another large segment of the pet trade involves tropical fish, which have generally been associated with fewer zoonotic diseases than other animals.

Much of the remainder of the pet trade, however, is in nontraditional pets, or species that are not domesticated and are captured from the wild or captive-bred to meet an increasing demand for unusual pets. Nontraditional pets include exotic species that are nonnative to the local ecosystem and native wildlife, which are local wildlife species. The number of wild animals, including reptiles and amphibians, captured in the United States for the pet trade each year is not precisely known but appears to be in the range of millions of animals.[7] This segment of the pet trade is extremely lucrative and mainly uses the Internet, specialty newsletters, swap meets, auctions, and private sales rather than pet shops. Such settings are largely unregulated and lack disease prevention and control methods such as quarantine or veterinary care and may contribute to species reduction. Currently, 22 states ban or regulate certain exotic pets.

Reptiles such as turtles and iguanas are popular pets (Figure 10-5). However, as subclinical carriers of *Salmonella*, they have been the source of many human illnesses.[8] A 1975 FDA ban on the sale of turtles with a carapace less than 4 inches is estimated to have prevented more than 100,000 infections.

The importation, trade, and ownership of wild-caught and exotic animals for pets enhances the risk of dissemination and transmission of novel, rare (hantavirus, rabies, lymphocytic choriomeningitis virus), emerging, and exotic

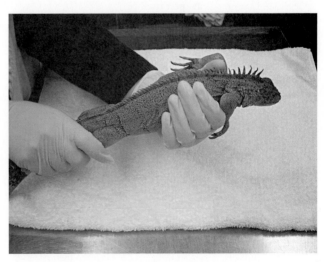

Figure 10-5 ■ Green iguana. (From Mitchell M, Tully TN Jr: *Manual of exotic pet practice*, St Louis, 2008, Saunders Elsevier.)

(Ebola, monkeypox, Nipah virus) pathogens. Human beings, domestic animals, and native wildlife are at risk.[9] Serious injuries are also a risk when handling wild or exotic animals because captivity and human companionship do not change natural behaviors or tame these animals. Many nonhuman primate pets have all their teeth removed but can still injure handlers.[10]

In addition to the zoonotic disease risk, some exotic and native wildlife species kept as pets are venomous and pose envenomation risks to other animals and pet owners (see Chapter 8).[11] Exotic venomous reptiles may produce venom for which antivenin may be not widely available.

INFECTIONS LINKED TO EXOTIC AND WILDLIFE PETS

Not surprisingly, the international trade in animals and the use of wildlife as pets have been linked to a number of zoonoses and other animal diseases. Table 10-5 shows documented examples of exotic and wildlife pets and diseases associated with them. Clearly the potential exists for injuries (trauma, envenomation), infections (viruses, bacteria, parasites, fungi) and allergies, although not specifically documented in the literature as a pet encounter.

These cases of reported disease illustrate the complexity of the issues surrounding nontraditional pets. The 1994 outbreak of *Salmonella* associated with African pygmy hedgehogs (Figure 10-6) involved captive-bred animals. Importation of hedgehogs from Africa had been banned

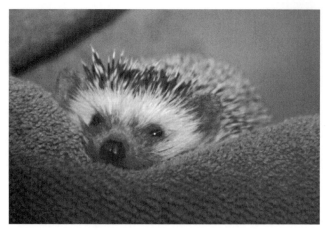

Figure 10-6   ▪   African hedgehog *(Atelerix albiventris).* (From Mitchell M, Tully TN Jr: *Manual of exotic pet practice,* St Louis, 2008, Saunders Elsevier.)

since 1991 because of concern about possible importation of foot and mouth disease.[23] Other exotic animals linked to salmonellosis include a komodo dragon at a zoo that infected 65 persons, mainly children, with contact to a temporary barrier around the exhibit.[24]

Spurred and leopard tortoises imported to Florida from Africa have been found to be infested with ticks of the genus *Amblyomma,* which can be a vector for heartwater, a serious livestock disease caused by the bacterium *Cowdria ruminantium.*[25] As a result, these African tortoises are currently banned in the United States. More recently, African vipers have been diagnosed with severe and even fatal tickborne disease related to a *Cowdria*-like organism.[26]

The 2003 multistate outbreak of monkeypox has received significant scientific and media attention and has a number of instructive points about imported zoonotic pathogens of wildlife. The outbreak was traced to the importation of wild-caught giant Gambian pouched rats (*Cricetomys gambianus;* Figure 10-7) and other rodents that had been recently imported from Africa for the pet trade.

Some of these exotic rodents were carriers of the monkeypox virus. When housed in dealer facilities, they

Table 10-5 ▪ Reported Infections Related to Nontraditional Pets

Nontraditional Pet Species	Associated Disease	Affected Species
Hedgehogs *(Atelerix albiventris)*[12]	Salmonellosis, dermatophytes, herpesvirus, yersiniosis, mycobacteriosis	Human beings
Leopard tortoises (*Geochelone pardalis*)[13]	Heartwater (found in *Amblyomma* ticks on tortoises)	Cattle
Various reptiles and amphibians[14–16]	Salmonellosis	Human beings
Gambian rat (*Cricetomys* spp.)	Monkeypox	Human beings, prairie dogs
Prairie dogs (*Cynomys* spp.)[17,18]	Tularemia, monkeypox	Human beings
Southern flying squirrel (*Glaucomys volans*)[19]	Leptospirosis	Human beings
Marmosets (*Callithrix jacchus*)[20]	Rabies	Human beings
Macaque monkeys (*Macaca* spp.)[21]	Herpes B	Human beings
Egyptian rousette bat (*Rousettus egyptiacus*)[22]	Lagos bat lyssa virus	Human beings

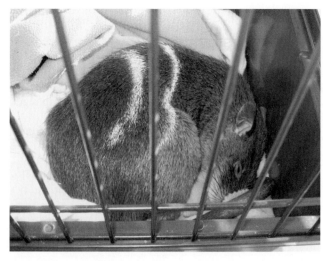

Figure 10-7   ▪   Gambian pouched rat. (From Wikipedia, http://en.wikipedia.org/wiki/Gambian_Pouch_Rat.)

were caged close to a susceptible native wildlife species, black-tailed prairie dogs *(Cynomys ludovicianus).* These prairie dogs then were sold as pets, and in the process 71 human beings, including pet owners, pet store workers, distributors, and veterinarians, contracted infection through contact with sick animals or their secretions (Figure 10-8).[27-29] Figure 10-9 shows the complex web of contact and distribution that resulted in human cases. The outbreak did not produce human fatalities but clearly showed the potential for a novel pathogen to cause outbreaks in the United States as a result of the global pet trade.

Examples of native wildlife used as pets and infecting their owners include a wild-caught prairie dog transmitting tularemia to an owner.[18] In Brazil, a new rabies virus variant was identified in human cases associated with pet marmosets *(Callithrix jacchus).*[20]

CONTROL EFFORTS

The magnitude and diversity of animal species being maintained as pets and the ongoing potential for novel and rare

zoonoses present challenges to health care providers and public health professionals. It appears that reduction of the rate of introduced pathogens can only be achieved by everyone at every level working on some aspect of the prevention

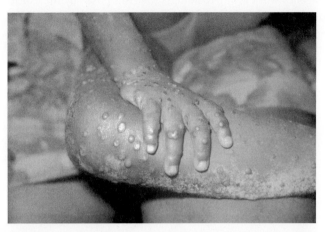

Figure 10-8 ▪ Monkeypox. (From the Centers for Disease Control and Prevention, Atlanta, Ga.)

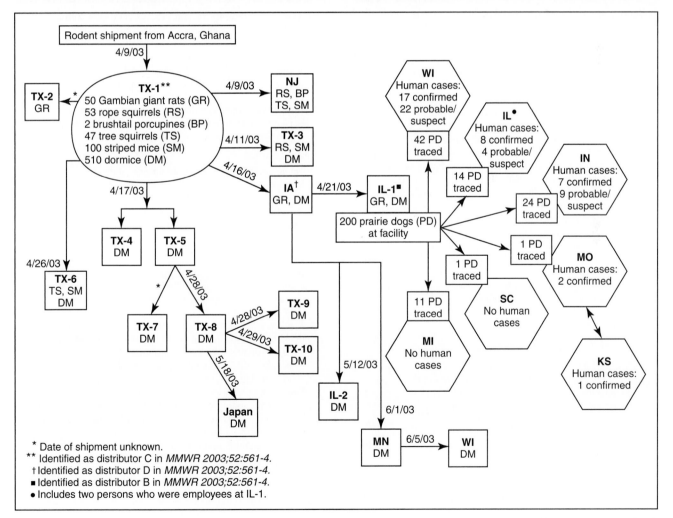

Figure 10-9 ▪ Movement of imported African rodents to animal distributors and distribution of prairie dogs from an animal distributor associated with human cases of monkeypox in 11 states (Illinois, Indiana, Iowa, Kansas, Michigan, Minnesota, Missouri, New Jersey, South Carolina, Texas, and Wisconsin) as of July 8, 2003. Japan is included among the locations having received shipment of rodents implicated in this outbreak. (This does not include one probable human case from Ohio.) (From Centers for Disease Control and Prevention: Update: multistate outbreak of monkeypox—Illinois, Indiana, Kansas, Missouri, Ohio, and Wisconsin, 2003, *MMWR Morb Mortal Wkly Rep* 52:642, 2003.)

and control—from local awareness of the problem to policy changes on a national or international level that restrict the trade in live animals.[2] NASPHV has joined with CSTE in developing position statements requesting a federal interagency work group to address the risks posed by the exotic animal trade (see Developing Importation and Importation Restrictions on Exotic and Native Wildlife with Potential Adverse Impact on Public Health, available online at http://www.cste.org/PS/2003pdfs/03-ID-13%20-%20FINAL.pdf).[30] In particular, NASPHV has called for the creation of an "approved species" list to reduce the threat of disease importation, more extensive inspection and quarantine of imported animals, and tracking of animals that have been imported. The AVMA is also on record discouraging exotic animals and wildlife as pets.[31] Although CDC regulations govern the importation of dogs, cats, turtles with a carapace of less than 4 inches, monkeys, bats, civets, birds from countries with H5N1 influenza, several species of African

rodents, and animal products capable of causing human disease,[32] only a small number of species (including the African rodents linked to the importation of monkeypox) are currently banned. In addition, most of the animals that are imported, with the exception of avian species, are neither quarantined nor tested for infectious disease agents before entering the country.

NASPHV has developed guidelines titled "Compendium of Measures to Prevent Disease Associated with Animals in Public Settings" to prevent spread of infections at public settings where animal contact could take place, including animal displays, petting zoos, animal swap meets, pet stores, zoological institutions, nature parks, circuses, carnivals, farm tours, livestock-birthing exhibits, county or state fairs, schools, and wildlife photo opportunities.[5] Key recommendations of these guidelines, as well as other recently published recommendations to reduce the risk of diseases related to nontraditional pets, are shown in Box 10-4.

BOX 10-4   *GUIDELINES FOR PREVENTION OF HUMAN DISEASES FROM NONTRADITIONAL PETS AT HOME AND EXPOSURE TO ANIMALS IN PUBLIC SETTINGS*

General

- Wash hands immediately after contact with animals, animal products, or their environment.
- Supervise handwashing for children younger than 5 years.
- Wash hands after handling animal-derived pet treats.
- Never bring wild animals home, and never adopt wild animals as pets.
- Teach children never to handle unfamiliar, wild, or domestic animals even if the animals appear friendly.
- Avoid rough play with animals to prevent scratches or bites.
- Children should not be allowed to kiss pets or put their hands or other objects into their mouths after handling animals.
- Do not permit nontraditional pets to roam or fly freely in the house or allow nontraditional or domestic pets to have contact with wild animals.
- Do not permit animals in areas where food or drink are prepared or consumed.
- Administer rabies vaccine to mammals as appropriate.
- Keep animals clean and free of intestinal parasites, fleas, ticks, mites, and lice.
- People at increased risk of infection or serious complications of salmonellosis (e.g., children younger than 5 years, older adults, and immunocompromised hosts) should avoid contact with animal-derived pet treats.

Animals Visiting Schools and Child-Care Facilities

- Designate specific areas for animal contact.
- Display animals in enclosed cages or under appropriate restraint.
- Do not allow food in animal contact areas.
- Always supervise children, especially those younger than 5 years, during interaction with animals.
- Obtain a certificate of veterinary inspection for visiting animals and/or proof of rabies immunization according to local or state requirements.
- Properly clean and disinfect all areas where animals have been present.
- Consult parents or guardians to determine special considerations needed for children who are immunocompromised or who have allergies or asthma.

- Animals not recommended in schools, child-care settings, and hospitals include nonhuman primates, inherently dangerous animals (lions, tigers, cougars, bears, wolf-dog hybrids), mammals at high risk of transmitting rabies (bats, raccoons, skunks, foxes, coyotes), aggressive animals or animals with unpredictable behavior, stray animals with unknown health history, reptiles, and amphibians.
- Ensure that people who provide animals for educational purposes are knowledgeable regarding animal handling and zoonotic disease issues.

Public Settings

- Venue operators must know about risks of disease and injury.
- Venue operators and staff must maintain a safe environment.
- Venue operators and staff must educate visitors about the risk of disease and injury and provide appropriate preventive measures.

Animal Specific

- Children younger than 5 years and immunocompromised people should avoid contact in public settings with reptiles, amphibians, rodents, ferrets, baby poultry (chicks, ducklings), and any items that have been in contact with these animals or their environments.
- Reptiles, amphibians, rodents, ferrets, and baby poultry (chicks, ducklings) should be kept out of households that contain children younger than 5 years, immunocompromised people, or people with sickle cell disease and should not be allowed in child-care centers.
- Reptiles, amphibians, rodents, and baby poultry should not be permitted to roam freely throughout a home or living area and should not be permitted in kitchens or other food-preparation areas.
- Disposable gloves should be used when cleaning fish aquariums, and aquarium water should not be disposed in sinks used for food preparation or for obtaining drinking water.
- Mammals at high risk of transmitting rabies (bats, raccoons, skunks, foxes, coyotes) should not be touched by children.

Adapted from Pickering LK, Marano N, Bocchini JA et al: Committee on infectious diseases: exposure to nontraditional pets at home and to animals in public settings: risks to children, *Pediatrics* 122:876, 2008.

References

1. Rosen T, Jablon J. Infectious threats from exotic pets: dermatological implications. *Dermatol Clin.* 2003;21(2):229–236.
2. Jenkins PT, Genovese K, Ruffler H. *Broken screens: the regulation of live animal importation in the United States.* Washington DC: Defenders of Wildlife; 2007.
3. Karesh WB, Cook RA, Bennett EL, et al. Wildlife trade and global disease emergence. *Emerg Infect Dis.* 2005;11(7):1000–1002.
4. Pickering LK, Marano N, Bocchini JA, et al. Committee on Infectious Diseases: Exposure to nontraditional pets at home and to animals in public settings: risks to children. *Pediatrics.* 2008;122(4):876–886.
5. National Association of State Public Health Veterinarians. Compendium of measures to prevent disease associated with animals in public settings, 2007. *MMWR Recomm Rep.* 2007;56(RR-5):1–14.
6. Kuehn BM. Wildlife pets create ethical, practical challenges for veterinarians. *J Am Vet Med Assoc.* 2004;225(2):171–173.
7. Reaser JK, Clark Jr EE, Meyers NM. All creatures great and minute: a public policy primer for companion animal zoonoses. *Zoonoses Public Health.* 2008;55(8–10):385–401.
8. Centers for Disease Control and Prevention. Reptile-associated salmonellosis—selected states, 1998–2002. *MMWR Morb Mortal Wkly Rep.* 2003;52(49):1206–1209.
9. Marano N, Arguin PM, Pappaioanou M. Impact of globalization and animal trade on infectious disease ecology. *Emerg Infect Dis.* 2007;13(12):1807–1809.
10. Johnson-Delaney CA. Safety issues in the exotic pet practice. *Vet Clin North Am: Exot Anim Pract.* 2005;8(3):515–524, vii.
11. Peterson ME. Toxic exotics. *Vet Clin North Am: Exot Anim Pract.* 2008;11(2):375–387, vii–viii.
12. Riley PY, Chomel BB. Hedgehog zoonoses. *Emerg Infect Dis.* 2005;11(1):1–5.
13. Burridge MJ, Simmons LA, Simbi BH, et al. Evidence of *Cowdria ruminantium* infection (heartwater) in *Amblyomma sparsum* ticks found on tortoises imported into Florida. *J Parasitol.* 2000;86(5):1135–1136.
14. Nagano N, Oana S, Nagano Y, et al. A severe *Salmonella enterica* serotype Paratyphi B infection in a child related to a pet turtle, *Trachemys scripta elegans. Jpn J Infect Dis.* 2006;9(2):132–134.
15. Schroter M, Roggentin P, Hofmann J, et al. Pet snakes as a reservoir for *Salmonella enterica* subsp. diarizonae (serogroup IIIb): a prospective study. *Appl Environ Microbiol.* 2004;70(1):613–615.
16. Greene S, Yartel A, Moriarty K, et al. *Salmonella kingabwa* infections and lizard contact, United States, 2005. *Emerg Infect Dis.* 2007;13(4):661–662.
17. Guarner J, Johnson BJ, Paddock CD, et al. Veterinary Monkeypox Virus Working Group: Monkeypox transmission and pathogenesis in prairie dogs. *Emerg Infect Dis.* 2004;10(3):426–431.
18. Avashia SB, Petersen JM, Lindley CM, et al. First reported prairie dog-to-human tularemia transmission, Texas, 2002. *Emerg Infect Dis.* 2004;10(3):483–486.
19. Chomel BB. *Wildlife zoonoses.* Michigan Veterinary Medical Association. http://www.michvma.org/documents/MVC%20Proceedings/Chomel. pdf.
20. Favoretto SR, de Mattos CC, Morais NB, et al. Rabies in marmosets *(Callithrix jacchus),* Ceara, Brazil. *Emerg Infect Dis.* 2001;7(6):1062–1065.
21. Ostrowski SR, Leslie MJ, Parrott T, et al. B-virus from pet macaque monkeys: an emerging threat in the United States? *Emerg Infect Dis.* 1998;4(1):117–121.
22. Chomel BB, Belotto A, Meslin FX. Wildlife, exotic pets, and emerging zoonoses. *Emerg Infect Dis.* 2007;13(1):6–11.
23. Centers for Disease Control and Prevention. African pygmy hedgehog–associated salmonellosis—Washington, 1994. *MMWR.* 1995;44(24): 462–463.
24. Friedman CR, Torigian C, Shillam PJ, et al. An outbreak of salmonellosis among children attending a reptile exhibit at a zoo. *J Pediatr.* 1998;132:802–807.
25. Burridge MJ, Simmons LA, Allan SA. Introduction of potential heartwater vectors and other exotic ticks into Florida on imported reptiles. *J Parasitol.* 2000;86(4):700–704.
26. Kiel JL, Alarcon RM, Parker JE, et al. Emerging tick-borne disease in African vipers caused by a *Cowdria*-like organism. *Ann N Y Acad Sci.* 2006;1081:434–442.
27. Reynolds MG, Davidson WB, Curns AT, et al. Spectrum of infection and risk factors for human monkeypox, United States, 2003. *Emerg Infect Dis.* 2007;13(9):1332–1339.
28. Croft DR, Sotir MJ, Williams CJ, et al. Occupational risks during a monkeypox outbreak, Wisconsin, 2003. *Emerg Infect Dis.* 2007;13(8):1150–1157.
29. Centers for Disease Control and Prevention. Update: multistate outbreak of monkeypox-Illinois, Indiana, Kansas, Missouri, Ohio, and Wisconsin, 2003. *MMWR Morb Mortal Wkly Rep.* 2003;52(27):642–646.
30. National Association of State Public Health Veterinarians. *Council of State and Territorial Epidemiologists: Joint statement: developing importation and exportation restrictions on exotic and native wildlife with potential adverse impact on public health, 2003.* http://www.cste.org/PS/2003pdfs/03-ID-13%20-%20FINAL.pdf. Accessed August 30, 2008.
31. American Veterinary Medical Association. *Birds, exotics and wild animals.* http://www.avma.org/careforanimals/animatedjourneys/petselection/birds.asp.
32. Centers for Disease Control and Prevention. *Global migration and quarantine.* http://www.cdc.gov/ncidod/dq/animal/index.htm. Accessed October 23, 2009.

IMMUNOCOMPROMISED INDIVIDUALS

Available evidence continues to suggest that the psychosocial support value of companion animals, particularly for the elderly or infirm,[1-3] outweighs the risk of acquiring a serious infection from such animals. Nevertheless, issues regarding hygiene and common sense practices must be addressed to support a healthy human-animal bond, especially among immunocompromised people or pets.

Key Points for Clinicians and Public Health Professionals

Public Health Professionals

- Provide public health guidance to reduce opportunistic infections among immunocompromised persons.

- Stress general hygiene principles, including handwashing, and ensure proper food preparation and safe water supplies.

Human Health Clinicians

- Understand the risks and considerable benefits of companion animal ownership among immunocompromised persons.
- Ensure that a thorough history is taken to best manage the patient's potential exposure to zoonotic disease.
- Be aware of the Guidelines for Preventing Opportunistic Infections among HIV-Infected Persons: Recommendations of the US Public Health Service and the Infectious Diseases Society of America (http://www.annals.org/cgi/content/full/137/5_Part_2/435).

- With an immunocompromised patient's permission, consider coordinating preventive interventions with the patient's veterinarian.
- Counsel immunocompromised patients with occupational exposure to animals about zoonotic infection risk and risk reduction measures.

Veterinary Clinicians

- Provide consultation about zoonotic disease risk reduction.
- Provide guidance on maintaining the health of immunocompromised animal patients, including a healthy environment.
- Maintain confidentiality of information regarding immunocompromised persons.

ETIOLOGY OF IMMUNOSUPPRESSION

Millions of people and companion animals in this country are living with less than a robust immune system. Immunosuppression can result from a number of etiologies, either from a primary or genetic malfunction (rare) or, more commonly, as a result of a secondary or acquired factor such as debilitation, immunosuppressive chemotherapy (Figure 10-10), human immunodeficiency virus (HIV) in human beings, or feline leukemia virus (FeLV) in cats (Table 10-6).

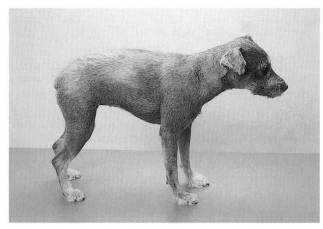

Figure 10-10 ▪ Alopecia in a 7-year-old Schnauzer undergoing doxorubicin and dacarbazine chemotherapy. (From Couto CG: Complications of cancer chemotherapy. In Nelson RW, Couto CG (eds): *Small animal internal medicine*, ed 4, St Louis, 2009, Mosby Elsevier.)

Table 10-6 ▪ Etiologies of Immunocompromise in Human Beings and Other Animals

	Examples (Breed Predilection)
Common to All Species	
Chemicals	Immunosuppressive medication (e.g., corticosteroids, cyclosporin, 6-mercaptopurine, methotrexate, azathioprine), mercury, PCBs
Radiation	Radiation therapy, excess radiation exposure
Neoplasia	Leukemia, other cancers
Other causes	Severe malnutrition, chronic diabetes, renal/hepatic/splenic failure, prematurity, advancing age
Human Beings	
Primary (genetic)	X-linked agammaglobulinemia, X-linked hyper-IgM syndrome, Wiskott-Aldrich syndrome, Ataxia telangiectasia, chronic granulomatous disease, SCID
Infections	HIV, other severe infections
Dogs	
Primary (genetic)[4]	X-linked severe combined immunodeficiency (Basset Hounds, Cardigan Welsh Corgis)
	Severe combined immunodeficiency disease (Jack Russell terriers)
	IgA deficiency (Beagles, German Shepherd dogs, Chinese Shar-Peis, English Cocker Spaniels, Irish Wolfhounds)[5]
	IgM deficiency (Doberman Pinschers)
	Thymic hypoplasia (dwarfed Weimaraners)
	Cyclic hematopoiesis (gray Collies)
	Leukocyte adhesion deficiency (Irish Setters)
	Complimentary deficiency (Brittany Spaniels)
	Bactericidal defect (Doberman Pinschers)
	Transient hypogammaglobulinemia (Samoyeds)
Chemicals	Organophosphate toxicity[6]
Cats	
Primary (genetic)	Chediak-Higashi syndrome (Persian cats)
Infectious	FIV/FeLV
Horses	
Primary (genetic)	SCID (Arabians)

PCBs, Polychlorinated biphenyls; *Ig*, immunoglobulin; *SCID*, severe combined immune deficiency.

In general, defects in humoral immunity (B-cell lines) can lead to increased susceptibility to bacterial infections; cell-mediated immunity (T-cell lines) defects to viral, fungal, or protozoal infections; and defects of phagocytosis or the complement system to disseminated infections.

IMPACT OF IMMUNODEFICIENCY STATES ON ANIMAL-HUMAN DISEASE TRANSMISSION

A large proportion of American households include pets,[7] and pet ownership among immunocompromised persons is common. For example, studies of patients with HIV infection have reported rates of pet ownership similar to that of the general population, with approximately half owning or living with pets.[8] In addition, on a global level, the HIV/AIDS pandemic has created large populations of individuals with compromised immune systems, many of whom may also be exposed to zoonotic diseases.[9,10] Human and veterinary clinicians are quite likely to encounter situations in which they may provide appropriate guidance for reducing animal sources of infectious diseases for human beings and vice versa by educating themselves and staff to provide the best available information.

There are at least three possible effects of human immunodeficiency on animal-human disease transmission:

1. An immunocompromised host is more susceptible to infection with opportunistic disease.
2. An immunocompromised host may transmit opportunistic disease to others.
3. A disease may be more severe in an immunocompromised host (e.g., toxoplasmosis, which causes asymptomatic or mild disease in most immunocompetent patients but can cause severe and even fatal systemic disease in immunocompromised individuals).

The knowledge level among immunocompromised persons and their health care providers about the risk of acquiring infections from pets could be increased with an appropriate educational strategy. In one study in which more than 400 patients with AIDS were interviewed—half of whom owned pets—only about 10% who were living with pets were given any information about zoonotic diseases from their health care provider, and one quarter of this information was incorrect or misunderstood (e.g., "fleas can give you rabies" or "cats can give you AIDS").[8] Because pet ownership is as common (and understanding of zoonoses as uncommon) among persons living with HIV as in the general population, human health care providers must be prepared to discuss with immunocompromised patients the risks of living with pets. Overly conservative approaches, including physician recommendations for their patients to relinquish pets, have largely been unheeded as owners often have strong bonds with their animals.[11] Armed with complete and accurate information, patients and their care providers can weigh these risks against the often substantial benefits of love, touch, social support, and companionship that accrue to pet owners. Zoonotic disease prevention is a shared responsibility among human, veterinary, and public health professionals. Improving communication among these persons will enhance zoonotic disease prevention.[12]

HUMAN HEALTH CARE PROVIDERS

Pet-owning human health care providers must be vigilant regarding nosocomial zoonoses, particularly if they are working with immunocompromised patients. In one situation, a common yeast pathogen of canine otitis externa (Figure 10-11) was introduced into a neonatal intensive care unit by a dog-owning health care worker, causing colonization in infants, some resulting in serious infections.[13,14] In another case, a cat on a geriatric ward was the likely suspect of staphylococcal infections (see Chapter 5).[15]

GENERAL GUIDELINES FOR THE PREVENTION OF ZOONOTIC DISEASE IN IMMUNOCOMPROMISED PATIENTS

Guidance From Both Human Health and Veterinary Health Care Providers

Hand and food hygiene is vital (Figures 10-12 and 10-13). Pets are not likely to be the most common source of zoonotic disease infection. More likely, contact with raw or undercooked meat or from an environmental infectious source is implicated in transmission. Unequivocally, immunocompromised individuals should avoid raw meat and eggs and unpasteurized dairy products. For example, although cats are the definitive host for *Toxoplasma gondii*, undercooked meat (less than 165° F) and inadequately washed, contaminated fruits and vegetables are likely the source for infection. See USDA food safety fact sheets: http://www.fsis.usda.gov/Factsheets/Keep_Food_Safe_Food_Safety_Basics/index.asp and http://www.fsis.usda.gov/Factsheets/At_Risk_&_Underserved_Fact_Sheets/index.asp.

Serologic or fecal evaluation of healthy cats for *Toxoplasma* infection is not recommended. Oocysts are shed transiently and are easily missed, and serologic evaluation does not predict cats shedding oocysts. Instead, prevention

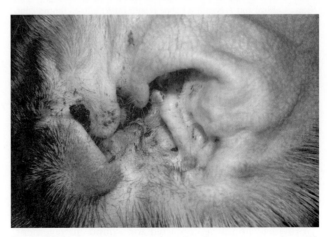

Figure 10-11 ■ Otitis externa in a dog. Brown, waxy exudate with a secondary yeast infection associated with an underlying allergy. (From Medleau L, Hnilica KA: *Small animal dermatology: a color atlas and therapeutic guide,* ed 2, St Louis, 2006, Saunders Elsevier.)

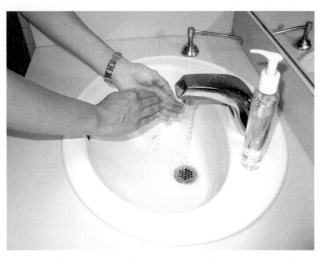

Figure 10-12 ■ Handwashing is critical to disease prevention. (From Centers for Disease Control and Prevention Public Health Image Library, Atlanta, Ga. Photo courtesy Kelly Thomas.)

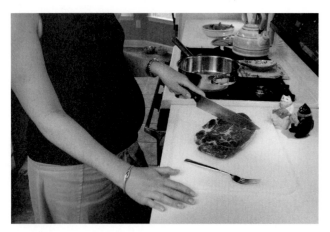

Figure 10-13 ■ Pregnant women and immunosuppressed patients can be at greater risk in acquiring foodborne illness and need to take additional precautions when handling raw food products. Cook meat, poultry, and eggs thoroughly. Using a thermometer to measure the internal temperature of meat is a good way to be sure that it is cooked sufficiently to kill bacteria. For example, ground beef should be cooked to an internal temperature of 160° F. Eggs should be cooked until the yolk is firm. (From Centers for Disease Control and Prevention Public Health Image Library. Photo courtesy James Gathany.)

of transmission of *Toxoplasma* directly from cats should focus on the following husbandry recommendations:

- Avoid contact with feces (have an immunocompetent person clean the litterbox or fecal accidents, or wear gloves followed by washing hands) (Figure 10-14).
- Pets should not be given prophylactic antibiotics without clinical signs of infection. For example, *Salmonella* carriage in reptiles cannot be eliminated. Use of antibiotics for this purpose has been unsuccessful and may favor development of antibiotic-resistant bacteria.[16]
- Any bite or wound from an animal should be flushed with copious amounts of soap and water and a health care provider should be contacted for wound management, including assessment for appropriate antibiotics, tetanus, and possible rabies postexposure prophylaxis (see Animal and Human Bites later in this chapter).

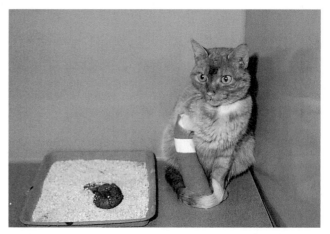

Figure 10-14 ■ Have an immunocompetent person clean the litterbox. (From Bunch SE: The exocrine pancreas. In Nelson RW, Couto CG (eds): *Small animal internal medicine*, ed 3, St Louis, 2003, Mosby Elsevier.)

- Review guidance to reducing exposure to selected opportunistic diseases among persons with HIV (see http://www.cdc.gov/mmwr/preview/mmwrhtml/rr5108a1.htm).
- Encourage questions about healthy living with companion animals and discourage kissing or face-to-face contact.
- Pet vaccines, including live attenuated strains, should be recommended and given as needed; they are not believed to present a human health hazard.[17]

Occupational or Recreational Risk Reduction

- Avoid contact with wild animals to reduce the risk of enteric disease, such as acquiring *Cryptosporidium* from wild birds.
- NEVER touch the feces of any animal.
- Avoid farm animals and petting zoos to decrease exposure to *Escherichia coli* in ruminants, *Bordetella bronchiseptica* in swine, and *Salmonella* in chicks and ducks.
- Occupational health care workers working with high-risk personnel such as veterinarians, veterinary staff, zookeepers, and pet shop workers should counsel immunocompromised workers about the risk of occupational of zoonotic disease infection and possible work restrictions to reduce risk for those with significant impairment of immunity.

Animal Selection Recommendations

- Select healthy, well-mannered dogs or cats 6 months or older to decrease the likelihood of exposure to enteric diseases and *Bartonella* from kittens.
- Avoid petting or handling free-roaming animals; when selecting a pet, choose one with a documented veterinary health history and current vaccinations.
- Avoid exotic or wild animals to reduce the likelihood of exposure to emerging infections (i.e., monkeypox in rodents) and known diseases such as herpes B infection from macaque monkeys and *Salmonella* from reptiles (Figure 10-15).

Cockatoos, like pigeons, may shed *Cryptococcus* in their feces. Transmission of this infection from a cockatoo to its owner who was chronically immunocompromised because

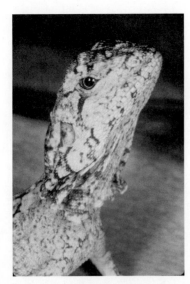

Figure 10-15 ▪ Immunocompromised persons should avoid selecting reptiles as pets, such as this frilled dragon *(Chlamydosaurus kingii)*. (From Mader DR: *Reptile medicine and surgery,* ed 2, St Louis, 2006, Saunders Elsevier.)

of a renal transplant has occurred.[18] Therefore some authors have recommended that immunocompromised patients not own cockatoos (Figure 10-16).[19]

A fatal outbreak of lymphocytic choriomeningitis virus (LCMV) in solid-organ transplant recipients was traced back to a pet hamster acquired by the organ donor 17 days before donation (Figure 10-17). The prevalence of this virus in rodent populations has led to recommendations that immunocompromised individuals (as well as pregnant women) should avoid owning pet rodents or having contact with wild or pet rodents.[20]

Have a veterinarian conduct a physical examination and fecal analysis on a new pet.

ANIMAL HUSBANDRY GUIDANCE

- Seek veterinary care early in the course of clinical disease of pets to limit chances for zoonotic disease exposure.

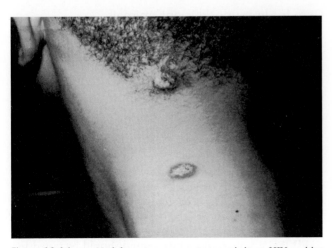

Figure 10-16 ▪ Nodular cutaneous cryptococcosis in an HIV-positive cockatoo owner. (From Rosen T, Jablon J: Infectious threats from exotic pets: dermatological implications, *Derm Clin* 21:229, 2003.)

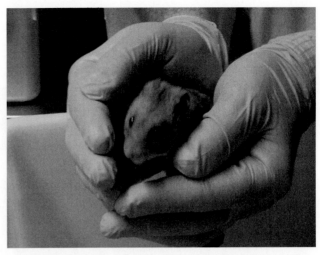

Figure 10-17 ▪ Pet rodents have been implicated in fatal LCMV infection in human beings. (From Sheldon CC, Sonsthagen T, Topel JA: *Animal restraint for veterinary professionals,* St Louis, 2006, Mosby Elsevier.)

- Keep pets indoors or leashed on walks to decrease the likelihood of engagement with other animals.
- Because of occasional cases of *Bordetella bronchiseptica* among immunocompromised persons,[21,22] avoid exposing dogs or owners to situations in which dogs are congregated, such as boarding kennels, grooming parlors, off-leash dog parks, or dog shows.
- Do not allow pets to hunt, scavenge, or eat feces to reduce the likelihood of exposure to enteric infections.
- Do not feed pets raw meat or egg diets or provide unpasteurized dairy products to limit exposure to enteric infections.
- Do not allow your pet to drink from the toilet.
- Keep animals and litterboxes out of food preparation areas.
- Avoid exposure to pet urine, feces, and saliva (don't allow your pet to lick your face or open lesions).
- Have a nonimmunocompromised household member remove a pet's solid waste and dispose daily by flushing down a toilet or discarding in the garbage or in a compost area (not to be spread on fruits or vegetables).
- Avoid animals with diarrhea. Have an immunocompetent household member clean soiled areas in the house of organic debris, followed by a 1:10 household bleach solution.
- Avoid rough play with the pet that could result in being bitten or scratched; keep pet's nails trimmed short.
- Remove and dispose of bird cage linings daily and use "wet" cleaning for the cage and utensils on a weekly basis. Wear gloves when handling items that are contaminated with bird droppings.
- Have a helper clean the fish tank (Figure 10-18) or wear disposable gloves during such activities, followed by washing hands thoroughly by rubbing hands together vigorously for 15 to 20 seconds with running water and soap.
- If assistance is required to care for your pet, contact local volunteer groups who may be willing to provide exercise, food, or foster care (e.g., during hospitalization).

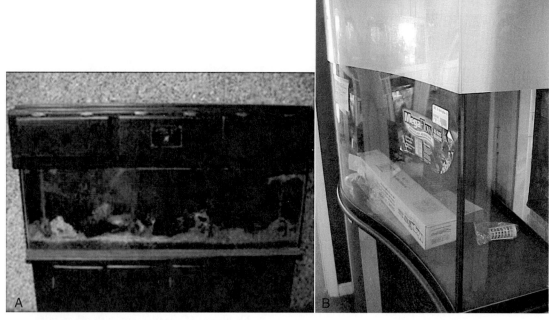

Figure 10-18 ▪ Types of fish tanks. (From Mitchell M, Tully TN Jr: *Manual of exotic pet practice*, St Louis, 2008, Saunders.)

U.S. PUBLIC HEALTH SERVICE GUIDELINES FOR PERSONS WHO ARE HIV POSITIVE

Although any zoonotic disease that occurs in immunocompetent individuals can also affect immunocompromised patients, the U.S. Public Health Service has highlighted a number of animal agents that pose a significant risk to HIV-infected persons. These include causes of enteritis (especially *Campylobacter, Salmonella,* and *Cryptosporidium*), and *Bartonella, Toxoplasma, Histoplasma,* and *Mycobacterium marinum.*

The evidence-based recommendations of the U.S. Public Health Service and the Infectious Diseases Society of America are listed in Table 10-7.

Although these guidelines recommend that human health care providers counsel their immunocompromised patients about zoonotic disease risk reduction, surveys of physicians have indicated that many believe that veterinarians are best equipped to provide such counseling and should therefore be involved in patient education of immunocompromised individuals.[12] Some authorities have stated that veterinarians are more qualified than physicians to advise pet owners and persons in high-risk professions about zoonotic risks.[23]

PUBLIC HEALTH ROLE OF THE VETERINARIAN: SAFER PET OWNERSHIP FOR IMMUNOCOMPROMISED PERSONS AND CARE OF IMMUNOCOMPROMISED PETS

In the veterinary setting, pet owners may be more willing to request information regarding safer pet ownership for immunocompromised persons if there are, for example, posters and handouts encouraging such client education or information in practice newsletters. Veterinarians can address high-risk persons during general discussions about zoonotic disease diagnosis, control, and prevention. Veterinarians should also emphasize among their staff the need for strict confidentiality regarding any personal information an animal owner happens to disclose about his or her own medical status (it is not recommended, for example, to document human medical information in the veterinary record).

Care for Pets of Immunocompromised Owners

- Neuter pets.
- Provide strict adherence to strategic deworming protocols and maintenance of appropriate vaccinations.
- Be prepared to discuss end-of-life planning for the pet's continued care (http://www.hsus.org/pets/pet_care/guidelines_ for_finding_a_responsible_home_for_a_pet.html).

Care for Immunodeficient Animals

- Do not administer modified live virus vaccines.
- Manage secondary and opportunistic infections (Color Plate 10-5).
- Provide supportive care.

Guidance for Owners of Immunodeficient Animals

- Animals with primary immunodeficiency disorders should not be bred.
- Cats with FIV or FeLV can spread the viruses to other cats, typically by bite wounds or close contact (FeLV) (Color Plate 10-6). Therefore separate household contacts that are FIV/FeLV negative. (All cats with unknown FIV/FeLV status with a bite wound should be tested for these viruses at the time of presentation and again 60 days later.)

Table 10-7 ▪ Guidelines for Preventing Opportunistic Infections Among HIV-Infected Persons

Topic	Recommendation	Strength of Recommendation*
General Pet-Related Recommendations		
	Health care providers should advise HIV-infected persons of the potential risk of pet ownership but should not routinely advise HIV patients to part with their pets.	DIII
	Seek veterinary care when pet develops diarrhea.	BIII
	Animals with diarrhea (and animals <6 months old) should be examined and stool tested for *Cryptosporidium*, *Salmonella*, and *Campylobacter*.	BIII
	When obtaining a new pet, avoid animals <6 months (1 year for cats) and animals with diarrhea. Avoid stray animals.	CIII
	Wash hands after handling pet, including before eating, and avoid contact with pet feces. Supervise handwashing in HIV-positive children.	BIII
	Avoid contact with reptiles (e.g., snakes, lizards, iguanas, turtles) as well as chicks and ducklings to reduce salmonellosis risk.	BIII
	Use gloves when cleaning aquarium to reduce risk of *Mycobacterium marinum* infection.	CIII
	Avoid contact with exotic pets (e.g., nonhuman primates).	BII
	Avoid exposure to calves and lambs and premises where calves and lambs are raised.	BII
Cat ownership	Discuss with HIV patient and caretakers that cat ownership increases risk of *Bartonella* and enteric infections.	CIII
	Patients acquiring a cat should adopt or purchase cat >1 year old and in good health; avoid acquiring a stray cat.	BII
Toxoplasmosis	Wash hands after working in a garden; wash all fruits and vegetables and ensure that raw meats are handled separately from raw food. Clean cat litterbox daily, preferably by HIV-negative, nonpregnant person (use gloves and wash hands afterwards), keep cat indoors, do not allow cat to hunt, do not feed cat undercooked meat.	BIII
	Testing cats for toxoplasmosis	EII (not recommended)
Bartonella infection	Declawing of cat not usually advised. Avoid activities resulting in bites or scratches.	BII
	Wash bites or scratches promptly.	CIII
	Do not allow cats to lick wounds.	BIII
	Flea control for cats.	CIII
	Testing cat for *Bartonella*.	DII (not recommended)
Occupational exposures	Occupations with animal contact may pose risk for cryptosporidiosis, toxoplasmosis, salmonellosis, campylobacteriosis, or *Bartonella*, but data are insufficient to recommend against patients with HIV working in such settings.	
	Follow recommendations and protocols for protective equipment and clothing.	BII
	Avoid contact with young farm animals, specifically those with diarrhea, to reduce cryptosporidiosis infection.	BIII
	Handwashing after gardening or soil contact to reduce risk of cryptosporidiosis and toxoplasmosis. In areas endemic for histoplasmosis, avoid risk activities including soil contact, cleaning chicken coops, disturbing soil beneath bird roosts, demolishing buildings, or cave exploring.	CIII
Birds	Screening healthy birds for *Cryptococcus neoformans*, *Mycobacterium avium*, or *Histoplasma capsulatum* is not recommended.	DIII

Adapted from Kaplan JE, Masur H, Holmes KK: Guidelines for preventing opportunistic infections among HIV-infected persons—2002. Recommendations of the U.S. Public Health Service and the Infectious Diseases Society of America, *MMWR Recomm Rep* 51(RR-8):1, 2002.

*System used to rate the strength of recommendations and quality of supporting evidence is as follows:

Rating strength of recommendation

A, Both strong evidence for efficacy and substantial clinical benefit support recommendation for use; should always be offered.

B, Moderate evidence for efficacy or strong evidence for efficacy but only limited clinical benefit; supports recommendation for use; should usually be offered.

C, Evidence for efficacy is insufficient to support a recommendation for or against use, or evidence for efficacy might not outweigh adverse consequences (e.g., drug toxicity, drug interactions) or cost of the chemoprophylaxis or alternative approaches; use is optional.

D, Moderate evidence for lack of efficacy or for adverse outcome supports a recommendation against use; should usually not be offered.

E, Good evidence for lack of efficacy or for adverse outcome supports a recommendation against use; should never be offered.

Rating quality of evidence supporting the recommendation

I, Evidence from ≥1 correctly randomized, controlled trials.

II, Evidence from ≥1 well-designed clinical trials without randomization, from cohort or case-controlled analytic studies (preferably from more than one center), or from multiple time-series studies, or dramatic results from uncontrolled experiments.

III, Evidence from opinions of respected authorities based on clinical experience, descriptive studies, or reports of consulting committees.

- Keep these animals indoors; do not allow pets to hunt, scavenge, or consume raw meat or egg diets or unpasteurized dairy products.
- Wash hands before and after handling the pet.
- Provide appropriate endoparasite and ectoparasite control.
- Avoid exposure to other ill animals.

CASE STUDIES

Case Study 1

A public health veterinarian working as an AIDS surveillance coordinator received a number of questions for which the human-animal bond was never more poignant. Indeed, one was from a gentleman who was recently diagnosed with AIDS and who owned a 4-year-old neutered male Golden Retriever. His family practitioner, concerned about any increased risk for opportunistic infections, advised him to find another home for his beloved pet. This man was heartbroken, trying to gather as much information as possible about what specifically he would face if he ignored his doctor's advice. Fortunately, with his permission, the veterinarian was able to contact his physician to discuss the relatively low risk as well as the benefits of owning a healthy pet (one that was receiving regular veterinary care) and encouraged the doctor to continue to contact public health practitioners for information as well as this pet owner's veterinarian (with permission) about the animal's preventive health care. Additionally, this pet owner happened to live in an area with an active volunteer organization that assisted with walking and feeding pets of persons living with AIDS. Armed with these resources, the patient was able to maintain a healthy pet.

Case Study 2

A public health veterinarian who was also a relief clinical veterinarian was presented with a 7-year-old neutered female cat for toxoplasmosis serologic testing and (reluctant) possible euthanasia of the cat. The cat's owner was the spouse of a cancer patient and was concerned that the spouse was on immunosuppressive chemotherapy and therefore at great risk for toxoplasmosis from their pet. The veterinarian explained the life cycle of toxoplasmosis, the epidemiology in people and cats, and that if the serology was positive it could actually be protective. The owner declined both serologic testing and euthanasia because the cat had never hunted in its lifetime, was indoors only, and was fed an exclusively commercial diet. There was no evidence of mice or rats in the house, decreasing the cat's likelihood of exposure to the parasite. However, the spouse enjoyed gardening—a much greater potential for exposure to toxoplasmosis. Fortunately the patient always wore gloves when doing so and thoroughly washed afterwards. The veterinarian and the cat owner discussed additional toxoplasmosis exposure reduction, including proper handling of raw meats and washing raw foods. The veterinarian and cat owner agreed that the owner would be the person cleaning the litterbox, schedule overall wellness examinations of the cat every 6 months, and would bring the cat in for evaluation and zoonotic disease prevention if diarrhea or signs of respiratory disease developed.

References

1. Raina P, Waltner-Toews D, Bonnett B, et al. Influence of companion animals on the physical and psychological health of older people: an analysis of a one-year longitudinal study. *J Am Geriatr Soc.* 1999;47(3):323–329.
2. Castelli P, Hart LA, Zasloff RL. Companion cats and the social support systems of men with AIDS. *Psychol Rep.* 2001;89(1):177–187.
3. Siegel JM, Angulo FJ, Detels R, et al. AIDS diagnosis and depression in the Multicenter AIDS Cohort Study: the ameliorating impact of pet ownership. *AIDS Care.* 1999;11:157–170.
4. Tilley LP, Smith FWK. *Blackwell's five-minute veterinary consult: canine and feline.* 3rd ed. Ames, IA: Blackwell; 2004.
5. Day MJ. Immunodeficiency disease in the dog. In: World Small Animal Veterinary Association World Congress Proceedings. 2004. http://www.vin.com/proceedings/Proceedings.plx?CID=WSAVA2004&PID=8598&O=Generic. Accessed May 3, 2009.
6. Sykora B, Tomsikova A. Kaposi's sarcoma in dog with acquired immunodeficiency after phosphate poisoning. *Folia Microbiol (Praha).* 1998;43(5):543–544.
7. American Veterinary Medical Association. *Market research statistics: U.S. pet ownership—2007.* http://www.avma.org/reference/marketstats/ownership.asp.
8. Conti L, Lieb S, Liberti T, et al. Pet ownership among persons with AIDS in three Florida counties. *Am J Public Health.* 1995;85(11):1559–1561.
9. Etter E, Donado P, Jori F, et al. Risk analysis and bovine tuberculosis, a re-emerging zoonosis. *Ann N Y Acad Sci.* 2006;1081:61–73.
10. Feldman RL, Nickell K. Avian influenza: potential impact on sub-Saharan military populations with high rates of human immunodeficiency virus/acquired immunodeficiency syndrome. *Mil Med.* 2007;172(7):753–758.
11. Angulo FJ, Glaser CA, Juranek DD, et al. Caring for pets of immunocompromised persons. *J Am Vet Med Assoc.* 1994;205(12):1711–1718.
12. Grant S, Olsen CW. Preventing zoonotic diseases in immunocompromised persons: the role of physicians and veterinarians. *Emerg Infect Dis.* 1999;5(1):159–163.
13. Chang HJ, Miller HL, Watkins N, et al. An epidemic of *Malassezia pachydermatis* in an intensive care nursery associated with colonization of health care workers' pet dogs. *N Engl J Med.* 1998;338(11):706–711.
14. Morris DO. *Malassezia pachydermatis* carriage in dog owners. *Emerg Infect Dis.* 2005;11(1):83–88.
15. Marcus LC, Marcus E. Nosocomial zoonoses. *N Engl J Med.* 1998;338(11):757–759.
16. Bradley T, Angulo FJ, Raiti P. Association of Reptilian and Amphibian Veterinarians guidelines for reducing risk of transmission of *Salmonella* spp. from reptiles to humans. *J Am Vet Med Assoc.* 1998;213:51–52.
17. Hemsworth S, Pizer B. Pet ownership in immunocompromised children—a review of the literature and survey of existing guidelines. *Eur J Oncol Nurs.* 2006;10(2):117–127.
18. Nosanchuk JD, Shoham S, Fries BC, et al. Evidence of zoonotic transmission of *Cryptococcus neoformans* from a pet cockatoo to an immunocompromised patient. *Ann Intern Med.* 2000;132(3):205–208.
19. Rosen T, Jablon J. Infectious threats from exotic pets: dermatological implications. *Dermatol Clin.* 2003;21(2):229–236.
20. Amman BR, Pavlin BI, Albarino CG, et al. Pet rodents and fatal lymphocytic choriomeningitis in transplant patients. *Emerg Infect Dis.* 2007;13(5):719–725.
21. Berkowitz DM, Bechara RI, Wolfenden LL. An unusual cause of cough and dyspnea in an immunocompromised patient. *Chest.* 2007;131(5):1599–1602.
22. Trevejo RT, Barr MC, Robinson RA. Important emerging bacterial zoonotic infections affecting the immunocompromised. *Vet Res.* 2005;36:493–506.
23. Nowotny N, Deutz A. Preventing zoonotic diseases in immunocompromised persons: the role of physicians and veterinarians. *Emerg Infect Dis.* 2000;6(2):208.

ANIMAL AND HUMAN BITES

Each year in the United States several million persons are bitten by animals. Although up to 80% of bites may never be reported, more than 300,000 emergency department visits occur each year for dog bites alone.[1] Approximately half of reported animal bite victims are children. Dogs are responsible for the majority of reported animal bite injuries to human beings in the United States, followed by cats and rodents.[2] Bites from human beings are rarer. With the increasing popularity of exotic pets, patients may present to emergency departments with bites from a wide range of species. In addition to trauma, infection (Color Plate 10-7) and envenomation (see Chapter 8) can be major concerns with animal bites. Animal bites can also result in allergy and anaphylaxis, which might be immediate or delayed (e.g., anaphylaxis has been reported after rodent bites and horse bites, even when the patient had a history of only mild allergic symptoms in the past[3,4]). In addition, the victim and/or animal owner might experience psychological trauma associated with either the bite incident itself or the consequent decisions that must be made regarding the biting animal. Animal (especially dog) bite fatalities in human beings are uncommon but occur at the rate of 1 to 2 dozen each year in the United States.[5]

Animal bites are common in companion animals and livestock as well (Figure 10-19), and fatalities in animals can occur if they are not systematically reported. The initial care

and treatment of animals bitten by other animals is similar to that for animal bites in human beings.

The optimal prevention and treatment of animal bites require good communication among veterinary, human health, and public health professionals. Often the veterinarian (and sometimes a zoologist) must provide critical information about the animal source of the bite, such as rabies risk status, whereas the public health professional may become involved in issues such as rabies prophylaxis and animal quarantine. As discussed in Chapter 12, animal bites are a major occupational risk of veterinarians, their staff, and other animal workers. This section covers key aspects of management and prevention of animal bites as well as bites by human beings.

Key Points for Clinicians and Public Health Professionals

Public Health Professionals

- Be aware of rabies risk in the community and be available for consultation with clinicians on postexposure prophylaxis.
- Provide public education to avoid feeding or handling wild or stray animals.
- Support community animal control efforts.
- Educate families to never leave a child alone with an animal.
- Be aware of educational resources for animal bite prevention, such as:
  - Humane Society of the U.S. (HSUS): http://www.hsus.org/pets/pet_care/dog_care/stay_dog_bite_free/index.html
  - CDC: http://www.cdc.gov/ncipc/duip/biteprevention.htm (Box 10-5)
  - AVMA: http://www.avma.org/press/publichealth/dog-bite/messpoints.asp.
  - US Postal Service: http://www.usps.com/communications/community/dogbite.htm.

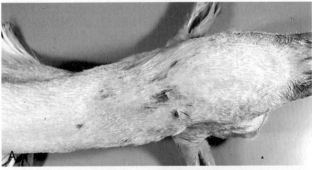
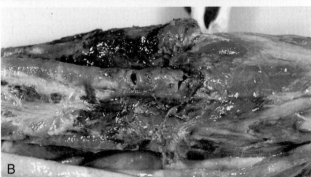

Figure 10-19 ■ **A,** This goat was attacked by dogs. Note bite wound on the ventral neck area. **B,** At postmortem, the skin has been removed to show the extensiveness of the injury; note tracheal defects and muscle lacerations. (From Fubini SL, Ducharme N: *Farm animal surgery,* St Louis, 2004, Saunders Elsevier. Courtesy John King, Cornell University.)

Human Health Clinicians

- Provide information on bite prevention to patients with animals and families with children.
- Counsel pregnant women and immunocompromised persons to avoid contact with rodents.
- Counsel patients on first-aid procedures to be taken in the event of a bite injury and to seek medical care for all bites.
- In caring for animal bite injuries, take a complete history regarding the animal, circumstances of the bite, history of allergies, and rabies and tetanus risk. Documentation that includes a drawing or photograph of the wound may be helpful because of legal implications.
- Systematically evaluate the need for antibiotic, rabies, and tetanus prophylaxis, consulting with veterinary and public health professionals as necessary.

BOX 10-5 CDC RECOMMENDATIONS FOR DOG-BITE PREVENTION

Things to Consider Before You Get a Dog

- Consult a professional (e.g., veterinarian, animal behaviorist, or responsible breeder) to learn about suitable breeds of dogs for your household.
- Dogs with histories of aggression are inappropriate in households with children.
- Be sensitive to cues that a child is fearful or apprehensive about a dog and, if so, delay acquiring a dog.
- Spend time with a dog before buying or adopting it. Use caution when bringing a dog into the home with an infant or toddler.
- Spay or neuter virtually all dogs (this frequently reduces aggressive tendencies).
- Never leave infants or young children alone with any dog.
- Do not play aggressive games with your dog (e.g., wrestling).
- Properly socialize and train any dog entering the household. Teach the dog submissive behaviors (e.g., rolling over to expose abdomen and relinquishing food without growling).

- Immediately seek professional advice (e.g., from veterinarians, animal behaviorists, or responsible breeders) if the dog develops aggressive or undesirable behaviors.

Preventing Dog Bites

- Teach children basic safety around dogs and review regularly.
- Do not approach an unfamiliar dog.
- Do not run from a dog and scream.
- Remain motionless (e.g., "be still like a tree") when approached by an unfamiliar dog.
- If knocked over by a dog, roll into a ball and lie still (e.g., "be still like a log").
- Do not play with a dog unless supervised by an adult.
- Immediately report stray dogs or dogs displaying unusual behavior to an adult.
- Avoid direct eye contact with a dog.
- Do not disturb a dog who is sleeping, eating, or caring for puppies.
- Do not pet a dog without allowing it to see and sniff you first.
- If bitten, immediately report the bite to an adult.

From Centers for Disease Control and Prevention: *Dog bite prevention.* http://www.cdc.gov/ncipc/duip/biteprevention.htm.

- Consider allergic, envenomation, and posttraumatic stress complications of an animal bite.
- Consider whether other family members or other human beings are at risk.
- Consult public health officials regarding the need for rabies postexposure prophylaxis in particular bite situations.

Veterinary Clinicians

- Counsel pet owners to appropriately socialize and train pets to be well mannered.
- Counsel clients and staff on proper handling precautions to minimize the risk of animal bites to human beings (see Box 10-5).
- Counsel clients and staff on proper first-aid to minimize the risk of animal bite infection.
- When dealing with animal behavioral problems such as aggression, fears, and phobias, assess risk of bites to human beings and whether modifications to the animal environment or handling practices are indicated or whether animal should be euthanized.
- Assist human health care providers in indentifying specific zoonotic disease risks from particular animal species.
- Neuter pets and practice preventative medicine (e.g., ensure all dogs, cats, and ferrets are current with rabies vaccination).
- Counsel cat owners to keep their pets indoors and dog owners to disallow their pets to hunt or garbage feed.
- Provide booster rabies vaccine to pets with animal bite wounds from known or suspected rabid animals and work with local public health officials concerning management for potential rabies exposure.
- Test pet cats with bite wounds for FeLV/FIV at time of presentation and again 6 months later.[6]

MANAGEMENT OF ANIMAL BITE INJURY IN HUMAN BEINGS

Prevention

Many animal bites can be prevented through avoidance of high-risk situations. Table 10-8 lists some risk factors for human animal bites from dogs and cats. These include factors affecting animal aggressiveness, characteristics of bitten human beings, and characteristics of injury events. Risk factors for animal aggressiveness include female gender in cats and male gender (especially unneutered) in dogs as well as particular dog breeds. Human victims of dog bites tend to be younger than victims of cat bites. Bite injuries are often associated with particular types of aggressive behavior in the biting animal. These include dominance aggression, in which an animal assert its social dominance over another animal (such as a child) that it perceives as being weaker (e.g., members of a wolf pack) and possessive aggression, in which an animal attacks to prevent an object such as a toy or food being taken away.

Education about reduction of animal bite risk can be incorporated into preventive health care counseling by both human health clinicians and veterinarians. Dog bite prevention recommendations by the CDC are summarized in Box 10-5. Other preventive steps include avoiding feeding or handling wild or stray animals (see Exotic and Wildlife Pets in this chapter), and keeping companion animals indoors except for daily, accompanied exercise.

History

The clinician caring for a human victim of an animal bite should determine and document in the chart how, where, and when the bite occurred; the species and distinguishing characteristics of the animal; whether the bite was provoked or

Table 10-8 ■ Epidemiologic Characteristics Associated With Dog- and Cat-Related Bites or Scratches

	Characteristics of Cats and Dogs Exhibiting Aggression	
	Cats	**Dogs**
Age	Insufficient data	<5 years (49%)
Sex	Female (67%)	Male (70%-79%)
Ownership status	Stray (57%)	Owned (a significant number of these aggressive dogs live in a household with at least one child)
Reproductive status	Insufficient data	Intact (not neutered)
Size	Insufficient data	Large dogs (>50 lb)
Breed	Insufficient data	Total annual number of bites: mixed breed and German Shepherds
		Bite rates: German Shepherds and Chow-Chows
		Highest rate of severe or fatal bites: Staffordshire Terriers (pit bulls), German Shepherds, Chow-Chows
Characteristics of People Injured by Cats and Dogs		
Age	25-34 years	<20 years, with significant occurrence in those 5-9 years
Sex	Females (59%)	Males (62%)
Relationship to animal	Victim does not own cat	Victim is family member or acquaintance to the owners. Dog owners are most frequently bitten by dogs but not necessarily their own dogs (family's dog, 30%; neighbor's dog, 50%)
Characteristic of the Injury Event (Common Scenario)		
Kinds of aggression	Fear-related aggression, play aggression, redirected aggression, "biting and petting syndrome"	Dominance aggression, possessive aggression, fear-related aggression, protective/territorial aggression, punishment-induced aggression, pain-elicited aggression
Time of year	May through August (warm weather)	May through August (warm weather)
Time of day	9:00 AM to noon	Late afternoon
Other factors	If the cat is owned, 50% of the victims are the owners	Unusually high incidence of bites by chained dogs who are restrained on their own property
Typical wound characteristics	80% of all bites require medical attention	20%-60% of all bites require medical attention
	50% of all wounds become infected	Insufficient data on number of wounds that become infected
	29% of all cat-bite victims return to doctor after initial visit because of complications	5% of all dog-bite victims return to doctor after initial visit because of complications
	Wounds consist of scratches (70%); punctures (27%) and tears (3%) to finger (21%), arm (18%), foot or leg (8%), face or neck (7%); and multiple body locations (3%)	Wounds consist primarily of puncture and tears to extremities (76%) and to face (15%). 70% fatal injuries to children <9 years. Highest death rate to neonates (<1 month old). Death rates of neonates 295/100 million; for children 1-11 months, 47/100 million.
Location of Bite Wounds (% Bites)		
Face, scalp, or neck	2	16
Trunk	0	2
Shoulder, arm, or forearm	23	12
Hand	63	50
Thigh or leg	9	16
Feet	3	4

From Greene CE: *Infectious diseases of the dog and cat*, ed 3, St Louis, 2006, Saunders Elsevier.

unprovoked; whether the animal is available for observation; its current location; and relevant veterinary information about the animal, including rabies vaccination status or any other known illnesses.

It is also necessary to determine the date of the human patient's most recent tetanus vaccination and any history of medical conditions placing them at increased risk of infection, such as immunocompromised conditions (e.g., HIV), cancer, diabetes, splenectomy, or immunosuppressive drugs. A history of prosthetic joints or heart valves is also an important risk factor for complications in human beings.[1] The human patient should be asked about any allergies to animals or medications. Finally, for both human beings and companion animals, if considering rabies postexposure prophylaxis, determine whether the patient has previously received rabies vaccination, including where and when.

Table 10-9 lists risk factors for animal bite infections. If these risk factors are present, antibiotic prophylaxis appears reasonable. If none of these risk factors is present, antibiotics may be withheld in many cases and the wound rechecked in 48 hours.

Physical Examination

A careful head-to-toe physical examination should be performed looking for other signs of trauma. The wound should be carefully explored to assess damage to deeper structures, including joints and bones. A detailed neurovascular examination should be performed to assess damage to nerves and blood vessels.

For human beings bitten by an animal, it may be worthwhile to draw a diagram or take a photograph of the wound because many animal bites result in litigation. Children bitten on the neck or head should have cervical immobilization until cervical fractures can be ruled out by radiological studies.[7]

Wound Culture

For fresh bite wounds, routine cultures are not necessary. However, if a wound later shows signs of infection such as redness, swelling, or discharge, cultures for both aerobic and anaerobic bacteria should be obtained (Figure 10-20).

Initial Wound Care, Irrigation, and Debridement

First-aid for an animal bite should involve control of bleeding and initial cleansing. Bleeding should be controlled with local pressure. Adequate cleaning and irrigation of a bite wound is critical to its management. Initial cleaning can be done immediately after the bite with soap and water. As soon as possible, copious irrigation of the wound with saline solution with an 18- or 19-gauge needle or catheter tip and large syringe should be performed. Many bite wounds involve damage to tissue at the wound edges. Therefore wound tissue that appears devitalized or necrotic should be carefully debrided.[1] In human patients, significant bites to the hand may require reconstructive surgery, and a detailed examination for possible injury to tendons, nerves, and other deeper tissues is warranted. A hand surgeon may need to be consulted, especially if there is any evidence of infection. If there are significant facial lacerations, a plastic surgeon consultation is appropriate.

Radiographs

If there is concern about involvement of joints and other bony structures, including facial bones and the skull, take radiographs (Figure 10-21) and obtain orthopedic consultation for possible surgical intervention.

Table 10-9 ▪ Risk Factors for Animal Bite Infection	
High-risk species	Cat Nonhuman primate Reptile Rat, other rodent Rabies vector species (raccoons, bats, skunks, foxes) Animal appearing sick Human being
Severity and location of bite	Hands, feet, wrist, neck, genital area Joints, bones Severe bites (involving large area, deep tissue structures, multiple bites) Puncture wounds Necrotic or poorly vascularized tissue Wounds where primary closure has been performed
Host factors	Immunocompromising medical conditions (e.g., HIV infection, FIV/FeLV infection, cancer chemotherapy, diabetes, steroids and other immunosuppressive medications, malnutrition, alcoholism, asplenia) Prosthetic joints or heart valves Infants or elderly
Other	Delays (more than several hours) in cleaning wound and seeking care High degree of contamination (extensive contact with animal saliva or other infectious material)

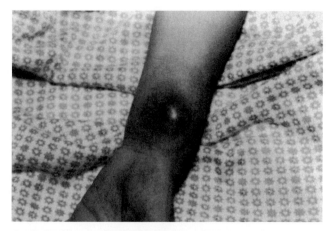

Figure 10-20 ▪ Cat-bite abscess of the wrist with presentation for care delayed 1 month after injury. *Pasteurella multocida* was isolated in pure culture. (From Long SS, Pickering LK, Prober CG: *Principles and practice of pediatric infectious diseases,* ed 3, Philadelphia, 2008, Saunders Elsevier.)

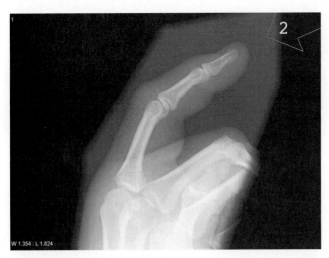

Figure 10-21 ▪ Radiograph of finger after a bite by a captive sub-adult Gila monster *(Heloderma suspectum)* after touching the lizard's tail. It took approximately 40 seconds to pry the reptile off with tongs. Immediately after, the patient complained of "10 out of 10" pain. Shortly after, he developed swelling and redness extending to his mid-forearm, as well as nausea and vomiting. A tooth was retained in the wound for more than 2 months before it was spontaneously expelled. (From Auerbach PS: *Wilderness medicine,* ed 5, Philadelphia, 2007, Mosby Elsevier. Courtesy Sean Bush.)

Wound Closure

Whether to close an animal bite wound with sutures or other technique is controversial. Considerations include risk factors for infection and cosmetic impact of the injury. Dog bites to the face rarely become infected and are often closed to reduce the possibility of disfiguring scars. Wounds that are at high risk of infection (e.g., from a high-risk species, in a high-risk area such as the hand, or in an immuno-compromised patient), are more than 24 hours old, or that are already infected generally should not be closed. Low-risk wounds can be closed, after thorough irrigation, with sutures, staples, or other techniques and observed closely for signs of infection.[8]

Antibiotic Prophylaxis and Therapy

Whether prophylactic antibiotics are indicated for an animal bite is also controversial, and data regarding the bites of many species are limited. A Cochrane review of antibiotic prophylaxis in uncomplicated dog and cat bites found no clear evidence of benefit.[9] Clinical decision making regarding antibiotic prophylaxis involves assessing the risk of infection. Risk factors include the species responsible for the bite, any information about the health of the animal, the severity and location of the bite, and whether the patient is immunocompromised or has other conditions that increase the risk of infection. High-risk bites include crush injuries that involve devascularized tissue and puncture wounds, hand involvement, significant edema, possible involvement of joints or bones, and proximity to genitalia or prosthetic joints nearby. Patients with very high-risk bites or evidence of tenosynovitis or deep infection should be admitted for parenteral antibiotics and hospital observation. Immunocompromised

individuals and those with asplenia or compromising medical conditions should receive prophylactic antibiotics for most animal bites. Table 10-10 provides recommendations for empiric antibiotic dosing for animal bites to human beings.

Dog bites usually do not become infected. Reported infection rates range from 5% to 15%.[10] Cat bites often involve deep puncture wounds that are prone to infection. Infection rates from cat bites may be as high as 80%.[11] The choice of antimicrobial prophylaxis for cat bites and high-risk dog bites should cover *Pasteurella, Streptococcus,* and *Staphylococcus.* A 5- to 7-day course of antibiotics should be administered. Ferret bites are increasing in frequency with their popularity as pets and their tendency to bite. Little is known about their microbial flora. Pig bites are considered to carry a high risk for infection.[12]

Alligators and related species tend to inflict severe bites and have polymicrobial flora that can lead to infection.[13] Many snake bites do not become infected.[7] Two controlled trials of prophylactic antibiotics for pit viper envenomation did not show a clinical benefit.[14,15] Nevertheless, snake bites should be monitored for potential infection.[16] Iguana bites can be severe and infection has been reported.[17]

Human bites to another human are considered high-risk bites for infection. In addition to bacterial pathogens (see Table 10-10), risk of infection with blood-borne pathogens such as HIV and hepatitis B should be considered.

Vaccinations

RABIES POSTEXPOSURE PROPHYLAXIS

The risk of rabies should be assessed in every animal bite situation in a human or pet, with rabies postexposure prophylaxis (PEP) for high-risk bites provided.[18] However, studies have shown that rabies PEP is often given inappropriately by clinicians treating bites in emergency care settings, such as when the biting animal is low risk or available for observation or testing (see Chapter 9).[19] The biting animal should be captured and monitored for 10 days for signs of rabies if it is a dog, cat, or ferret; for 14 days if livestock; or euthanized and tested if a rabies vector species (e.g., bat, raccoon, skunk, fox) or other wild carnivore such as a river otter (Figure 10-22). If animal rabies testing is positive or if the animal is not available for observation or testing and is a high-risk rabies species, PEP should be provided to the patient.

TETANUS

Tetanus status should be determined in all human bite patients. A booster should be provided for a low-risk bite if the patient was not vaccinated within the past 10 years and for a high-risk bite if the patient was not vaccinated within the past 5 years. If there is not a history of at least 3 tetanus vaccinations in the past (for an adult), tetanus immune globulin should also be given. Table 10-11 details these recommendations.

Table 10-10 ▪ Pathogens Complicating Animal Bites to Human Beings and Recommended Empiric Therapy

Species	Reported Pathogens	Empiric Antibiotic Therapy Primary	Alternative
Dogs	Usually polymicrobial, mixed aerobic and anaerobic organisms[1] Aerobic bacteria: *Pasteurella (P. canis, P. multocida multocida, P. multocida septica), Streptococcus* spp. *(S. immitis, S. mutans, S. pyogenes), Staphylococcus (S aureus, S. epidermidis, S. intermedius[7]), Moraxella, Corynebacteria, Bergeyella zoohelcum, Capnocytophaga* spp. Anaerobes: *Fusobacterium, Bacteroides, Porphyromonas, Prevotella*[1]	Amoxicillin-clavulanate 875/125 mg bid or 500/125 mg PO tid[30]	Clindamycin 300 mg PO qid + fluoroquinolone (adults) or Clinda + Trimethoprim sulfa (children)[30]
Cats	Often polymicrobial, mixed aerobic and anaerobic organisms[31] Aerobic bacteria: *Pasteurella multocida multocida, P. multocida septica, Streptococcus* spp. *(S. mitis, S. mutans), Staphylococcus (S. epidermidis, S. warneri, S. aureus), Moraxella, Corynebacteria, Bergeyella zoohelcum, Bacillus, Capnocytophaga* spp. Anaerobes: *Fusobacterium, Bacteroides, Porphyromonas, Prevotella*[1] *Sporothrix schenckii*	Amoxicillin-clavulanate 875/125 mg bid or 500/125 mg PO tid[30]; itraconazole	Cefuroxime axetil 0.5 gm PO q12h or doxycycline 100 mg PO bid; do not use cephalexin[30]
Human beings	*Streptococcus viridans, Staphylococcus epidermidis, Corynebacterium, Staphylococcus aureus, Eikenella, Bacteroides, Peptostreptococcus*	Early: amoxicillin-clavulanate 875/125 mg bid ×5 days Infected: ampicillin/sulbactam 1.5 g IV q6h	Cefoxitin 2 g IV q8h, *or* ticarcillin-clavulanate 3.1 g IV q6h *or* piperacillin-tazobactam 3.375 g IV q6h *or* 4-hour infusion 3.375 g q8h (x-rays for clenched fist injuries)[30]
Ferrets	Not well documented; consider rabies risk	As for cat and dog bites[32]	
Horses	*Pasteurella caballi*[38], *S. aureus, Neisseria*, and other anaerobic gram-negative bacilli[33]	As for dog	
Sheep	*Actinobacillus*, others[33]	As for dog	
Rats	*Streptobacillus moniliformis* (North America, Europe), *Spirillum minus* (Asia), *Leptospira*	Amoxicillin-clavulanate 875/125 mg bid[30]	Doxycycline 100 mg PO bid
Pigs	Polymicrobial: gram-positive cocci, gram-negative bacilli, anaerobes, *Pasteurella* spp.[30]	Amoxicillin-clavulanate 875/125 mg bid[30]; some recommend adding ciprofloxacin[34]	Third-generation cephalosporin or ticarcillin-clavulanate or ampicillin-sulbactam or imipenem[30]
Rabbits	*Pasturella multocida*[35] (rabies has been reported[29])	As for dog and cat	
Nonhuman primates (e.g., macaque)	Consider risk for herpes B virus *(Herpes simiae)*	Valacyclovir	Acyclovir[26]
Hamsters	*Francisella tularensis*,[36] *Pasteurella* spp.	See rat	
Reptiles (e.g., iguanas, snakes, alligators)	*Pseudomonas aeruginosa, Proteus, Clostridium, Bacteroides fragilis, Salmonella* groups IIIa and IIIb,[13,37] *Serratia marescens*[17]	Ceftriaxone (infected wounds)[30]	
Bats, raccoons, skunks, foxes	*Staphylococcus* and *Streptococcus* spp. (skin flora)	Amoxicillin-clavulanate 875/125 mg bid or 500/125 mg PO tid[30]	Doxycycline 100 mg PO bid[30]
	Rabies virus	Assess for rabies postexposure prophylaxis	
Seal	Marine *Mycoplasma* (sealpox; see Chapter 12)	Tetracycline ×4 weeks[30]	

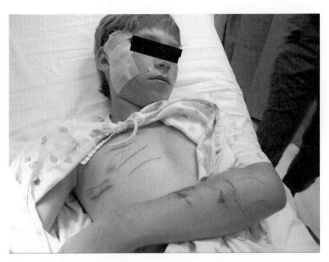

Figure 10-22 ▪ Victim of river otter attack. (From Auerbach PS: *Wilderness medicine*, ed 5, Philadelphia, 2007, Mosby Elsevier. Photo courtesy Jill Hanna.)

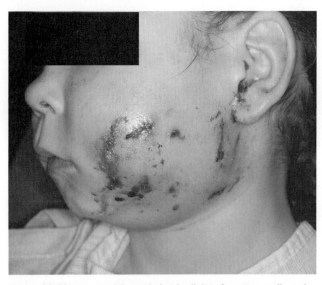

Figure 10-23 ▪ A toddler with facial cellulitis from *Pasteurella multocida* after a dog bite. (From Long SS, Pickering LK, Prober CG: *Principles and practice of pediatric infectious diseases*, ed 3, Philadelphia, 2008, Saunders Elsevier. Courtesy J. H. Brien.)

SPECIFIC BITE INFECTIONS

Clinicians should be familiar with a number of specific bite-associated infections.

Pasteurella Infection

Pasteurella multocida is the most common agent isolated from infected dog and cat wounds (Figure 10-23). It causes cellulitis and can cause bacteremia with sepsis, meningitis, and hemorrhagic complications. *Pasteurella* wound infections tend to develop rapidly, producing swelling, redness, tenderness, and discharge at the wound area within 12 to 24 hours after the bite.[20] Tenosynovitis and osteomyelitis can develop and should be aggressively treated with parenteral antibiotics.

Rat-Bite Fever

Rat-bite fever from *Streptobacillus moniliformis* in human beings was traditionally a disease of inner-city children

bitten by peridomestic rodents. With the popularity of rats as pets and the use of rats in laboratories, cases now occur in pet store employees, pet owners, and laboratory animal workers. The disease causes a rash (Color Plate 10-8) that may be petechial, hemorrhagic, or purpuric, as well as fever, and systemic symptoms including arthralgias. Without treatment, the case fatality rate can be 10%. Most domestic and wild rats carry the causative agent, *S. moniliformis*, in their oral flora. Up to an estimated 10% of rat bites can become infected.[21] Patients with rat bites need to be counseled about the signs and seriousness of this disease, and prophylactic antibiotics should be considered for infection-prone bites.

S. moniliformis in guinea pigs causes cervical lymphadenitis or granulomatous pneumonia; in mice, purulent lesions and acute septicemia; and endocarditis or septic arthritis in nonhuman primates.

Table 10-11 ▪ Indications for Tetanus Prophylaxis in Wounds				
	Clean, Minor Wound		**All Other Wounds***	
History of Absorbed Tetanus Toxoid (Doses)	**Tdap or Td†**	**TIG**	**Tdap or Td†**	**TIG**
Unknown or <3	Yes	No	Yes	Yes
≥3	No‡	No	No§	No

From Kretsinger K, Broder KR, Cortese MM et al: Preventing tetanus, diphtheria, and pertussis among adults: use of tetanus toxoid, reduced diphtheria toxoid and acellular pertussis vaccine recommendations of the Advisory Committee on Immunization Practices (ACIP) and recommendation of ACIP, supported by the Healthcare Infection Control Practices Advisory Committee (HICPAC), for use of Tdap among health-care personnel, *MMWR Recomm Rep* 55(RR-17):1, 2006.

*Such as, but not limited to, wounds contaminated with dirt, feces, soil, and saliva; puncture wounds; avulsions; and wounds resulting from missiles, crushing, burns, and frostbite.

†Tdap is preferred to Td for adults who have never received Tdap. Td is preferred to TT for adults who received Tdap previously or when Tdap is not available. If TT and TIG are used, tetanus toxoid absorbed rather than tetanus toxoid for booster use only (fluid vaccine) should be used.

‡Yes, if ≥10 years since the last tetanus toxoid–containing vaccine dose.

§Yes, if ≥5 years since the last tetanus toxoid–containing vaccine dose.

Capnocytophaga Infection

Capnocytophaga canimorsus is found in dog and cat saliva (especially the former). In asplenic and immunocompromised human beings, it can produce septicemia with meningitis, endocarditis, and eye involvement.[22] Serious infections have also been reported in persons with no apparent risk factors.[23] The first known animal with a *Capnocytophaga*-infected dog bite wound, a pet rabbit, was successfully treated.[24]

Herpes B Infection

Herpes B infection causes an often fatal viral meningo-encephalitis that can be transmitted to human beings from Old World monkeys of the genus *Macaca* (Figure 10-24; see Chapter 12).[25] Although there have been no controlled trials of prophylaxis, the B Virus Working Group recommends antiviral prophylaxis for high-risk bites (or other exposures) from these monkeys. The recommended prophylactic regimen is 1 g valacyclovir three times a day for adults, excluding pregnant women. An alternative regimen is 800 mg acyclovir five times a day. Prophylaxis should begin as soon as possible after exposure. If signs of herpes B infection appear, systemic treatment with antivirals and hospitalization are necessary.[26]

Lymphocytic Choriomeningitis

LCMV can be present in the saliva of rodents, especially mice, and can pose a risk after a bite (see Chapter 9). Fetal complications can occur in pregnant women and severe disease in immunocompromised persons. Therefore pregnant women and immunocompromised individuals should avoid rodent exposure.

Sporotrichosis

Sporotrichosis is a fungal disease (Color Plate 10-9) that can produce ulcerating skin nodules and systemic infection (rare). It is usually acquired from contact with plants or soil but has been reported in association with cat bites and scratches (with an outbreak of more than 1000 cats and 500 persons in Brazil[27]) and after a squirrel bite.[28] Veterinarians are at increased risk of occupational infection. *Sporothrix schenckii* has also been reported in horse and dog lesions.

Cat-Scratch Fever

Bartonella infection can be transmitted by cat bites and scratches (see Chapter 9).

MANAGEMENT OF BITES IN ANIMALS

As in human beings, immunocompromised conditions (such as FIV/FeLV in feline patients) predispose an animal to bite-related infection. Pet dogs, cats, and ferrets that are bitten by potentially or known rabid animals should be managed according to their rabies vaccination status. If they are currently vaccinated, a booster vaccine should be immediately administered and the pet should be observed for 45 days for signs of rabies. If the pet is unvaccinated, it should be euthanized or held in strict isolation for 180 days and provided a rabies vaccine 1 month before release from quarantine. Certain domestic animals such as rabbits are at risk of wildlife rabies if caged outside or allowed to roam outside.[29]

Table 10-12 provides recommended antibiotic therapy for animal bite infections in dogs and cats. Depending on the severity of the bite, other treatment modalities, including physical therapy, may be required for rehabilitation of the animal (Figure 10-25).

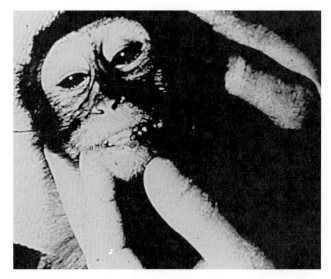

Figure 10-24 ■ A lower lip ulceration in a rhesus monkey caused by herpes B virus infection. (From Mandell GL, Bennett JE, Dolin R: *Principles and practice of infectious diseases,* ed 6, New York, 2005, Churchill Livingstone Elsevier.)

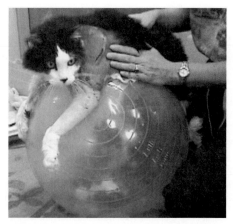

Figure 10-25 ■ Cat relaxing on ball after surgery to repair dog bite wound. (From Gaynor JS, Muir WW 3d: *Handbook of veterinary pain management,* ed 2, St Louis, 2008, Mosby Elsevier.)

Table 10-12 ▪ Recommended Therapy for Bite Infections in Cats and Dogs

Drug	Species	Dose (mg/kg)	Route	Interval (hr)	Antibacterial Spectrum
Amoxicillin-clavulanate	D	10-20	PO	8	Most gram-positive and gram-negative aerobes and anaerobes; first-choice drug for most bite wounds
	D	13.75	PO	12	
	C	10-20	PO	12	
Ampicillin (amoxicillin)	B	22	PO	8	Some gram-positive and gram-negative aerobes
	B	11-22	SC, IV	6–8	
Ticarcillin	D	20-50	IV	6–8	Gram-positive and gram-negative aerobes and anaerobes
Cefotaxime	B	15-30	IV, IM, SC	6–8	Sepsis from bite wounds caused by gram-negative aerobes or anaerobes
Doxycycline	D	5	PO, IV	12	Some aerobes and anaerobes; mycoplasmas
Clindamycin	B	5-11	PO	8–12	Gram-positive aerobes and anaerobes
Enrofloxacin	D	5	PO, SC	12–24	Gram-negative aerobes
Difloxacin	D	5-10	PO	24	Gram-negative aerobes
Orbifloxacin	D	2.5-7.5	PO	24	Gram-negative aerobes
Marbofloxacin	D	2-4	PO	24	Gram-negative aerobes
Azithromycin	D	20	PO	24	Gram-positive aerobes; mycoplasmas and mycobacteria
Chloramphenicol	D	25-50	PO, IV, IM, SC	8	Some anaerobes; variable with gram-positive and gram-negative aerobes
Metronidazole	B	10	PO, IV	8	Anaerobes

From Greene CE: *Infectious diseases of the dog and cat*, ed 3, St Louis, 2006, Saunders Elsevier.
D, Dog; *C*, cat; *B*, dog and cat; *PO*, by mouth; *SC*, subcutaneous; *IV*, intravenous; *IM*, intramuscular.

References

1. Taplitz RA. Managing bite wounds. Currently recommended antibiotics for treatment and prophylaxis. *Postgrad Med.* 2004;116(2):49–52, 55–56, 59.
2. Langley RL. Animal bites and stings reported by United States poison control centers, 2001–2005. *Wilderness Environ Med.* 2008;19(1):7–14.
3. Guida G, Nebiolo F, Heffler E, et al. Anaphylaxis after a horse bite. *Allergy.* 2005;60(8):1088–1089.
4. Lim DL, Chan RM, Wen H, et al. Anaphylaxis after hamster bites—identification of a novel allergen. *Clin Exp Allergy.* 2004;34(7):1122–1123.
5. Garth AP, Harris NS. *Bites, animal.* http://www.emedicine.com/emerg/topic60.htm. Accessed April 16, 2009.
6. Journal of the American Veterinary Medical Association. 2001 *Feline practitioners recommend new FIV and FeLV testing guidelines, initiate public awareness campaign.* http://www.avma.org/onlnews/javma/apr01/s041501g.asp. Accessed April 16, 2009.
7. Morgan M. Hospital management of animal and human bites. *J Hosp Infect.* 2005;61(1):1–10.
8. Auerbach PS. *Wilderness medicine.* 5th ed. Philadelphia: Mosby Elsevier; 2007.
9. Medeiros IM, Saconato H. Antibiotic prophylaxis for mammalian bites. *Cochrane Database Syst Rev.* 2001;(2):CD001738.
10. Moran GJ, Talan DA, Abrahamian FM. Antimicrobial prophylaxis for wounds and procedures in the emergency department. *Infect Dis Clin North Am.* 2008;22(1):117–143.
11. Louisiana State University School of Veterinary Medicine. *What you should know about animal bites.* http://www.vetmed.lsu.edu/animal_bites.htm.
12. Barnham M. Pig bite injuries and infection: report of seven human cases. *Epidemiol Infect.* 1988;101(3):641–645.
13. Hertner G. Caiman bite. *Wilderness Environ Med.* 2006; 17(4):267–270.
14. Kerrigan KR, Mertz BL, Nelson SJ, et al. Antibiotic prophylaxis for pit viper envenomation: prospective, controlled trial. *World J Surg.* 1997;21(4):369–372.
15. LoVecchio F, Klemens J, Welch S, et al. Antibiotics after rattlesnake envenomation. *J Emerg Med.* 2002;23(4):327–328.
16. Wu CH, Hu WH, Hung DZ, et al. Snakebite complicated with *Vibrio vulnificus* infection. *Vet Hum Toxicol.* 2001;43(5):283–285.
17. Hsieh S, Babl FE. *Serratia marcescens* cellulitis following an iguana bite. *Clin Infect Dis.* 1999;28(5):1181–1182.
18. Manning SE, Rupprecht CE, Fishbein D, et al. Advisory Committee on Immunization Practices Centers for Disease Control and Prevention: Human rabies prevention—United States, 2008: recommendations of the Advisory Committee on Immunization Practices. *MMWR Recomm Rep.* 2008;57(RR-3):1–28.
19. Conti LA, Wiersma S, Hopkins R. Evaluation of state-provided rabies post-exposure prophylaxis (PEP), Florida, July-September 1997 and July-September 1998. *Southern Med J.* 2002;95(2):225–230.
20. Kristinsson G. *Pasteurella multocida* infections. *Pediatr Rev.* 2007;28(12): 472–473.
21. Elliott SP. Rat bite fever and *Streptobacillus moniliformis.* *Clin Microbiol Rev.* 2007;20(1):13–22.
22. Jolivet-Gougeon A, Sixou J-L, Tamanai-Shacoori Z, et al. Antimicrobial treatment of *Capnocytophaga* infections. *Int J Antimicrob Agents.* 2007;29(4):367–373.
23. Ball V, Younggren BN. Emergency management of difficult wounds: part I. *Emerg Med Clin North Am.* 2007;25(1):101–121.
24. van Duijkeren E, van Mourik C, Broekhuizen M, et al. First documented *Capnocytophaga canimorsus* infection in a species other than humans. *Vet Microbiol.* 2006;118(1–2):148–150.
25. Andersen E. B virus—the risks in monkey business. *AAOHN Journal.* 2005;53(9):385–387.

26. Cohen JI, Davenport DS, Stewart JA, et al. the B Virus Working Group. Recommendations for prevention of and therapy for exposure to B virus (Cercopithecine Herpesvirus 1). *Clin Infect Dis.* 2002;35(10):1191–1203.

27. Schubach A, Schubach TM, Barros MB, et al. Cat-transmitted sporotrichosis, Rio de Janeiro, Brazil. *Emerg Infect Dis.* 2005;11(12):1952–1954.

28. Saravanakumar PS, Eslami P, Zar FA. Lymphocutaneous sporotrichosis associated with a squirrel bite: case report and review. *Clin Infect Dis.* 1996;23(3):647–648.

29. Eidson M, Matthews SD, Willsey AL, et al. Rabies virus infection in a pet guinea pig and seven pet rabbits. *J Am Vet Med Assoc.* 2005;227(6): 932–935, 918.

30. Gilbert DN, Moellering RC, Eliopoulos GM, et al. *Sanford guide to antimicrobial therapy 2009.* 39th ed. Sperryville, VA: Antimicrobial Therapy Inc; 2009.

31. Talan DA, Citron DM, Abrahamian FM, et al. Bacteriologic analysis of infected dog and cat bites. *New Engl J Med.* 1999;340(2):85–92.

32. Applegate JA, Walhout MF. Childhood risks from the ferret. *J Emerg Med.* 1998;16(3):425–427.

33. Angoules AG, Lindner T, Vrentzos G, et al. Prevalence and current concepts of management of farmyard injuries. *Injury.* 2007;38(suppl 5):S27–S34.

34. Morgan MS. Treatment of pig bites. *Lancet.* 1996;348(9036):1246.

35. Silberfein EJ, Lin PH, Bush RL, et al. Aortic endograft infection due to *Pasteurella multocida* following a rabbit bite. *J Vasc Surg.* 2006;43(2):393–395.

36. Centers for Disease Control and Prevention (CDC). Tularemia associated with a hamster bite—Colorado, 2004. *MMWR.* 2005;53(51):1202–1203.

37. Quirk EK. Human and animal bites. In: Starlin R, ed. *Infectious diseases subspecialty consult (the Washington Manual subspecialty consult).* Philadelphia: Lippincott Williams & Wilkins; 2005.

38. Escande F, Vallee E, Aubart F. *Pasteurella caballi* infection following a horse bite. *Zentralbl Bakteriol.* 1997;285(3):440–444.

Foodborne Illness

11

Peter M. Rabinowitz and Lisa A. Conti

The Centers for Disease Control and Prevention (CDC) estimates that each year in the United Sates 76 million persons experience foodborne illness, leading to 300,000 hospitalizations and 5000 deaths. Although most of these cases are attributable to infectious etiologies, exposure to foodborne toxins occurs as well.[1] Companion animals are also believed to commonly experience foodborne illness, with signs including acute gastritis or diarrhea, although the actual incidence of animal foodborne illness is not known.

In the United States the Foodborne Diseases Active Surveillance Network of the CDC (FoodNet) performs active surveillance for nine pathogens in selected states (*Campylobacter, Cryptosporidium, Cyclospora, Listeria, Salmonella, Shiga* toxin–producing *Escherichia coli* [STEC] O157, *Shigella, Vibrio,* and *Yersinia*). Clinicians can access recent reports at http://www.cdc.gov/FoodNet/reports.htm. Despite ongoing prevention efforts on the part of both public health and agricultural health authorities, the rates of *Campylobacter, Listeria, Salmonella, Shigella,* STEC O157, *Vibrio,* and *Yersinia* infections do not appear to have declined in recent years, whereas the rate of cryptosporidiosis has increased. The rate of *Salmonella* infection was the furthest from public health goals. It is clear that controlling or eliminating foodborne illness will require comprehensive efforts from farm to fork.[2] The production of safe, healthy food for the expanding world population has increased the complexity and globalization of the process. There are multiple potential interactions between human and animal health at a number of steps of the food chain (Table 11-1).

Dog and cat food sales were close to $17 billion in the United States in 2008 (Figure 11-1).[3] Although many human health care providers may be unaware of the magnitude of the pet food industry, the human health relevance of foodborne illness in companion animals is becoming more evident. Human outbreaks of salmonellosis have been linked to contact with contaminated pet food. Similarly, the outbreak of melamine contamination in human infant formula in China was presaged by an outbreak of disease in cats and dogs traced to a similar melamine contamination of pet food imported from the same country.

Clearly, then, food safety and foodborne illness are issues that human health and animal health care providers cannot ignore. They cross any artificial barriers between human health and animal health practice and require increased cooperation and communication across disciplines. This chapter presents a systems approach to foodborne illness at different levels of the food chain and outlines principles of the evaluation and management of foodborne illness in human beings and other animals.

Key Points for Clinicians and Public Health Professionals

Public Health Professionals

- Educate farmers, retailers, and consumers about food safety at all stages of the food production chain (see National Food Safety Programs at http://www.food-safety.gov).
- Support preventive strategies such as hazard analysis and critical control point process principles.
- Support food sustainability measures.
- Ensure that local farms and retailers comply with food safety guidelines.
- Consider cases of disease in food industry workers as potential sentinel events for inadequate preventive measures.
- Support uniform standards and practices across federal, state, and local levels.
- Educate human health and veterinary care providers regarding the detection and reporting of foodborne illness in human beings and animals.

Human Health Clinicians

- Consider foodborne illness in all patients presenting with gastrointestinal symptoms or unexplained fever. Take adequate history of food-related exposures.
- In evaluating a patient with suspected foodborne illness, ask whether other human beings or animals in the vicinity are also sick.
- Report suspected cases of foodborne illness to the health department.
- If diagnosing foodborne illness in a farm worker or food industry worker, provide that information to the

Table 11-1 ▪ Risks Along the Food Chain

Level	Risks to Animals	Risks to Human Beings	Preventive Steps
Animal feed, manure, and other animal waste for plant crops	Direct poisoning or infection, antibiotic resistance	Occupational exposure through handling of feed or manure	Limit use of antibiotics, hormones, and pesticide treatments in feed; use appropriate water source; safely handle of livestock wastes
Farm and field	Infection in animals, animal-animal transmission	Occupational exposure to infected animal, animal-human transmission	Farm management, veterinary surveillance, traceback, occupational surveillance
Harvest and processing	NA	Occupational exposure to infected animal; animal-human transmission through butchering, handling	Personal protection, pasteurization, refrigeration, occupational surveillance of processor workers
Retail	NA	Occupational exposure to infected meat handling, live animal market exposures	Personal protection
Consumer	Pet food contaminated with infectious or toxic agents or low-level antibiotic; hormone exposures	Meat and dairy products contaminated with infectious or toxic agents; low-level antibiotic; hormone exposures; vegetables, grains, or fruit contaminated with pathogens or chemicals	Home and food safety practices and recalls; clinicians and public health: detect and investigate sentinel events, traceback

NA, Not applicable.

local health department to consider whether other workers or animals may be at risk.

- Counsel patients about food safety in the home for human beings and companion animals (Box 11-1).

Veterinary Clinicians

- In evaluating an animal with suspected foodborne illness, ask whether other animals or nearby human beings are also sick.
- Consider contacting the local or state health department regarding suspected cases of foodborne illness in animals.
- Counsel clients about food safety in the home for companion animals and human beings (see Box 11-1).

RISKS ALONG THE FOOD CHAIN

Foodborne risks and food safety can be thought of conceptually in terms of a chain of production from animal feed or plant fertilizer to consumer.[4,5] At each stage in the chain there are certain risks for both human beings and other animals. At each stage are also opportunities for prevention and control. The Center for Veterinary Medicine of the Food and Drug Administration (FDA) has recommended applying hazard analysis and critical control point (HACCP) principles to the food manufacturing processes to detect and reduce risks.[6]

Animal Feed and Plant Fertilizer

The first stage of food production involves supplying safe feed for food animals and safe fertilizer for plant crops. The

two concepts are interrelated. Animal feed may include both plant and animal products, and plant fertilizer may contain livestock manure and other animal wastes.[7] At this stage of the production chain, the health risks are primarily to the food animals, with some risk also to agricultural workers

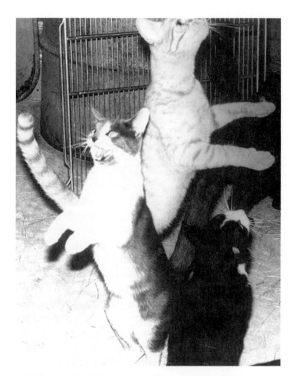

Figure 11-1 ▪ Bipedal posture used to request food. (From Beaver BV: *Feline behavior,* ed 2, St Louis, 2003, Saunders Elsevier.)

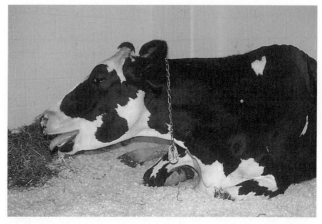

Figure 11-2 ▪ Open-mouth breathing in a 5-year-old cow. (From Divers TJ, Peek SF: *Rebhun's diseases of dairy cattle,* ed 2, St Louis, 2008, Saunders Elsevier.)

directly handling animal feed and fertilizer. Risks to animals include both toxic and infectious agents. Examples of toxic exposures have included dioxin contamination in pigs[8] and poultry; exposure of cattle to the fire retardant PBB (polybrominated biphenyl) through inadvertent contamination of feed; and heavy metal poisoning from cadmium, lead, or mercury contamination of fertilizers applied to crops and pastures.[9] Infectious agents threatening the human and animal food supply include bovine spongiform encephalopathy, which appeared in cattle and other animals after being fed meat and bone meal prepared from animals infected with transmissible spongiform encephalopathy (TSE) (see Chapter 9). This risk has been greatly reduced through animal feeding bans. Less clear cut are the risks from the use of antibiotics and hormones in animal feed. Such additives may be used to reduce infection and increase meat or dairy product production (growth promoters).[10] There is evidence that these practices can increase the development of antibiotic-resistant pathogens.[11] However, most animals treated with such agents show no ill effects and may have increased meat and dairy product output.

Not all animals who have ingested either toxicants or infectious agents show evidence of disease and therefore may pass the risks along the food production chain. A pathogen that has proved difficult to control is *Salmonella,* many strains of which are adapted to a wide number of animal hosts (see Chapter 9). There is evidence that *Salmonella* may enter the food supply chain through rendered animal protein used as animal feed.[6]

Occupational exposure to animal feed and manure fertilizers can result in disease in agricultural workers and persons engaged in small-scale (backyard) food production. Manure used as fertilizer on fields may come from animals who shed pathogens in their feces. Such contaminated feces can then be a risk to workers. For example, contact with infected chicken manure for use in a backyard garden has been linked to a fatal human case of avian influenza.[12] Commercial farm workers who have direct contact with infected human or animal wastes used as fertilizer on crops may also be at risk of infection.[13] Another hazard of animal feed to workers is allergic and other reactions to grain, which can include "farmer's lung," grain mite allergy, and endotoxin exposure (see Chapters 7 and 12). Stored silage can be a source of toxic nitrogen dioxide. This gas forms nitric acid when in contact with the respiratory mucosa and creates acute lung damage,

known as *silo filler's disease.* This is also a risk for livestock housed near silage; outbreaks of respiratory disease and death in cattle from silo gases have been reported (Figure 11-2), potentially providing warning to human beings of the toxic risk (see Chapter 12).[14]

A number of measures can be implemented to prevent disease at the level of feed and manure production. In the case of bovine spongiform encephalopathy, banning the use of animal protein for cattle feed effectively reduced the incidence of new cases of the disease. Similarly, weighing the risks and benefits of feed additives that include hormones and antibiotics is an ongoing assessment process between agricultural and public health agencies. Inspections of animal feed can further improve the safety at this stage.

On a clinical level, surveillance for sentinel disease in both farm animals by veterinarians and workers handling feed and manure by occupational medicine professionals can detect emerging problems at this stage of the food production chain.

Farm and Field

In the farm environment, animal-animal, animal-human, and human-animal transmission of infectious agents can occur. In addition to the feed and manure exposures listed, environmental exposures (e.g., water, mosquitoes, and other vectors) and contact with wildlife can introduce pathogens into the food chain if meat is consumed raw or undercooked or if dairy products are unpasteurized. For example, a recent multistate outbreak of salmonellosis in Serrano peppers was traced to contaminated irrigation water in Mexico.[15] Rift Valley fever is an example of a vector-borne disease in which infected cattle can then pose an occupational risk to abattoir (slaughterhouse) workers.

At this stage of the food production chain, preventive care by veterinarians is crucial to improved herd health and also improved public health for both workers and future consumers. Early detection, prevention, and treatment of disease in herds are key. Agricultural extension services and other veterinary preventive services can encourage improved biosecurity in farming methods that reduce potential for disease outbreaks.

Harvest and Processing

When animals are slaughtered and processed for human and pet consumption, any pathogens that have entered the food chain can be spread to contaminate other carcasses and pose a risk to abattoir workers and butchers. Meat inspection at this point often may involve both veterinary and agricultural professionals as well as public health inspectors. Occupational medicine professionals and other human health clinicians can play an important role in providing medical surveillance of abattoir workers and detecting sentinel cases of disease that have implications for both animal and human health.

Although most processing of animal meat in industrialized countries occurs in specialized facilities with infection control policies and adequate refrigeration, food animals in other countries are slaughtered in backyards or households, farmyards, or open air markets. In these settings biosecurity is low, meat inspection and refrigeration are often not available, and the potential for infection consequently is greater. In addition, hunting for subsistence bushmeat consumption as well as hunting of deer, waterfowl, and other game often involves both slaughter and dressing of the wild animal carcass in a field or other improvised location. Such activities, even in developed countries, may take place without availability of running water or the use of gloves or other types of personal protection. Transmission of simian viruses has been documented in bushmeat hunters,[16] and toxoplasmosis, tularemia, and brucellosis have been reported in U.S. hunters who field-dressed their carcasses without personal protection. In these informal settings there is generally no process of organized inspection or medical surveillance of at-risk individuals. Recently there has been a call for improved surveillance of bushmeat hunters[17] to detect emerging pathogens and other foodborne diseases that could trigger disease outbreaks in human beings. Occupational medicine surveillance of farmers and workers in processing facilities and marketing retail chains can help detect sentinel health events in human beings (e.g., a Q fever or brucellosis outbreak),[18] indicating the presence of the disease in the livestock as well and a likely problem with food safety (see Chapter 12).

To reduce the possibility of disease transmission, dairies generally use pasteurization methods on waste milk fed to calves. Although milk pasteurization for human consumption occurs at the farm level in farms that produce milk and milk products, most U.S. dairies ship milk for human consumption to processing plants, where it is pasteurized and then shipped to distributors.[19] Pasteurization practices may vary between farms and regions. Although there is a consumer market for unpasteurized dairy products, which are considered by some to be more "natural," such products have resulted in a number of foodborne illness outbreaks.[20,21]

Retail

In the retail sector, handling of meat carries a risk of pathogen exposure similar to that faced by workers in abattoirs, although exposures tend to be lower and reported disease cases are fewer. If vegetables (e.g., peppers contaminated with *Salmonella* and spinach contaminated with *E. coli*)[22] and fruit (e.g., raspberries with *Cryptosporidium*)[23] have been contaminated with pathogens from animal manure, there is some risk of retail workers becoming sickened by handling such produce.

A special case of retail exposure is the live animal market, many of which exist even in developed countries such as the United States. In these markets animals of different species are often housed in the same or immediately adjacent cages, allowing pathogen spread among species and to human beings. In addition, contamination of such markets with feces, feathers, and other animal waste can be an indirect source of exposure for market workers (as well as consumers visiting the markets). Animal slaughter taking place in such markets exposes workers to the same pathogens faced by workers in abattoirs but with less potential for biosecurity measures.

Agricultural agencies have an important role to play in such markets by veterinary surveillance of live animals and animal products. Workers in such markets should also receive ongoing medical surveillance for infectious diseases as well as training in risk reduction measures. The occurrence of a zoonotic disease in a market worker is sometimes an important sentinel health event indicating the presence of risk for diseases such as avian influenza. Unfortunately, such workers may not be included in ongoing preventive programs.

Consumer

By the time that food is prepared and served for consumption in the home or restaurant, it has ideally been monitored all along the food production chain to reduce the chance of causing illness. The fact that outbreaks tied to residential and restaurant food consumption continue to occur makes it clear that food may contain pathogens as well as certain toxicants. For example, in 2007, 9% of sampled chicken broilers, 17% of ground turkey, and 26% of ground chicken samples were positive for *Salmonella*.[24] The USDA Food Safety and Inspection Service (FSIS), through its Pathogen Reduction: Hazard Analysis and Critical Control Point (PR/HACCP) rule, has set a priority of reducing the prevalence of *Salmonella* in broiler chicken carcasses.

Pet foods also can contain significant contamination. This can pose a risk to both the pet as well as the owner who handles the food. For example, a multistate outbreak of *Salmonella* was traced to dry dog food.[25] Outbreaks in North America have also been tied to pet treats, including pig ears and dried beef.[26] *Salmonella*-contaminated pet food has also been shown to persist as a contaminant on the surface of dog feed bowls, posing an ongoing environmental infection risk.[27]

Because food entering the home must therefore be assumed to possibly contain foodborne pathogens, food safety measures in the home are critical (Figure 11-3). These also need to involve pet food and pet food dish handling. A number of Web sites provide guidelines to consumers regarding safe food handling and preparation, including http://www.foodsafety.gov, http://www.fightbac.org, and http://www.cdc.gov/healthypets. The Partnership for Food Safety's Fight Bac program to reduce risk of bacterial contamination of foods includes four basic steps: clean, separate, cook, and chill.[28] These four steps are explained in Box 11-1.

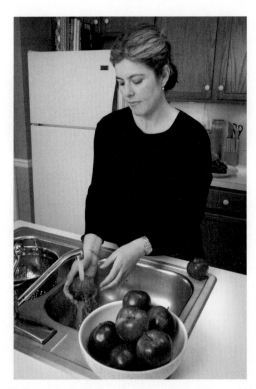

Figure 11-3 ▪ A pregnant woman washing an apple to avoid acquiring a possible foodborne illness. (From Centers for Disease Control and Prevention Public Health Image Library, Atlanta, Ga. Photo courtesy James Gathany.)

Clinicians have an important role to play in the detection of outbreaks of foodborne disease. Detection of such disease can lead to improved treatment outcomes for the animals and human beings, link to other reported cases, and allow for traceback to discover the source of common-source outbreaks.

SPECIFIC FOODBORNE ILLNESSES

Because of public health interventions of sewage treatment, water disinfection, and milk pasteurization, previously common foodborne illnesses such as typhoid fever, cholera, and bovine tuberculosis are rarely reported in the United States. However, vigilance must be maintained as emerging pathogens are now recognized as causing foodborne illness (e.g., *Vibrio vulnificus, E. coli*) O157:H7, and *Cyclospora cayetanensis*).[29]

Clinicians should always maintain a heightened awareness of foodborne illness in both human beings and other animals. A key point is that susceptibility to particular foodborne illnesses varies significantly between species. For some conditions such as staphylococcal food poisoning, it is not clear that animals are susceptible. Therefore it is unlikely that both human beings and animals would be affected in an outbreak. In other situations, such as melamine contamination of food, both animals and human beings have shown susceptibility and outbreaks in animals have provided warning about human risk. Table 11-2 lists the clinical presentation of a number of specific agents in human beings and other animals. Several of these agents are covered in Chapters 8 and 9. Others are described in the following paragraphs.

Botulism

Botulism is caused by seven different toxins (types A-G) produced by *Clostridium botulinum,* an anaerobic spore-forming bacteria. The bacteria are found in soil as well as the digestive tract of a wide range of mammals, fish, and birds. Foodborne illness can occur when spores germinate in carcasses and decaying vegetation and the bacteria begin producing toxin, which is then ingested. Alternatively, ingesting spores could lead to intestinal toxin production—or wound infection can occur, leading to bacterial growth and toxin production. The toxin causes muscle paralysis, which can result in respiratory failure. Most botulism in animals is due to type C, whereas type A is more common in human beings. Cattle become sick from eating contaminated feed (Figure 11-4). Massive die-offs can occur in waterfowl. Dogs are relatively resistant but can occasionally develop weakness.[39]

Clostridial Food Poisoning

Clostridium perfringens is a gram-positive sporogenic bacillus that produces extracellular toxins. There are several types of *C. perfringens* (A-F). *C. perfringens* type A is found in soil and as normal flora in the gastrointestinal tract of human beings and other animals. When allowed to grow in food that is not adequately cooked or refrigerated, *C. perfringens* type A produces an alpha toxin that can cause acute foodborne illness in human beings marked by diarrhea and abdominal discomfort. Clostridial food poisoning from type A toxin is not well described in animals, but types B, C, D, and E can cause infection and hemorrhagic enteritis in calves, sheep, pigs, and other livestock.[36] There is some evidence that *C. perfringens* infection can cause diarrhea in dogs and cats.[35,45] *C. perfringens* type A is being increasingly recognized as a cause of necrotizing enteritis in chickens.[46]

Listeriosis

Listeria monocytogenes is a gram-positive coccobacillus bacterium found in soil and the intestines of a wide range of animals, including mammals, birds, fish, and insects. Contaminated food, including pasteurized dairy products, undercooked meat, and drinking water, can be a source of infection for human beings. Human infection during pregnancy can cause miscarriages, stillbirth, and neonatal sepsis. Older and immunocompromised individuals can develop meningitis and other complications. It also can cause encephalitis, vomiting, septicemia, and neonatal death in ruminants (Figure 11-5).[36]

Staphylococcal Food Poisoning

Staphylococcus aureus is a gram-positive bacterium that is part of the microbial flora of the skin, nose, and throat in a wide range of animals, including human beings (see Chapter 9). When food is contaminated with a toxin-producing strain of *S. aureus,* a toxin is produced that is heat resistant and can cause the rapid onset of nausea, vomiting, cramping, and diarrhea. Animals do not appear to be susceptible to staphylococcal food poisoning.[39]

Table 11-2 ■ Presentation and Management of Selected Foodborne Illnesses in Human Beings and Other Animals

Agent	Incubation Period (Human Beings)[1]	Human Beings	Dogs	Cats	Other Animals	Principles of Treatment
Bacteria						
Campylobacter jejuni	2-5 days	Diarrhea, cramps, fever (neurologic sequelae may occur)	Diarrhea, usually mild, possibly with mucus or blood (enteritis is more common in young animals)		Calves: diarrhea with blood and mucus, fever Chick hatchlings: acute enteritis and death	Supportive care, antibiotics in severe cases
Clostridium botulinum (botulism toxin)[30]	12-72 hours	Usually type A, B, or E: vomiting, diarrhea, cranial nerve signs (diplopia, blurred vision), muscle weakness	Rare; usually type C, possibly type D (after eating contaminated bird or fish carcasses): cranial nerve involvement, weakness	Type C reported after eating contaminated bird or fish carcasses[31]	Waterfowl and other bird die-offs (especially type C; also A or E): paralysis, drowning Horses: type C and B Cattle: type C and D: weakness, drooling, incoordination	Supportive treatment, gastric lavage, *Botulinum* antitoxin given early
Clostridium perfringens (preformed toxin)[32]	8-16 hours	Watery diarrhea, abdominal pain (toxin produced by type A growing in food)	Clostridial food poisoning not well described; infection possible[33-35]	Clostridial food poisoning not well described[33-35]	Calves, lambs: hemorrhagic enteritis (types B, C, D, and E)[36] Chickens: necrotic enteritis (types A and C)	Food poisoning in human beings: supportive care Treat animals with clinical signs
Escherichia coli O157:H7	1-8 days	Severe diarrhea, possibly bloody; vomiting, abdominal pain; hemolytic uremic syndrome may develop	Acute enteritis, idiopathic cutaneous vasculopathy of Greyhounds		Cattle, sheep, goats, pigs, deer, poultry do not have clinical signs	Supportive care, monitor hematologic and renal status
Enterotoxigenic *E. coli*	1-3 days	Watery diarrhea, cramps, vomiting				Supportive care, antibiotics often not needed
Listeria	9-48 hours (invasive disease after 2-6 weeks)	Neonatal sepsis, miscarriage, stillbirth, meningitis	Rare: generalized neurologic signs[37]; tonsillitis reported[38]	Not reported	Septicemia, abortion, encephalitis, mastitis in ruminants	Antibiotics
Salmonella	1-3 days	Diarrhea, fever, vomiting	Malaise, fever, diarrhea, abortion	Fever without diarrhea, abortion	Pregnant, young, and lactating animals are most susceptible	Supportive care, antibiotics for sepsis and *S. typhi*, *S. paratyphi*, extraintestinal infection NSAIDs to decrease the effects of endotoxemia
Staphylococcus aureus (toxin)	1-6 hours	Vomiting, nausea, cramps; possible diarrhea and fever	Animals do not appear to be susceptible to staphylococcal food poisoning[39]			Supportive care

Yersinia enterocolitica (yersiniosis)	24-48 hours	Abdominal pain (pseudoappendicitis), fever, diarrhea, vomiting	Subclinical infection		Supportive care, antibiotics for invasive disease
Parasites					
Taeniasis	8-12 weeks	Abdominal discomfort, bloating, anal discomfort	Animals resistant to infection with adult parasite[40]		
Cryptosporidium	2-10 days	Watery diarrhea, cramps, nausea	Usually subclinical	Calves 1-3 weeks old most susceptible; diarrhea, weight loss	Supportive care, antibiotics for severe cases; hyperimmune bovine colostrum in calves
Giardia	1-2 weeks	Diarrhea, cramps, bloating	Puppies, kittens, calves, and lambs may have diarrhea, poor haircoat, flatulence, weight loss		Antibiotics fenbendazole, albendazole, metronidazole
Toxoplasma	5-32 days	Flulike illness, lymphadenopathy, severe disease in immunocompromised individuals	Generalized infection in puppies and immunocompromised dogs, fever, weight loss, diarrhea, encephalitis	Usually subclinical; Abortion in sheep, hogs, and goats; fever and dysphagia	Supportive care and antibiotics in pregnancy and immunocompromised individuals (antibiotics do not destroy bradyzoites or eliminate infection)
Trichinella	1-2 days for initial signs and symptoms	Variable; possible fever, muscle pain, eye swelling, diarrhea[41]	Mild vomiting, diarrhea	Mild vomiting, diarrhea[42]	Antibiotics mebendazole or albendazole in human beings; mebendazole or fenbendazole in dogs[42]
Toxicants					
Lead (see Chapter 8)	Acute or chronic	Abdominal pain, weakness	Vomiting, anorexia		Removal from exposure, chelation in severe cases
Melamine and other protein additives		Renal failure in infants fed contaminated formula	Renal toxicity[43]		
Vomitoxin	Minutes to hours	Headache, nausea, vomiting	Vomiting, anorexia[44]	Cows, sheep, pigs: fever, abortion[44]	Supportive care

NSAIDs, Nonsteroidal antiinflammatory drugs.

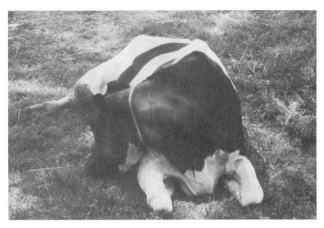

Figure 11-4 ■ An adult cow with generalized weakness from botulism. She was one of several that became affected when a new grass silage that had not been properly fermented was fed. The cow was recumbent for nearly 30 days but recovered with supportive care. (From Divers TJ, Peek SF: *Rebhun's diseases of dairy cattle,* ed 2, St Louis, 2008, Saunders Elsevier.)

Yersiniosis

Yersinia enterocolitica is a gram-negative rod that is classified in the same genus as the agent of plague (*Yersinia pestis;* see Chapter 9). Many animals carry *Yersinia* in their intestinal flora and shed bacteria in their feces. Human beings can become infected by ingesting contaminated water or food. Often the source of infection is not clear, but pigs are believed to be the reservoir for many human infections. Occupational groups such as butchers may be at increased risk. *Yersinia* infection in human beings can range from mild

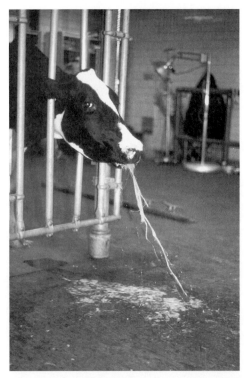

Figure 11-5 ■ Vomiting and depression were the most noticeable clinical signs in this adult cow with listeriosis. (From Divers TJ, Peek SF: *Rebhun's diseases of dairy cattle,* ed 2, St Louis, 2008, Saunders Elsevier.)

gastroenteritis to septicemia and abdominal pain that can mimic appendicitis. *Yersinia* appears to only rarely cause disease in animals; enteritis has been reported in a number of species.[36]

Taeniasis/Cysticercosis

Cestode tapeworms *Taenia solium* (pork tapeworm) and *T. saginata* (beef tapeworm) cause a unique foodborne illness in that human beings are the definitive host for these parasites. Infected human beings with adult tapeworms in their intestine may have few symptoms but can release gravid proglottids in feces, which then release eggs. If human beings have defecated in pastures or other areas frequented by swine or cattle, the animals can become infected through ingestion of the tapeworm eggs. When ingested by animals, the tapeworms form larval cysts (cysticerci) in tissues. Human beings can become infected by eating undercooked pork or beef (Figure 11-6). Veterinary inspection in slaughterhouses can reduce the risk of human infection.

Symptoms in human beings include abdominal pain, nausea and bloating, and anal discomfort. Infection with *T. solium* is more common in developing countries where human beings live closely with swine, and is rare in developed countries where intensive swine rearing prevents access of swine to human feces. Infection with *T. saginata* from undercooked beef is more widely distributed.

Cysticercosis infection in human beings occurs when human beings ingest viable eggs of *T. solium* that have been shed in human feces (Figure 11-7). The most serious complication of human infection is neurocysticercosis. Symptoms include headache, psychiatric disturbances, and seizures. Ocular involvement and painful muscle cysts can also occur.[40] Cysticercosis infection in pigs is usually subclinical. Dogs will occasionally manifest signs of neurocysticercosis that can resemble rabies.[40]

Trichinellosis

Trichinellosis is a foodborne disease caused by parasitic roundworms of the genus *Trichinella,* including *T. spiralis* (found in pigs and rodents; Figure 11-8), *T. murelli* (found in wild game), and *T. nativa* (found in bears, foxes, wolves, walrus, and other cold-climate mammals).[39] Most human cases are from consumption of undercooked meat. Infection can produce muscle swelling, pain, and headache. In severe cases encephalitis can develop. Although pigs and many other animals show no signs of infection, dogs and cats may show vomiting, diarrhea and, in rare cases, muscle stiffness and muscle pain.[42]

The fact that the encysted larval form can be detected by microscopic inspection of muscle tissue allowed nineteenth-century researchers to link trichinellosis to the consumption of pork and the development of veterinary control over the slaughter of animals for food consumption.[47]

Control measures include education of consumers about not eating raw meat, inspection of both domestic meat and relevant wild game meat such as wild boar, prohibitions on feeding animal carcasses or raw waste to swine, and prevention of contact between domestic swine and infected rodents or wildlife.[48]

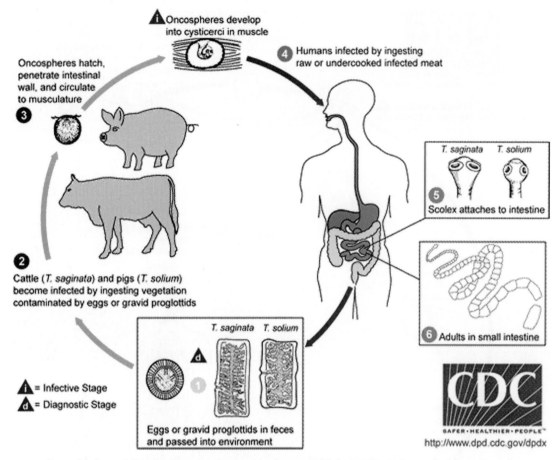

Figure 11-6 ▪ Life cycle of *Taeniasis* (pork and beef tapeworm) infection. (From Centers for Disease Control and Prevention, Laboratory of Parasites of Public Health Concern, Atlanta, Ga.)

Vomitoxin

Vomitoxin (deoxynivalenol) is a trichothecene mycotoxin found in moldy grain. Because it is heat stable, it will persist even after cooking. It is a widespread contaminant in grain supply and is particularly associated with fungal infection in the field. It can cause vomiting and anorexia in animals, including cattle, hogs, dogs, and cats. Its effects on human beings are not well understood but are believed to include nausea and vomiting.

EVALUATION OF SUSPECTED FOODBORNE ILLNESS

History

In taking a history from a patient with suspected foodborne illness, it is important to determine when symptoms began, the particular constellation of symptoms, and whether any other human beings or animals in the vicinity are experiencing illness. The reported time interval between exposure and illness onset, as well as the pattern of symptoms, can help the clinician sort through the differential diagnosis.

The presence or absence and the volume of vomiting, diarrhea, and hematuria should be determined, as well as whether the diarrhea is bloody or contains mucus (a sign of large-bowel disease). The clinician should inquire about any other symptoms, including neurologic signs. A detailed food and exposure history should be obtained, including whether the patient has visited farms, petting zoos, what type of pets are owned (especially asking about reptiles, puppies, kittens, ducklings, and any animals with diarrhea), any current health problems, consumption of unpasteurized dairy products, recent travel, day care center exposures, camping trips or other exposure to untreated water, attendance at events where food was served, and whether any persons with similar exposures also have symptoms.

Physical Examination

Determine the degree of dehydration and whether hospitalization for intravenous hydration is indicated. Particular attention should be paid to the abdominal exam and whether a surgical consult should be obtained.

Laboratory Tests

When foodborne illness is suspected in human beings, appropriate lab testing supports the diagnosis, yet hospitals and laboratories may vary in their testing protocols. If the patient is immunocompromised or has fever, bloody diarrhea, severe

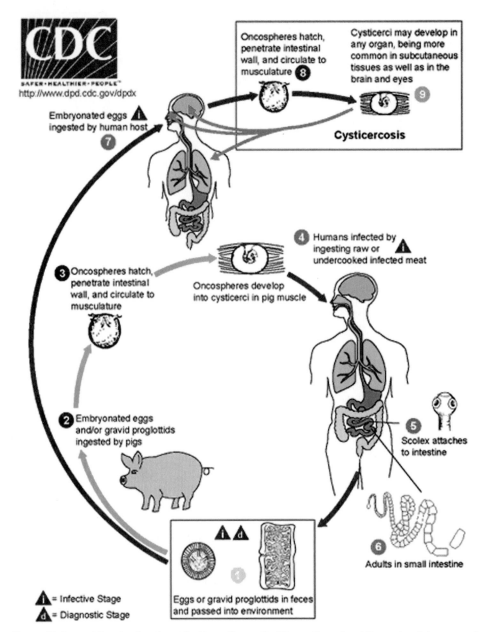

Figure 11-7 ▪ Lifecycle of cysticercosis. (From Centers for Disease Control and Prevention, Laboratory of Parasites of Public Health Concern, Atlanta, Ga.)

abdominal pain, or severe or persistent illness, or if fecal leukocytes are present, fecal cultures are indicated.[49] Many laboratories limit fecal culture screening to *Salmonella, Shigella,* and *Campylobacter* species. If infection with *Vibrio, Yersinia,* or *E. coli* O157:H7 is suspected, it may be necessary to contact the laboratory to arrange special culture media or incubation. If diarrhea is chronic or does not respond to antimicrobial therapy or there is a suggestive history of travel or other risk factors (such as immunocompromised status or an ongoing outbreak), fecal examination should include testing for parasitic infection.

Blood cultures should be obtained if septicemia is suspected. Samples of vomitus may be obtained in particular cases, such as suspected toxic ingestion.

If a particular food is suspected to be the cause of illness, samples should also be obtained and submitted for culture (and possible toxic analysis). The public health department should be able to assist with such analysis.

EVALUATION OF SUSPECTED FOODBORNE ILLNESS IN ANIMALS

The veterinarian evaluating an animal with suspected foodborne illness should ask the caretaker about routine foods eaten (including animal treats and food "toys") and whether unusual foods have been eaten recently. Whether a cat or dog is allowed to roam outside and could have eaten

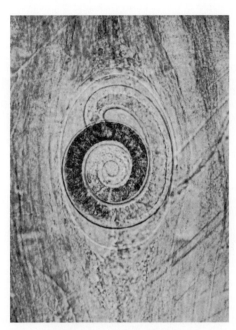

Figure 11-8 ■ *Trichinella spiralis* cyst in a fresh squash preparation of pork muscle (magnification ×160). (From Bowman DD: *Georgi's parasitology for veterinarians*, ed 8, 2003, St Louis, Saunders Elsevier.)

garbage, an animal carcass, or a source of toxins such as mushrooms should also be determined. A history of any other animals or nearby human beings with clinical illness should also be obtained. In addition to asking about signs of diarrhea, anorexia, and vomiting, the veterinarian should also inquire about muscle weakness and spasms, which could indicate neurologic involvement.

Physical Examination

The physical examination should always include a careful abdominal exam to palpate for masses, distension, and tenderness, which could indicate obstruction.

Laboratory Tests

As with the evaluation of human beings, the choice of laboratory testing depends on the clinical scenario. Feces can be submitted for bacterial culture as well as for parasites if suspected. A fecal enterotoxin assay by enzyme-linked immunosorbent assay is available.[42] In particular situations, samples of food, blood, or vomitus may be submitted for analysis.

TREATMENT

Rehydration is essential and may be accomplished with oral subcutaneous or intravenous fluids.

The use of antibiotics depends on the severity of illness and the specific pathogen. In some mild cases (such non-typhi or paratyphi species of *Salmonella*) antibiotics may be avoided to minimize the development of a chronic carrier state.

In animals, most foodborne illness involves removal of exposure and supportive care. In certain cases, antibiotics are indicated (see Table 11-2).

REPORTING OF FOODBORNE ILLNESS

Because foodborne illnesses occurring in a human or animal can signal a problem with food safety affecting potentially large populations, it is essential that cases be reported in a timely manner to the appropriate public health authority. Infection with *Salmonella, Shigella, E. coli* O157:H7, other *Shiga* toxin–producing *E. coli*, hemolytic uremic syndrome (HUS), and hepatitis A are reportable almost everywhere in the United States. Infection with other pathogens may also be reportable.[50] The CDC's Foodborne Disease Outbreak Response and Surveillance Team conducts national surveillance for outbreaks and assists states in investigations. A number of national and international reporting mechanisms are in place in addition to the FoodNet system previously described. Many foodborne pathogens are reportable to local and state health departments (see Chapter 13). The GeoSentinel system of the International Society of Travel Medicine, in cooperation with the CDC, reports on illnesses occurring in travelers, including foodborne illness. The World Health Organization is working to strengthen the capacity of its member states in the surveillance and control of major foodborne diseases.

Private veterinary practitioners can become certified through a voluntary accreditation program with the USDA to control exported animal diseases from entering another state or country.[51] The certification of animals for national and international movement is one important part of veterinary accreditation. Accredited veterinarians work cooperatively with federal veterinarians and state animal health officials and are the backbone of many U.S. regulatory programs for livestock and poultry diseases. All veterinarians are required to report animal cases of disease of agricultural importance that are notifiable or foreign to the state veterinarian or USDA veterinarian. This information is then compiled at the national level through the USDA National Animal Health Policy and Programs staff or through the National Animal Health Reporting System maintained by the USDA.[52] Many states also require selected diseases in animals to be reported to the public health system to prevent human disease from occurring (see Chapter 13). The World Organization for Animal Health (OIE) tracks reports of disease outbreaks in animals with trade and food safety implications. OIE member countries are required to report to the OIE the status of OIE reportable diseases in their country and on events that may require immediate reporting. Veterinarians diagnosing animals with suspected disease that could pose a risk to other animals or people should contact their state veterinarian, state public health veterinarian, or USDA veterinarian.

References

1. American Medical Association, et al. Diagnosis and management of foodborne illnesses: a primer for physicians and other health care professionals. *MMWR Recomm Rep.* 2004;53(RR-4):1–33.
2. Centers for Disease Control and Prevention. Preliminary FoodNet data on the incidence of infection with pathogens transmitted commonly through food—10 states, 2007. *MMWR Morb Mortal Wkly Rep.* 2008;57(14):366–370.
3. The Pet Food Institute. *Pet food data.* http://www.petfoodinstitute.org/index.cfm?page=uspetfoodsales. Accessed October 20, 2009.
4. Mumford EL, Kihm U. Integrated risk reduction along the food chain. *Ann N Y Acad Sci.* 2006;1081:147–152.

5. D'Mello JPF. *Contaminants and toxins in animal feeds.* http://www.fao.org/docrep/article/agrippa/x9500e04.htm. Accessed July 14, 2008.

6. Franco DA. A survey of *Salmonella* serovars and most probable numbers in rendered-animal-protein meals: inferences for animal and human health. *J Environmental Health.* 2005;67(6):18–22.

7. Haapapuro ER, Barnard ND, Simon M. Review—animal waste used as livestock feed: dangers to human health. *Prev Med.* 1997;26(5 Pt 1):599–602.

8. European Food Safety Authority. Statement of EFSA on the risks for public health due to the presence of dioxins in pork from Ireland. *EFSA J.* 2008;911:1–15.

9. O'Keefe PW. Formation of brominated dibenzofurans from pyrolysis of the polybrominated biphenyl fire retardant, FireMaster FF-1. *Environ Health Perspect.* 1978;23:347–350.

10. Chopra I, Roberts M. Tetracycline antibiotics: mode of action, applications, molecular biology, and epidemiology of bacterial resistance. *Microbiol Mol Biol Rev.* 2001;65(2):232–260.

11. Garofalo C, Vignaroli C, Zandri G, et al. Direct detection of antibiotic resistance genes in specimens of. *N Engl J Med.* 2006;355(21):2186–2194.

12. Kandun IN, Wibisono H, Sedyaningsih ER, et al. Three Indonesian clusters of H5N1 virus infection in 2005. *N Engl J Med.* 2007;356:1375.

13. Centers for Disease Control and Prevention. *Guidance for controlling potential risks to workers exposed to class B biosolids.* http://www.cdc.gov/niosh/docs/2002-149/2002-149.html. Accessed July 14, 2008.

14. Verhoeff J, Counotte G, Hamhuis D. Nitrogen dioxide (silo gas) poisoning in dairy cattle. *Tijdschr Diergeneeskd.* 2007;132(20):780–782.

15. U.S.Food and Drug Administration. FDA extends consumer warning on Serrano peppers from Mexico. http://www.fda.gov/NewsEvents/Newsroom/PressAnnouncements/2008/ucm116929.htm. Accessed September 7, 2008.

16. Wolfe ND, Heneine W, Carr JK, et al. Emergence of unique primate T-lymphotropic viruses among central African bushmeat hunters. *Proc Natl Acad Sci USA.* 2005;102(22):7994–7999.

17. Wolfe ND, Dunavan CP, Diamond J. Origins of major human infectious diseases. *Nature.* 2007;447(7142):279–283.

18. Rodriguez Valin ME, Pousa Ortega A, Pons Sanchez C, et al. Brucellosis as occupational disease: study of an outbreak of air-born transmission at a slaughter house[in Spanish]. *Rev Esp Salud Publica.* 2001;75(2):159–169.

19. Bruntz S. *Personal communication.* 2008.

20. Centers for Disease Control and Prevention. Outbreak of *Campylobacter jejuni* infections associated with drinking unpasteurized milk procured through a cow-leasing program—Wisconsin, 2001. *MMWR Morb Mortal Wkly Rep.* 2002;51(25):548–549.

21. Cornell University; Milk quality improvement program. disease outbreaks associated with milk products. http://www.milkfacts.info/Milk%20Microbiology/Disease%20Outbreaks.htm.

22. Jay MT, Cooley M, Carychao D, et al. *Escherichia coli* O157:H7 in feral swine near spinach fields and cattle, central California coast. *Emerg Infect Dis.* 2007;13(12):1908–1911.

23. Smith HV, Caccio SM, Cook N, et al. *Cryptosporidium* and *Giardia* as foodborne zoonoses. *Vet Parasitol.* 2007;149(1–2):29–40.

24. United States Department of Agriculture Food Safety and Inspection Service. Progress report on *Salmonella* testing of raw meat and poultry products, 1998–2007, 2008 http://www.fsis.usda.gov/science/progress_report_salmonella_testing/index.asp. Accessed April 20, 2009.

25. Centers for Disease Control and Prevention. Multistate outbreak of human *Salmonella* infections caused by contaminated dry dog food—United States, 2006–2007. *MMWR Morb Mortal Wkly Rep.* 2008;57(19):521–524.

26. Centers for Disease Control and Prevention. Human salmonellosis associated with animal-derived pet treats-United States and Canada, 2005. *MMWR.* 2006;55:702–705.

27. Weese JS, Rousseau J. Survival of *Salmonella* Copenhagen in food bowls following contamination with experimentally inoculated raw meat: effects of time, cleaning, and disinfection. *Canadian Veterinary J.* 2006;47(9):887–889.

28. Partnership for Food Safety Education. *Safe food handling.* http://www.fightbac.org/content/view/6/11/. Accessed July 14, 2008.

29. Tauxe RV. Emerging foodborne diseases: an evolving public health challenge. *Emerg Infect Dis.* 3(4):425–434, 1997.

30. Center for Food Security and Public Health. *Botulism.* http://www.cfsph.iastate.edu/Factsheets/pdfs/botulism.pdf. Accessed April 20, 2009.

31. Elad D, Yas-Natan E, Aroch I, et al. Natural *Clostridium botulinum* type C toxicosis in a group of cats. *J Clin Microbiol.* 2004;42(11):5406–5408.

32. FDA/Center for Food Safety and Applied Nutrition. *Foodborne pathogenic microorganisms and natural toxins handbook: Clostridium perfringens.* http://www.cfsan.fda.gov/~mow/chap11.html.

33. Brooks WC. *The pet health library: Clostridium perfringens.* http://www.veterinarypartner.com/Content.plx?P=A&A=2239&S=1&SourceID=42.

34. Sasaki J, Goryo M, Asahina M, et al. Hemorrhagic enteritis associated with *Clostridium perfringens* type A in a dog. *J Vet Med Sci.* 1999;61(2):175–177.

35. Cassutto BH, Cook LC. An epidemiological survey of *Clostridium perfringens*–associated enterotoxemia at an army veterinary treatment facility. *Mil Med.* 2002;167(3):219–222.

36. Acha PN, Szyfres B. *Zoonoses and communicable diseases common to man and animals, Vol. I: Bacterioses and mycoses.* 3rd ed. Washington DC: Pan American Health Organization; 2003.

37. Schroeder H, van Rensburg IB. Generalised *Listeria monocytogenes* infection in a dog. *J S Afr Vet Assoc.* 1993;64(3):133–136.

38. Laikko T, Baverud V, Danielsson-Tham ML, et al. Canine tonsillitis associated with *Listeria monocytogenes.* *Vet Rec.* 2004;154(23):732.

39. Colville J, Berryhill D. *Handbook of zoonoses: identification and prevention.* St Louis: Mosby; 2007.

40. Acha PN, Szyfres B. *Zoonoses and communicable diseases common to man and animals: vol. III: chlamydioses, parasitoses.* 3rd ed. Washington DC: Pan American Health Organization; 2003.

41. Heymann DL, ed. *Control of communicable diseases manual.* 18th ed. Washington DC: American Public Health Association; 2004.

42. Barr SC, Bowman DD. *The 5-minute veterinary consult clinical companion: canine and feline infectious diseases and parasitology.* Ames, IA: Blackwell; 2006.

43. Dobson RL, Motlagh S, Quijano M, et al. Identification and characterization of toxicity of contaminants in pet food leading to an outbreak of renal toxicity in cats and dogs. *Toxicol Sci.* 2008;106(1):251–262.

44. Gupta RC, ed. *Veterinary toxicology: basic and clinical principles.* New York: Academic Press; 2007.

45. Marks SL, Kather EJ, Kass PH, et al. Genotypic and phenotypic characterization of *Clostridium perfringens* and *Clostridium difficile* in diarrheic and healthy dogs. *Journal of Veterinary Internal Medicine.* 2002;16(5):533–540.

46. Van Immerseel F, De Buck J, Pasmans F, et al. *Clostridium perfringens* in poultry: an emerging threat for animal and public health. *Avian Pathology.* 2004;33(6):537–549.

47. Pozio E, Darwin Murrell K. Systematics and epidemiology of *Trichinella.* *Adv Parasitol.* 2006;63:367–439.

48. Gamble HR, Bessonov AS, Cuperlovic K, et al. International Commission on Trichinellosis: recommendations on methods for the control of *Trichinella* in domestic and wild animals intended for human consumption. *Vet Parasitol.* 2000;93(3–4):393–408.

49. American Medical Association, et al. Diagnosis and management of foodborne illnesses: a primer for physicians. *MMWR Recomm Rep.* 2001;50(RR-2):1–69.

50. Centers for Disease Control and Prevention. *Reporting a foodborne illness—healthcare professionals.* http://www.cdc.gov/foodborneoutbreaks/reporting_professionals.htm. Accessed July 14, 2008.

51. United States Department of Agriculture. *Animal and Plant Health Inspection Service: Veterinary accreditation.* http://www.aphis.usda.gov/animal_health/vet_accreditation. Accessed July 14, 2008.

52. United States Department of Agriculture. *Animal and Plant Health Inspection Service: Animal health monitoring and surveillance.* http://www.aphis.usda.gov/vs/ceah/ncahs/nahrs. Accessed July 14, 2008.

Occupational Health of Animal Workers

12

Ben Hur P. Mobo, Peter M. Rabinowitz, Lisa A. Conti, and Oyebode A. Taiwo

Some of the most intensive human-animal interactions occur in the occupational setting. Animal workers may encounter hundreds to thousands of animals each day, which increases the risk of exposure to biological, physical, and chemical hazards. In recent years a number of emerging infectious diseases have first appeared—as deadly outbreaks among workers with animal exposures. In addition to zoonotic disease risks, high rates of allergic disease, physical injuries, and psychological stress have also been reported in animal handlers. Many animal workers in both developing and developed countries are not enrolled in formal occupational safety and health programs or may receive medical care from human health care providers who are not familiar with the occupational risks these workers face.

Veterinarians have a special role to play in the development of occupational safety and health strategies for animal workers because they are intimately familiar with animal diseases and the necessary procedures involved in animal care and handling. Therefore improving occupational health and safety among animal workers represents a global health challenge that will require increased communication and cooperation between human health and animal health care providers.

This chapter outlines the occupational health hazards that animal workers encounter, presents a One Health team approach to worker health and safety that involves both human and animal health professionals, and suggests preventive health programs for particular worker groups.

Key Points for Clinicians and Public Health Professionals

Public Health Professionals

- Identify occupational groups in the community that have significant exposures to animals and work to educate them, local medical providers, and veterinary providers to ensure they receive appropriate preventive health services.
- Work with local petting zoos, county fairs, pet stores, and other organizations involved in human contact with animals in public settings to ensure that the guidelines of the National Association of Public Health Veterinarians (NAPHV) for Animals in Public Settings (http://www.nasphv.org/Documents/AnimalsInPublicSettings.pdf) are being followed. This will help protect both the public and workers in such settings.

Human Health Care Providers

- Ask patients whether they work with animals. If they do, assess their occupational risks.
- If asked to provide medical services (such as a preplacement physical) for a worker with animal contact, consider contacting the veterinarian responsible for the health of the animals in the workplace to discuss specific occupational risks.
- When evaluating a worker with an animal-related exposure (e.g., bite, scratch, mucous membrane contact), ensure that all potential zoonotic pathogens are being considered in the risk assessment and that prophylactic medication is started as necessary if indicated.
- When evaluating animal workers with acute or chronic illnesses, including asthma, dermatitis, and other allergic conditions, determine whether work exposures could play a causative role.
- If contracting to provide occupational health services to a group of workers with animal contact, employ a team approach to preventive care. The team should ideally include the veterinarian providing care to the animals as well as experts in exposure reduction such as an infection control/biosafety specialist and/or an industrial hygienist. This team approach will help ensure that relevant health risks in the workplace are being identified and addressed with adequate preventive services, including engineering controls, training, vaccination, postexposure protocols, and surveillance.
- Counsel immunocompromised and pregnant workers about particular risks of animal handling.
- Safeguard the confidentiality of any medical information about animal workers, including medical records and any information regarding immunocompromising conditions.

- If managing a clinical practice, ensure that policies and procedures are in place so that veterinary staff receive adequate preventive health services.
- If providing veterinary services to a facility such as a zoo, animal shelter, research laboratory, or pet store, advise management about the need for adequate preventive health services for the animal workers.
- Help inform human health care providers in the community who will be performing preplacement and follow-up examinations of workers about the occupational health risks and needs of animal workers.
- Respect the confidentiality of any medical information about animal workers, including medical records and any information regarding immunocompromised individuals.

TYPES OF ANIMAL WORKERS

More than 2 million people in the United States are engaged in a wide range of occupational activities that involve animals.[1] These include approximately 750,000 persons involved with livestock confinement; 500,000 involved with dairy farming[2]; 200,000 workers employed in animal care and services as kennel attendants, groomers, stable hands, zoo keepers, and animal trainers[3]; and 125,000 researchers and animal handlers involved with laboratory animal research.[4] Globally, as much as 49% of the world's population is estimated to be involved in agriculture, which often involves animal husbandry and animal-associated health risks.[5] Some of these workers are formally employed in full-time positions in animal-related care and may receive preventive health services (such as described in this chapter) through their workplace. However, many individuals who work part-time or full-time with animals may receive little or no preventive health services related to their work exposures. For example, staff at pet swap meets, pet store employees, volunteers at zoos and county fair animal exhibits, wildlife rehabilitators, wildlife biologists, volunteer animal rescue workers, individuals engaged in home slaughter of animals for family consumption, and subsistence (bushmeat) hunters may all face significant "occupational" health risks related to their contact with animals, yet may never receive preplacement examinations, prophylactic vaccinations, or follow-up surveillance examinations to prevent or detect work-related disease. If they do see a medical provider for care of a work-related injury or illness, that medical provider may not be aware of the range of health risks these workers face, and therefore the treatment or recommendations for prevention may not be optimal.

OCCUPATIONAL HEALTH APPROACH

The majority of occupational health services in the United States are provided by family physicians and other clinicians without specialized training.[6] However, when using a team approach these individuals can learn to provide adequate occupational health services to animal workers.

The components of an occupational health approach are simple and adaptable to a wide range of work settings. They involve identification and control of hazardous exposures, medical services such as careful screening of workers at baseline, vaccination, surveillance of workers' health, identification of sentinel health events, and management of necessary work restrictions and work-related problems. Although such preventive services may be viewed by some employers as an unnecessary expenditure of resources, they can be cost effective in the long run by preventing potentially compensable work-related illness and injury and promoting worker well-being. Box 12-1 illustrates this approach.

OCCUPATIONAL HEALTH TEAM

Because of the diversity of the hazards encountered by animal workers, providing effective occupational health services to such workers is best accomplished through a team approach. Such a team can include a medical provider to provide screening and management of medical problems, a veterinarian who is familiar with zoonotic disease risks, industrial hygienists to identify and evaluate hazardous exposures and help devise engineering and work practice controls to reduce them, and biosafety/infection control specialists to focus on zoonotic disease transmission risks. Figure 12-1 diagrams the ideal components of an occupational health team that provides preventive health care to animal workers.

Actively involving a designated human health care provider in an occupational health approach for animal workers also has many advantages. Such involvement can lead to the medical provider becoming more knowledgeable about the specific health risks faced by animal workers. Ongoing communication between the medical provider and the veterinarian helps ensure that injured workers are properly managed, workers at increased risk of illness (e.g., immunocompromised persons) and injury are adequately counseled, and preventable hazards in the workplace are identified and addressed.

Veterinarians can play key roles in an occupational health team. The veterinarian is the source of knowledge about relevant animal diseases and the necessary procedures of animal handling and typically has regular contact with the animals, the workplace, and the animal workers. In animal research facilities, the veterinarian is often the administrative

---

BOX 12-1   COMPONENTS OF OCCUPATIONAL HEALTH APPROACH TO WORKPLACE HEALTH HAZARDS

- Hazard identification
- Hazard control using hierarchy of controls
- Preplacement screening of workers
- Preventive vaccines and training
- Medical surveillance
- Acute injury/illness management; identification of sentinel health events
- Management of work restriction, job modification, and return to work
- Confidential management of records and medical information

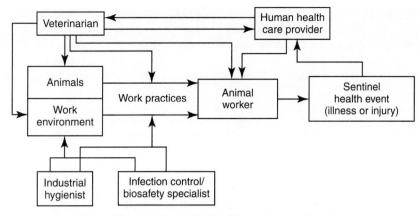

Figure 12-1 ▪ Occupational health team for animal workers.

supervisor of the animal care workers. In veterinary hospitals the veterinarian may be both the chief clinician and the practice director. For wildlife rehabilitation facilities, animal shelters, zoos, and many other settings, the consulting veterinarian may be the principal point of contact with the medical providers as well as the chief source of medical information about occupational health and safety hazards of the workplace. The veterinarian may be the health professional who is most familiar to the workers and with whom the workers have established a trusting relationship. The veterinarian may also be in regular contact with the employer or worksite supervisor and be able to advocate for the provision of occupational health services for the workers. For all these reasons the veterinarian may be the most appropriate professional to assemble and help lead the occupational health team as well as ensure that the services provided to workers are appropriate for the work setting.

Industrial hygienists have training in the identification and engineering control of a wide range of workplace hazards, including chemical, physical, and biological agents. Consultation from such individuals can help an occupational health team design safe strategies for the handling of hazardous chemicals such as cleaning agents and anesthetic gases, control of noise, and methods to reduce dust exposures that can cause allergy and infection.

Infection control and biosafety specialists are professionals who specialize in the prevention of infectious disease transmissions in workplaces and other settings. They can play a consulting role in the occupational health team by identifying specific infectious disease hazards and helping design strategies to reduce both animal-animal and animal-human transmission of disease. This may involve the design of ventilation systems and work policies such as disposal of infectious waste and use of personal protective equipment.

HAZARD IDENTIFICATION

Animal workers face a wide number of potential occupational health hazards that can be classified as biological, chemical, physical, or psychosocial. These hazards and their control are listed in Table 12-1.

Biological Hazards

ALLERGENS

As discussed in Chapter 7, many animal proteins are potential allergens in human beings. Although guinea pigs, mice, rats, and cats are common causes of allergy, virtually any species, including primates, larger domestic animals (such as horses and cattle), and reptiles can also pose an allergic risk to workers.[7,8] Exposure to insects such as roaches, flies, and mites as well as insect parts, shellfish (e.g., snow crabs, king crab, lobster, shrimp, scallops), and fish species (e.g., salmon, trout, pilchard, anchovy, hake) has also been associated with allergic reactions.[9] Other animal-related sources of allergens in the workplace include molds and thermophilic bacteria that infect animal foods (including hay and prepared animal food) and cause asthma, rhinitis, dermatitis, and hypersensitivity pneumonitis.[10]

In addition to animal allergens, other allergen exposures for animal workers may include latex gloves, allergenic chemicals such as disinfecting agents (e.g., glutaraldehyde), other cleaning agents and detergents, and organic dusts (e.g., red cedar shavings used as animal bedding).

Not surprisingly, allergic reactions are a well-recognized health problem among animal workers.[11] In some settings almost half of animal workers have been reported to develop allergy-related symptoms such as rhinitis, conjunctivitis, asthma, contact urticaria, and other types of allergic dermatitis.[1,4,12,13] Risk factors for developing allergic responses to antigens include the intensity and duration of exposure to specific antigens[4,13] and a history of atopy (allergic predisposition).[14] Allergic exposures can pose a difficult problem for sensitized workers because even low levels of exposure to an allergen may provoke a response in a previously sensitized individual. In addition, personal protective equipment may not adequately protect them from further allergic reactions.

ZOONOTIC PATHOGENS

As described in Chapter 9, a large number zoonotic pathogens can pose a hazard to animal workers, who generally have increased exposures to zoonotic diseases compared with the general public. Many of these individual zoonotic

TABLE 12-1 ▪ Occupational Hazards Encountered by Animal Workers and Relevant Hierarchy of Control Strategies

Hazard	Elimination	Substitution	Engineering Controls	Administrative/ Work Practice Controls	Personal Protective Equipment
Biological					
Allergens, endotoxin	Eliminate particular allergenic source	Work with different species/ gender with less allergenic potential; substitute bedding material that is less allergenic or dusty	Adequate ventilation in work areas; reduce dust generation; clean frequently; reduce animal density	Avoid wearing street clothes while working with animals[1]; perform animal manipulations in safety hood if possible; job modification or restriction for sensitized employees	Masks/respirators, gloves, gowns to reduce allergen exposure
Zoonoses[41]	Vaccinate or otherwise eliminate disease in animals (preventive veterinary care)	Work with different species with less zoonotic potential	Nonporous surfaces; appropriate use of disinfectants; separation of patient areas from staff break areas; physical isolation of sick animals; disposal containers for infectious waste; needlestick prevention devices	Written infection control plan; hand hygiene; bite and other injury prevention; worker vaccination; restrict eating and drinking in care areas; consider job modification/restriction for immunocompromised or pregnant workers	Gloves, sleeves when handling fluids, infected animals, necropsy, dental procedures, resuscitation, obstetrics, diagnostic specimens, tick removal Facial protection for splash or spray Respirator use for abortions, poultry deaths, other aerosol risk Footwear and head cover when gross contamination is suspected
Pathogenic fungi	Prevent bats and birds from roosting in buildings		Control aerosolized dust, disinfect contaminated material, dispose of waste safety	Warn workers of risk	Disposable footwear and clothing, respirator use, gloves
Live vaccines	Avoid use of live vaccines	Substitute vaccine with less risk to human beings	Needlestick prevention systems, sharps disposal containers	Needlestick prevention training, avoid recapping needles, report exposures; use tick repellant, perform frequent tick checks	Gloves, sleeves, leg coverings
Arthropods	Control mites, ticks, fleas in animals			Use of tick repellant, frequent tick checks	Protective clothing
Physical					
Bites, crush injuries	Avoid acquiring dangerous animals	Substitute less-dangerous animals	Rooms, corrals with adequate exits	Allow only trained individuals near dangerous or large animals; bite prevention	Impermeable gloves for certain tasks
Lifting animals, carrying heavy loads			Design ergonomic solutions (mechanical lifts, storage solutions that reduce need for lifting)	Training in injury prevention; housekeeping training and maintenance	Footwear selection
Slip, trip, and fall	Eliminate fall risks		Floor material selection	Control access to areas with slippery environment and provide appropriate signage	

Continued

TABLE 12-1 ■ Occupational Hazards Encountered by Animal Workers and Relevant Hierarchy of Control Strategies—cont'd

Hazard	Elimination	Substitution	Engineering Controls	Administrative/ Work Practice Controls	Personal Protective Equipment
Noise	Eliminate noisy machines	Substitute less-noisy machines or processes	Noise shielding/ barrier	Motivate/train regarding use of hearing protection; limit time in noisy areas	Hearing protection
Radiation	Eliminate need for on-site x-rays, other radiation	Substitute equipment with less radiation hazard	Appropriate radiologic housing facility	Training in radiation safety, sun exposure protection; restrict access to radiologic facilities	Use of sunscreen, protective clothing, and radiation shielding (lead gowns, gloves, etc.)
Chemical					
Anesthetic gases		Substitute less-toxic compounds	Adequate scavenging systems	Follow MSDS with chemical-specific guidelines	Gloves, respirators when indicated
Disinfectants, cleaners, pesticides		Substitute safer chemicals	Adequate ventilation when cleaning; safe application systems	Safety policies to restrict use to trained individuals	Gloves, respirators when indicated
Nitrogen dioxide, H_2S, ammonia (farms)			Silage management, manure management	Safety policies regarding entry into silos, manure storage areas	Air respirators, other respirators as indicated
Psychosocial					
Stress of euthanasia, compassion fatigue, burnout; fear of trauma, isolation		Work with different species	Safety equipment, injury prevention as above	Support groups, coping skills training, animal handling skills training	

MSDS, Material Safety Data Sheet.

diseases with occupational exposure potential are covered in Chapter 9. Selected pathogens of relevance to particular worker groups are described in the sections that follow. For example, occupational cases of *Campylobacter* and *Chlamydophila psittaci* infection have been documented among poultry workers[15,16] and reported human plague cases have been reported among veterinary staff attending to infected cats.[17] With the increasing focus on emerging infectious diseases, it should be remembered that many such diseases appear first or with greatest intensity in the occupational setting. The first recognized (index) human case for the epidemic of severe acute respiratory syndrome (SARS) that began in China was a chef who had extensive exposure to wild game animals in his work.[18] Nipah virus, another deadly emerging viral pathogen, first broke out among Malaysian pig farm workers.[19] Human outbreaks of Ebola virus infection in Africa are believed to originate at least in part from exposures to nonhuman primates and other wildlife during bushmeat hunting and butchering.[20] A strain of highly pathogenic avian influenza (HPAI) has caused fatal work-related infection in a veterinarian, and human cases of H5N1 HPAI remain strongly associated with working in animal markets, poultry rearing, slaughtering, defeathering, and preparing infected birds for consumption.[21] Rift Valley fever, another emerging viral disease, often occurs in human

beings as an occupational disease among herdsmen engaged in activities such as assisting with cattle birthing and caring for sick animals.[22]

Direct routes of exposure for zoonotic pathogens include a bite or scratch from an infected animal, exposure to infected fluids through splashes to the eye or mucous membranes, touching of contaminated surfaces, needlestick or other sharp instrument injuries, or inhalation of infectious particles in dusts. Vector-borne transmission can also occur in certain workplaces (see arthropod exposures later in this chapter).

In addition to animal-human transmission, some zoonotic diseases can be "reverse zoonoses," potentially transmitted from human beings to animals in the occupational setting. Examples include tuberculosis, which may be transmitted by human beings to nonhuman primates,[23] elephants,[24] and dogs.[25]

Live Vaccines

Accidental autoinoculation of live vaccines for diseases with zoonotic potential has been reported to result in worker infections. An example is the vaccine for *Brucella abortus* strain RB51.[26] A 1995 survey of veterinarians found that 23% of large animal veterinarian respondents reported accidental self-inoculation with live *Brucella* vaccine.[27]

ENDOTOXIN AND ORGANIC DUSTS

Endotoxin is a biological hazard consisting of lipopolysaccharide compounds from the cell walls of gram-negative bacteria that can grow in animal bedding or feed. When the bedding or feed is disturbed, dusts are generated that can have endotoxin concentrations of 3000 nanograms per meter cubed (ng/m^3), in excess of a proposed guideline[2] of 9 ng/m^3. Adverse respiratory effects such as bronchitis and airway obstruction have been reported in workers who inhale such dusts, especially when working in confined areas with less than adequate ventilation.[28] Organic dusts from moldy grain used for animal feed can cause organic dust toxic syndrome (ODTS), a self-limited disease with symptoms including fever, cough, myalgias, headache, and shortness of breath.[2]

PATHOGENIC FUNGI

A hazard related to work around areas of bird or bat droppings is the exposure to potentially pathogenic fungi including *Histoplasma, Cryptococcus,* and *Blastomyces. Histoplasma capsulatum* is a fungus that exists in two forms: a mold form in the soil environment and a yeast form that develops when human beings or other animals inhale or ingest the spores. Although many infected human beings are asymptomatic, some may develop complications ranging from mild flulike illness to chronic lung and eye infections and pericarditis.[29] Skin infection can also occur. Immunocompromised individuals are at increased risk of severe disease. The nutrients in bird or bat guano can encourage the growth of spores in the environment. Therefore areas of pigeon and other bird roosting where bird droppings accumulate may be more likely to have high levels of *H. capsulatum* spores that can lead to inhalation or ingestion by human beings. Poultry litter can also contain *Histoplasma* spores. Farmers, construction workers, forestry workers, and other workers exposed to disturbed soil or poultry guano can be at risk of infection, especially if individuals are immunocompromised. Unlike birds, bats appear to shed infectious *Histoplasma* in their droppings. Caves and other areas where bat guano accumulates have been associated with human cases of histoplasmosis.[30] The National Institute for Occupational Safety and Health (NIOSH) has published guidelines for reduction of occupational risk of *Histoplasma* infection that also can be applied to the risk of other fungal pathogens such as *Cryptococcus* and *Blastomyces.* These guidelines include the use of respiratory protection, disposable protective clothing and shoe coverings, and gloves that avoid skin trauma to reduce the risk of skin infection. The types of respirators that should be worn during occupational activities with exposures to spore-contaminated dusts depend on intensity of exposure. In low-risk situations (e.g., site surveys of bird roosts), disposable, filtering facepiece respirators may be adequate, whereas extremely dusty work such as removing accumulated bird or bat manure from an enclosed area such as a barn or attic may require full-facepiece, powered air-purifying respirators.[31]

Cryptococcus is another genus of potentially pathogenic fungi found in soil. Like *Histoplasma,* high concentrations of *Cryptococcus* spores can be found in soil enriched by bird droppings. *Cryptococcus neoformans* is found worldwide and can cause significant infections, including meningitis, in immunocompromised individuals. However, *C. neoformans* has not been extensively associated with occupational or environmental exposures. In contrast, *Cryptococcus gatii* infection (a species formerly thought to be confined to the tropics) has been tied to environmental and occupational exposures to disturbed contaminated soil in both human beings and domestic animals (including cats, a ferret, and a llama) in North America. In these recent outbreaks, human *C. gatii* infection has involved both chronic pulmonary manifestations as well as meningitis.[32]

Another fungus associated with environmental exposures is *Blastomyces,* which can cause chronic lung disease in human beings and other animals as well as extrapulmonary manifestations. The typical human case of blastomycosis related to occupational or environmental exposure is a male who works or recreates outdoors where there is wildlife activity. A history of a pet dog with the disease helps support the diagnosis because dogs appear to act as sentinels for environmental exposure risk.[33]

ARTHROPOD EXPOSURES

Animal workers may be exposed to ticks, mites, and other arthropods that may be attached to animals or in the vicinity. Such exposures can lead to transmission of zoonotic pathogens as well as bites and allergic reactions. Grain mites are a cause of allergy among agricultural workers.

Chemical Hazards

Exposure to chemical hazards can occur in workers with animal contact, especially among laboratory animal research staff and veterinary workers. Anesthetic gases are a significant risk to veterinary personnel and are discussed below. Other chemicals include immobilizing agents, disinfectants, animal-related pesticides (see Chapter 8), rodenticides, and protocol-specific chemicals in animal research.[34] These chemicals can cause a wide range of health effects from skin and mucous membrane irritation to neurological effects and adverse pregnancy outcomes (e.g., miscarriage from anesthetic exposures).[35] A Materials Safety Data Sheet (MSDS) on the hazards, safe handling, and exposure management of specific chemicals should be available to all animal workers encountering chemicals in the workplace. Depending on the particular exposure, specific types of decontamination and acute medical care may be needed. In addition, inspection of the workplace should be considered in coordination with the industrial hygienist and other safety personnel.

Farm workers, especially those working in animal confinement facilities with large numbers of animals such as swine, may be exposed to pesticides as well as high levels of ammonia and hydrogen sulfide levels related to animal waste. These irritating chemical fumes can cause toxic chemical pneumonitis and bronchitis.[10] Hydrogen sulfide, produced by decaying organic waste, is a mitochondrial toxin that can cause acute loss of consciousness, respiratory arrest, and death.[36]

Cattle silage can be a source of nitrogen dioxide toxicity causing "silo filler's disease," an acute syndrome characterized by pulmonary edema, respiratory distress, and death in sufficiently high exposures.[37]

Physical Hazards

Common physical hazards faced by animal workers include bites and crush injuries from animals; acute and chronic musculoskeletal strain from handling animals and equipment; slip, trip, and fall injuries; and, in certain settings, exposure to noise, extremes of temperature, and radiation.[38]

Psychosocial Stressors

Although there are many psychosocial benefits of human-animal interaction (see Chapter 5), animal workers may face particular psychosocial stressors. These can include fear of attack and injury; fear of infectious disease; emotional reactions to performing euthanasia, necropsies, slaughtering, or other procedures; compassion fatigue[39]; and professional burnout.[40]

HAZARD CONTROLS

Once workplace hazards are identified, the goal is to reduce exposures to these hazards. Taking an occupational health approach to such hazards involves using a hierarchy of controls that range from most effective to least effective methods to reduce the health risks to workers. This hierarchy is listed in Table 12-2. Many hazards can be eliminated at the source, or a less-dangerous substance or process can be substituted. Engineering controls include physical methods to reduce exposures such as improved ventilation and use of nonporous surfaces on counters that can be easily disinfected. Administrative and work practice controls involve job restrictions for susceptible persons, limiting individual worker exposure times in high-exposure areas, and preventive practices such as hand hygiene. Reliance on personal protective equipment such as gloves, gowns, and respirators is considered to be the least effective and often most cumbersome approach to hazard control.

Table 12-1 shows examples of such controls for handling biological, chemical, physical, and psychosocial hazards in animal work. Obviously the most effective controls vary by the specific type of hazard, and the occupational health team must consider the most feasible type of control for each particular hazard. Although they may require a greater upfront investment, controls at the top of the hierarchy, such as elimination, substitution, or engineering controls, may be most cost effective at preventing work-related health problems. For example, eliminating a zoonotic disease (such as brucellosis) in an animal population through vaccination and other preventive veterinary care may be more cost effective over time than relying on personal protective equipment such as respirators and gloves for animal workers. Similarly, substituting a less-toxic cleaning agent (see Chapter 8) may be more cost effective in reducing health complaints of eye and throat irritation among exposed workers than the use of gloves and respirators.

OCCUPATIONAL MEDICINE SERVICES

Because not all health hazards in the workplace can be eliminated or completely controlled by the methods listed above, animal workers may require occupational medicine services to prevent and treat work-related illnesses and injuries. Such services may involve both human health care providers and other members of the occupational health team.

Preplacement Screening

Preplacement examination (or post–job offer evaluation) is a medical evaluation conducted to determine if a newly hired worker is able to safely perform the essential functions of the job with or without accommodation. Such examinations can present an ideal opportunity for preventive risk assessment and counseling as well as prophylactic vaccination. However, for many animal workers such examinations are not required by law and may not be provided because an employer believes they are not necessary. Even when animal workers do have such clearance examinations, the service may be provided by a personal physician or other health care provider who is not familiar with the health risks of animal work. As a result, there may be many missed opportunities for prevention.

The content of the preplacement examination can vary depending on the particular job type and set of exposure risks but often involves a screening medical history, physical examination, and diagnostic testing, if indicated, to identify important preexisting conditions that might place an individual at increased risk of injury or illness, including immunocompromising conditions[41] or history of allergy. A history of previous animal contacts and whether animals are kept in the home may provide useful information. The use of standardized history and physical forms may assist in this process. Figure 12-2 shows an example of an animal worker questionnaire that might be appropriate for a worker in an animal care facility or a veterinary practice.

If workers will be using respiratory protection involving N-95 respirators or other types of respirators, they should complete the Occupational Safety and Health Administration (OSHA) respirator questionnaire as part of the respirator medical clearance required under the OSHA Respirator Standard 1910.134 (available at http://www.osha.gov/pls/oshaweb/owadisp.show_document?p_table=STANDARDS&p_id=9783). If latex is used in the workplace, workers should be asked about any previous reactions to latex, including rash, hives, nasal or eye inflammation, breathing difficulties, or anaphylaxis.

TABLE 12-2 ▪ Hierarchy of Controls for Workplace Hazards	
Control Strategy	**Effectiveness**
1. Eliminate the hazard	Most effective
2. Substitute for the hazard	
3. Engineering controls	
4. Administrative/work practice controls	
5. Use of personal protective equipment (e.g., gloves, masks)	Least effective

Confidential Risk Assessment and Medical Questionnaire for Animal Workers

Name: _____ Gender: ☐Male ☐Female Date of Birth: _____

Occupational exposure to animals and animal tissue:

Please state whether you work with live animals or animal tissue and which species you work with.

☐ Amphibian ☐ Bird ☐ Cat ☐ Cattle ☐ Dog ☐ Ferret ☐Fish ☐Goat ☐Horse ☐ Insect

☐ Nonhuman primate ☐ Pig ☐ Rabbit ☐ Reptile ☐ Rodent ☐ Sheep ☐Wildlife species (please list): _____

_____ ☐ Other (please specify): _____

☐ No animal or animal tissue contact

Other hazardous exposures:

☐ Human blood/tissue ☐ Chemicals (please list): _____

☐ Dust ☐Noise ☐ Radiation ☐ Heavy lifting ☐Other (please specify): _____

Personal protective equipment worn:

☐ Mask/respirator (type): _____ ☐Gloves ☐Other (please specify): _____

Pets, other nonoccupational animal exposures:

Please state whether outside of work you have contact with any of the following:

☐ Bird ☐Cat ☐Dog ☐ Ferret ☐Fish ☐ Horse ☐ Rabbit ☐ Reptile ☐ Rodent ☐Other (please list): _____

_____

Medical conditions:

Please list known allergies to medications, animals, or other environmental allergens: _____

_____

Please list whether you have any of the following:

☐ Asthma ☐Rhinitis ☐ Eczema ☐Other skin disease ☐ Diabetes ☐Cancer ☐Recurrent infections ☐Other medical conditions that could compromise immune system ☐Heart murmur ☐Hepatitis ☐Back problems ☐Other musculoskeletal problems ☐ Depression or anxiety

Please list current medications (prescription, over-the-counter, and supplements): _____

_____

Symptoms:

Please check if you have any of the following symptoms:

☐ Cough ☐Shortness of breath ☐Wheezing ☐Runny/itchy eyes ☐Runny/itchy/congested nose/sneezing ☐Skin rash

☐ Musculoskeletal pain ☐ Persistent diarrhea ☐Weight loss ☐Unexplained fevers ☐Depression or anxiety ☐Other

(please list): _____

Do you feel any of your symptoms are related to work? ☐Yes ☐No

Immunizations/tuberculosis testing:

Please state your most recent immunizations and tuberculosis (TB) test and date:

Immunization	Date
Tetanus	
Rabies	
Influenza	
Hepatitis B	
TB testing	

Figure 12-2 ▪ Sample medical questionnaire for animal workers.

In addition to the history and physical, other baseline testing may be indicated. Audiometry at baseline is required by OSHA if the worker will be exposed to noise at levels of 85 A-weighted decibels (dBA) or higher for an 8-hour time-weighted average. Testing of lung function (spirometry) is recommended for individuals with potential exposure to respiratory allergens, including veterinary workers and workers in animal facilities. Allergy testing is not usually performed routinely at baseline but may be warranted if the history suggests sensitization to particular allergens found in the work setting. In certain settings baseline serology or serum banking may be indicated to detect immunologic response to zoonotic pathogens.

Based on the findings of the preplacement examination, the medical provider can perform a risk assessment for the individual and decide whether the individual can safely do the job with or without accommodation. To do this, the medical provider may need to consult a veterinarian, biosafety professional, or other members of the occupational health team to learn more about specific risks of the job. For example, a person with valvular heart disease may need to be restricted from working in a research facility with pregnant sheep because of the risk of Q fever. A worker who developed allergy to mice or rats in a previous job may need to be restricted from future contact with such animals. In discussing disease risks with other professionals, it is important (although sometimes a challenge) to keep medical information about the worker confidential and prevent possible workplace discrimination because of a medical condition. If work restrictions are necessary, they can be indicated on a work status form that can be given to the employer to outline such restrictions without revealing confidential health information about the employee. In general, confidential health information on employees should not be shared with the employer, supervisor, or other management personnel by the human health clinician evaluating the worker.[42]

Vaccinations

A number of preventive vaccinations may be indicated for animal workers. Previous vaccination history should be assessed at the preplacement evaluation and the need for additional vaccination determined. As with other aspects of the preplacement risk assessment, consultation with a veterinarian may be advisable or clear instructions conveyed to the health care provider regarding necessary vaccinations. All animal workers should be up to date with respect to tetanus vaccination. Table 12-3 lists vaccines to consider for particular groups of workers. Rabies vaccination is indicated for a number of workers.[43] Table 12-4 shows recent recommendations for which individuals should receive preexposure rabies vaccine.

Training

Training at the time of job entry is recommended by the National Association of Public Health Veterinarians (NAPHV) for workers in veterinary facilities[41] and is relevant for other animal workers as well. Aspects of such training include education about zoonotic disease risks, infection control practices, use of personal protective equipment, safe chemical handling techniques, and injury prevention, with emphasis on proper animal handling, restraints, and recognition of behavioral cues in animals. Such training should be provided by an individual familiar with the risks of a particular workplace and the safety policies in place, such as a safety officer. Training should be documented. Follow-up training in health and safety can take place on a regular basis with animal workers to identify and mitigate hazards, address institutional occupational health policies (including record keeping), address personal hygiene, provide points of contact for more information or for when to seek medical

attention for work-related problems, review unit inspection standards, and evaluate future training needs.

Medical Surveillance

Depending on the degree of occupational risk, animal workers should receive periodic evaluations to detect evidence of work-related disease, reassess risk factors for occupational illness and injury, and ensure that vaccinations are current. Table 12-1 suggests medical surveillance that may be appropriate for different types of animal workers.

Questionnaires should ask about new health problems that have developed since the last examination, including symptoms of allergy or infection that could indicate increased risk of disease or the occurrence of work-related disease or injury. A key aspect of such history is whether the symptoms show a temporal relation with work exposures. Box 12-2 shows characteristic symptom patterns suggesting work-related occupational asthma. Similar temporal relations may occur with other occupational diseases.

Based on the results of screening questions, further testing may be indicated, such as serial peak flow diaries, spirometry, and methacholine testing of lung function in a worker reporting shortness of breath. Another example of periodic medical surveillance testing is annual audiometry, which is required by OSHA for workers exposed to noise and enrolled in hearing conservation programs.

Management of Acute Injuries, Exposures, and Illnesses

When an animal worker seeks medical attention for an acute illness or injury that may be work related, the health care provider should be familiar with the worker's occupational hazards. As previously stated, many medical providers in emergency departments or clinics may not be aware of the zoonotic or other disease risks faced by animal workers. It may therefore be advisable for workers with acute work-related injuries or illnesses to carry a card listing relevant zoonotic disease exposures and other work hazards and be able to show the card to the health care provider. An example of such a card is shown in Figure 12-3. This type of card should be customized to the specific work setting.

If an animal worker has an acute exposure, illness, or injury the work supervisor should document and report the incident. This documentation should include the date, time, location; persons injured or exposed; other persons present; description of the incident; the species, breed, and health status (vaccination history, clinical signs, diagnostic testing) of any involved animals; contact with public health and health care providers; and follow-up plans.[41] If possible, pertinent documentation of the incident should be made available to the treating medical provider. Because work-related injuries and illnesses must be reported on the employer's OSHA 300 Log, attending clinicians will need to provide a medical opinion and rationale on the work-relatedness of the injury, illness, or exposure.[44]

A key part of the evaluation of any work-related illness or injury is determining whether it represents a sentinel health event indicating a problem with existing hazard controls and potentially representing an index case in terms of other workers and possibly animals being at risk. This may require

TABLE 12-3 ▪ Occupational Medicine Services for Animal Workers

Category of Medical Service	Specific Medical Services Indicated	Types of Animal Workers Requiring Occupational Medicine Services
Preplacement screening	Questionnaire regarding immune compromise, musculoskeletal problems, pets and other animal contacts Physical examination	All
	Respirator clearance questionnaire, spirometry	Workers exposed to respiratory hazards, workers who will be using respirators
	Audiometry	Noise-exposed workers
	HIV and TB screening	Animal research and workers in contact with nonhuman primates
	Consider serum banking	Zoological, wildlife, or research workers; others with zoonotic exposures
Vaccination	Rabies	See Table 12-4
	Tetanus (every 10 years)	All
	Annual influenza vaccine	All (especially poultry and swine workers)
	Anthrax	Laboratory workers routinely working with concentrations of anthrax or aerosol potential[87]
	Q fever (consider)*	Laboratory workers, researchers working with pregnant sheep, slaughterhouse workers[70]
	Hepatitis A and B, measles, polio	Workers in contact with chimpanzees and other nonhuman primates
Training	Veterinary standard precautions, anesthetic safety, bite and injury prevention, OSHA training, safe chemical handling	All
Medical surveillance	Periodic questionnaire about allergy/respiratory symptoms	NIOSH recommendations in all animal workers with allergen exposures
	Reassess zoonotic disease risk	All animal workers with change in medical status
	OSHA respirator questionnaire; spirometry; further evaluation in positive responses to questionnaire	Workers using respirators
	TB testing (skin test or interferon assay)	Animal workers with nonhuman primate and/or elephant contact (see Figure 12-2)
	Annual audiometry	Workers with noise exposures ≥85 dBA (8-hour average)
Acute injury and illness management	Treat acute problem, determine if work related, identify sentinel health events indicating problem with hazard control and risk to other workers and/or patients Consider whether human being with a zoonotic disease is a sentinel for animal health problem as well as indicator of occupational risk to other workers Determine source of infectious exposure and consider prophylactic treatment for exposure (e.g., rat-bite fever, leptospirosis)	All
	Herpes B exposure prophylactic treatment[65]	Workers with exposure to nonhuman primates
Confidential medical record management	Protect confidentiality of medical records	All

*Not commercially available in the United States. Persons wishing to be vaccinated should first have a skin test to determine a history of previous exposure. Individuals who have previously been exposed to *C. burnetii* should not receive the vaccine because severe reactions, localized to the area of the injected vaccine, may occur.
HIV, Human immunodeficiency virus; *TB,* tuberculosis; *OSHA,* Occupational Safety and Health Administration; *dBA,* decibels (acoustic).

communication between the health care provider and the veterinarian and/or other members of the occupational health team (see Figure 12-1).

After an episode of acute injury or illness, or because of results of a periodic surveillance evaluation, the employee may not be able to resume full duties immediately. In this case the medical provider should specify the necessary job restrictions that would allow the worker to safely return to work and how long those restrictions are expected to be required. Again, making appropriate recommendations may require a team approach involving the veterinarian and other professionals. As with preplacement evaluations, it is

TABLE 12-4 ▪ Rabies Preexposure Prophylaxis Guide

Risk Category	Nature of Risk	Typical Population	Preexposure Recommendations
Continuous	Virus present continuously, often in high concentrations; specific exposures likely to go unrecognized; bite, nonbite, or aerosol exposure	Rabies research laboratory workers; rabies biologics production workers	Primary course*; serologic testing every 6 months; booster vaccination if antibody titer is below acceptable level
Frequent	Exposure usually episodic and with source recognized, but exposure also may be unrecognized; bite, nonbite, or aerosol exposure	Rabies diagnostic lab workers, spelunkers, veterinarians and staff, animal control and wildlife workers in rabies-endemic areas; all persons who frequently handle bats	Primary course; serologic testing every 2 years; booster vaccination if antibody titer is below acceptable level
Infrequent	Exposure nearly always episodic with source recognized; bite or nonbite exposure	Veterinarians and terrestrial animal control workers in areas where rabies is uncommon to rare; veterinary students; travelers visiting areas where rabies is enzootic and immediate access to appropriate medical care, including biologics, is limited	Primary course; no serologic testing or booster vaccination
Rare (population at large)	Exposure always episodic with source recognized; bite or nonbite exposure	U.S. population at large, including persons in rabies-epizootic areas	No vaccination necessary

From Manning SE et al, Centers for Disease Control and Prevention: Human rabies prevention–United States, 2008: recommendations of the Advisory Committee on Immunization Practices, *MMWR Recomm Rep* 57(RR-3):1-28, 2008.
*Primary vaccination: three 1.0-mL injections of HDCV or PCEC vaccine should be administered intramuscularly (deltoid area)–one injection per day on days 0, 7, and 21 or 28.

BOX 12-2 ▪ *PATTERN OF SYMPTOMS OF WORK-RELATED ASTHMA*

- Symptoms of asthma develop after a worker starts a new job or after new materials are introduced on a job (a substantial period of time may elapse between initial exposure and development of symptoms).
- Symptoms develop within minutes of specific activities or exposures at work.
- Delayed symptoms occur several hours after exposure, during the evenings of workdays.
- Symptoms occur less frequently or not at all on days away from work and on vacations.
- Symptoms occur more frequently on returning to work.

From National Institute for Occupational Safety and Health (NIOSH): *NIOSH alert: preventing asthma in animal handlers, DHHS (NIOSH) Publication No. 97-116.* http://www.cdc.gov/Niosh/animalrt.html.

Name: _____
Job title: _____
Name and telephone number of supervisor: _____
In case of an emergency, please be aware that the holder of this card, by virtue of work involving animals, is exposed to certain zoonotic diseases. These include rabies, Q fever, leptospirosis, toxoplasmosis, tularemia, psittacosis, cat-scratch fever, rat-bite fever, *Pasteurella multocida, Capnocytophaga canimorsus,* viral encephalitis, Rocky Mountain spotted fever, and herpes B. When possible, review the specific animal exposure of this worker. Consult with local infectious disease specialists, public health authorities, and other resources for appropriate management.

Figure 12-3 ▪ Example of hazard card for animal workers seeking medical care for acute illness or exposure (to be customized to particular work setting).

important that the worker's privacy and the confidentiality of medical information be respected during this process.

Management of Confidential Medical Records and Information

Medical evaluations of workers must uphold standards of privacy and confidentiality in the provision of care and in record keeping. In agreement with the Health Information Portability and Accountability Act (HIPAA), the American College of Occupational and Environmental Medicine has published a position paper in support of confidentiality of medical information in the workplace.[45] Results of baseline and periodic questionnaires and physical examinations (including, but not limited to, information about immuno-compromised conditions) represent medical information that should be treated with the same confidentiality as information in a hospital and not shared with the employer. Such information should be kept in a secure chart in a medical office and not placed in an employee's personnel file in the workplace.

Table 12-3 summarizes occupational medical services for different groups of animal workers.

OCCUPATIONAL HEALTH IN SPECIFIC SETTINGS

Veterinary Personnel

As a group, veterinarians and their staff are at increased risk for work-related injuries and illnesses. A study of 10,000 veterinary practices in Europe found that the rate of work accidents and occupational disease was almost three times as great as that of general medical practitioners and their staff, and the rate of severe accidents resulting in lost work time was nine times greater. The most common occupational diseases reported were skin disorders (39%), followed by allergic respiratory diseases (31%) and infectious diseases (19%).[46] In the United States federal law requires veterinary practices to implement a workplace plan to comply with OSHA Hazard Communication Standards (http://www.avma.org/ issues/policy/workplace_hazards.asp). It also appears that veterinarians may be held liable for harm if their employees develop a work-related illness such as a zoonotic infection.[47] It is not clear how many workers in veterinary practices receive occupational medicine services from human health care providers or have access to members of the occupational health team, such as industrial hygienists or infection control specialists. Many veterinary offices are located in rural or other areas where shortages of occupational medicine providers exist.[48] The practice director, who is often a veterinarian, or another staff member may have to perform a number of functions such as identifying hazards and designing control strategies. The National Association of State Public Health Veterinarians (NASPHV) has published a compendium of veterinary standard precautions that provides useful practice guidelines as well as a model infection control plan (Figure 12-4).[41] The veterinarian may need to educate local medical providers to ensure adequate and confidential preplacement screening, medical surveillance, and acute injury/ illness follow-up of veterinary care workers. Having a designated medical provider as well as a designated emergency medical care facility that is aware of the special exposures of the veterinary workers can help ensure improved preventive and acute care of exposure-related health problems.

Allergens

A survey of California veterinarians found that 40% reported animal-related allergic symptoms, especially to cats and dogs.[49] Allergens identified as hazards in veterinary practice include animal hair and dander, feathers, latex, mites, organic dust, and amniotic fluid. Fortunately, a study of skin allergy in veterinarians found that most sensitized individuals were allergic to only one species of animal.[50]

Hypersensitivity pneumonitis has been reported in veterinarians from exposure to antigens in animal feeds.[46]

Latex allergy is also a risk among veterinary personnel who use latex gloves and other latex equipment.

Measures to control these hazards in veterinary practices include frequent cleaning of facilities and adequate ventilation. Personal protective devices such as gloves and respirators can reduce allergen exposure. Box 12-3 shows the recommendations for animal handler allergen control published by NIOSH that target veterinary and research animal workers.

However, even with these measures, sensitized individuals may have difficulty working around animals to which they are allergic. Job modification may be necessary; there may be areas of the building with a lower allergy load that a sensitized individual could tolerate. Allergy desensitization should be considered as part of the management of some allergic conditions.

Zoonoses

Many different zoonotic infections, including fatal cases, have been reported in veterinarians.[41] In a European study of work-related claims by veterinary workers, the most frequent infections were ringworm, brucellosis, Lyme disease, and psittacosis.[46] A survey of American veterinarians found that the occupational infections of current greatest concern to small-animal veterinarians were ringworm, gastrointestinal bacteria, gastrointestinal parasites, leptospirosis, rabies, toxoplasmosis, and unknown or emerging pathogens. Large-animal veterinarians were concerned about ringworm, gastrointestinal bacteria, leptospirosis, brucellosis, gastrointestinal parasites, and rabies. Despite these concerns, most veterinarians responding to the survey reported low rates of personal protective equipment use and other protective behaviors currently recommended to protect against zoonotic disease transmission.[51]

Veterinarians and their staff have been identified as a group at increased risk for many other zoonotic infections, including Q fever, salmonellosis, methicillin-resistant *Staphylococcus aureus,* avian influenza,[51] cat-associated plague, animal bite infections including pasteurellosis, other bacterial infections, and cat-associated sporotrichosis (see Chapter 10).

The NASPHV *Veterinary Standard Precautions for Zoonotic Disease Prevention in Veterinary Personnel* includes a model infection control plan for veterinary offices.[41] Figure 12-4 shows this model plan.

This NASPHV document recommends engineering controls such as single-purpose isolation rooms for sick animals; separate rooms for patient care and employee breaks; designated sharps containers; the use of nonporous, easily cleaned surface materials in areas where animals are housed, examined, or treated; and sealing up of rodent entry portals. Recommended work practice controls include training new employees in practices such as hand hygiene before and after each patient encounter and after contact with body fluids, secretions, or excretions as well as after eating, drinking, smoking, using lavatories, and cleaning animal areas. Additional work practices include bite prevention and avoidance of needlesticks by not recapping needles. Bite prevention could include physical or chemical restraints, muzzles, and bite-resistant gloves. Personal protective equipment recommendations include gloves or sleeves and facial protection with a mask or goggles when splashes or sprays are expected. An N-95 respirator should be worn when evaluating abortions in small ruminants, poultry deaths, sick psittacine birds, and other situations with the risk of aerosolized pathogens.[41] The NASPHV document also recommends that immunocompromised individuals and pregnant workers be counseled about their increased risk of zoonotic disease, especially when working with high-risk animals such as young animals and animals that are parturient, unvaccinated, stray or feral, housed in shelters or crowded conditions, fed raw meat diets, or with parasites; wildlife; reptiles and amphibians; and exotic or nonnative species.[41] Such counseling should ideally be done by a health care professional who is aware of the zoonotic disease risks faced by the worker. For this reason the NASPHV document recommends that all workers inform their health care providers

National Association of State Public Health Veterinarians (NASPHV)

Veterinary Infection Control Committee (VICC)

This plan should be adapted to your practice in keeping with local, state, and federal regulations. A modifiable electronic version is available on the NASPHV Web site (www.nasphv.org). Please refer to the full compendium of veterinary standard precautions for complete information and guidance (also available at www.nasphv.org).

Clinic: _____

Date of plan adoption: _____

Date of next review: _____

Infection control officer: _____

This plan will be followed as part of our practice's routine procedures. The plan will be reviewed at least annually and as part of new employee training.

PERSONAL PROTECTIVE ACTIONS AND EQUIPMENT

Hand hygiene: Wash hands before and after each patient encounter and after contact with feces, blood, body fluids, secretions, excretions, exudates, or articles contaminated by these substances. Wash hands before eating, drinking, or smoking; after using the toilet; after cleaning animal cages or animal-care areas; and whenever hands are visibly soiled. Alcohol-based rubs may be used if hands are not visibly soiled, but handwashing with soap and running water is preferred. Keep fingernails short. Do not wear artificial nails or hand jewelry when handling animals. Keep handwashing supplies stocked at all times.

Staff responsible: _____

Correct handwashing procedure:

- Wet hands with running water
- Place soap in palms
- Rub hands together to make a lather
- Scrub hands vigorously for 20 seconds
- Rinse soap off hands
- Dry hands with disposable towel
- Turn off faucet using the disposable towel as a barrier

Use of gloves and sleeves: Gloves are not necessary when examining or handling normal, healthy animals. Wear gloves or sleeves when touching feces, blood, body fluids, secretions, excretions, exudates, and nonintact skin. Wear gloves for dentistry, resuscitations, necropsies, and obstetric procedures; when cleaning cages, litter boxes, and contaminated environmental surfaces and equipment; when handling dirty laundry; when handling diagnostic specimens (e.g., urine, feces, aspirates, swabs); and when handling an animal with a suspected infectious disease. Change gloves between examination of individual animals or animal groups (e.g., a litter of puppies) and between dirty and clean procedures performed on the same patient. Gloves should be removed promptly and disposed of after use. Disposable gloves should not be washed and reused. Hands should be washed immediately after glove removal.

Facial protection: Wear facial protection whenever exposure to splashes or sprays is likely to occur. Facial protection includes a face shield or a surgical mask worn with goggles. Wear facial protection for the following procedures: lancing abscesses, flushing wounds, dentistry, nebulization, suctioning, lavage, obstetric procedures, and necropsies.

Protective outerwear: Wear a protective outer garment such as a lab coat, smock, nonsterile gown, or coveralls when attending animals and when conducting cleaning chores. These should be changed whenever soiled, after handling an animal with a known or suspected infectious disease, after working in an isolation room, and after performing a necropsy or other high-risk procedure. Shoes or boots should have thick soles and closed toes and be impermeable to water and easily cleaned. Disposable shoe covers should be worn when heavy quantities of infectious materials are present or expected. Impermeable outerwear should be worn during obstetric procedures and necropsies and whenever substantial splashes or large quantities of body fluids may be encountered. Keep clean outer garments available at all times.

Staff responsible: _____

Figure 12-4   ▪   NASPHV model infection control plan for veterinary practices, 2008. (Adapted from National Association of State Public Health Veterinarians: *NASPHV compendia.* http://www.nasphv.org/documents-Compendia.html.

Bite and other animal-related injury prevention: Take precautions to prevent bites and other injuries. Identify aggressive animals and alert clinic staff. Use physical restraints, muzzles, bite-resistant gloves, and sedation or anesthesia in accordance with practice policies. Plan an escape route when handling large animals. Do not rely on owners or untrained staff for animal restraint.

- If there is concern for personal safety, notify: _____
- When injuries occur, wash wounds with soap and water, then immediately report incident
  to: _____ (infection control officer)
- If medical attention is needed contact: _____ (health care provider)
- Bite incidents will be reported to: _____ (public health agency)
  as required by law. Telephone number: _____

PROTECTIVE ACTIONS DURING VETERINARY PROCEDURES

Intake: Avoid bringing aggressive or potentially infectious animals through the reception area. If they must come through the main entrance, carry the animal or place it on a gurney so that it can be taken directly to a designated examination room.

Examination of animals: Wear appropriate protective outerwear and wash hands before and after examination of individual animals or animal groups (e.g., a litter of puppies). Potentially infectious animals will be examined in a designated examination room and remain there until diagnostic procedures and treatments have been performed.

Injections, venipuncture, and aspiration procedures: Wear gloves while performing venipuncture on animals suspected of having an infectious disease and when performing soft tissue aspirations.

Needlestick injury prevention: Do not recap needles except in rare instances when required as part of a medical procedure or protocol. Do not remove an uncapped needle from the syringe by hand or place a needle cap in the mouth. Dispose of all sharps in designated containers. After injection of live-organism vaccines or aspiration of body fluids, dispose of used syringes with attached needles in a sharps container. Otherwise, remove the needle with forceps or the needle removal device on the sharps container, and throw the syringe away in the trash. Do not transfer sharps from one container to another. Replace sharps containers before they are completely full.

Staff responsible: _____

Dental procedures: Wear protective outerwear, gloves, and facial protection when performing dental procedures or when in range of splashes or sprays (such as when monitoring anesthesia).

Resuscitation: Wear gloves and facial protection.

Obstetrics: Wear gloves or shoulder-length sleeves, facial protection, and impermeable outerwear.

Necropsy: Wear cut-resistant gloves, facial protection, and impermeable outerwear. Only necessary personnel are allowed in the vicinity of the procedure. Wear a respirator when using a band saw or other power equipment. If an animal is suspected of having a notifiable infectious or foreign animal disease, consult the state veterinarian before proceeding with a necropsy. Contact information for state veterinarian's office: _____

Diagnostic specimen handling: Wear protective outerwear and gloves. Discard gloves and wash hands before touching clean items (e.g., medical records, telephone). Eating and drinking are not allowed in the laboratory.

ENVIRONMENTAL INFECTION CONTROL

Isolation of infectious animals: Animals with a contagious or zoonotic disease will be housed in isolation as soon as possible. Clearly mark the room or cage to indicate the patient's status and describe additional precautions. Keep only the equipment needed for the care and treatment of the patient in the isolation room, including dedicated cleaning supplies. Disassemble and thoroughly clean and disinfect any equipment that must be taken out of the room. Discard gloves after use. Leave other personal protective equipment (e.g., gown, mask) in the isolation room for reuse. Clean and disinfect or discard protective equipment between patients and whenever contaminated by body fluids. Place potentially contaminated materials in a bag before removal from the isolation room. Use a disinfectant footbath before entering and leaving the room. Limit access to the isolation room. Keep a sign-in log of all people (including owners and other nonemployees) having contact with an animal in isolation. Monitor air pressure daily while the room is in use.

Staff responsible: _____

Figure 12-4—cont'd.

Cleaning and disinfection of equipment and environmental surfaces: First, clean surfaces and equipment to remove organic matter, then use a disinfectant according to the manufacturer's instructions. Minimize dust and aerosols when cleaning by first misting the area with water or disinfectant. Clean and disinfect animal cages, toys, and food and water bowls between uses and whenever visibly soiled. Clean litter boxes once a day. Wear gloves when cleaning and wash hands afterwards. There is a written checklist for each area of the facility (e.g., waiting room, examination rooms, treatment area, kennels) that specifies the frequency of cleaning, disinfection procedures, products to be used, and staff responsible.

Handling laundry: Wear gloves when handling soiled laundry. Wash animal bedding and other laundry with standard laundry detergent and machine dry. Use separate storage and transport bins for clean and dirty laundry.

Decontamination and spill response: Immediately spray a spill or splash of blood, feces, or other potentially infectious substance with disinfectant and contain it with absorbent material (e.g., paper towels, sawdust, cat litter). Put on gloves, mask, and protective clothing (including shoe covers if the spill is large and may be stepped in) before beginning the clean-up. Pick up the material, seal it in a leak-proof plastic bag, and clean and disinfect the area. Keep clients, patients, and employees away from the spill area until disinfection is completed.

Veterinary medical waste: *Insert here your local and state ordinances regulating disposal of animal waste, pathology waste, animal carcasses, bedding, sharps, and biologics. Refer to the US Environmental Protection Agency Web site for guidance:* www.epa.gov/osw/nonhaz/industrial/medical/index.htm.

Rodent and vector control: Seal entry portals and eliminate clutter and sources of standing water; keep animal food in closed metal or thick plastic, covered containers; and dispose of food waste properly to keep the facility free of wild rodents, mosquitoes, and other arthropods.

Other environmental controls: There are designated areas for eating, drinking, smoking, application of cosmetics, and similar activities. These activities should never occur in animal-care areas or in the laboratory area. Do not keep food or drink for human consumption in the same refrigerator as food for animals, biologics, or laboratory specimens. Dishes for human use should be cleaned and stored away from animal-care and animal food-preparation areas.

EMPLOYEE HEALTH

Infection control and employee health management: The following personnel are responsible for development and maintenance of the practice's infection control policies, record keeping, and management of workplace exposure and injury incidents.

Staff responsible: _____

Record keeping: Current emergency contact information will be maintained for each employee. Records will be maintained on vaccinations, rabies virus antibody titers, and exposure and injury incidents. Report and record changes in health status (e.g., pregnancy) that may affect work duties.

Preexposure rabies vaccination: All staff with animal contact must be vaccinated against rabies, followed by periodic titer checks and rabies vaccine boosters, in accordance with the recommendations of the Centers for Disease Control and Prevention (CDC) Advisory Committee on Immunization Practices.

Tetanus vaccination: Tetanus immunizations must be up to date. Report and record puncture wounds and other incidents. Consult a health care provider regarding the need for a tetanus booster.

Seasonal influenza vaccination: Unless contraindicated, veterinary personnel are encouraged to receive the current seasonal influenza vaccine. Refer to the CDC Web site for guidance (www.cdc.gov).

Staff training and education: Infection control training and education will be documented in the employee health record.

Documenting and reporting exposure incidents: Report incidents that result in injury or potential exposure to an infectious agent to _____ . The following information will be collected for each exposure incident: date, time, location, person(s) injured or exposed, other persons present, description of the incident, whether a health care provider was consulted, the status of any animals involved (e.g., vaccination history, clinical condition, diagnostic information), and plans for follow-up.

Figure 12-4—cont'd.

Pregnant and immunocompromised personnel: Pregnant and immunocompromised employees are at increased risk from zoonotic diseases. Inform _____ if you are concerned about your work responsibilities so that accommodations may be made. Consultation between the supervising veterinarian and a health care provider may be needed.

The following information is attached to the Infection Control Plan:

- Emergency services telephone numbers: fire, police, sheriff, animal control, poison control, etc.
- Reportable or notifiable veterinary diseases and where to report
- State Department of Agriculture or Board of Animal Health contact information and regulations
- State and local public health contacts for consultation on zoonotic diseases
- Public Health Laboratory services and contact information
- Environmental Protection Agency (EPA)-registered disinfectants
- Occupational Safety and Health Administration (OSHA) regulations
- Animal waste-disposal and biohazard regulations
- Rabies regulations
- Animal control and exotic animal regulations and contacts
- Other useful resources

Figure 12-4—cont'd.

BOX 12-3   *PREVENTING ASTHMA IN ANIMAL HANDLERS*

WARNING! Exposure to animals or animal products in the workplace can cause asthma and allergies. Animal handlers should take steps to protect themselves from exposure to animals and animal products.
- Perform animal manipulations within ventilated hoods or safety cabinets when possible.
- Avoid wearing street clothes while working with animals.
- Leave work clothes at the workplace to avoid potential exposure problems for family members.
- Keep cages and animal areas clean.
- Reduce skin contact with animal products such as dander, serum, and urine by using gloves, lab coats, and approved particulate respirators with face shields.
- Employers of animal handlers should take steps to protect workers from exposure to animals and animal products.
- Modify ventilation and filtration systems:
  - Increase the ventilation rate and humidity in the animal housing areas.
  - Ventilate animal housing and handling areas separately from the rest of the facility.
  - Direct airflow away from workers and toward the backs of the animal cages.
- Install ventilated animal cage racks or filter-top animal cages.
- Decrease animal density (number of animals per cubic meter of room volume).
- Keep cages and animal areas clean.
- Use absorbent pads for bedding. If these are not available, use corncob bedding instead of sawdust bedding.
- Use an animal species or sex that is known to be less allergenic than others.
- Provide protective equipment for animal handlers: gloves, lab coats, and approved particulate respirators with face shields.
- Provide training to educate workers about animal allergies and steps for risk reduction.
- Provide health monitoring and appropriate counseling and medical follow-up for workers who have become sensitized or have developed allergy symptoms.

From National Institute for Occupational Safety and Health (NIOSH): *NIOSH alert: preventing asthma in animal handlers, DHHS (NIOSH) Publication No. 97-116.* http://www.cdc.gov/Niosh/animalrt.html.

---

of their work activities, but additional direct communication between a health care provider and a veterinarian about disease risks may be advisable. However, as previously mentioned, such communication needs to respect patient privacy and confidentiality of medical information (see Chapter 2).

CHEMICAL HAZARDS

Chemical hazards in veterinary practices include disinfectant chemicals, pesticides (see Chapter 8), and anesthetic gases. These chemicals are capable of allergic, irritant, and other toxic effects. Chemical irritant effects such as irritant contact dermatitis and eye irritation have been associated with the use of chemical disinfectants.[52] Table 12-5 lists disinfectant chemicals commonly used in veterinary practices. As can be seen among the list of disadvantages, a number of these chemicals are highly irritating to skin, eyes, and mucous membranes. If a particular disinfectant chemical is causing adverse effects in workers, substitution should be considered.

Approximately 50,000 veterinary workers in the United States risk potential exposure to anesthetic agents, including nitrous oxide and halogenated agents, mostly through significant inhalation and accidental injections in veterinary operating rooms.[53,54] Many of these workers are women of childbearing age. Adverse reproductive outcomes, such as spontaneous abortion, have also been reported among workers exposed to these anesthetic agents.[54] Control of anesthetic hazards involves ensuring 100% fresh air and 100% exhausted air for dilution of waste gases and odors in animal rooms, filtering of supplied air prior to recirculation, and institution of a scavenging system for waste anesthetic gases and vapors. This scavenging system should be checked periodically to ensure it is working properly. Air levels of anesthetic gases can also be monitored periodically.[55]

PHYSICAL HAZARDS

Physical hazards in veterinary practices include bites and crush injuries from animals; lifting hazards related to equipment and patients; and slip, trip, and fall injuries. A survey of 2800 Australian veterinarians found that more than half had sustained a significant work injury.[56] Animals have been reported to be the most common cause of occupational accidental injuries, with cats and dogs causing the most accident-related injuries in small-animal practices and horses and cows causing the most injuries in large-animal practices. Large animal accidents were more likely to cause broken bones.[46] Some of the major causes of accidents involving animals are dangerous animal behaviors, such as panic, male dominance aggression, fear aggression, and maternal aggression. Control of these physical hazards includes bite prevention, proper animal handling and restraint, training animals to voluntarily cooperate with veterinary procedures,[57] and inadequate barriers or animal handling facilities to protect workers.

Repetitive trauma from carrying and handling animals and cages as well as acute trauma from lifting and carrying can result in musculoskeletal injuries such as acute and chronic low back injury, carpal tunnel syndrome, and tendonitis.

Barking dogs, other noisy animals, and noisy machinery can cause significant noise exposure to animal workers. Veterinary staff can be exposed to significant noise, especially during the cleaning of cages with power washers. Noise levels above 85 dBA over an 8-hour period require inclusion of workers in a hearing conservation program that complies with the OSHA standard on occupational noise exposure.[58] If a person has to shout to converse with another person at arm's length, the noise is likely to exceed 85 dBA.

Radiation is another physical hazard for staff in veterinary practices where radiographs are taken. Although evidence of adverse effects in veterinary staff from radiation exposure is limited, staff performing radiography should be monitored for radiation exposure.

PSYCHOSOCIAL STRESSORS

Psychosocial hazards of veterinary work include the stress of euthanizing animals, compassion fatigue, and professional burnout.[39] Increased rates of suicide have been reported for veterinarians.[59] There is little published evidence of successful interventions to reduce psychosocial stressors in veterinary practice, but strategies used in other occupational groups include job rotation and increased time off, coping skills training, support groups, and stress-reduction techniques.[60]

OCCUPATIONAL MEDICINE SERVICES FOR VETERINARY PERSONNEL

As previously described, human health care providers who care for workers in a veterinary facility may not be familiar with the particular occupational health risks faced by such workers. Such practitioners may need to be provided with information about the disease risks and the preventive services required. Table 12-3 outlines some suggested occupational services for veterinary staff, including preplacement evaluation, vaccination, and management of acute injuries and illnesses.

Preplacement Screening. Because all veterinary workers encounter the risk of allergic reactions, preplacement examination should focus on history of skin, respiratory, or other allergies and any history of asthma or other underlying respiratory conditions as well as medical conditions associated with immunocompromised status. The OSHA Respirator Medical Evaluation questionnaire previously mentioned should be part of this baseline health history for any worker who will be using respiratory protection.[61]

Along with a thorough physical examination, baseline testing can include spirometry for anyone with allergen exposures. Even nonclinical personnel such as office staff could be exposed to allergens in waiting rooms or other parts of the facility.

Baseline vaccination should include a rabies preexposure series if not previously vaccinated against rabies (see Table 12-4). All veterinary staff should have a current tetanus vaccination and be encouraged to have an annual influenza vaccination. If the veterinary practice cares for pregnant sheep and goats, baseline titers for the etiologic agent of Q fever (*Coxiella burnetii*) should be considered. Other components of the preplacement evaluation can be tailored depending on the specific type of veterinary practice and the expected hazards.

Medical Surveillance. After a baseline medical evaluation, there are few guidelines for periodic examination of veterinary personnel by a medical provider. However, NIOSH recommends that veterinary workers receive periodic monitoring for the development of allergy and asthma. Such monitoring could be accomplished with a screening questionnaire (see Figure 12-2) that could also assess any reported infectious disease symptoms or diagnoses that could be work related (such as febrile illnesses, diarrhea, and/or skin infections) as well as newly developed medical conditions that could affect risk of zoonotic disease. If workers use respirators, repeat medical evaluations may be required under the OSHA Respiratory Protection standard if a change occurs in workplace conditions. NASPHV also recommends that veterinary personnel who have a change in their health status, such as pregnancy, should discuss their work exposures with their medical providers. They should also see their medical providers periodically for follow-up rabies vaccine boosters. Workers enrolled in a hearing conservation program because of excessive noise exposures require annual audiometry.

TABLE 12-5 ■ Disinfectants Used in Veterinary Practices

	Alcohols	Aldehydes	Biguanides	Halogens: Hypochlorites	Halogens: Iodine Compounds	Oxidizing Agents	Phenols	QACs
Sample trade names	Ethyl alcohol Isopropyl alcohol	Formaldehyde Glutaraldehyde	Chlorhexidine Nolvasan Virosan	Bleach	Betadyne Providone	Hydrogen peroxide Peracetic acid Virkon S Oxy-Sept 333	One-Stroke Environ Pheno-Tek II Tek-Trol	Roccal DiQuat D-256
Mechanism of action	Precipitates proteins; denatures lipids	Denatures proteins; alkylates nucleic acids	Alters membrane permeability	Denatures proteins	Denatures proteins	Denature proteins and lipids	Denatures proteins; alters cell wall permeability	Denatures proteins; binds phospholipids of cell membrane
Advantages	Fast acting; leaves no residue	Broad spectrum	Broad spectrum	Broad spectrum; short contact time; inexpensive	Stable in storage; relatively safe	Broad spectrum	Good efficacy with organic material; noncorrosive; stable in storage	Stable in storage; nonirritating to skin; effective at high temperatures and high pH (9 to 10)
Disadvantages	Rapid evaporation, flammable	Carcinogenic mucous membrane and tissue irritation; only use in well-ventilated areas	Only functions in limited pH range (5 to 7); toxic to fish (environmental concern)	Inactivated by sunlight; requires frequent application; corrodes metals; mucous membrane and tissue irritation	Inactivated by QACs; requires frequent application; corrosive; stains clothes and treated surfaces	Damaging to some metals	Can cause skin and eye irritation	
Precautions	Flammable	Carcinogenic		Never mix with acids; toxic chlorine gas will be released			May be toxic to animals, especially cats and pigs	

Vegetative bacteria	Effective	Effective	Effective	Effective	Effective	Effective	Yes, gram-positive; limited, gram-negative
Mycobacteria	Effective	Effective	Variable	Effective	Limited	Effective	Variable
Enveloped viruses	Effective	Effective	Limited	Effective	Effective	Effective	Variable
Nonenveloped viruses	Variable	Effective	Limited	Effective	Limited	Effective	Not effective
Spores	Not effective	Effective	Not effective	Variable	Limited	Variable	Not effective
Fungi	Effective	Effective	Limited	Effective	Effective	Variable	Variable
Efficacy with organic matter	Reduced	Reduced	?	Rapidly reduced	Rapidly reduced	Variable	Inactivated
Efficacy with hard water	?	Reduced	?	Effective	?	?	Inactivated
Efficacy with soap/detergents	?	Reduced	Inactivated	Inactivated	Effective	?	Inactivated

The use of trade names does not in any way signify endorsement of a particular product.
For additional product names, please consult the most recent Compendium of Veterinary Products.
Adapted from Linton AH, Hugo WB, Russel AD: *Disinfection in veterinary and farm practice*, Oxford, UK, 1987, Blackwell Scientific; Quinn PJ, Markey BK: Disinfection and disease prevention in veterinary medicine. In Block SS, ed: *Disinfection, sterilization and preservation*, ed 5, Philadelphia, Lippincott, 2001, Williams & Wilkins.
?, Information not available. QACs, quaternary ammonium compounds.

Acute Injury, Illness, or Exposure Evaluation and Follow-up.

As with other animal workers, it is ideal that the health care provider treating veterinary workers for acute work-related injuries and illnesses be familiar with the hazards in the workplace. Medical providers providing such care should take a careful history of occupational exposures. Common acute injuries in veterinary personnel are animal bites (see Chapter 10). In such situations use of a zoonotic disease risk card (see Figure 12-3) may help guide the medical care provider to adequately consider zoonotic disease risks. Care of animal bites in veterinary workers involves a review of rabies risk from the bite and rabies vaccination status (see Chapter 9), as well as consideration of antibiotic treatment.

Any acute injury or illness in a veterinary worker can be considered a sentinel event indicating a hazard in the workplace that has not been adequately controlled. Therefore communication between the medical care provider and the veterinarian or other members of the occupational health team can help turn an acute illness or injury event into an opportunity to identify and reduce workplace hazards. In addition, the medical care provider will need to consider whether and when the worker can safely return to work and whether job modification or restriction is necessary. Again, this may require communication between the medical provider and a work supervisor or veterinarian. Individuals with suspected allergy should be evaluated and may need to be restricted from exposure to the animal to which they are sensitized (see Chapter 7). Individuals with musculoskeletal injuries may need temporary job modification while they recover. The possibility of posttraumatic stress should be considered in all employees returning to work after an acute work-related injury or illness.

Workers in Animal Research Facilities

Because many animal research facilities have affiliation with larger institutions, there is often a designated industrial hygienist and/or infection control specialist to help design and implement preventive workplace hazard controls. There is also often a designated medical care provider for the employees working in such facilities and a formal occupational health and safety program. In 1997 the Committee on Occupational Safety and Health in Research Animal Facilities, Institute of Laboratory Animal Resources, published *Occupational Health and Safety in the Care and Use of Research Animals,* which outlines guidelines for occupational health programs for research animal workers.[62]

ALLERGENS

As with veterinary workers, allergy can be a significant problem in workers in research animal facilities. Allergy to rodents is common, resulting in the spectrum of allergic rhinitis, dermatitis, and asthma. Rodent allergy may be species specific; individuals sensitized to mice may be able to work safely with rats.

Control of allergens in animal facilities can involve engineering controls including adequate fresh air ventilation, filtering of any recycled air, and airflow of ventilation to blow air to the back of cages from the aisles to reduce worker exposures (see Box 12-3).[63] Control by substitution may be feasible in some situations because male rats are more allergenic than female rats, and species such as rabbits are less allergenic than rats.[1]

ZOONOSES

Several zoonoses are of particular concern to animal facility workers who work with nonhuman primates and rodents.[64] Some can result in death. Therefore occupational exposures are considered medical emergencies. Unlike veterinary hospitals where elimination of zoonotic hazards is not possible, the control of many zoonotic diseases in animal facilities often involves control at the source through screening and eliminating disease in the animal colony. Separation of species prevents interspecies transmission, and signage helps increase awareness of risks among employees. Use of instruments and equipment with safety features such as retractable needles can help prevent bloodborne pathogen exposures.

Herpes B.

Cercopithecine herpesvirus 1 infection, herpes B, is endemic in monkeys of the genus *Macaca.* This group of Asiatic monkeys includes rhesus macaques, pigtailed macaques, and cynomolgus monkeys. Human beings who work with these monkeys can be infected by bites, scratches, needlesticks, and mucocutaneous exposure.[65] In monkeys herpes B can be subclinical or cause lesions on the oral mucosa. In human beings herpes B can result in fatal encephalomyelitis. Although rare, death has been reported in up to 80% of cases. Workers dealing with these nonhuman primates must be informed of the risk of herpes B infection and receive training in proper use of appropriate personal protective equipment, including gowns, gloves, masks, and face shields and the maintenance of a safe workplace. They should seek medical care immediately if an exposure occurs because early prophylaxis with antiviral agents has resulted in favorable outcomes.[66] The Centers for Disease Control and Prevention (CDC) has developed guidelines for assessment and medical management of monkey scratches and bites, wound contaminations, cage scratches, and other potential exposures.[67]

Simian Retroviruses.

A number of simian retroviruses, including simian immunodeficiency virus and simian foamy virus, are found in a variety of nonhuman primates. Cases of transmission of these viruses to laboratory workers with nonhuman primate exposure have been reported. Prevention is similar to that for herpes B infection.[68]

Measles.

Measles (rubeola), a paramyxovirus infection, is primarily a disease of human beings. The primary concern for laboratory animal workers is therefore reverse zoonosis (anthropozoonosis) when working with nonhuman primates because measles can cause lethal infection in these animals. Outbreaks of measles in captive nonhuman primates usually originate from an infectious human animal handler.[69] Therefore animal workers with contact with nonhuman primates must have documented measles vaccination and receive booster vaccinations if necessary.

Viral Hepatitis.   Hepatitis A, B, and C are primarily viral diseases of human beings. However, chimpanzees and other nonhuman primates have been experimentally infected.[70] Therefore there is risk of reverse zoonosis. Workers in animal facilities who have direct contact with nonhuman primates should be immunized against hepatitis A and B,[64] have baseline serology for protective hepatitis B antibodies (HbSAb), and consider having baseline serology for hepatitis C.

Tuberculosis.   Nonhuman primates are susceptible to infection with *Mycobacterium tuberculosis* (TB) and can transmit the disease to human beings by the respiratory route. Likewise, human beings infected with TB can potentially infect nonhuman primates. All animal workers with nonhuman primate contact should have skin testing for TB at baseline and annually. New employees who have not had a TB skin test in the previous 5 years should be tested with a two-step technique (retesting after 1 week if the first test is negative) to detect boosted immunity from previous infection. Alternative testing methods include an assay for interferon specific to TB (see Chapter 9).[71] Workers with positive TB tests should be evaluated medically. Such evaluation may include a chest radiograph to exclude active disease and a determination of the need for treatment with antituberculous medication.[72]

Rat-Bite Fever (Streptobacillosis).   Rat-bite fever is caused by infection with the bacterium *Actinobacillus muris* (formerly *Streptobacillus moniliformis*), usually as a result of a rat bite or contact with rat saliva or urine. The incubation period is between 3 and 10 days. Symptoms include the acute onset of fever, headache, and muscle pain, followed by the development of a maculopapular rash on the extremities over the next several days. In untreated cases complications can include endocarditis, parotitis, and abscesses.

Doxycycline or penicillin can be used as a prophylactic treatment after a rat bite. Cases of infection are treated with penicillin or tetracyclines (see Chapter 10).[70]

Lymphocytic Choriomeningitis Virus.   Lymphocytic choriomeningitis virus (LCMV) is an arenavirus infection found especially in mice but also hamsters (see Chapter 9). Infected animals shed the virus in urine, saliva, and feces. Nude mice, used in some animal research laboratories, appear to shed increased amounts of LCMV.[70] Transmission to human beings can involve contact of secretions with broken skin or oral or respiratory contact with dust or contaminated food. Handling contaminated surfaces and objects is considered a risk factor for infection.[70] Infection in human beings can range from mild flulike symptoms to severe meningoencephalitis. Diagnosis involves viral cultures and serology. Cerebrospinal fluid can show lymphocytosis and decreased glucose level. The disease is usually self-limiting in immunocompetent individuals. Immunocompromised individuals are at increased risk of severe disease, sometimes with hemorrhagic complications and fatal outcomes. There is no specific treatment. Control measures include screening of laboratory animals for infection (see Chapter 9).

Q Fever.   Laboratory animal personnel engaged in research with pregnant sheep and goats are at risk for infection with Q fever (see Chapter 9). High-risk individuals include immunocompromised individuals and persons with valvular heart disease.

Human Immunodeficiency Virus.   Another human disease with potential to be a reverse zoonosis in nonhuman primates is human immunodeficiency virus (HIV), and some research facilities using nonhuman primates have adopted policies requiring anonymous periodic HIV testing be part of the job requirement. These HIV-related policies should include outlining the steps undertaken to safeguard each individual worker's privacy.

CHEMICAL HAZARDS

Chemical exposures in laboratory animal facilities include disinfectants and anesthetics, as previously mentioned. Protocol-specific chemicals such as medications and toxins used in research can pose additional risks from a wide variety of chemicals. Eyewash stations and showers may be necessary for immediate decontamination by some agents.

Control of anesthetic gases and disinfectant chemical risks is similar to that for veterinary personnel.

PHYSICAL HAZARDS

Physical hazards for workers in animal care facilities are similar to those of veterinary workers and include ergonomic risks for musculoskeletal injury, noise, and radiation. Sources of radiation exposure may include both diagnostic and protocol-related radiation.[73]

PSYCHOSOCIAL STRESSORS

Work-related stress, anxiety, uneasiness, and depression have been reported in laboratory animal handlers. Particular psychosocial stressors include developing strong attachments to laboratory animals, having strong sentiments about "sacrificing" the animals, having friends and acquaintances who are critical of animal experimentation, and having doubts about the clinical value of animal research.[74]

OCCUPATIONAL MEDICINE SERVICES FOR ANIMAL RESEARCH FACILITY WORKERS

As previously mentioned, many animal research facilities have designated medical providers for both preventive and acute care services.

Preplacement Screening.   Preplacement evaluations are similar to those for veterinary personnel. Particular work restrictions to consider based on the preplacement evaluation include the risk of previously sensitized persons working with animal allergens, the increased risk of immunocompromised persons working with rodents possibly infected with LCMV as well as other zoonotic risks, and risks to women of childbearing age from working with pregnant sheep and goats (Q fever). Baseline testing often includes spirometry, serology to document immunity, and HIV and TB skin testing for primate workers.

Vaccination services include ensuring that primate workers are current with measles, hepatitis B, hepatitis A, and polio immunizations. If wild stock animals that could carry rabies (such as stray dogs) are used in the facility, rabies vaccine should be considered for workers exposed to such animals.[75]

Medical Surveillance.   Many research animal workers are enrolled in periodic medical surveillance on a yearly basis. Periodic screening may include a questionnaire that inquires about allergic and infectious symptoms. For primate workers, HIV and TB testing is often repeated on a regular (every 6 months or annual) basis.

Acute Injury, Exposure, and Illness Evaluation and Follow-up.   Special issues in the acute care of animal care workers include management of exposures to nonhuman primates and the need for possible herpes B prophylaxis. Workers with rodent exposures should ensure that acute febrile episodes are evaluated by medical providers for the possibility of rat-bite fever and LCMV. As with veterinary workers, all acute injuries and illnesses should be considered possible sentinel health events with implications for the health of coworkers as well as the laboratory animals.

Issues regarding job modifications and restrictions after acute injuries and illnesses are similar to those of veterinary personnel.

Zoo and Aquarium Workers

Although zoo and aquarium employees share many of the same occupational health issues as veterinary and animal research workers, there are particular challenges for occupational health programs targeting these workers. Depending on the zoo, the diversity of species may far exceed that encountered by most other animal workers. Workers are employed in only one area of the zoo or aquarium, and therefore their occupational health needs may differ widely. Although the animals in a particular collection are likely captive bred, some have originated in the wild, where potential for zoonotic infections could be greater. Many zoos and aquariums are also open to the outdoor environment, allowing contact between wild animals and the captive specimens, with the possibility of disease introduction. For example, outbreaks of highly pathogenic animal influenza (HPAI) have been reported in captive birds in zoos after contact with wild birds. Cases of avian influenza have also occurred in captive felids, presumably as a result of feeding on infected poultry carcasses. Both of these introductions posed infectious risks to zoo workers. For these reasons, zoo workers (as well as zoo animals) may serve as sentinels of emerging infectious disease threats. For example, primate workers in zoos have been found to have evidence of possible infection with simian viruses considered to have potential for emergence.[76] A special issue with zoo and aquarium workers is the significant number of volunteers working in many facilities who may not receive medical screening or prophylactic vaccinations.

Surveys of zoos have reported high rates of occupational injury and illness among zoo veterinarians, with more than

60% reporting significant animal-related injury, more than 30% reporting animal allergies, and more than 30% reporting zoonotic infections. Formalin exposures and insect allergies have also been reported as significant concerns.[77] A survey of marine mammal workers found that 50% reported suffering injuries from marine mammals (one third of which were considered severe), and 23% reported skin rashes or reactions.[78]

ALLERGENS

Zoo workers are exposed to allergens in both indoor and outdoor environments. Aquariums may have additional challenges with controlling mold. Control of allergens is similar to that for veterinary personnel.

ZOONOSES

Because of the diversity of species and the possibility of introduction of infectious agents from contact between captive and wild animals, zoo and aquarium workers are exposed to perhaps the widest variety of zoonotic diseases compared with any other animal workers (see the species chart in Chapter 9). Guidelines for occupational health programs for zoo workers have been published by the American Association of Zoo Veterinarians.[79] Zoonotic risks to nonhuman primate handlers resemble those of workers in primate research facilities. The care of wild ruminants may expose workers to livestock pathogens such as brucellosis and Q fever. Reptile keepers are at risk of *Salmonella* infection and envenomations, and bird workers are at risk of *Chlamydophila* infection. Other enteric disease risks to zookeepers include campylobacteriosis and shigellosis. Elephant handlers and staff working with nonhuman primates are at risk of TB exposure (Figure 12-5). Zoonotic risk prevention and control in zoo workers are similar to that in veterinary facilities.

Aquarium workers are at risk of *Mycobacterium marinum* from tropical fish tanks. Other dermal exposure risks worthy of mention for aquarium workers include erysipeloid and *Vibrio vulnificus*.

Erysipeloid.   Erysipeloid is an infection from contact with *Erysipelothrix rhusiopathiae*, a gram-positive rod bacterium found in fish as well as birds and pigs. The bacteria usually enter through broken skin. The most common manifestation is local erythema and wound infection (Color Plate 12-1). Although rare, bacteremia and endocarditis can occur.[80]

Vibrio Vulnificus.   *Vibrio vulnificus* is a marine bacteria that can be encountered while handling tanks and marine animals. It may infect wounds and cause local wound infections in immunocompetent individuals and fatal septicemia (Color Plate 12-2) in immunocompromised persons.[81] Careful hand hygiene after handling tanks and aquatic animals is essential.

Aquarium workers may also be at risk of exposure to pathogens in marine mammals during regular care as well as veterinary care and necropsies. Potential pathogens include leptospirosis, brucellosis, and "seal finger" from

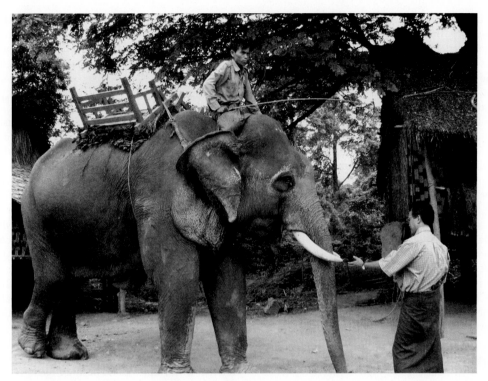

Figure 12-5 ▪ Elephant being examined by a veterinarian. (From Fowler ME: *Zoo and wild animal medicine current therapy,* ed 6, St Louis, 2007, Saunders Elsevier.)

bites or other direct contact with seals and other pinnipeds. Seal finger is believed to be caused by infection with *Mycoplasma phocacerebrale*[82] and is characterized by pain, cellulitis, and joint swelling (Color Plate 12-3). Treatment is with tetracycline.

CHEMICAL HAZARDS

Disinfectant chemicals are used widely in zoos and aquariums and may be capable of inducing irritation and allergy. If a veterinary facility is present in the zoo, anesthetic exposures may resemble those in other veterinary facilities.

Envenomations from reptiles, insects, fish, and other marine organisms represent a significant hazard to reptile handlers and aquarium workers. Emergency procedures for treating envenomations should be in place, including a stockpile or other resources to ensure the availability of antivenin for specific species housed at the facility (see Chapter 8).

PHYSICAL HAZARDS

Zoo and aquarium workers may have regular contact with captive wild animals capable of inflicting serious and fatal trauma, including large felids, bears, sharks, and elephants. Numerous other ergonomic risks exist, including transport of feed and bedding.

Risks can be controlled by design of enclosures and training of zoo workers in safe procedures for working near dangerous animals as well as engineering solutions for transport of heavy materials, such as ergonomically designed wheelbarrows and hoists. Special training is also needed for injury prevention for workers handling dangerous animals and equipment.

PSYCHOSOCIAL STRESSORS

Zoo and aquarium workers may share psychosocial stressors with other animal workers, including grief after an animal death and fear of attack by dangerous animals. They also may develop stress related to encounters with the general public.

OCCUPATIONAL MEDICINE SERVICES FOR ZOO AND AQUARIUM WORKERS

Because of the diversity and complexity of the occupational exposures, it would seem advisable that zoos and aquariums designate a medical provider or group of providers for both routine and emergency medical services. This designated provider should be familiar with both the infectious and noninfectious hazards that such workers face.

Preplacement Screening. Preplacement evaluations of zoo and aquarium workers should consider the range of species with which the worker is expected to have contact. Otherwise, baseline evaluations resemble those for veterinary and research animal workers.

Primate handlers should be screened for vaccination status as listed for laboratory primate workers. Nonhuman primate handlers and elephant handlers should be screened for TB. Stool cultures and stool tests for ova and parasites have been recommended at baseline for zoo workers. Such cultures should include *Salmonella, Shigella,* and *Campylobacter.*[79]

Audiometry at baseline should be performed for workers entering noisy jobs. Because of the wide range of infectious disease exposures, some with implications for disease emergence, it has been recommended that zoo workers bank serum at baseline and receive follow-up serology periodically to detect zoonotic infections.[83] Such serum banking should be done under strict protocols to preserve confidentiality of workers and should be under the supervision of the consulting medical provider.

Medical Surveillance.   Medical surveillance for zoo and aquarium workers is similar to that for veterinary and animal research workers.

Acute Injury, Illness, or Exposure Evaluation and Follow-up.   Management of acute injuries and illnesses in zoo workers resembles that for veterinary and research animal workers. Designated emergency facilities should have protocols for antivenin treatment of reptile and other envenomations (see Chapter 8). Nonhuman primate exposures should be handled as emergencies, as with animal research workers, because of the risk of herpes B infection.

Pet Store Workers

Pet store employees share many of the exposures of zoo and aquarium workers yet are rarely enrolled in formal occupational health programs and may not have access to medical providers with a knowledge of the particular risks of the workplace. Compared with zoos, veterinary practices, and animal research facilities, there is a lack of published guidelines for occupational health services for this worker population. Despite this, the pet store industry is large and growing and employs thousands of workers nationwide. The recent multistate outbreak of monkeypox associated with importation of African rodents underscored the potential for disease emergence in pet stores and distribution facilities related to trade in exotic pets (see Chapter 10). Pet stores are generally required by local and federal regulations to have a designated veterinarian. Such an individual could be in a position to advocate for preventive health services for the employees. NASPHV has developed a compendium of measures to prevent disease associated with animals in public settings, which gives general guidelines for infection control in areas where the public has contact with animals, including pet stores, but does not provide detailed guidance on the occupational health of pet store workers.[84]

HAZARDS AND THEIR CONTROL IN THE PET STORE SETTING

The hazards and principles of hazard control are similar to those in zoos and veterinary offices, with the exception that veterinary care procedures are not likely to take place. Consequently, exposures to anesthetics and radiation are not expected. Ventilation systems and cleaning of the facility may be geared to the retail setting, with less attention to health concerns. There also is potential for inadequate ventilation and consequent increased risk of airborne allergy.

Zoonotic disease risks depend on the species of animals sold in the facility but generally encompass risks seen in

veterinary, animal research, and zoo settings, with the difference being the lack of invasive procedures performed on animals. Chemical and physical hazards to pet store workers are similar to those of other animal workers described.

OCCUPATIONAL MEDICINE SERVICES FOR PET STORE WORKERS

Preplacement Screening.   As previously mentioned, many pet store workers do not receive occupational health services, including preplacement examinations. It would seem reasonable, however, to offer such workers preplacement examinations that resemble those for veterinary workers. At the least, pet store workers should inform their health care providers, if they have one, about their work activities. The health care provider could then assess whether the individual is at increased risk of zoonotic infection because of an immunocompromised condition or is at risk of developing allergic reactions from work exposures. As with other animal worker occupational health issues, this requires that the health care provider be aware of the health risks related to animal work or can consult a veterinarian to be updated about such risks.

Vaccination.   Vaccination for all workers should include tetanus if not up to date. Because ferrets can be susceptible to human influenza, influenza vaccine should be encouraged for workers with ferret contact.

Medical Surveillance.   Ongoing medical surveillance of pet store workers is generally not performed. However, as with other animal handlers, NIOSH has recommended periodic monitoring for allergic symptoms with a symptom questionnaire and follow-up of positive responses as indicated. Such a screening questionnaire could cover infectious disease risk as well. Annual audiometry should be performed on workers with significant noise exposures.

Acute Injury, Illness, or Exposure Evaluation and Follow-up.   A wide range of acute infectious conditions can present in pet store workers and should be considered in the differential diagnosis of ill employees. Animal bites and scratches should be treated according to the pathogens associated with particular species. In workers with bird contact who report respiratory symptoms, *Chlamydophila* infection and hypersensitivity pneumonitis (see Chapter 7) should be considered. Job restrictions and modifications after acute illnesses and injuries are similar to those of zoo and veterinary workers.

Farm Animal Workers

Agricultural workers with animal contact may work in settings ranging from backyard farms with a small number of animals to intensive confinement facilities with hundreds of thousands of animals. Therefore their work status may vary from informal laborers without written job contracts to registered employees in large and well-organized facilities. Job activities may range from feeding to manure management to slaughtering. The informal and varied settings may make use of personal protective equipment difficult, and there may be budgetary and other limitations to implementing engineering controls. There are few comprehensive occupational health guidelines for farm animal workers as well as a lack of OSHA standards directly targeting this setting. Farm managers may therefore be reluctant to see any value in developing relationships with members of an occupational health team or arranging for preplacement and periodic worker evaluations. Although veterinarians are often involved in the care of farm animals, some of the first-aid and other medical treatment may be accomplished by the farmers themselves. Some of the occupational exposures may resemble those of workers in zoos, yet the high density of animals in some production facilities can present unique exposure situations.

Technological changes in swine and poultry production have increased the efficiency of husbandry operations over the past several decades. A single concentrated animal feeding operation (CAFO) facility may house hundreds of pigs or more than 50,000 chickens or other poultry.[2] Such facilities produce high concentrations of airborne dusts and gases, large quantities of manure, as well as the potential for rapid spread of diseases among animals and workers.

ALLERGENS

A large variety of animal allergens on farms can pose a significant health hazard to animal workers. Allergy from pigs, horses, chickens, cattle, goats, and other domestic animals is well recognized (see Chapter 7). The development of occupational allergy to such allergens may cause significant difficulties in workers who are skilled in working with one particular type of animal, such as horses. Control strategies include wetting dusts to avoid airborne exposures, frequent washing of animals, and use of respirators and gloves when around animals. Workers may want to consider allergen desensitization to allow them to continue working with particular animal species.

Other significant antigens around farms include those produced by thermophilic bacteria growing on moldy hay or silage and in other moist environments that can cause hypersensitivity pneumonitis (farmer's lung; see Chapter 7), which can produce chills, fever, cough, and shortness of breath. A survey of dairy farmers found antibodies to such antigens in 75% of farmers tested and a history of symptoms consistent with farmer's lung in 17%.[2]

ENDOTOXIN AND ORGANIC DUSTS

Farm workers in CAFOs have some of the highest exposure to endotoxins and organic dusts, which can cause obstructive airway changes and the febrile syndrome known as *organic toxic dust syndrome* (ODTS).[28] These organic dusts may contain plant material from bedding and feed; animal particulates, including feces, feathers, hair, skin cells, and urine; bacteria; pathogenic fungi; endotoxins; antibiotics and other feed additives; and chemicals including pesticides, ammonia, hydrogen sulfide, and methane. Significant rates of OTDS have been reported among swine CAFO workers.[2] Wetting dusts and regular cleaning of bedding as well as improved ventilation and manure management may reduce worker exposure to organic dusts. When exposures are not able to be controlled, the use of respiratory protection may be necessary.

ZOONOSES

Many diseases of domestic livestock and poultry are potentially communicable to workers. Table 12-6 shows some of these pathogens.

Contact with rodents near animal operations can increase the risk of hantavirus and other rodent-borne infections. Control of zoonotic disease risks involves many of the preventive measures mentioned for veterinary and research animal workers, including control of disease in animals, handwashing practices, disinfection of surfaces, and use of personal protective equipment as necessary. Rodent management and tick control can further reduce zoonotic risks, as can reducing contact between farm animals and wildlife.

CHEMICAL HAZARDS

Chemical hazards encountered by farm animal workers include animal pesticides such as tick dips, oxides of nitrogen causing silo filler's lung from decomposing silage, and ammonia and hydrogen sulfide from manure waste in swine CAFO facilities.[28] Silo filler's lung is a toxic pneumonitis that develops hours to days after a filling a silo and inhaling the irritating oxides of nitrogen gas. This exposure can result in acute respiratory distress syndrome (ARDS) and death in severe cases. Hydrogen sulfide can also cause

TABLE 12-6 ▪ Specific Occupational Pathogens Associated With Animal Husbandry

Type of Production	Pathogens	High-Risk Activities
Poultry	*Salmonella, Campylobacter fetus, Chlamydophila,* avian influenza virus, Newcastle disease virus, *Erysipelothrix, Histoplasma*	Slaughtering, meat processing, close contact with sick animals
Swine	*Salmonella, Campylobacter, Streptococcus suis, Brucella, Erysipelothrix rhusiopathiae,* vesicular stomatitis virus, hepatitis E virus, Nipah virus, influenza	
Cattle	*Brucella, B. anthracis*	Butchering meat, contact with birthing products, skinning, inadequate cooking of meat
Sheep	Orf virus, *Coxiella, B. anthracis*	Skinning, butchering, marketing
Bushmeat, wild game	*Francisella, Trichinella,* other emerging pathogens, primate viruses (non-U.S.)	

ARDS and death in human beings and animals, often after pumping liquid manure out of a pit. Ammonia fumes can be highly irritating to the respiratory tract. These chemical risks can be reduced by substitution of less-toxic pesticides, proper silage and manure management, improvements in ventilation, and personal protective equipment for short-term, high-exposure tasks.

PHYSICAL HAZARDS

Work with large domestic animals carries a significant risk of crush and other traumatic injuries from kicking, biting, and other direct contact. Other physical hazards include noise and traumatic injuries from farm machinery, ultraviolet radiation, and musculoskeletal strains from lifting objects and animals. Certain tasks such as animal slaughter and processing may involve repetitive motions and result in overuse injuries. Animal slaughter and butchering can also result in injuries from knives and other sharp tools.

PSYCHOSOCIAL STRESSORS

Psychosocial stressors in working with farm animals include fear of trauma or infection. There may also be feelings of isolation for farmers working in rural locations.[85]

OCCUPATIONAL MEDICINE SERVICES FOR FARM ANIMAL WORKERS

As previously mentioned, many farm animal workers are not currently enrolled in preventive occupational medicine screening and follow-up programs. Nonetheless, the following components of preventive occupational medicine services for such workers should be considered based on the level of hazardous exposure. Sometimes screening is necessary after an outbreak of disease among either workers or animals; this process would be greatly simplified if baseline medical information were obtained on all workers.

Preplacement Screening.
Because of the risk of allergy, workers on farms should be screened for allergic symptoms at baseline and periodically thereafter. Baseline spirometry is advisable. Workers with immunocompromised status are at increased risk of zoonotic transmission, and farm animal workers, especially if zoonotic diseases are endemic, should be screened and counseled for the risk of transmission in immunocompromised individuals. Musculoskeletal problems at baseline should be identified and a preventive plan implemented to prevent injuries. If a respirator will be used, the OSHA respirator medical evaluation and questionnaire should be completed.

Vaccination.
Vaccinations for all farm animal workers should include tetanus and seasonal influenza vaccine (especially for swine and poultry workers). Periodic examinations should inquire about allergic and infectious disease symptoms as well as problems related to contact with chemicals or physical hazards.

Acute Injury, Illness, or Exposure Evaluation and Follow-up.
The acute care of farm animal workers should consider zoonotic and allergic risks as well as the possibility of hypersensitivity pneumonitis. Cases of zoonotic disease in an animal worker should be considered a sentinel health event with relevance to both co-workers and herd health. Communication back to the veterinarian responsible for the health of the farm animals should occur, perhaps mediated by the public health department. The veterinarian may be simultaneously managing an outbreak in the domestic animals, and close communication between animal and human health professionals is critical. Infectious disease exposures requiring prophylaxis and follow-up may include anthrax and *Mycobacterium bovis*. Similarly, acute exposures to chemicals could be a sign that other workers and animals are at risk. Acute injuries from animals and other physical factors should also be viewed as opportunities to review possible breakdowns in safety measures and ways to further improve safety. Decisions about job restriction and modification and confidentiality issues are similar to those for other animal workers.

Wildlife Rehabilitators, Hunters, and Other Workers With Wildlife Contact

Although often not included in discussions of occupational risks to animal workers, several groups with significant exposure to wild animals through informal or formal work activities deserve mention. Wildlife rehabilitators are often volunteers who care for injured and sick wild animals in a variety of settings, including wildlife sanctuaries and their homes. Hunters may be amateur or professional and have intimate contact with blood and other body fluids of animals while butchering and skinning mammals and defeathering birds, in addition to the consumption of wild game meat. Other workers with potential wildlife contact include zoologists, who may be trapping, dissecting, and otherwise coming in contact with a wide variety of wild animals; forestry workers; and animal control officers and wildlife management biologists, who may be involved in the immobilization and transportation of wild animals and who are at risk of zoonotic disease through direct contact as well as exposure to vectors, including ticks and mosquitoes.

HAZARDS WITH WILDLIFE CONTACT

Hazards faced by these groups include a wide range of zoonotic disease exposures similar to those of zoo personnel and vary according to the species encountered. Examples include Lyme disease, ehrlichioses, brucellosis, tularemia, plague, rabies, giardiasis, and hantavirus.[86] Vector-borne diseases are a greater threat to these individuals compared with many other animal workers. Wildlife rehabilitators face allergen and chemical exposures similar to those in veterinary practice or zoos. Individuals working around areas of bird and bat roosting, including caves, bridges, and abandoned buildings, are at risk for exposure to pathogenic fungi, including *Histoplasma, Cryptococcus,* and *Blastomyces.* Chemical exposures for wildlife management professionals may include inadvertent exposure to immobilizing (tranquilizer) agents and envenomations from reptiles and arthropods. Physical exposures for wildlife biologists include sun exposure, cold, and heat stress. Individuals working with wild animals face physical hazards of attacks and bites. Hunters risk similar hazards as well as the risk of noise exposure from firearms and acute injuries and bloodborne disease transmission during skinning and butchering game.

OCCUPATIONAL HEALTH SERVICES FOR PERSONS WITH WILDLIFE CONTACT

Occupational medical services for wildlife workers are often less formalized than for other worker groups such as research animal workers. Depending on the level of exposure, baseline medical screening that includes screening for allergy, immunocompromised status and other major medical conditions, and counseling about ways to reduce risk of exposure to zoonotic pathogens and avoid animal-related injury would appear to be indicated. If individuals have contact with rodents in a hantavirus-endemic area, they should undergo respirator medical clearance and respirator fit testing as required under the OSHA respirator standard. Serum banking should be considered for individuals at high risk of zoonotic disease exposure. Immunizations should include tetanus prophylaxis as well as vaccine rabies for individuals working with bats, raccoons, skunks, or other potentially rabid animals. Personal protective equipment should include respirators (Figure 12-6) and gloves for working with rodents in hantavirus-endemic areas. In other areas, gloves and masks are advisable when handling rodents. Hunters should use adequate hearing protection while hunting and impermeable gloves while preparing carcasses.

Ongoing monitoring for allergy and infectious disease symptoms can be done periodically by using a screening questionnaire, as with other animal workers. Having an identified health care provider for these individuals could be of benefit both for ongoing prevention as well as for appropriate management of acute illnesses and injuries, which may involve unusual zoonotic diseases, envenomations, or other animal-related medical conditions with which many human health clinicians will be less familiar.

ONLINE RESOURCES

- The National Institute for Occupational Safety and Health (NIOSH): http://www.cdc.gov/NIOSH
- Occupational Safety and Health Administration (OSHA): http://www.osha.gov
- Committee on Occupational Safety and Health in Research Animal Facilities, Institute of Laboratory Animal Resources, Commission on Life Sciences, National Research Council: *Occupational health and safety in the care and use of research animals,* Washington DC: National Academy Press; 1997. Available at http://books.nap.edu/openbook.php?isbn=0309052998

References

1. National Institute for Occupational Safety and Health. *NIOSH Alert: Preventing asthma in animal handlers.* DHHS (NIOSH) Publication No. 97–116. http://www.cdc.gov/Niosh/animalrt.html.
2. Rosenstock L, Cullen MR, Brodkin CA, et al. eds, *Textbook of clinical occupational and environmental medicine.* 2nd ed. Philadelphia: Saunders Elsevier; 2005.
3. Bureau of Labor Statistics. Animal care and service workers. *In Occupational outlook handbook, 2008–2009 edition.* http://www.bls.gov/oco/ocos168.htm#outlook. Accessed May 27, 2008.
4. Seward JP. Occupational allergy to animals. *Occup Med.* 1999;14:285–302.
5. Stellman JM, ed. *Encyclopedia of occupational health and safety.* Vol. 4. 4th ed. Geneva: International Labour Office; 1998.
6. Harber P, Mummaneni S, Crawford L. Influence of residency training on occupational medicine practice patterns. *J Occup Environ Med.* 2005;47:161–167.
7. Lincoln TA, Bolton NE, Garrett AS. Occupational allergy to animal dander and sera. *J Occup Med.* 1974;16:456–469.
8. Bush RK. Mechanism and epidemiology of laboratory animal allergy. *ILAR Journal.* 2001;42:4–11.
9. Gordon S, Bush RK, Newman-Taylor AJ. Laboratory animal, insect, fish and shellfish allergy. In: Bernstein IL, Chan-Yeung M, Malo JL, et al, eds. *Asthma in the workplace.* 3rd ed. New York: Taylor and Francis Group; 2006.
10. Von Essen S, Donham K. Illness and injury in animal confinement workers. *Occup Med.* 1999;14:337–350.
11. Matsui EC, Diette GB, Krop EJ, et al. Mouse allergen-specific immunoglobulin G and immunoglobulin G4 and allergic symptoms in immunoglobulin E-sensitized laboratory animal workers. *Clin Exp Allergy* 2005;35(10):1347–1353.
12. Chan-Yeung M, Malo JL. Aetiological agents in occupational asthma. *Eur Respir J.* 1994;7:346–371.
13. Hunskaar S, Fosse RT. Allergy to laboratory mice and rats: a review of the pathophysiology, epidemiology and clinical aspects. *Lab Anim.* 1990;24(4):358–374.
14. Seward JP. Medical surveillance of allergy in laboratory animal handlers. *ILAR Journal.* 2001;42:47–54.
15. Wilson IG. Airborne *Campylobacter* infection in a poultry worker: case report and review of the literature. *Commun Dis Public Health.* 2004;7(4):349–353.
16. Tiong A, Vu T, Counahan M, et al. Multiple sites of exposure in an outbreak of ornithosis in workers at a poultry abattoir and farm. *Epidemiol Infect.* 2007;135(7):1184–1191.
17. Gage KL, Dennis DT, Orloski KA, et al. Cases of cat-associated human plague in the Western US, 1977–1998. *Clin Infect Dis.* 2000;30(6):893–900.

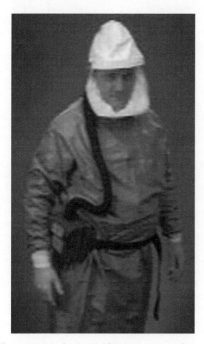

Figure 12-6 ■ Powered air purifying respirator for working with rodents in a hantavirus-endemic area. (From Centers for Disease Control and Prevention: *Respirators as a precaution for hantavirus infection.* http://www.cdc.gov/ncidod/diseases/hanta/hps/noframes/prevent7.htm.)

18. Cheng VC, Lau SK, Woo PC, et al. Severe acute respiratory syndrome coronavirus as an agent of emerging and reemerging infection. *Clin Microbiol Rev.* 2007;20(4):660–694.

19. Centers for Disease Control and Prevention. Update: outbreak of Nipah virus–Malaysia and Singapore, 1999. *MMWR Morb Mortal Wkly Rep.* 1999;48(16):335–337.

20. Wolfe ND, Prosser TA, Carr JK, et al. Exposure to nonhuman primates in rural Cameroon. *Emerg Infect Dis.* 2004;10(12):2094–2099.

21. Mumford E, Bishop J, Hendrickx S, et al. Avian influenza H5N1: risks at the human-animal interface. *Food Nutr Bull.* 2007;28(suppl 2): S357–S363.

22. Wilson ML, Chapman LE, Hall DB, et al. Rift Valley fever in rural northern Senegal: human risk factors and potential vectors. *Am J Trop Med Hyg.* 1994;50(6):663–675.

23. Michel AL, Huchzermeyer HF. The zoonotic importance of *Mycobacterium tuberculosis:* transmission from human to monkey. *J S Afr Vet Assoc.* 1998;69(2):64–65.

24. Michalak K, Austin C, Diesel S, et al. *Mycobacterium tuberculosis* infection as a zoonotic disease: transmission between humans and elephants. *Emerg Infect Dis.* 1998;4(2):283–287.

25. Hackendahl NC, Mawby DI, Bemis DA, et al. Putative transmission of *Mycobacterium tuberculosis* infection from a human to a dog. *Am Vet Med Assoc.* 2004;225(10):1573–1577 1548.

26. Berkelman RL. Human illness associated with use of veterinary vaccines. *Clin Infect Dis.* 2003;37(3):407–414.

27. Langley RL, Pryor WH, O'Brien KF. Health hazards among veterinarians: a survey and review of the literature. *J Agromedicine.* 1995;2:23–52.

28. Mitloehner FM, Calvo MS. Worker health and safety in concentrated animal feeding operations. *J Agric Saf Health.* 2008;14(2):163–187.

29. Mandell GL, Bennett JE, Dolin R. *Principles and practice of infectious diseases.* 6th ed. New York: Churchill Livingstone; 2005.

30. Huhn GD, Austin C, Carr M, et al. Two outbreaks of occupationally acquired histoplasmosis: more than workers at risk. *Environ Health Perspect.* 2005;113(5):585–589.

31. National Institute for Occupational Safety and Health. *Histoplasmosis–protecting workers at risk. NIOSH Publication No. 2005–109.* http://www.cdc.gov/niosh/docs/2005-109/. Accessed January 1. 2009.

32. MacDougall L, Kidd SE, Galanis E, et al. Spread of *Cryptococcus gattii* in British Columbia, Canada, and detection in the Pacific Northwest, USA. *Emerg Infect Dis.* 2007;13(1):42–50.

33. Bradsher Jr RW. Pulmonary blastomycosis. *Semin Respir Crit Care Med.* 2008;29(2):174–181.

34. Meggs WJ. Chemical hazards faced by animal handlers. *Occup Med.* 1999;14:213–223.

35. Study links occupational exposures with risk of miscarriage. Anesthetic gases, radiation, pesticides are areas of concern for pregnant workers. *J Am Vet Med Assoc.* 2008;232(10):1445–1447.

36. Gerasimon G, Bennett S, Musser J, et al. Acute hydrogen sulfide poisoning in a dairy farmer. *Clin Toxicol (Phila).* 2007;45(4):420–423.

37. Zwemer Jr FL, Pratt DS, May JJ. Silo filler's disease in New York State. *Am Rev Respir Dis.* 1992;146(3):650–653.

38. Jeyaretnam J, Jones H. Physical, chemical and biological hazards in veterinary practice. *Aust Vet J.* 2000;78(11):751–758.

39. Cohen SP. Compassion fatigue and the veterinary health team. *Vet Clin North Am Small Anim Pract.* 2007;37(1):123–134.

40. Managing stress and avoiding burnout. A self-care primer for overly compassionate and overworked veterinarians. *J Am Vet Med Assoc.* 2004;225(4):492–493.

41. Elchos BL, Scheftel JM, Cherry B, et al. Compendium of veterinary standard precautions for zoonotic disease prevention in veterinary personnel. *J Am Vet Med Assoc.* 2008;233(3):415–432.

42. American College of Occupational and Environmental Medicine. *ACOEM code of ethical conduct.* http://www.acoem.org/codeofconduct.aspx. Accessed November 7, 2008.

43. National Association of State Public Health Veterinarians, Inc., Centers for Disease Control and Prevention. Compendium of animal rabies prevention and control, 2008. *MMWR.* 2008;57(RR-2):1–9.

44. Occupational Safety and Health Administration. *OSHA recordkeeping handbook.* http://www.osha.gov/recordkeeping/handbook/index.html. Accessed July 24, 2008.

45. American College of Occupational and Environmental Medicine. *Confidentiality of medical information in the workplace.* http://www.acoem.org/guidelines.aspx?id=3538. Accessed July 2, 2008.

46. Nienhaus A, Skudlik C, Seidler A. Work related accidents and occupational diseases in veterinarians and their staff. *Int Arch Occup Environ Health.* 2005;78:230–238.

47. Babcock S, Marsh AE, Lin J, et al. Legal implications of zoonoses for clinical veterinarians. *J Am Vet Med Assoc.* 2008;233(10):1556–1562.

48. Castorina JS, Rosenstock L. Physician shortage in occupational and environmental medicine. *Ann Intern Med.* 1990;113(12):983–986.

49. Susitaival P, Kirk JH, Schenker MB. Atopic symptoms among California veterinarians. *Am J Ind Med.* 2003;44(2):166–171.

50. Susitaival P, Kirk J, Schenker MB. Self-reported hand dermatitis in California veterinarians. *Am J Contact Dermatitis.* 2001;12(2):103–108.

51. Wright JG, Jung S, Holman RC, et al. Infection control practices and zoonotic disease risks among veterinarians in the United States. *J Am Vet Med Assoc.* 2008;232(12):1863–1872.

52. Bulcke DM, Devos SA. Hand and forearm dermatoses among veterinarians. *J Eur Acad Dermatol Venereol.* 2007;21(3):360–363.

53. National Institute of Occupational Safety and Health. *A recommended standard for occupational exposure to waste anesthetic gases and vapors.* Cincinnati, DHHS (NIOSH) Publication No. 77–140, 1977.

54. Meyer RE. Anesthesia hazards to animal handlers. *Occup Med.* 1999;14:225–233.

55. Panni MK, Corn SB. Scavenging in the operating room. *Curr Opin Anaesthesiol.* 2003;16(6):611–617.

56. Fritschi L, Day L, Shirangi A, et al. Injury in Australian veterinarians. *Occup Med (Oxford).* 2006;56(3):199–203.

57. Grandin T. Safe handling of large animals. *Occup Med.* 1999;14:195–212.

58. OSHA: CFR occupational noise exposure. In: *Hearing conservation amendment (final rule), in 48 Federal Register.* http://www.osha.gov/pls/oshaweb/owadisp.show_document?p_table=STANDARDS&p_id=9735.

59. Miller JM, Beaumont JJ. Suicide, cancer, and other causes of death among California veterinarians, 1960–1992. *Am J Ind Med.* 1995;27(1): 37–49.

60. Rogelberg SG, DiGiacomo N, Reeve CL, et al. What shelters can do about euthanasia-related stress: an examination of recommendations from those on the front line. *J Appl Anim Welf Sci.* 2007;10(4):331–347.

61. Occupational Safety and Health Administration. OSHA respirator medical evaluation questionnaire. http://www.osha.gov/pls/oshaweb/owadisp.show_document?p_table=STANDARDS&p_id=9783.

62. Committee on Occupational Safety and Health in Research Animal Facilities. Institute of Laboratory Animal Resources, Commission on Life Sciences, National Research Council. *Occupational health and safety in the care and use of research animals.* Washington, DC: National Academy Press; 1997.

63. Rahija RJ. Animal facility design. *Occup Med.* 1999;14:407–422.

64. Van Rhijn DJ. Occupational health for animal research facility. *Chem Health Safety.* 2004;11:24–27.

65. Centers for Disease Control and Prevention. *B virus (Cercopithecine herpesvirus 1) infection.* http://www.cdc.gov/ncidod/diseases/bvirus.htm.

66. Cohen JI, Davenport DS, Stewart JA, et al. Recommendations for prevention of and therapy for exposure to B virus (Cercopithecine herpesvirus 1). *Clin Infect Dis.* 2002;35:1191–1203.

67. Centers for Disease Control and Prevention. Fatal Cercopithecine herpesvirus 1 (B virus) infection following a mucocutaneous exposure and interim recommendations for worker protection. *MMWR.* 1998;47(49):1073–1076.

68. Centers for Disease Control and Prevention. Nonhuman primate spumavirus infections among persons with occupational exposure–United States, 1996. *MMWR Morb Mortal Wkly Rep.* 1997;46(6):129–131.

69. Wachtman LM, Mansfield KG. Opportunistic infections in immunologically compromised nonhuman primates. *ILAR J.* 2008;49(2):191–208.

70. Heymann DL. ed. *Control of communicable diseases manual.* 19th ed. Washington DC: American Public Health Association; 2008.

71. Mazurek GH, Jereb J, Lobue P, et al. Guidelines for using the QuantiFERON-TB Gold test for detecting *Mycobacterium tuberculosis* infection, United States. *MMWR Recomm Rep.* 2005;54(RR-15):49–55.

72. Jensen PA, Lambert LA, Iademarco MF, et al. CDC guidelines for preventing the transmission of *Mycobacterium tuberculosis* in health-care settings, 2005. *MMWR Recomm Rep.* 2005;54(RR-17):1–141.

73. Langley R. Physical hazards of animal handlers. *Occup Med.* 1999;14:181–194.

74. Arluke A. Uneasiness among laboratory technicians. *Occup Med.* 1999;14:305–316.

75. Lang YC. Animal exposure surveillance: a model program. *AAOHN Journal.* 2005;53(9):407–412.

76. Engels EA, Switzer WM, Heneine W, et al. Serologic evidence for exposure to simian virus 40 in North American zoo workers. *J Infect Dis.* 2004;190(12):2065–2069.

77. Hill DJ, Langley RL, Morrow WM. Occupational injuries and illnesses reported by zoo veterinarians in the United States. *J Zoo Wildlife Med.* 1998;29(4):371–385.

78. Hunt TD, Ziccardi MH, Gulland FM, et al. Health risks for marine mammal workers. *Dis Aquat Organ.* 2008;81(1):81–92.

79. American Association of Zoo Veterinarians. *Guidelines for zoo and aquarium veterinary medical programs and veterinary hospitals* (Appendix 6) 1998.

80. Brooke CJ, Riley TV. *Erysipelothrix rhusiopathiae:* bacteriology, epidemiology and clinical manifestations of an occupational pathogen. *J Med Microbiol.* 1999;48(9):789–799.

81. Hsueh PR, Lin CY, Tang HJ, et al. *Vibrio vulnificus* in Taiwan. *Emerg Infect Dis.* 2004;10(8):1363–1368.

82. Baker AS, Ruoff KL, Madoff S. Isolation of *Mycoplasma* species from a patient with seal finger. *Clin Infect Dis.* 1998;27(5):1168–1170.

83. Wolfe ND, Dunavan CP, Diamond J. Origins of major human infectious diseases. *Nature.* 2007;447(7142):279–283.

84. National Association of State Public Health Veterinarians, et al. Inc. Compendium of measures to prevent disease associated with animals in public settings, 2007. *MMWR Recomm Rep.* 2007;56 (RR-5):1–14.

85. Hovey JD, Seligman LD. The mental health of agricultural workers. In: Lessinger JE, ed. *Agricultural medicine: a practical guide.* Porterville, CA: Springer; 2006.

86. Guidotti TL, Naidoo K. Hunting, trapping and wilderness-related work. *Clin Occup Environ Med.* 2002;2:651–661.

87. Use of anthrax vaccine in the United States: recommendations of the Advisory Committee on Immunization Practices. *J Toxicol Clin Toxicol.* 2001;39(1):85–100.

Public Health and Human-Animal Medicine

13

Peter M. Rabinowitz, Lisa A. Conti, and Hugh M. Mainzer

Both the human and veterinary medical oaths address the need for the promotion of public health. This chapter deals with human-animal health situations in which population health duties take primacy and where human and veterinary clinicians perform many functions that place them together on the front line of public health practice (Color Plate 13-1).

In ancient Greece, Asclepius, Apollo's son, was charged by the gods with caring for the mortals of Greece (the classic symbol of medicine is Asclepius' staff, around which is wound one snake).* His two daughters were Hygeia (Figure 13-1), the guardian of health and champion of common sense practices as the basis of wellness ("cleanliness is next to godliness"), and Panacea, whose occupation was to cure individuals already sick, one at a time. Mortals remained healthier when they followed Hygeian principles, creating a healthy environment and preventing disease. Individuals who lost their health sought Panacea.

Although in today's culture, human and veterinary clinicians are more likely to practice solely as the hand of Panacea, the "one health" concept—drawing human, veterinary, and population health practices together—is focused on providing a comprehensive approach to disease control and prevention and wellness promotion.

Key Points for Clinicians and Public Health Professionals

Public Health Professionals

- Facilitate communication between human health care providers and veterinary health care providers.
- Recognize that veterinary and human health clinicians perform many functions that place them on the front lines of public health practice.

---

*Commercial, military, and American medical organizations use the caduceus of Hermes (rod entwined by two snakes and topped by a pair of wings) as their symbol. Most medical associations around the world, including the World Health Organization and the veterinary profession, use the staff of Asclepius, which has a single serpent encircling a staff.

- Educate clinicians on ways to refocus clinical activities toward prevention and to understand the links among environment, host, and agent.
- Consider surveillance of animals as well as human beings for early detection of disease risk.

Human Health Clinicians

- At a minimum, clinicians are required to report "notifiable diseases" to the state or local health department. It is critical to contact the health department if an issue of public health importance is even suspected.
- Practice preventive medicine.

Veterinary Clinicians

- All veterinary clinicians must recognize that they are essential parts of the public health system, with responsibility to protect and improve the health of human as well as animal populations. What the veterinarian observes, diagnoses, and treats in the clinical setting can have a far-reaching population health impact.
- It is important to contact the health department (in addition to requirements for reporting to agriculture officials) if an issue of public health importance is suspected to discuss the situation. For example, if leptospirosis is diagnosed in an animal, the public health department can provide guidance for preventing human cases and be on the watch for human cases. Contacting the health department regarding a communicable disease or other environmental health hazard can also increase communication between veterinarians and human health clinicians in the community.
- Practice preventive medicine.

THE 10 ESSENTIAL PUBLIC HEALTH SERVICES

In 1994, the U.S. Public Health Service assembled and tasked the Public Health Functions Steering Committee to develop a working definition of public health and a guiding

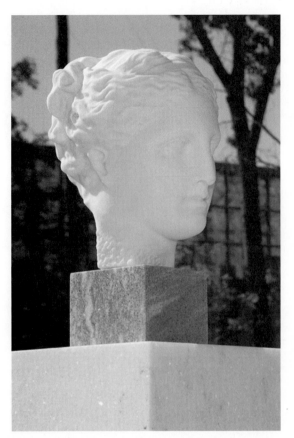

Figure 13-1 ■ The bust of the Greek muse of health, Hygeia, on the CDC's Roybal campus in Atlanta, Ga. (From Centers for Disease Control and Prevention Public Health Image Library. Photo courtesy John P. Anderton.)

framework for the responsibilities of local public health systems.[1] The resulting 10 Essential Public Health Services are the following:

1. Monitor health status to identify and solve community health problems.
2. Diagnose and investigate health problems and health hazards in the community.
3. Inform, educate, and empower people about health issues.
4. Mobilize community partnerships and action to identify and solve health problems.
5. Develop policies and plans that support individual and community health efforts.
6. Enforce laws and regulations that protect health and ensure safety.
7. Link people to needed personal health services and ensure the provision of health care when otherwise unavailable.
8. Ensure a competent public and personal health care workforce.
9. Evaluate effectiveness, accessibility, and quality of personal and population-based health services.
10. Research for new insights and innovative solutions to health problems.

The actions of public health professionals as well as human and veterinary clinicians that are mentioned in many sections of this book encompass these 10 core responsibilities.

DISEASE SURVEILLANCE AND INFORMATION FLOW BETWEEN HUMAN AND ANIMAL HEALTH PROFESSIONALS

Much of this book discusses the need for enhanced communication between animal health and human health professionals. Not always evident is the key role that public health professionals and the public health system play in such communication.

The first three core functions of public health systems are to monitor the status of the health of the community; to diagnose and investigate health problems and health hazards affecting communities; and inform, educate, and empower communities to improve health. To accomplish these functions, accurate information is required on the prevalence and incidence of disease events and risk factors as well as the extent of environmental health hazards. A major method of obtaining this information is from surveillance data gathered through mandated reporting systems. These data, reported by clinicians, laboratories, and others, are used to identify emerging diseases, plan for disasters, track trends, and evaluate progress of intervention strategies. Reportable disease events in animals could be sentinel events for human health hazards, and vice versa.

In the United States each state can set its own priorities for disease reporting. The Council of State and Territorial Epidemiologists (CSTE; http://www.cste.org) and National Association of State Public Health Veterinarians (NASPHV; http://www.nasphv.org) provide guidance for such reportable condition criteria and for both communicable and noncommunicable conditions. State and local health departments then provide selected data to the Centers for Disease Control and Prevention (CDC).[2] Most states have required animal disease reporting of agricultural importance to agricultural agencies as well (see state requirements at http://www.biosecuritycenter.org/reportDisease.php). Box 13-1 lists the human infectious diseases that are nationally notifiable to the public health system. One animal disease, rabies, is also required to be reported. For a complete listing of nationally notifiable diseases and other conditions of public health importance (including injury and lead), see http://www.cdc.gov/ncphi/disss/nndss/phs/files/NNDSS_event_code_list_January_2008.doc.

In individual states, additional diseases may also be reportable to state health and/or agriculture departments.

In the United States veterinarians may be required to report selected clinical conditions to either public health authorities, who may perform further disease investigations to protect human health, or to their state veterinarian at the state department of agriculture for the protection of animal and human health. Ideally, the public health and agriculture authorities then communicate. State veterinarians provide selected data to the U.S. Department of Agriculture (USDA). Every 6 months the USDA reports to the World Organization for Animal Health (OIE) regarding the presence or absence of reportable animal diseases in the United States.[3] Box 13-2 lists reportable diseases tracked by the OIE.

When veterinarians report clinical illness in animals to public health authorities, public health professionals can assist with providing prevention guidance to minimize

BOX 13-1   *NATIONALLY NOTIFIABLE INFECTIOUS DISEASES, UNITED STATES, 2009*

AIDS
Anthrax
Arboviral neuroinvasive and nonneuroinvasive diseases
- California serogroup virus disease
- Eastern equine encephalitis virus disease
- Powassan virus disease
- St. Louis encephalitis virus disease
- West Nile virus disease
- Western equine encephalitis virus disease

Botulism
- Foodborne
- Infant
- Other (wound and unspecified)

Brucellosis
Chancroid
Chlamydia trachomatis, genital infections
Cholera
Coccidioidomycosis
Cryptosporidiosis
Cyclosporiasis
Diphtheria
Ehrlichiosis/anaplasmosis
- *Ehrlichia chaffeensis*
- *Ehrlichia ewingii*
- Anaplasma phagocytophilum
- Undetermined

Giardiasis
Gonorrhea
Haemophilus influenzae, invasive disease
Hansen disease (leprosy)
Hantavirus pulmonary syndrome
Hemolytic uremic syndrome, postdiarrheal
Hepatitis, viral, acute
- Hepatitis A, acute
- Hepatitis B, acute
- Hepatitis B virus, perinatal infection
- Hepatitis, C, acute

Hepatitis, viral, chronic
- Chronic hepatitis B
- Hepatitis C virus infection (past or present)

HIV infection
- Adult/adolescent (age ≥13 years)
- Child (age ≥18 months and <13 years)
- Pediatric (age <18 months)

Influenza-associated pediatric death
Legionellosis
Listeriosis
Lyme disease
Malaria
Measles
Meningococcal disease

Mumps
Novel influenza A virus infections
Pertussis
Plague
Poliomyelitis, paralytic
Poliovirus infection, nonparalytic
Psittacosis
Q Fever
- Acute
- Chronic

Rabies
- Animal
- Human

Rocky Mountain spotted fever
Rubella
Rubella, congenital syndrome
Salmonellosis
Severe acute respiratory syndrome–associated coronavirus (SARS-CoV) disease
Shiga toxin–producing *Escherichia coli*
Shigellosis
Smallpox
Streptococcal disease, invasive, group A
Streptococcal toxic-shock syndrome
Streptococcus pneumoniae, drug resistant, invasive disease
Streptococcus pneumoniae, invasive disease, non–drug resistant, in children <5 years

Syphilis
- Primary
- Secondary
- Latent
- Early latent
- Late latent
- Latent, unknown duration
- Neurosyphilis
- Late, nonneurologic
- Syphilitic stillbirth

Syphilis, congenital
Tetanus
Toxic-shock syndrome (other than streptococcal)
Trichinellosis (trichinosis)
Tuberculosis
Tularemia
Typhoid fever
Vancomycin-intermediate *Staphylococcus aureus*
Vancomycin-resistant *Staphylococcus aureus*
Varicella (morbidity)
Varicella (deaths only)
Vibriosis
Yellow fever

From Centers for Disease Control and Prevention: *National notifiable infectious diseases.* Available at http://www.cdc.gov/ncphi/disss/nndss/phs/infdis.htm. Accessed April 8, 2009. *AIDS,* Acquired immunodeficiency syndrome; *HIV,* human immunodeficiency virus.

human risk of disease. In addition, an inquiry into possible associated human cases may ensue.

Both human medical reporting requirements and agricultural requirements vary from state to state, but the nationally notifiable diseases and the OIE list represent a minimum dataset for which ongoing surveillance is conducted.

Surveillance for disease can be both passive and active. Passive surveillance involves tracking the number of diagnosed cases of disease in a community that are reported to public health authorities. Active surveillance involves performing surveys or other systematic investigations to detect cases not reported through passive systems. Active surveillance can take place for both human and animal diseases.

Multiple Species Diseases

Anthrax
Aujeszky's disease
Bluetongue
Brucellosis
- *Brucella abortus*
- *Brucella melitensis*
- *Brucella suis*
Crimean Congo hemorrhagic fever
Echinococcosis/hydatidosis
Foot and mouth disease
Heartwater
Japanese encephalitis
Leptospirosis
New world screwworm (*Cochliomyia hominivorax*)
Old world screwworm (*Chrysomyia bezziana*)
Paratuberculosis
Q fever
Rabies
Rift Valley fever
Rinderpest
Trichinellosis
Tularemia
Vesicular stomatitis
West Nile fever

Cattle Diseases

Bovine anaplasmosis
Bovine babesiosis
Bovine genital campylobacteriosis
Bovine spongiform encephalopathy
Bovine tuberculosis
Bovine viral diarrhea
Contagious bovine pleuropneumonia
Enzootic bovine leukosis
Hemorrhagic septicemia
Infectious bovine rhinotracheitis/infectious pustular vulvovaginitis
Lumpy skin disease
Malignant catarrhal fever (wildebeest only)
Theileriosis
Trichomonosis
Trypanosomosis (tsetse-transmitted)

Sheep and Goat Diseases

Caprine arthritis/encephalitis
Contagious agalactia
Contagious caprine pleuropneumonia
Enzootic abortion of ewes (ovine chlamydiosis)
Maedi-visna
Nairobi sheep disease
Ovine epididymitis (*Brucella ovis*)
Peste des petits ruminants
Salmonellosis (*Salmonella abortus ovis*)
Scrapie
Sheep pox and goat pox

Equine Diseases

African horse sickness
Contagious equine metritis
Dourine
Equine encephalomyelitis (Eastern)
Equine encephalomyelitis (Western)
Equine infectious anemia
Equine influenza
Equine piroplasmosis
Equine rhinopneumonitis
Equine viral arteritis
Glanders
Surra (*Trypanosoma evansi*)
Venezuelan equine encephalomyelitis

Swine Diseases

African swine fever
Classical swine fever
Nipah virus encephalitis
Porcine cysticercosis
Porcine reproductive and respiratory syndrome
Swine vesicular disease
Transmissible gastroenteritis

Avian Diseases

Avian chlamydiosis
Avian infectious bronchitis
Avian infectious laryngotracheitis
Avian mycoplasmosis (*Mycoplasma gallisepticum*)
Avian mycoplasmosis (*Mycoplasma synoviae*)
Duck virus hepatitis
Fowl cholera
Fowl typhoid
Highly pathogenic avian influenza and low-pathogenic avian influenza in poultry*
Infectious bursal disease (Gumboro disease)
Marek's disease
Newcastle disease
Pullorum disease
Turkey rhinotracheitis

Lagomorph Diseases

Acarapisosis of honey bees
American foulbrood of honey bees
Bee diseases
European foulbrood of honey bees
Myxomatosis
Rabbit hemorrhagic disease
Small hive beetle infestation (*Aethina tumida*)
Tropilaelaps infestation of honey bees
Varroosis of honey bees

Fish Diseases

Epizootic hematopoietic necrosis
Epizootic ulcerative syndrome
Gyrodactylosis (*Gyrodactylus salaris*)
Infectious hematopoietic necrosis
Infectious salmon anemia
Koi herpesvirus disease
Red sea bream iridoviral disease
Spring viremia of carp
Viral hemorrhagic septicemia

Mollusk Diseases

Abalone viral death
Infection with *Bonamia exitiosa*
Infection with *Marteilia refringens*
Infection with *Perkinsus marinus*
Infection with *Perkinsus olseni*
Infection with *Xenohaliotis californiensis*
Infection with *Bonamia ostreae*

Continued

BOX 13-2 *ANIMAL DISEASES REPORTABLE TO THE WORLD ORGANIZATION FOR ANIMAL HEALTH—Cont'd*

Crustacean Diseases

Infectious hypodermal and hematopoietic necrosis
Spherical baculovirosis (*Penaeus monodon*–type baculovirus)
Taura syndrome
Tetrahedral baculovirosis (*Baculovirus penaei*)
White spot disease
Yellowhead disease

Crayfish plague (*Aphanomyces astaci*)
Infectious myonecrosis
White tail disease

Other Diseases

Camelpox
Leishmaniosis

As of January 21, 2008.
From World Organisation for Animal Health: *OIE listed diseases.* http://www.oie.int/eng/maladies/en_classification2008.htm?e1d7. Accessed March 3, 2008.
*Per Chapter 2.7.12 of the Terrestrial Animal Health Code.

For specific diseases, public health authorities may create and maintain surveillance systems using animal sentinels. Examples are the use of sentinel chickens for West Nile virus and other encephalitis viruses (Figure 13-2) and routine tick and mosquito surveillance for Lyme disease and West Nile virus, respectively.

Ongoing monitoring for the appearance of disease outbreaks in both human beings and other animals takes place on local, state, national, and international levels. Figure 13-3 depicts some of the mandated and potential information flow between animal and human health. As with any system of such complexity, there is potential for information to be lost or for miscommunication to occur. Public health professionals can play an important role in facilitating communication between human health and animal health care providers. However, for nonreportable conditions, and even in the case of conditions that have reporting requirements, veterinarians and human health clinicians should consider contacting each other in addition to the relevant authorities, while respecting patient confidentiality (see Chapter 14).

Fostering such communication in a community is an example of the fourth public health function—to "mobilize community partnerships and action to identify and solve health problems." Such information is fundamental to the ability for the public health service to "develop policies and plans that support individual and community health efforts," the fifth essential service.

OUTBREAKS

When outbreaks of disease occur in human or other animal populations, they are ideally detected by the surveillance systems described above. Such detection can lead to a response on both the public health and clinical levels (Figure 13-4). If an outbreak involves both human and animal health, communication and coordination between human and animal health professionals becomes critical. Specific roles for clinicians and public health professionals are mentioned in many chapters of this book.

The occurrence of a disease outbreak in human beings or other animals can be a sign of an emerging health hazard in the environment. Examples include an unintentional release of a toxic chemical such as chlorine gas from a tanker truck, which could sicken both human beings and animals, or the introduction of a novel pathogen into an ecosystem.

Public health systems need to be alert to the possibility of intentional releases of pathogens or chemicals as in a biological or chemical terrorism attack. In such scenarios, there is potential for animals to serve as sentinels for human beings if they develop signs of illness before it is recognized in human populations. As Table 13-1 shows, in the event of a bioterrorism attack in the United States, different animal species may either provide early warning to human beings, serve as indicators of ongoing risk in the environment or, in

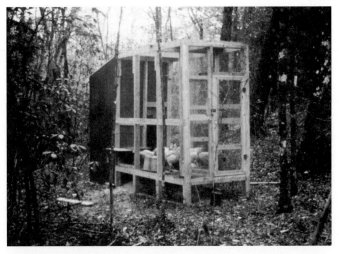

Figure 13-2 ■ A caged sentinel chicken flock used to detect the presence of a specific arbovirus. (From Centers for Disease Control and Prevention Public Health Image Library, Atlanta, Ga.)

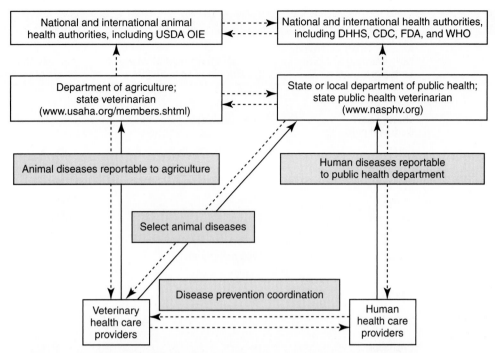

Figure 13-3 ▪ Flow of disease information between animal health and human health. *Solid line,* Mandated reporting; *hatched line,* recommended communication.

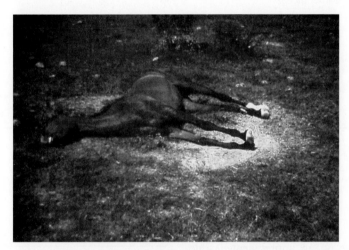

Figure 13-4 ▪ This victim of Venezuelan equine encephalitis was reported and permitted public health authorities to alert the community to take precautions against mosquito bites. (From Centers for Disease Control and Prevention Public Health Image Library, Atlanta, Ga. Courtesy James Stewart.)

some situations, help spread or maintain an outbreak though propagation of infection in an animal population.

Similarly, animals could provide early warning of an intentional release of chemical warfare agents.[4,5] For animals to serve as effective sentinels for either biological or chemical classes of agents, there must be adequate surveillance systems in place (particularly for animal populations) and working channels of communication between human and animal health, with the public health system playing a vital role in such channels.

An example of the use of electronic animal surveillance for public health benefit occurred after the unintentional release of propyl mercaptan (a chemical with a strong onionlike odor and potential for irritant effects)

from an industrial facility in Georgia. In the days after the release, electronic records from pet hospitals in the area showed that respiratory signs in cats, gastrointestinal signs in dogs, and eye inflammation signs in dogs and cats increased significantly in areas of greater chemical exposure. These signs were consistent with chemical irritation, and such data provided information about high-risk exposure areas for both animals and human beings in the vicinity.[6]

The prospect for another global pandemic of human influenza derived from a highly pathogenic animal strain has strengthened existing partnerships and created new ones in the human, veterinary, and public health realms. Surveillance of wild birds for subclinical viral carriage, as well as morbidity

Table 13-1 ■ Public Health Implications of Animals Exposed to Bioterrorism Agents*

Agent/Disease	Animals That Can Provide Early Warning of Acute Bioterrorism Attack	Animals That Could Be Markers for Ongoing Exposure Risk	Animals That Can Propagate or Maintain Epidemic
Category A			
Anthrax	Sheep, cattle‡ Dogs and pigs*	Sheep, cattle‡	
Plague	Cats*	Dogs, cats*; multiple species†	Cats, camels, goats‡
Tularemia	None‡	Rodents† Horses, cows†	Ticks, rodents, prairie dogs†
Botulism	None‡	None‡	None‡
Filovirus infection	Unknown	Unknown	Wildlife‡
Category B			
Q fever	Sheep*	Wild hogs, goats†	Cats, sheep, goats, cattle‡
Brucellosis	None‡	Cattle†	Wildlife, cattle, dogs‡
Foodborne illness: *Salmonella* spp., *Shigella* spp., *Cryptosporidium* spp., etc.	Cattle‡	Unknown	Unknown
Glanders	Unknown	Horses†	Horses†
Alphaviruses (VEE/EEE)	Horses‡	Birds*	Wild birds†
Rift Valley fever	Cattle, sheep‡	Sheep*	Mosquitoes, rodents*
Ricin toxin	Unknown	Unknown	Unknown
Epsilon toxin	Unknown	Unknown	Unknown
Category C (Emerging Diseases)			
Nipah virus	Unknown	Multiple species‡	Pigs*
Hantavirus	None†	Multiple species†	Rodents†
Flavivirus (WN, JE)	Wild birds‡	Mosquitoes, birds†	Birds*

From Rabinowitz P, Gordon Z, Chudnov D, et al: Animals as sentinels of bioterrorism agents, *Emerg Infect Dis* 12:647, 2006.
*Level 1 evidence available; experimental or cohort study or randomized clinical trial.
†Level 2 evidence available: case-control or cross-sectional study.
‡Level 3 evidence available: Case reports or case series, expert opinion.
Unknown, Insufficient evidence found; *VEE/EEE*, Venezuelan equine encephalitis/Eastern equine encephalitis; *WN*, West Nile; *JE*, Japanese encephalitis.

and mortality, is taking place on an unprecedented scale through efforts such as the Global Avian Influenza Network for Surveillance (GAINS)[7] and the Highly Pathogenic Avian Influenza Early Detection Data System (HEDDS).[8] Reports of disease events in animals are being collected on a real-time basis by the Emergency Prevention System for Transboundary Animals and Plant Pests and Diseases (EMPRES), coordinated by the United Nations Food and Agriculture Organization (FAO).[9] Such efforts may provide the first clue to possible impending human outbreaks of highly pathogenic avian influenza.

The public health response to outbreaks can involve a number of measures to control the spread of disease. These include environmental health measures to ensure clean air, water, food supplies, and housing as well as elimination of specific hazards, vector control, and public health messaging regarding risk reduction measures for affected populations. Specific control measures are mentioned in many of the disease-specific sections of this book.

INSPECTIONS AND REGULATIONS OF FACILITIES

A number of clinical conditions discussed in this book are related to facilities such as petting zoos, pet stores, and veterinary clinics, where members of the public come in contact with animals. It can often be confusing to the clinician regarding which agency has responsibility for the inspection and regulation of particular facilities, an example of the sixth essential public health service. Table 13-2 lists a number of different types of facilities, and whether animal health or human health officials tend to be involved in inspections and regulations. In some of these settings, such as food processing, both animal health and human health agencies may be involved. In certain situations, local animal control divisions are also often involved; this division is usually separate from both public health departments and departments of agriculture.

Table 13-2 ▪ Inspection and Regulation of Various Settings Involving Human Animal Contact			
Type of Facility or Scenario	Public Health Inspections/ Regulations	Local Animal Control Officer	Department of Agriculture Inspections/Regulations
Pet store, petting zoo, country fair with animal exhibits, pet swap meets	Recommendations for handwashing facilities and other infection control measures, zoonoses investigation		Ensures animal health
Beaches (pet policies)	Beach water monitoring for pathogens	Enforces pet policies	
Veterinary clinics	Occupational health of veterinary staff and biomedical waste		Management of reportable diseases
Quarantine of dog or cat after bite to human being	Oversees quarantine	Ensures dog or cat is quarantined	
Farms	Occupational health of workers		Health of animals, biosecurity, management of reportable diseases
Food processing facilities/ abattoirs/live bird markets	Occupational health of workers, food safety (including FDA)		Food safety
Building with lead contamination	Oversees screening of persons, remediation		

Local regulations and scope of jurisdiction may vary.
FDA, Food and Drug Administration.

DISASTERS AND HUMAN-ANIMAL MEDICINE

In a disaster situation, there is a need to coordinate services for animals as well as human beings. The seventh and eighth public health services, linking people to health care and ensuring a competent workforce are never more critical than during a disaster. People often keep themselves in harm's way if their pets' safety and health needs are not addressed. Recent experience with hurricanes has demonstrated that some directly in the path of these storms would not leave their homes when there was no place to take their pets. The extended public health community is now addressing this. The Pets Act authorizes the Federal Emergency Management Agency (FEMA) to provide shelter for the animals belonging to those persons beings sheltered, at least close enough in proximity so that they can have access to the animals.[10] States have animal emergency response teams that can be and have been mobilized to address animal emergency management issues, including assisting with the movement of animals to emergency shelters and caring for the animals in the shelters. They often collaborate extensively with local communities as well as a number of nongovernmental organizations working to provide shelter and care of human and animal populations.

Box 13-3 shows that many of the health risks that occur after a natural disaster are shared by both human beings and other animals.

Both human health clinicians and veterinarians can volunteer for clinical roles in disaster response, including caring for individuals and animals in shelters. Opportunities include the medical reserve corps of Health and Human Services Office of the Surgeon General as well as the Disaster Medical Assistance Team (DMAT; http://www.hhs.gov/aspr/opeo/ndms/teams/dmat.html)* and the National Veterinary Response Team (http://www.dhhs.gov/aspr/opeo/ndms/teams/vmat.html).†

The USDA has its own emergency response unit, the National Animal Health Emergency Response Corps, which can address herd health or flock health issues such as outbreaks of foot and mouth disease, Newcastle's disease of poultry, or avian influenza (see http://www.aphis.usda.gov/emergency_response). Such efforts may involve mass vaccination, culling, or quarantine.

---

*The National Response Framework (NRF) uses the National Disaster Medical System (NDMS), a part of the U.S. Department of Health & Human Services. Under the NRF, NDMS serves as a component of Emergency Support Function #8 (ESF-8), Health and Medical Services. The National Veterinary Response Team (NVRT) is a cadre of individuals within the NDMS system who have professional expertise in areas of veterinary medicine, public health, and research. In addition to supporting the NRF mission requirements of NDMS under ESF-8, operational support may also be rendered by the NVRT to other federal partners such as the U.S. Department of Agriculture (USDA) under ESF-11, Agriculture, and Federal Emergency Management Act (FEMA) under ESF-6, Mass Care, in the support of the Pets Evacuation and Transportation Standards Act (PETS Act). The NVRT provides assistance in identifying the need for veterinary services after major disasters, emergencies, and public health or other events requiring federal support and in assessing the extent of disruption to animal and public health infrastructures. The NVRT is a fully supported federal program.

†Under the National Response Framework, USDA is a primary agency for Emergency Support Function #11, Agriculture and Natural Resources. The Animal and Plant Health Inspection Service (APHIS) is expected to play a significant role in a wide variety of emergency incidents. APHIS' Veterinary Services program safeguards U.S. poultry and livestock from the introduction, establishment, and spread of foreign animal diseases. Veterinary Services National Center for Animal Health Emergency Management develops strategies and policies for effective incident management, and coordinates incident responses.

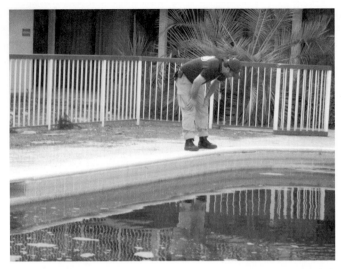

Figure 13-5 ■ Abandoned pools are a source for emerging mosquito populations.

- Bites from injured or stray animals
- Rodent infestation and rodent-borne disease
- Mosquito-borne disease after flooding (Figure 13-5)
- Leptospirosis after floods
- Potential for occupational exposures of persons working in emergency human and animal shelters
- Posttraumatic stress in animal owners who have lost pets
- Heat or cold stress, depending on the disaster
- Food or waterborne illness
- Carbon monoxide poisoning from generators
- Envenomations from displaced animals

Guidelines for Management of Animals After a Disaster

The CDC, in cooperation with the American Veterinary Medical Association, has prepared a set of detailed guidelines for animal health professionals managing animals in emergency shelters and other facilities after a natural disaster (Figure 13-6).[11] These guidelines are provided in Box 13-4.

The care of displaced domestic animals in emergency shelters can present occupational health hazards for individuals handling such animals. The National Institute for Occupational Safety and Health (NIOSH) has published guidelines for the prevention of occupational injury and illness among emergency first responders and animal rescue workers handling animals during a disaster.[12] Identified health and safety hazards include animal bites and scratches, rabies and other zoonoses, sharps-related injuries, heavy lifting, skin rashes and other dermatologic conditions, animal allergy, latex allergy, noise, and pesticide exposure. Recommended steps to reduce these risks are shown in Box 13-5.

The last two essential public health services—evaluate effectiveness, accessibility, and quality of personal and population-based health services and research for innovative

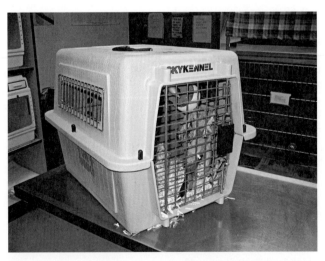

Figure 13-6 ■ A bird in a pet carrier. (From Mitchell M, Tully TN Jr: *Manual of exotic pet practice,* St Louis, 2008, Saunders Elsevier.)

These interim guidelines have been developed by consultation between the American Veterinary Medical Association and the CDC and are advisory in nature. They are intended to provide guidance for the care of animals entering shelters and for persons working with or handling the animals in response to natural disasters.

Animals arriving at shelters as a result of a natural disaster need special care. Because they may have been exposed to contaminated water and may not have had access to safe food and fresh water, many are stressed and dehydrated and some may be injured and/or ill. Stressed animals may or may not show signs of illness and may also exhibit behavioral disorders. Following some simple animal management and disease control guidelines can help improve animal health and reduce the risk of disease transmission and injury between animals and people.

What follows are some recommendations for pets arriving at animal shelters.

Animal Health History, Examinations, and Identification

- Each animal should be examined at a triage site. Particular attention should be paid to hydration status, cuts and abrasions, paw/hoof/foot health (e.g., pads and claws, area between toes), ear health (e.g., redness, discharge), oral injuries (may have occurred if animal was foraging for food), vomiting and/or diarrhea, respiratory disease, and evidence of parasite infestation.
- Animals should be bathed upon entry, particularly if they may have been in contact with contaminated flood water. Commercial dish soap can remove petroleum and some other toxic chemicals, but care should be taken with use on sensitive species (e.g., horses). Those bathing the animals should wear protective clothing (e.g., rain suits, ponchos), gloves, and a face shield or goggles with a surgical mask to avoid mucous membrane contact with droplets and splashes that may contain toxic materials.
- Intake personnel should ask whether the pet has been in the custody of the owner since the beginning of the evacuation and should inquire about the animal's health and vaccination history, paying particular attention to any current medical needs or chronic health problems (e.g., diabetes, which would signal a need for insulin injections). In addition, owners should be questioned about the animal's usual temperament (e.g., whether the animal can safely be housed with others of the same species, whether it might be aggressive toward caretakers).
- A health record for each animal should be created and updated as needed. Identification information for the animal should correspond to that for the owner so that animals and their owners can be reunited. Owned animals should be clearly marked as "owned" and not "abandoned" to reduce the risk of mix-ups. Photographs should be taken, if possible. Collars (leather or nylon, not choke chains) containing readily legible identification information should be placed on all animals. Ideally, all animals should be microchipped.
- Cages should be clearly labeled so that newly arriving personnel are easily apprised of the health status and temperament of sheltered animals.
- Animals arriving without owners should be scanned for microchip identification. Microchips are most often placed between the shoulder blades, but earlier models were prone to migration, so animals should be scanned from the shoulder blade down to the ventral chest. All scanners are not capable of reading all microchips, so if multiple types of scanners are available, scan with each type before declaring an animal to be microchip-free. Animals without microchips should be checked

for other forms of identification such as a tag or tattoo. Tattoos on dogs may correspond to an AKC registration number and this information should be used to trace the animal, if possible.

Animal Health Management and Prevention and Treatment of Zoonotic and Nosocomial Diseases

Intestinal Parasitism

- Dogs should be treated prophylactically for internal parasites, including *Giardia*, roundworms, hookworms, and whipworms.
- Exposure to mosquitoes in flood-ravaged areas presents an increased risk of heartworm disease. If possible, dogs should be tested for heartworms and appropriate preventatives or treatment should be administered.

External Parasitism

- Dogs and cats should be examined for flea or tick infestation and treated appropriately.
- Preventive flea and tick treatments should be considered for all dogs and cats housed in shelters.

Vaccinations

- While the American Veterinary Medical Association normally recommends that vaccination programs be customized to individual animals, in disaster situations vaccination status may be difficult, if not impossible, to determine. For this reason, administration of "core" vaccines to animals upon admission to shelters when vaccination status is unavailable or not current is considered appropriate. Vaccines take some time to become effective and will not address preexisting exposures, so personnel are cautioned to be alert for clinical signs of disease.
- A rabies vaccination should be administered to dogs, cats, and ferrets. This is especially important for dogs and cats housed in group settings. Personnel should be aware that rabies vaccines may take as long as 28 days to become effective.
- Additional core vaccinations for dogs include distemper, hepatitis, and parvovirus.
- Additional core vaccinations for cats include feline viral rhinotracheitis, panleukopenia, and calicivirus. Vaccination against feline leukemia should be considered for young kittens that will be housed in contact with other cats.
- Vaccination (intranasal) against *Bordetella bronchiseptica* and parainfluenza should be considered for all dogs to reduce the incidence of kennel cough.
- Because leptospirosis risk is higher in flood-ravaged areas and because the disease is zoonotic, vaccination should be considered. Personnel are cautioned that leptospirosis vaccines are serovar specific and that the potential for adverse reactions may be higher than for some other vaccines.

Diarrheal Disease

- Animals presenting with (or developing) diarrhea should be separated from healthy animals.
- Nosocomial agents of concern that may be transmitted by feces include parvovirus, panleukopenia, *Giardia*, and intestinal parasites.
- Zoonotic agents of concern for small animals include *Campylobacter* and *Salmonella*, which are highly infectious and have been associated with outbreaks in shelters and veterinary clinics.

Ill Birds

- Ill birds are usually lethargic, depressed, and inappetent. Care should be taken when handling ill birds because they may be infected with the zoonotic bacteria *Chlamydophila psittaci*, which causes psittacosis. Face masks should be worn when handling birds of unknown origin that are exhibiting signs of illness.

Continued

BOX 13-4   *CDC GUIDELINES FOR ANIMAL HEALTH AND CONTROL OF DISEASE TRANSMISSION IN PET SHELTERS—cont'd*

Behavioral Concerns

- Fear, panic, separation anxiety, noise and storm phobias, and other behavioral disorders are common problems in displaced animals. Animals that have never had these problems may develop them, and preexisting problems are likely to worsen.
- Providing housed animals with fresh food and water on a regular basis and establishing other familiar routines will help animals adjust to their new environment. Food and water should be provided at multiple smaller and dispersed stations, rather than a few large clumped stations, to minimize fear competition and fighting among unfamiliar animals.
- Animals without a prior history of aggression may snap, bite, or hiss as a result of fear or uncertainty. Shelter personnel should approach rescued animals calmly, but cautiously. Only experienced personnel should handle animals that exhibit significant behavioral disorders.

- Behavioral exercises and behavioral medications may be administered short or long term, as required, to help animals recover. Shelters are encouraged to seek assistance from qualified animal and veterinary behaviorists who can assist them in meeting these needs.

Euthanasia

- Animals that are irreversibly ill or exhibiting intractable signs of aggression should be euthanized. Records should be kept of animals euthanized.
- Animals that have been previously associated with transmission of monkeypox (i.e., prairie dogs, African rodents) are under legal restrictions for movement except to a veterinarian for care. If one of these high-risk species is presented for veterinary care at a shelter, it must be kept isolated from other animals and housed in a separate cage. If this cannot be accomplished, these animals must be humanely euthanized.

From Centers for Disease Control and Prevention: *Disaster recovery information: Interim guidelines for animal health and control of disease transmission in pet shelters*. http://www.bt.cdc.gov/disasters/animalhealthguidelines.asp. Accessed April 8, 2009.

BOX 13-5   *GUIDANCE TO PREVENT INJURIES AND ILLNESSES FROM WORKING WITH DISPLACED DOMESTIC ANIMALS*

Recommendations for Workers

Workers can reduce their risk of occupational hazards associated with displaced domestic animals by taking the following steps:

Sanitation and Hygiene

- Wash your hands frequently with soap and water:
  - Before and after handling animals.
  - After coming in contact with animal saliva, urine, feces, or blood.
  - After cleaning cages or equipment.
  - Before eating, drinking, smoking, taking breaks, or leaving work.
  - After removing gloves.
- Use alcohol-based hand sanitizers for cleaning hands when soap and water are not available.
- Change into clean clothing before leaving the workplace.
- Wear disposable outerwear or clothing that can be removed before leaving the workplace if clean clothing or laundry facilities are not available.
- Keep your nails trimmed to 1/4 inch and do not use artificial nails.
- Use personal protective clothing and equipment.
  - Wear medical examination gloves that provide your skin with a protective barrier when handling animals, animal waste, cages, equipment, and pesticides.
  - Wear two pairs of gloves if one pair alone might tear.
  - Make sure that latex gloves are reduced-protein, powder-free gloves to reduce exposure to allergy-causing proteins.
  - Use nonlatex gloves if you need or want to avoid latex.
  - Wear cotton or leather work gloves as the outer pair when heavy work gloves are needed.
  - Remember that cotton, leather, and other absorbent gloves are not protective when worn alone.
  - Wear protective eyewear (safety glasses with side shields) or face shields if there is a risk of spitting or splashing of contaminated material.

- Wear sturdy clothing and protective footwear with nonslip soles; tennis shoes or sneakers do not provide protection from bite, puncture, or crush injuries.
- Wear hearing protection if you must raise your voice to talk to someone an arm's length away (e.g., when working in enclosed spaces with barking dogs).

Animal Bites and Scratches

- Complete the rabies preexposure vaccination series before directly handling dogs, cats, ferrets, or other mammals that may be infected with rabies.
- Thoroughly clean all bite wounds and scratches with soap and water.
- Report any bite injury to your supervisor.
- Immediately receive medical evaluation of any bite wound and the need for possible rabies postexposure treatment.

Other Hazards

- Take precautions when using scalpels, forceps, and other sharp instruments.
  - Dispose of sharp devices in labeled, puncture-resistant, leak-proof sharps disposal containers immediately after use.
  - Do not recap, bend, or remove contaminated needles and sharps.
  - Do not shear or break contaminated needles.
- Take precautions when lifting heavy or awkward loads.
  - Use proper lifting techniques.
  - Reduce the weight of loads when possible.
  - Work together to lift loads that are unsafe for one person to handle.
- Pregnant or immunocompromised workers should avoid contact with cat feces and pet rodents to reduce their risk of zoonotic disease.
- Immediately report to the supervisor:
  - Any needlestick or other sharps-related injury.
  - Any symptoms of infectious disease or zoonosis.
  - Any other workplace injury or illness.
- Consult a health care provider about any occupational injury or illness.

BOX 13-5 *GUIDANCE TO PREVENT INJURIES AND ILLNESSES FROM WORKING WITH DISPLACED DOMESTIC ANIMALS—cont'd*

Recommendations for Employers

Employers should protect their workers from the hazards associated with working with displaced domestic animals by taking the following steps.

- Provide training in:
  - Workplace-specific hazards, including bites and scratches, zoonoses, sharps-related injuries, heavy lifting, dermatologic conditions, allergies, excessive noise, and pesticide exposure.
  - Good housekeeping, sanitation, hygiene, and infection control procedures.
  - Animal handling procedures and use of equipment.
  - The use and maintenance of personal protective clothing and equipment.
- Provide handwashing and sanitation facilities.
  - Provide alcohol-based hand sanitizers for cleaning hands when soap and water are not available.
- Provide appropriate personal protective clothing and equipment.
  - Provide disposable outerwear or clothing if laundry facilities are not available.

- Provide medical examination gloves that provide workers' skin with barrier protection.
- Provide nonlatex gloves for those workers who need or want to avoid latex.
- Provide heavy work gloves or restraints for use with aggressive animals.
- Provide hearing protection for workers when needed.
- Provide preexposure rabies vaccination for workers with direct animal contact; only workers who have completed the preexposure rabies vaccination series should work with dogs, cats, ferrets, or other mammals that may be infected.
- Provide a medical surveillance system that monitors and records all occupational injuries and illnesses.
- Stress to workers the importance of reporting all work-related injuries and illnesses as soon as possible.
- Ensure that any worker with a bite injury is immediately evaluated by a health care provider for rabies risk and possible postexposure treatment and vaccination.

Modified from National Institute for Occupational Safety and Health: *NIOSH interim guidance on health and safety hazards when working with displaced domestic animals.* http://www.cdc.gov/niosh/topics/flood/pdfs/displacedanimals.pdf. Accessed September 22, 2008.

continuous system improvement. This cannot happen without the partnerships, the communication, and the feedback from the human, veterinary, and public health communities' coordinated approach to animal and human health.

References

1. Centers for Disease Control and Prevention. *National Public Health Performance Standards Program: ten essential public health services.* http://www.cdc.gov/od/ocphp/nphpsp/EssentialPHServices.htm. Accessed March 3, 2008.
2. Centers for Disease Control and Prevention. *National notifiable infectious diseases.* http://www.cdc.gov/ncphi/disss/nndss/phs/infdis.htm. Accessed March 3, 2008.
3. World Organisation for Animal Health. *OIE listed diseases.* http://www.oie.int/eng/maladies/en_classification2008.htm?e1d7. Accessed March 3, 2008.
4. Rabinowitz P, Gordon Z, Chudnov D, et al. Animals as sentinels of bioterrorism agents. *Emerg Infect Dis.* 2006;12(4):647–652.
5. Rabinowitz P, Wiley J, Odofin L, et al. Animals as sentinels of chemical terrorism agents. *Clin Toxicol (Phila).* 2008;46(2):93–100.
6. Maciejewski R, Glickman N, Moore G, et al. Companion animals as sentinels for community exposure to industrial chemicals: the Fairburn, GA, propyl mercaptan case study. *Public Health Rep.* 2008;123(3):333–342.
7. Global Avian Influenza Network for Surveillance. http://www.gains.org. Accessed September 23, 2008.
8. Highly Pathogenic Avian Influenza Early Detection Data System. *What does the HEDDS system do?* http://wildlifedisease.nbii.gov/ai/abouthedds.jsp. Accessed September 23, 2008.
9. Food and Agriculture Organization of the United Nations. *Emergency Prevention System.* http://www.fao.org/ag/AGAinfo/programmes/en/empres/home.asp. Accessed September 23, 2008.
10. Public Law 109-308. *Pets evacuation and transportation standards act of 2006.* http://www.animallaw.info/statutes/stusfd2006pl109_308.htm. Accessed September 7, 2008.
11. Centers for Disease Control and Prevention. *Interim guidelines for animal health and control of disease in pet shelters.* http://www.bt.cdc.gov/disasters/pdf/petshelterguidelines.pdf. Accessed March 3, 2008.
12. National Institute for Occupational Safety and Health. NIOSH interim guidance on health and safety hazards when working with displaced domestic animals. http://www.cdc.gov/niosh/topics/emrs/pdfs/displacedanimals.pdf. Accessed October 21, 2009.

Shared Strategies to Maximize Human and Animal Health

14

Peter M. Rabinowitz and Lisa A. Conti

This textbook has outlined numerous scenarios in which the health of human beings and other animals is closely aligned. The majority of the health conditions discussed are considered preventable. Key prevention roles for human health care providers, veterinarians, and public health professionals are outlined in each section.

These professionals traditionally have worked in parallel, seeing different parts of the human-animal medicine picture and responding to the issues that fell within one particular domain (see Chapter 1). However, the growing convergence of human and animal health and interest in a "one health" approach to human-animal disease issues suggest that more direct communication and cooperation among veterinarians, physicians and other human health care providers, and public health officials will become increasingly important to better prevent disease threats. This chapter presents steps to facilitate such cooperation. Some of the case scenarios are based on actual cases. They illustrate the concept of veterinarians and human health care providers making formal patient referrals to each other, just as specialty consultation referrals are routinely made between members of the same profession. Although local public health authorities may be a conduit for information flow between human health care providers and animal health care providers in a community, there is a role for direct communication as well. In doing so, care must be taken to both convey necessary information and also respect patient privacy considerations, including HIPAA (see Chapters 2 and 3). The use of standardized forms may facilitate such communication. Forms shown in the case scenarios that follow are suggested examples of communication templates for transmitting information.

The focus of many of the chapters of this book has been the clinical recognition of shared environmental health risks facing both human beings and other animals. Enhanced clinical awareness, communication, and improved history taking can gather important information about environmental health risks. A preventive risk assessment checklist can add to such information. Home or other site visits provide an opportunity to gain detailed information about clinically relevant environmental risks. This chapter outlines mechanisms for preventive risk assessments geared toward maximizing the health of human beings and animals living in proximity.

Key Points for Clinicians and Public Health Professionals

Public Health Professionals

- Include veterinarians in public health outreach efforts in the community.
- Adopt a "one health" model and maximize the role of the public health department in enhancing communication between human health care providers and animal health care providers.

Human Health Clinicians

- Identify opportunities for direct referrals to veterinarians while respecting patient privacy.
- Encourage other direct communication with veterinarians, including shared efforts to improve environmental health risks.
- Use the health department as a means for communicating with animal health professionals regarding environmental health problems and other shared health risks.
- For patients with pets and farm animals, perform preventive disease risk assessments.

Veterinary Clinicians

- Identify opportunities for direct referrals to physicians and other health care providers while respecting patient privacy.
- Use the health department as a means for communicating with human health care providers regarding environmental health problems and other shared health risks.
- Educate human health care providers about the importance of the human-animal bond and alternatives to giving up a pet for health reasons.
- For owners with pets and farm animals, perform preventive disease risk assessments.
- Use home visits as an opportunity for a preventive risk assessment.

REFERRALS FROM HUMAN HEALTH CARE PROVIDERS TO VETERINARIANS

At times a busy physician or other human health care provider may suspect that a patient's clinical condition may be affected by contact with animals in the home or vicinity. However, clinicians are limited by time and experience at addressing such issues in depth. At such times the health care provider can advise the patient to consult his or her veterinarian. A direct referral from the health care provider to the veterinarian may facilitate this process. One example is an immunocompromised patient who reports having companion animals. Such a patient is in need of a detailed discussion of zoonotic disease risks (see Chapter 10). Studies have shown that human health care providers do not feel comfortable providing in-depth counseling about zoonotic disease risk reduction and believe veterinarians are best suited to do so.[1] Mechanisms by which human health care providers could make direct referrals of patients to a veterinarian for zoonotic disease risk reduction assessment and counseling are therefore appropriate. Box 14-1 shows the possible components of such a referral visit.

Many medical insurance plans pay for preventive medicine counseling sessions, but whether a veterinarian's services would be compensable at this point by such human health insurance plans is not clear. However, if such consultations become increasingly frequent, this situation could change. In addition, some pet insurance policies may cover such referrals from a human health care provider as preventive visits under either a wellness rider (e.g., routine care, including vaccinations and parasite testing) or the illness portion for medical coverage if the pet was suspected of having or exhibiting clinical signs of a zoonosis.[2]

Case Scenario: Referral for Zoonotic Disease Counseling and Risk Reduction

A nephrologist is providing ongoing care for a patient (Mr. Doe) who has been on dialysis in the past but who just recently received a kidney transplant. The patient is now taking a number of immunosuppressive medications to prevent transplant rejection. At a follow-up visit, the patient asks whether there is any risk of infection from the animals in the house. The physician suspects that the risk of zoonotic disease could be increased but is interested in having the family veterinarian review this issue and provide recommendations. The physician is particularly concerned about the patient's cat, since she knows that toxoplasmosis can be a severe disease in immunocompromised persons. The physician

asks Mr. Doe's permission to contact the family veterinarian to request a consultation, and Mr. Doe agrees. The physician writes a note of referral to the veterinarian that does not mention the patient's medical condition (Box 14-2).

The veterinarian evaluates the patient's exposure to the patient's pets, other animals that may be in the household, and other potential animal exposures. It is not necessary for the veterinarian to know details about the patient's medical condition. Preventive services are provided to the pets during the visit. The veterinarian writes a consultation letter back to the physician (Box 14-3).

This communication illustrates the possibility of cooperation between human health care providers and veterinarians regarding the care of immunocompromised patients without needing to share confidential medical data (see Chapter 2).

Another situation in which the human health care provider may want to directly refer a patient to a veterinarian is the occurrence of dermatophytes (see Chapter 9). Some animals remain subclinically infected and may contribute to clinical disease in human beings. The following case scenario illustrates this.

Case Scenario: Dermatophyte Associated With Animal in the Home

A physician diagnoses a 9-year-old with ringworm and cultures Microsporum canis *as the causative agent (Figure 14-1). During the history taking, the mother reports that for the past 2 years there has been a cat living in the house and the family is attached to the cat. The mother has not noticed skin problems in the cat. In addition to prescribing symptomatic medication, the physician suggests that the mother contact the veterinarian to determine if the cat's condition is associated with the child's infection. The mother requests a letter that she can take to the veterinarian. The physician writes the veterinarian the referral letter shown in Box 14-4.*

Again, this form demonstrates the possibility of direct communication between human health and animal health professionals without sharing confidential medical information about individuals. In this case the veterinarian can respond to the human health care provider, with the owner's permission,

---

BOX 14-1 *COMPONENTS OF A MEDICAL REFERRAL VISIT FOR PREVENTIVE RISK REDUCTION COUNSELING BY A VETERINARIAN*

- Inventory animal contacts in home and around home.
- Review animal husbandry practices.
- Review biosafety measures taken.
- Identify specific infectious disease risks.
- Provide counseling on disease risk reduction.
- Provide a summary of recommendations to human health care provider (see Box 14-3).

BOX 14-2 *REFERRAL OF PATIENT TO VETERINARIAN FOR ZOONOTIC RISK REDUCTION COUNSELING*
Human-Animal Medicine Consultation Referral Form

Anytown Nephrology Associates
48 Medical Drive, Anytown, State, 10001
Phone 000-000-0000, Fax 111-222-3333

Patient Name: Mr. John Doe

Date of referral: November 7, 2009

To: Preventive Family Veterinary Associates

Referring Provider: Alan O. Pathic, MD

Reason for referral: Zoonotic disease risk reduction with Mr. Doe's permission

Services requested: Please provide counseling on zoonotic risk reduction, including the types of pets in the house and risks associated with each type.

BOX 14-3   *SAMPLE CONSULTATION LETTER SENT FROM VETERINARIAN TO PHYSICIAN REGARDING ZOONOTIC DISEASE RISK REDUCTION*
Human-Animal Medicine Consultation Report (Zoonotic Disease Prevention)

Preventive Family Veterinary Associates
100 Urban Street, Anytown, State, 10001
Phone 000-00-000, Fax 111-222-3333

To: Alen O. Pathic, MD
Anytown Nephrology Associates
48 Medical Drive, Anytown, State, 10001

Dear Dr. Pathic,

Thank you for referring Mr. Doe to me for zoonotic disease risk assessment and preventive counseling in regard to reducing his risk of zoonotic disease. He was seen in our office on December 12, 2009. His evaluation consisted of an inventory of animal contacts in the home and peridomestic environment, a review of animal husbandry and biosafety practices in the home, and a discussion of specific risk reduction measures. I also examined his puppy and cat and performed their preventive care. I am writing this summary evaluation with Mr. Doe's permission.

Mr. Doe and his wife live in a one-story single-family dwelling on a city lot. There is a lawn outside and a park nearby. They recently acquired a puppy in addition to their cat and iguana.

The puppy is currently 9 weeks old and is a Labrador–German Shepherd cross. According to the records Mr. Doe provided, the puppy received its core vaccinations at 6 weeks of age, along with deworming, and did not reportedly have any health problems when they acquired it from the city animal shelter. It is eating a puppy diet of dried food, but Mr. Doe also reported that he likes to feed it "special puppy treats." It has a bed in the kitchen, and Mr. Doe reports that he likes to sit in a chair and read a book with the puppy in his lap. He also reports that he likes to let the puppy lick his face. Handwashing after handling the puppy is inconsistent. The puppy is still being housebroken. Mr. Doe and his wife take turns cleaning up after the puppy and dispose of the waste in the trash. During the past week, Mr. Doe reports that the puppy's feces have "been a little loose" but without blood or mucus. Mr. Doe takes the puppy for a short walk twice a day in the backyard. If the puppy defecates on the lawn, he picks up the feces with a plastic bag. The puppy's physical examination was unremarkable. I did not see evidence of abnormal behavior or other signs of illness. A fecal flotation test was negative for ova and parasites, and I submitted a fecal sample for culture. I administered core vaccination boosters and deworming and scheduled a rabies vaccination to be provided when the puppy is 12 weeks.

The cat is a domestic short-hair that is 2 years old and has been previously seen by a veterinarian. Mr. Doe reported that it is allowed in the kitchen on counters and is an indoor-outdoor cat, spending several hours visiting the neighborhood park before returning for an evening meal of a commercial wet diet. There is a litterbox in the corner of the kitchen that Mr. Doe and his wife take turns cleaning every 3 days. The cat also appeared healthy and was negative for feline leukemia virus and feline immunodeficiency virus but positive for roundworms. It was dewormed and provided its core vaccinations. Because I recommended that the cat not go outdoors (see below), we trimmed the nails.

The pet iguana lives in a conservatory room off the living room, and it sometimes likes to sit on a person's shoulder. Mr. Doe's wife is responsible for cleaning and feeding the iguana.

Mr. Doe denies other pets or animal contacts, including petting zoos, other farm exposures, caged birds, or fish.

Mr. Doe is obviously attached to his puppy and cat, and they provide him with a great deal of emotional comfort and satisfaction.

In general, the risk of zoonotic disease from these animals is low. However, there are several important risks that should be addressed:

1. Puppies are at increased risk of infection with a number of zoonotic disease agents, including *Salmonella*, *Giardia*, and *Cryptosporidium*. Therefore it would be better for anyone at increased risk of infection to avoid any contact with puppy feces and to use careful handwashing precautions around the animal. I communicated this to Mr. Doe. Allowing the puppy to lick one's face is not advisable, and Mr. Doe was counseled about this. I recommended that they discontinue feeding the special puppy treats because the ingredients included raw meat, which can be a source of *Salmonella* or *E. coli*.

2. Overall, many authorities consider that the positive health benefits of a pet such as the family cat, in terms of the human-animal bond, greatly outweigh any risk of infection. To reduce disease transmission risk, I have recommended that they move the litterbox from the kitchen. We discussed methods to train the cat to stay off kitchen counters and to keep the cat indoors only. I also recommended that an immunocompetent person take responsibility for changing the cat litter, removing solids daily, and washing the box on a weekly basis. These steps will greatly reduce any potential risk of toxoplasmosis. Another risk to consider is *Bartonella* infection, although this disease in human beings is generally associated with kittens. Nevertheless, I trimmed the cat's nails and provided a flea prevention treatment that will reduce this risk further.

3. Reptiles, such as the pet iguana, can be carriers for *Salmonella* infection and are not advised for families with children younger than 5 years or with immunocompromised persons. If Mr. Doe is at increased risk of zoonotic infection, he and his wife should seriously consider finding another home for this pet.

Mr. Doe was provided printed information about zoonotic disease risk reduction. He has a return appointment for his puppy in 3 weeks when it is the appropriate age for rabies vaccination, and I will revisit these issues at this time.

Thank you again for the referral of this pleasant gentleman. If you have any questions regarding this report, please do not hesitate to contact me. I will let you know the results of the puppy fecal culture when it is available next week.

Sincerely,

Jane Q. Veterinarian

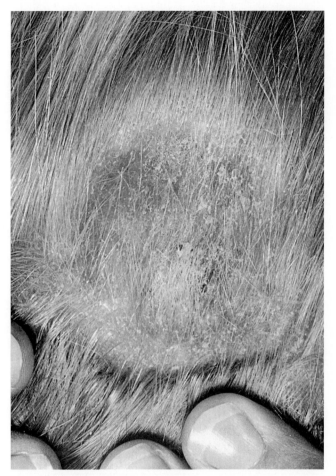

Figure 14-1 Scalp ringworm in which an ectothrix infection of the hair is caused by *Microsporum canis*. (From Mandell GL, Bennett JE, Dolin R: *Principles and practice of infectious diseases*, ed 6, New York, 2005, Churchill Livingstone Elsevier.)

that the cat was cultured (Figure 14-2) and treated appropriately and that recommendations were made regarding cleaning the environment. The veterinarian can also educate the physician about the therapeutic importance of the human-animal bond between the family and the pet.

REFERRALS FROM VETERINARIANS TO HUMAN HEALTH CARE PROVIDERS

As discussed in Chapter 2, veterinarians are restricted by scope of practice guidelines from providing human medical advice to owners and other clients. At the same time, there may be liability if they do not adequately communicate information about zoonotic and other health risks to their clients. In the following case scenario, the veterinarian suspects an environmental health risk and brings it to the attention of the health care provider.

Case Scenario: Shared Environmental Toxic Risk

The family cat is diagnosed with malignant lymphoma by the veterinarian. Despite treatment, the cat dies. The family is upset about the loss of the pet and asks if the veterinarian has any ideas about what caused the cancer. In talking with the family,

BOX 14-4 *COMMUNICATION FROM MEDICAL PROVIDER TO VETERINARIAN*
Communication to Veterinary Provider Regarding Human-Animal Medicine Issue

Alice O. Pathic, MD
242 Medical Drive, Anytown, USA
Phone 111-112-1111, Fax 111-112-1112

John Q. Veterinarian:

  With permission of the owner, I am contacting you regarding a potential zoonotic disease or other shared health issue. In particular, I am requesting an:

  ☐ Evaluation of pet(s) for internal parasites, especially_____
  ☐ Evaluation report of health problems in pet(s)
  ☐ Evaluate risks from specific pet for: _____
    dermatophyte_____(name health concern)
  ☐ Other_____

  Reason for communication: There is concern that the family cat may be the source of dermatophyte infection for people in the house. Please evaluate the cat and advise the family whether there is anything they can do to reduce zoonotic transmission if the cat is infected.

  Please call if you need more information and/or want to discuss.
Health department contacted?   Yes   No
Person contacted:
Date of contact:

Sincerely,
Alice O. Pathic, MD
02/20/09

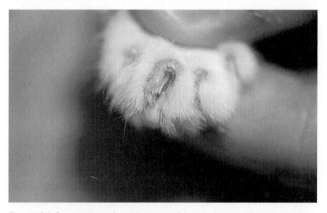

Figure 14-2 Dermatophytosis. Paronychia in a cat caused by *Microsporum canis*. The nailbed is erythematous and alopecic. (From Medleau L, Hnilica KA: *Small animal dermatology: a color atlas and therapeutic guide*, ed 2, St Louis, 2006, Saunders Elsevier.)

the veterinarian finds that there are two smokers living in the house. In discussion, the veterinarian mentions that second-hand cigarette smoke has been linked to malignant lymphoma in cats.[3] In this case, the cat may be a sentinel for the health risk of second-hand smoke to human beings in the household. The two smokers in the family decide they want to start a smoking cessation program but are not sure how to start. The veterinarian suggests that they contact their family physician. The family requests that the veterinarian write a letter about the cat's cancer that they can share with the physician. The veterinarian writes the letter shown in Box 14-5.

BOX 14-5   *LETTER FROM VETERINARIAN TO PHYSICIAN REGARDING ANIMAL SENTINEL EVENT FOR ENVIRONMENTAL TOXIC RISK*
Human-Animal Medicine Communication to Medical Provider

John Q. Veterinarian, DVM
200 Parkside Road, Anytown, State
Phone 111-111-1111, Fax 111-111-1112

Alice O. Pathic, MD:
An evaluation was recently performed on animals that may have been in contact with one of your patients.
Findings: Family cat has developed malignant lymphoma.
Reason for communication: According to mother in household, the husband and nephew living in the house are heavy smokers. Exposure to secondhand smoke could have played a role in the development of the cat's neoplasia. The family has asked that I provide you with this documentation because they are interested in participating in smoking cessation. Please contact me if you have any questions.

Health department contacted?   Yes   No
Person contacted:
Date of contact:

Thank you for your collaboration.
John Q. Veterinarian, DVM
02/20/09

BOX 14-6   *LETTER FROM VETERINARIAN TO HUMAN HEALTH CARE PROVIDER REGARDING DOG OBESITY*
Human-Animal Medicine Communication to Medical Provider

Preventive Family Veterinary Associates
100 Urban Street, Anytown, State, 10001
Phone 000-00-000, Fax 111-222-3333

Alan O. Pathic, MD:
An evaluation was recently performed on animals that may have been in contact with one of your patients.
Findings: Family dog is obese
Reason for communication: Owner reports not taking his dog on walks. I have recommended that the dog get more exercise. Owner is interested in starting exercise program with the dog but mentions he has medical questions. Please evaluate. I have suggested a nearby dog park as an exercise area because there are no sidewalks in the neighborhood near his house. Please contact me if you would like to discuss this further.

Health department contacted?   Yes   No
Person contacted:
Date of contact:

Thank you for your collaboration.
Jane Q. Veterinarian
03/21/09

The physician, receiving this letter, is able to use it in motivating the husband and nephew to start a smoking cessation program.

Such direct communication between veterinarians and human health care providers can lead to further cooperative efforts, as shown in the following case scenario.

Case Scenario: Shared Behavioral Risks

A veterinarian is seeing a 3-year-old dog for a routine checkup. She notices that the dog has gained 10 pounds over the past 18 months and is now significantly overweight. The owner is also overweight. In asking about exercise routines for the dog, the veterinarian learns that the dog spends most of the time in a small yard and is rarely walked. The veterinarian asks whether the owner has considered getting more exercise himself. The owner says yes, that he used to jog regularly, but in the suburban development where they live there are currently no sidewalks. The veterinarian agrees that this makes taking walks more difficult, but tells the owner about a nearby dog park within a 10-minute drive that has a walking path around the perimeter. The veterinarian recommends a modified diet for the dog and also advises the owner to get evaluated by his health care provider before starting an exercise program. With the owner's permission, she writes a communication to the health care provider (Box 14-6).

The next week the veterinarian receives a phone call from the patient's nurse practitioner, who has seen the patient and is grateful that the veterinarian helped motivate him to start an exercise program. The nurse practitioner and the veterinarian agree to set goals for exercise and weight loss for both the patient and the dog and to separately provide reinforcement for the healthy change in behavior. They also agree to co-write a letter to the town mayor pointing out the need for construction of a walking path in the patient's neighborhood to benefit the health

of both human beings and companion animals in the community. It takes some time, but eventually, due in part to the efforts of the health professionals, the walking paths are constructed.

HEALTH DEPARTMENT COORDINATION OF CARE BETWEEN HUMAN AND ANIMAL HEALTH

As outlined in Chapter 13, public health professionals can play a key role in coordinating preventive actions between human and animal health care providers. Public health departments are dedicated to improving the environmental health of communities, and these efforts can obviously benefit the health of both human beings and nonhuman animals, as shown in the following scenario.

Case Scenario: Shared Environmental Exposure to Lead

A self-employed painter is seen in an emergency department for abdominal pain and nausea. His blood test shows anemia. The physician assistant seeing the patient suspects lead poisoning and orders a test of venous lead. The level comes back several days later markedly elevated (112 mcg/dL). The painter is seen in follow-up and reports that he has been sanding paint on the exterior an old house that is being renovated and that a couple is living in the house. The health department is contacted and investigates the house. The environmental health officer for the health department contacts the couple living in the house and asks whether they have any children who could have been exposed to paint dust from the renovation. The couple reports that they do not have any children, but that their two cats have been acting strangely, refusing to eat, and appearing drowsy. The health department recommends that they take the cats to the veterinarian for evaluation for possible lead poisoning. The environmental health officer contacts the veterinarian personally to inform him of the toxic risk. It is determined that the cats are suffering from severe lead toxicosis (see Chapter 8) and require chelation treatment. Meanwhile, the environmental health department supervises the cleanup of the lead-contaminated environment around the house. Based on this case, the health department starts an educational initiative with both medical providers and veterinarians in the community to raise awareness of lead poisoning risks.

Box 14-7 shows text from a sample brochure produced as part of this educational initiative. This type of document could be distributed to both human health care and veterinary offices in the community.

Case Scenario: Shared Environmental Exposure to Tickborne Disease

A state health department is engaged in tracking tickborne disease risk and alerting clinicians and the general public to areas and seasons of increased risk. To do this, the health department decides to use data from a large companion animal database of electronic records of pets seen in animal hospitals around the state. Such databases have already been developed for this pur-

pose.[5] *This database captures the occurrence of ticks detected during physical examination of pets and reports this as an incidence rate based on the number of animals examined.[6] Increases in the incidence of ticks found on the animals are thereby able to provide early warning of risk of Lyme disease and other tickborne illness to both animals and human beings. The health department uses this information to send out alerts to both veterinary and human health clinicians about the tickborne disease risk in the community.*

PREVENTIVE ENVIRONMENTAL RISK ASSESSMENTS FOR HUMAN BEINGS AND OTHER ANIMALS

A cornerstone of prevention is ensuring that health threats in the environment are recognized and minimized, and that living environments are designed and maintained to foster optimal health status. Direct assessment of environments are often not performed as part of clinical care but can have a positive effect on outcomes.

An example of a commercially available form for assessing disease risk in dogs is shown in Figure 14-3.

This disease risk assessment process can be expanded into a comprehensive assessment of the home environment.

Healthy Home Environments

As discussed throughout this book, homes shared by human beings and other animals can be healthy and nurturing environments, but the risks of zoonotic disease transmission and shared environmental health risks must be addressed and minimized. National programs such as the Healthy Homes initiative (http://www.uwex.edu/healthyhome/tool) provide information about toxic hazards in homes, but it is also important to assess other human-animal medical issues related to home environments.

Figure 14-4 gives an example of a home environment risk assessment checklist. Such a form can be given to patients by their medical care providers or their veterinarians. The information provided can supplement the basic medical history forms included in Chapter 3.

While clinicians can ask questions about environmental health hazards during a medical history (see Chapter 8), home visits can provide even greater information. Although physicians are less likely to make home visits, a number of other health care providers routinely visit homes, including visiting nurse and physical therapy services. Some veterinarians and public health workers routinely make home visits. Most of these professionals should be able to make a cursory assessment and decide if further evaluation and/or counseling is needed. It is useful to identify a network of health professionals who are comfortable performing in-depth home environmental health assessments that include pets and other animals if the situation seems more complex.

Figure 14-4 reviews steps that should be in place in a household to ensure that the risk of disease transmission is reduced. This checklist can be given to patients and clients to fill out or be used by visiting nurses, other home health or public health personnel, and veterinarians performing home visits.

BOX 14-7 **EXAMPLE OF PUBLIC HEALTH COMMUNICATION TO HUMAN AND ANIMAL HEALTH CARE PROVIDERS, PATIENTS, AND CLIENTS**

Lead—It's Everywhere: Facts for Families, Human Health Care Providers, and Veterinarians

Sources of Lead in the Environment
- Peeling paint (houses built before 1978)
- Dust and dirt contaminated with lead
- Lead pipes
- Toys, cans, other household objects containing lead

Lead Is Harmful to People
- 310,000 children aged 1 to 5 years in the United States have elevated blood lead levels.[4]
- Children are particularly vulnerable to lead poisoning and are exposed by ingesting paint chips, lead objects, and dirt and dust contaminated with lead.
- Some children show no obvious symptoms; others may develop anemia, developmental delay, abdominal pain and, in high doses, seizures.
- Talk to your medical provider about getting screened for lead exposure.

Lead Is Harmful to Pets
- Pets get lead poisoning, too. Dogs and cats may have physical contact with dust and dirt contaminated with lead. They then lick their fur and ingest even more lead. Sometimes they develop signs before human beings do.
- Signs to look for include fatigue, vomiting, and weight loss.
- Talk to your veterinarian about getting pets screened for lead exposure.

Questions about lead? Call the Environmental Health Division at 111-222-3333.

Anytown Department of Health, Division of Environmental Health

Canine Disease Risk Assessment Form

Being a dog is risky business. Disease risks vary by region and individual animal. Answering these questions will help your veterinary team develop a disease protection plan that's right for *your* dog.

Date: _____

Your name: _____

Your dog's age: _____

Your dog's name: _____

Part 1: Risk assessment (to be completed by veterinary technician and pet owner)

	Y	N
Does your dog go outdoors unsupervised?	☐	☐
Do you have multiple pets?	☐	☐
Does your dog come in contact with other people's pets?	☐	☐
Other than visiting the clinic, does your dog ever leave your premises?	☐	☐
Is there wildlife in your area, including deer, mice, squirrels, birds, opossums, raccoons, rats, or skunks?	☐	☐
Have you seen ticks on your dog recently?	☐	☐
Do you frequently see mosquitoes near where your dog goes outdoors?	☐	☐
Has your dog been spayed or neutered?	☐	☐
Does your dog have an opportunity to drink from water outdoors (ponds, puddles, water bowls, etc.)?	☐	☐
Do you ever take your dog to a groomer or boarding facility?	☐	☐
Do you ever take your dog to dog shows?	☐	☐
Do you hunt with your dog?	☐	☐
If your dog is on monthly heartworm preventative, have you ever missed a dose by more than 2 weeks?	☐	☐
Does your dog have any known diseases?	☐	☐
Is your dog on any medications?	☐	☐
Has your dog ever become sick after a vacation?	☐	☐

Figure 14-3   Example of disease risk assessment for dogs. Courtesy Fort Dodge Animal Health, Madison, NJ.

It is also important to assess if the animals are being taken care of properly in terms of mental and social well being (e.g., appropriate exercise, attention, appropriate discipline). Mental or physical neglect can be signs of social or psychiatric dysfunction in the home (see Chapters 3 and 5).

Healthy Backyards and Neighborhoods

If there is a yard connected to the house, or if the house is located in a suburban area that may be encroaching on wildlife habitat, further steps can also be taken to reduce risk of disease transmission between local wildlife and domestic pets and people. The checklist shown in Figure 14-5 can be given to patients and families to make their own assessments of the animal-associated health risks in their backyard and what can be done to reduce them.

Healthy Farms

Individuals living in proximity to farm animals have additional environmental health and occupational health issues to consider in a preventive risk assessment (see Chapter 12).[7] Figure 14-6 is a checklist of farm-related health issues for patients and animal owners to complete and return to their clinicians or for completion by a veterinarian during a farm visit. In the United States many issues related to the health of farm animals are managed by state and federal departments of agriculture. Therefore efforts to improve environmental health around farms require close cooperation between animal and human health care providers.

OTHER PARTNERSHIPS

Following are other recent examples of successful clinical veterinary-human medical partnerships that are expanding the horizons of medical care.

Case Scenario: Development of Novel Surgical Procedure for the Care of a Pet Dog

A pet dog is found to have a congenital heart defect that is not treatable with traditional veterinary cardiac surgical techniques. The veterinary cardiologist contacts a human pediatric cardiac surgeon to discuss the case. The cardiac surgeon has experience in the performance of a particular surgical technique designed to cure similar cardiac defects in human beings but has not attempted an operation on the type of lesion that

Healthy Home with Animals Checklist (Check All the Following That Apply):

Pets in household (list numbers):

Adult dogs _____ Puppies _____ Adult cats _____ Kittens _____ Birds _____ Reptiles _____ Rodents _____ Fish _____

Farm animals _____ Other (please identify) _____

Local wildlife being fed or living in close proximity_____

Name of veterinarian(s): _____

Name of human health care provider(s): _____

Type of home: Apartment _____ Single-family house _____ Trailer _____ Other (please describe) _____

Urban _____ Suburban _____ Rural _____

☐ Separation between pets and any food preparation

☐ Separation between storage of animal food and toys and human food

☐ Separation between storage of animal medications and human medications

☐ Family does not smoke inside the house

☐ Absence of peeling paint that could represent a risk of lead poisoning

☐ Family has a smoke alarm

☐ Family has a carbon monoxide alarm

☐ Household cleaners and other toxic chemicals are out of reach of children, dogs, and other pets

☐ Household pets are kept inside and, when taken outside, are supervised and prevented from having direct contact with wildlife or unfamiliar domestic animals

☐ Family has a policy of handwashing after handling all animals and their food and bedding

☐ Pets are up to date with appropriate vaccinations, are regularly screened for ectoparasites and endoparasites, and are placed on a proper preventative medicine plan

☐ Flea and tick medications are low toxicity (list chemicals)_____

☐ Family physician or other primary care provider is aware of pets in house

☐ Any persons with immunodeficiency are taking extra precautions with pet contact

☐ Pets are restricted from bedroom(s) of individual(s) with allergies

☐ Family regularly cleans cages, litter boxes, shed hair, etc.

☐ Animal waste is immediately disposed of in a sanitary manner and animals are discouraged from relieving themselves in inappropriate places (e.g., uncovered sandboxes)

Figure 14-4   Healthy home with animals checklist.

the dog has because such a specific procedure has not yet been developed for human beings. With the appropriate consents and approvals, arrangements are made for the pediatric cardiac surgeon to perform a novel procedure on the dog in partnership with the veterinary cardiologist. The procedure proves to be lifesaving for the dog. In the process, the veterinary cardiologist learns skills that could allow him to help other animals in the future, and the pediatric surgeon gains experience to better perform the novel procedure on children with congenital heart disease.[8]

Case Scenario: Echocardiography for Zoo Primates

After several nonhuman primates (tamarins) in a zoo die of apparent heart failure, the zoo veterinarian contacts a cardiologist at a nearby medical school. The cardiologist agrees to perform echocardiograms on the tamarins. Working collaboratively, the cardiologist and the veterinarian detected evidence of cardiomyopathy and heart failure in a number of animals in the captive colony. The cardiologist helped the veterinarian develop clinical treatment protocols for the animals. When another tamarin dies, the heart is examined by both a veterinary pathologist and a human pathologist, who agree on the diagnosis of sclerosing cardiomyopathy. The cardiologist learns from zoo veterinarians that animals can suffer from "capture myopathy" as a result of stress. This condition has been recognized in animals for several decades. The cardiologist notes the similarity to a recently described condition in human beings (Tako-Tsubo, or stress cardiomyopathy),[9] which could be underdiagnosed. This overlap of clinical conditions between animals and human beings impels the physician to search the medical literature to find other disease syndromes in human beings and nonhuman animals that could benefit from increased communication between human health care providers and animal health care providers.[10]

Healthy Backyard and Neighborhood Checklist (Check all the Following That Apply):

Date: _____ Person completing form: _____

Address of the house/apartment: _____

1. Outside the house:

☐ Wildlife (deer, raccoons, skunks, coyotes, etc.) are restricted from coming near the house, and garbage and pet food containers are secured to not attract wildlife.

☐ Any feces is cleaned up and disposed in the trash can quickly.

☐ Sandbox is covered when not in use.

☐ Any bird feeder is regularly cleaned and away from the house to not attract rats and mice.

☐ If in area where ticks are a problem, vegetation is kept cut short around the house.

☐ There is no standing water (e.g., old tires, clogged gutters, pots, toys, buckets or barrels filled with water) that could be a breeding area for mosquitoes.

☐ Firewood is kept at least 100 feet from house (it can attract rodent nests).

2. In the neighborhood:

☐ There are adequate walking paths and other exercise areas for people and pets.

☐ There are policies on cleaning up after pets in playgrounds and other public areas.

☐ There are no recognized toxic hazards in the neighborhood that could be a risk to animals or people.

Comments: _____

Figure 14-5   Healthy backyard and neighborhood checklist.

Healthy Farms Checklist (Check all the Following That Apply)

☐ Individuals working with horses, cows, and other large animals are aware of injury prevention.

☐ Species are separated as appropriate.

☐ Diseased animals are isolated.

☐ Food bins are secured against vermin and other scavenging animals and are away from toxic chemicals.

☐ Adequate handwashing facilities are available.

☐ Food product handlers are aware of safety and hygiene procedures for all animal products (eggs, milk, etc.).

☐ Dairy products are pasteurized.

☐ If home slaughter for meat production, meat is cooked or cured adequately to destroy parasites.

☐ Wells are properly constructed to prevent contamination from livestock, human, and wildlife wastes.

☐ Farm has a manure management and animal disposal plan. Animal waste and carcasses are disposed of in ways that do not leak into water supply or attract scavengers.

☐ Workers are using adequate and appropriate personal protective equipment.

☐ Wildlife are kept from contact with farm animals.

☐ Animals have proper access to preventive and acute veterinary care (vaccines, parasite control, reproductive care, injuries, infections, etc.).

☐ Workers have access to preventive occupational health care for injuries, allergies, infectious diseases, and other occupational health risks.

☐ Workers have access to adequate personal protective equipment.

Figure 14-6   Farm animal safety and health checklist.

References

1. Grant S, Olsen CW. Preventing zoonotic diseases in immunocompromised persons: the role of physicians and veterinarians. *Emerg Infect Dis.* 1999;5(1):159–163.

2. Dr. J. Stephens. Personal communication. November 19, 2008.

3. Bertone ER, Snyder LA, Moore AS. Environmental tobacco smoke and risk of malignant lymphoma in pet cats. *Am J Epidemiol.* 2002;156(3):268–273.

4. Centers for Disease Control and Prevention. Lead: topic home. http://www.cdc.gov/lead/. Accessed November 15, 2008.

5. Glickman LT, Moore GE, Glickman NW, et al. Purdue University-Banfield National Companion Animal Surveillance Program for emerging and zoonotic diseases. *Vector Borne Zoonotic Dis.* 2006;6(1):14–23.

6. Raghavan M, Glickman N, Moore G, et al. Prevalence of and risk factors for canine tick infestation in the United States, 2002–2004. *Vector Borne Zoonotic Dis.* 2007;7(1):65–75.

7. Will LA. Shared human-animal diseases. *Safe Farm Fact Sheet.* Ames, IA: Iowa State University Extension; 1994. http://www.cdc.gov/nasd/docs/d001001-d001100/d001073/d001073.pdf.

8. Carey S. *Human, animal doctors report success in dog's open heart surgery.* University of Florida Health Science Center News. http://news.health.ufl.edu/news/story.aspx?ID=3487. Accessed May 5, 2009.

9. Prasad A, Lerman A, Rihal CS. Apical ballooning syndrome (Tako-Tsubo or stress cardiomyopathy): a mimic of acute myocardial infarction. *Am Heart J.* 2008;155(3):408–417.

10. Cima G. One-health wonders. *J Am Vet Med Assoc.* 2008;233(7):1026.

Index

Note: Page numbers followed by *f* indicate figures; *t*, tables; and *b*, boxes.

395